ATOPIC DERMATITIS

ATOPIC DERMATITIS
Second Edition

edited by

Thomas Bieber
University of Bonn
Bonn, Germany

Donald Y.M. Leung
National Jewish Medical & Research Center
Denver, Colorado, USA

informa
healthcare

New York   London

First published in 2009 by Informa Healthcare, Telephone House, 69-77 Paul Street, London EC2A 4LQ, UK.

Simultaneously published in the USA by Informa Healthcare, 52 Vanderbilt Avenue, 7th Floor, New York, NY 10017, USA.

Informa Healthcare is a trading division of Informa UK Ltd. Registered Office: 37–41 Mortimer Street, London W1T 3JH, UK. Registered in England and Wales number 1072954.

A CIP record for this book is available from the British Library.

Library of Congress Cataloging-in-Publication Data available on application

ISBN-13: 9781420077988

Orders may be sent to: Informa Healthcare, Sheepen Place, Colchester, Essex CO3 3LP, UK
Telephone: +44 (0)20 7017 5540
Email: CSDhealthcarebooks@informa.com
Website: http://informahealthcarebooks.com/

For corporate sales please contact: CorporateBooksIHC@informa.com
For foreign rights please contact: RightsIHC@informa.com
For reprint permissions please contact: PermissionsIHC@informa.com

Preface

Atopic dermatitis is one of the most common inflammatory skin diseases found in the general population. This disease has a major impact on the quality of life of affected patients and a substantial socioeconomic burden. Since the first edition of this book in 2002, there has been enormous progress in our understanding of the epidemiology, breakthrough discoveries in genetics, and new milestones in immunologic research, contributing to a novel view of the pathophysiology and the management of this complex disease. Therefore, there was a great need to update this widely read book.

In this second edition, we have again gathered a panel of international experts who have provided important contributions in atopic dermatitis research and were willing to share their view on its progress with the readers of this book. This new edition is divided into several parts, presenting the various scientific and clinical aspects of atopic dermatitis. Part I addresses the definition and general mechanisms underlying the disease, including the new advances in genetics and epidermal barrier dysfunction. Part II provides an overview of the cellular aspects and the complex cytokine and chemokine network as well as the pathophysiology of itching. Part III focuses on the immunologic triggers (foods, inhalants, bacteria, and fungi). The final part of the book is dedicated to all aspects of management of atopic dermatitis with a particular focus on the topical calcineurin inhibitors and new developments such as the biologics and the revival of specific immunotherapy.

The information included in this new edition should help clinicians from many specialties including dermatologists, allergists, family practitioners, and pediatricians in their daily practice. Also, physician scientists, medical students, and experimental investigators will benefit from this work, which reflects the progress underlying the modern view of the pathophysiology and its consequences in the management of atopic dermatitis.

Thomas Bieber
Donald Y.M. Leung

Contents

Contributors

Werner Aberer Department of Dermatology, University of Graz, Graz, Austria

Cezmi A. Akdis Swiss Institute of Allergy and Asthma Research (SIAF), Davos, Switzerland

Mübeccel Akdis Swiss Institute of Allergy and Asthma Research (SIAF), Davos, Switzerland

Bruce G. Bender National Jewish Health, Denver, Colorado, U.S.A.

Thomas Bieber Department of Dermatology and Allergy, University of Bonn, Bonn, Germany

Mark Boguniewicz National Jewish Health and University of Colorado School of Medicine, Denver, Colorado, U.S.A.

Franck Boralevi Pediatric Dermatology Unit and Department of Dermatology, Centre Hospitalier Universitaire of Bordeaux, Bordeaux, France

Burkhard Brosig Department of Psychosomatic Medicine, Justus Liebig University Giessen, Giessen, Germany

Reto Crameri Swiss Institute for Allergy and Asthma Research SIAF, Davos, Switzerland

Ulf Darsow Department of Dermatology and Allergy Biederstein, Technische Universität München and Division of Environmental Dermatology and Allergy Helmholtz Center/TUM, München, Germany

Carsten Flohr Centre of Evidence Based Dermatology, University of Nottingham, Nottingham, U.K.

Regina Fölster-Holst Department of Dermatology, University of Kiel, Kiel, Germany

Richard L. Gallo Division of Dermatology, University of California, San Diego, California, U.S.A.

Uwe Gieler Department of Psychosomatic Medicine, Justus Liebig University Giessen, Giessen, Germany

Gerald J. Gleich Departments of Dermatology and Medicine, University of Utah, Salt Lake City, Utah, U.S.A.

Tissa R. Hata Division of Dermatology, University of California, San Diego, California, U.S.A.

Bernhard Homey   Department of Dermatology, Heinrich-Heine-University, Düsseldorf, Germany

Anne-Marie Irani   Virginia Commonwealth University, Richmond, Virginia, U.S.A.

Alan D. Irvine   Paediatric Dermatology, Our Lady's Children's Hospital, Crumlin, and Trinity College Dublin, Dublin, Ireland

Heidi Jacobe   Department of Dermatology, University of Texas, Southwestern Medical Center, Dallas, Texas, U.S.A.

Jens-Michael Jensen   Department of Dermatology, University of Kiel, Kiel, Germany

Kristin M. Leiferman   Departments of Dermatology and Medicine, University of Utah, Salt Lake City, Utah, U.S.A.

Donald Y. M. Leung   Division of Pediatric Allergy-Immunology, National Jewish Health, and Department of Pediatrics, University of Colorado Denver Health Sciences Center, Denver, Colorado, U.S.A.

Thomas A. Luger   Department of Dermatology, University of Münster, Münster, Germany

Volker Niemeier   Department of Psychosomatic Medicine, Justus Liebig University Giessen, Giessen, Germany

Natalija Novak   Department of Dermatology and Allergy, University of Bonn, Bonn, Germany

Peck Y. Ong   Division of Clinical Immunology and Allergy, Children's Hospital Los Angeles, and Department of Pediatrics, University of Southern California Keck School of Medicine, Los Angeles, California, U.S.A.

Cevdet Ozdemir   Swiss Institute of Allergy and Asthma Research (SIAF), Davos, Switzerland and Marmara University, Division of Pediatric Allergy and Immunology, Istanbul, Turkey

Margot S. Peters   Rochester, Minnesota, U.S.A.

Douglas A. Plager   Department of Dermatology, Mayo Clinic and Mayo Foundation, Rochester, Minnesota, U.S.A.

Ehrhardt Proksch   Department of Dermatology, University of Kiel, Kiel, Germany

Johannes Ring   Department of Dermatology and Allergy Biederstein, Technische Universität München and Division of Environmental Dermatology and Allergy Helmholtz Center/TUM, München, Germany

Elke Rodriguez   Division of Environmental Dermatology and Allergy, Helmholtz Zentrum München and ZAUM-Center for Allergy and Environment, Technische Universität München (TUM), Munich, Germany

Hugh A. Sampson   Department of Pediatrics, Jaffe Food Allergy Research Institute, Mount Sinai School of Medicine, New York, U.S.A.

Peter Schmid-Grendelmeier   Allergy Unit, Department of Dermatology, University Hospital, Gloriastr, Zuerich, Switzerland

Lawrence B. Schwartz   Virginia Commonwealth University, Richmond, Virginia, U.S.A.

Sonja Ständer   Department of Dermatology and Competence Center Pruritus, University of Münster, Münster, Germany

Martin Steinhoff   Department of Dermatology, University of Münster, Münster, Germany

Alain Taïeb   Pediatric Dermatology Unit and Department of Dermatology, Centre Hospitalier Universitaire of Bordeaux, Bordeaux, France

Julie Wang   Department of Pediatrics, Jaffe Food Allergy Research Institute, Mount Sinai School of Medicine, New York, U.S.A.

Stephan Weidinger   Department of Dermatology and Allergy Biederstein, Technische Universität München (TUM), Munich, Germany

Thomas Werfel   Department Immunodermatology and Allergy Research, Hannover Medical School, Hannover, Germany

Hywel C. Williams   Centre of Evidence Based Dermatology, University of Nottingham, Nottingham, U.K.

Klaus Wolff   Department of Dermatology, University of Vienna, Vienna, Austria

Travis Vandergriff   Department of Dermatology, University of Texas, Southwestern Medical Center, Dallas, Texas, U.S.A.

Sabine Zeller   Swiss Institute for Allergy and Asthma Research SIAF, Davos, Switzerland

1 Atopic Dermatitis: One or Several Diseases?

Thomas Bieber

Department of Dermatology and Allergy, University of Bonn, Bonn, Germany

INTRODUCTION

As a consequence of the substantial progress made in biomedical sciences, many of the most common diseases have experienced a reappraisal of their pathophysiologic mechanisms. As for type 1 diabetes or psoriasis vulgaris, which are now considered more as autoimmune diseases (1), this kind of progress has lead to a fundamental revision of many established dogmas and will have profound consequences on the management of these conditions. Similarly, eczema, a common chronic inflammatory skin disease, has greatly benefited from the scientific efforts in the last years, and the knowledge gained so far, on one hand, contributed to complicate our initial and rather simplistic view of this disease but, on the other hand, gives us the opportunity to reconsider the great diversity in pathophysiologic and clinical aspects of this complex disease under a new light (2). Most of the recent developments have been addressed in the present book, and each chapter provides detailed information on the topics it deals with.

Basically, at least two dogmas have been put forward to explain the pathophysiologic origin of eczema. First, the keratinocyte-based dogma where the intrinsic defect is supposed to reside in the epithelial cells, leading to the known altered epidermal barrier function. Here, immunologic aspects including allergic sensitization have been considered only as epiphenomena and not of primary relevance. The second dogma, on the other hand, postulates that the primum movens resides in yet-to-be-defined immunologic deviations, and the epithelial dysfunction was displaced as an event secondary to the local inflammation. This has largely contributed to question the definition of atopic dermatitis (AD), suggesting at least a dichotomic viewpoint on this disease.

Taking into consideration the recent progress in the field of epidemiology, genetics, and immunology of eczema, this chapter tries to put the scientific arguments for a rational discussion concerning the identity of AD and addresses the debated issue (3–5) of possible heterogeneity of this condition.

THE NEED FOR A STRINGENT DEFINITION OF THE CLINICAL PHENOTYPE

According to the classical dogma, eczema has been considered as a synonymous for atopic dermatitis (AD) or atopic eczema (AE) and contributes together with allergic rhino-conjunctivitis and allergic asthma to the so-called atopic diathesis. However, as it is the case for asthma, it is well accepted that at least 20% to 30% of the adult patients presenting skin lesions typical for AD do not exhibit any sign of IgE-mediated sensitization, thus strongly implying that the atopic background is not a pathophysiologic prerequisite for the development of this disease (6,7). This observation was made already more than 30 years ago by Wüthrich et al. and lead these authors define this condition as the intrinsic form of AD. This dichotomic view persists since then, and this particular form has been granted with several names, that is, intrinsic form, non–IgE-associated form, non-AD/eczema, and lastly atopiform dermatitis (8).

In an effort to council this important aspect, the World Allergy Organization (WAO) has proposed a new classification where the presence of IgE-mediated sensitization is a *conditio sine qua non* for the definition of an atopic disease (9). According to this definition, the term eczema is now to be considered for the skin disease with typical clinical aspects of AD but without any signs of atopic sensitization, while AD/AE should be restricted to those forms associated with IgE-mediated sensitization. The term eczema will therefore be used in this chapter. Bos has suggested that eczema/non-AD (intrinsic AD) should be renamed as atopiform dermatitis (8) and be considered as a distinct disease. The study on which this assumption was based provided (10) a series of clinical and biologic parameters but suffers from some paradoxical aspects because the group of atopiform dermatitis patients included a substantial number of individuals who definitely had a personal history of associated atopic diseases such as allergic rhinitis and asthma and should therefore be considered as atopic individuals. Furthermore, it is likely that some patients may have specific IgE to allergens not included in the panel tested in most of the allergologic routine work up (11) or even to allergens that have not yet been identified. The concept of AD and atopiform dermatitis proposes two separate entities but does not consider the possibility of eczema as a transient status in the course of atopic march. This, however, may be of particular importance in infants and small children where the proof of sensitization by detection of elevated total IgE and/or the presence of specific IgE can be timely delayed, for example, several years (12). The design of future epidemiologic, genetic, pathophysiologic, and therapeutic studies should, however, take into account the clinical heterogeneity for the recruitment to increase the quality of the clinical phenotyping.

LESSONS FROM EPIDEMIOLOGY

As mentioned above, 20% to 30% of adult patients presenting skin lesions compatible with AD lack any sign of atopic sensitization (and should be considered as eczema but not as AD/AE patients) and forces the question whether this dichotomic view, which is the result of a cross-sectional analysis in the adult population, is an established and stable situation during the natural history of the disease. It is well known that typical eczematous lesions appear during the first two months of life and longitudinal studies have unraveled an important aspect in the natural history of the disease. Indeed the majority of the children who have been diagnosed as AD/AE at the age of four to six years did not exhibit any sign of IgE-mediated sensitization during the first two to four years of their life, that is, at the initial phase of the disease (12). Most of the sensitization, which then occurs far later after the first skin lesions, is directed against food allergens and subsequently against environmental allergens such as pollens or house dust mite allergens. Several important conclusions can be drawn from these observations: (*i*) IgE-mediated sensitization is not a prerequisite for the development of AD/AE, (*ii*) eczema can persist until the adult age in up to one-third of the patients, and (*iii*) eczema in infants can be a transient and starting condition on which sensitization and AD/AE may develop subsequently. Here, beside the putative genetic background, the risk factors for developing sensitization during infantile phase are increasingly recognized and include most prominently distinct foodstuffs such as peanuts, egg, or milk (13,14) and exposure to environmental factors such as cigarette smoke.

Intriguingly, older children and adults with eczema are predominantly females (up to 100% in our own cohort) but no plausible explanation could be provided so far for this phenomenon (15). Also whether the spontaneous remission observed around the adolescents in about the half of eczema or AD/AE children is related to the sensitization profile or other yet-to-be-defined factors remains debatable and should be addressed by epidemiologists in the near future.

Another important aspect to be considered in this context is the putative role of eczema versus AD/AE in the so-called atopic march (16,17) or atopic carrier, which has been postulated. According to this concept, children with AD/AE but not eczema are at a higher risk to subsequently develop allergic rhinitis and allergic asthma. It is well accepted that (*i*) epithelial barrier function is disturbed in the gut, skin, and airways of atopic individuals and (*ii*) chronic inflammation primarily localized in the skin may have substantial repercussion on systemic immunologic mechanisms (2). More recent genetic studies have highlighted the association of variants and mutations of the filaggrin encoding gene and the high risk for developing allergic diseases of the airways, that is, rhinitis and asthma (18–21). Therefore, we suggest that chronic skin inflammation when occurring in the context of atopic predisposition (see section lessons from genetics), that is, dominant Th2 response, may facilitate the emergence of sensitization including those to food allergens. This is further supported by the fact that the highest total IgE levels and specific IgE to allergens are observed in patients with long-lasting eczematous skin lesions.

LESSONS FROM GENETICS

Atopic eczema is considered as paradigmatic genetic complex disease where gene–gene and gene–environment interactions will dictate the emergence and the phenotype including the severity of the disease. This has been already postulated in the 1970 s on the basis of twin studies, which showed a relative risk of nearly 80% in homozygotous twins but only 20% in dizygotous twins. Modern approaches based on genome-wide scans, using microsatellite genotyping and linkage analysis as well as genome-wide association studies (GWAS) in nuclear families, have been applied for the mapping of genes putatively responsible for complex diseases. Initially, the three linkage studies performed in atopic eczema showed a distinct set of loci without overlapping with the loci identified for asthma. This finding is rather surprising with regard to the concept of atopic march, which postulates that children affected by atopic eczema are at high risk to develop allergic asthma later on. Even more intriguing is the fact that the above-mentioned loci in AE match with the chromosomal regions identified for psoriasis—another chronic inflammatory skin disease— although both diseases have been postulated to be nearly mutually exclusive. More recent studies on AE have focused on 1q21, which harbor a set of genes of the so-called epidermal differentiation complex (EDC) involved in the epidermal barrier function thus supporting the concept of a primary epidermal defect.

As dry and scaly skin is a clinical aspect shared by AD and ichthyosis vulgaris (OMIM #146700), an autosomal recessive common disease of keratinization, it has been postulated that both diseases may overlap genetically. As filaggrin (FLG; chr. 1q21.3)—a key protein in terminal differentiation of the epidermis—has been identified as the gene responsible for ichthiosis vulgaris, subsequent analysis in patients with AD have confirmed this hypothesis, showing several loss-of-function mutations (R501X, 2282del4, R2447X, S3247X, 3702delG) of the profilaggrin/ filaggrin gene in European populations (18–21). Interestingly, distinct FLG mutations, S2554X and 3321del A, have been reported in a Japanese cohort of AD patients (22). Mutations of the filaggrin gene correlate to the early onset of the disease, being a predictive marker in terms of AD predisposing and finally leading to asthma, the so-called atopic march (23,24). However, there is no correlation between loss of function of filaggrin and allergic airway disease without AD and there is also a strong correlation between filaggrin mutation and nonatopic eczema. It is expected that further yet-to-be-defined genetic variants of other epidermal structures such as those localized in the epidermal differential complex on chr. 1q21, for example, the stratum corneum tryptic enzyme (SCCE) may also play a role in these phenomena (25). These findings provide an important support for the well-known impairment of the physical epidermal barrier observed in AD.

Finally, in search of candidate genes related to the immunologic aspects underlying AD and other atopic diseases, several candidate genes have been identified in recent years, notably on chromosome 5q31–33, all containing genes for cytokines involved in the regulation of IgE synthesis such as interleukin (IL)-4, IL-5, IL-12, IL 13, and granulocyte-macrophage colony-stimulation factor (GM-CSF) as well as CD14 (26). Further studies identified functional mutations of the promoter region of the chemokine RANTES (17q11) (27) and gain-of-function polymorphisms in the alpha subunit of the IL-4 receptor (16q12) (28). Interestingly, the only study addressing the issue of genetic differences between eczema and AD highlights the putative role of gene variants of the IL-4 receptor (29). A disbalance between Th1- and Th2-immune responses in AD may be explained by polymorphisms of the IL-18 gene (30). Association of polymorphisms in genes encoding for receptors of the innate immune system such as CD14 and TLR have also been reported but have not yet been confirmed in larger cohorts. More recently, Weidinger et al. reported an association between high IgE level and the gene encoding for the alpha of the high-affinity receptor for IgE (FcERIA).

Overall, it appears that AD emerges on the genetic background of two major sets of genes: (*i*) penetration and sensitization of not only skin-related genes encoding for epidermal structural proteins, such as FLG, but also of many other structures involved in the epidermal barrier function and (*ii*) genes encoding for major players of the immunologic concert. It is tempting to speculate, based on this concept, that patients suffering from eczema may have genetic variations leading to rather minimal dysfunction of the epidermal barrier, which are not related to FLG mutations and/or lack one or several key genetic components mandatory for the sensitization phenomenon (Fig. 1).

LESSONS FROM IMMUNOLOGY

During the last decade, our attention has been focused on the complex interaction of the old and evolutionary conserved innate immunity and the more specifically and finally tuneable adaptive immune system. It rapidly became clear that effective cross-talking mechanisms between both immune systems are mandatory for healthy individuals. As an organ at the interface with the environment, these mechanisms are exquisitely regulated in the skin and can also be subjected to substantial defects as exemplified in AD.

The epidermal barrier function can be regarded as an integral part of the skin innate immunity (31), which is, however, finely regulated by genetic variation as

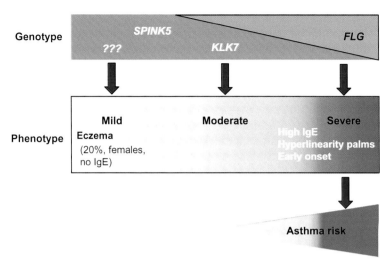

FIGURE 1 Genetic variants of the epidermal barrier-related genes determine the degree of sensitization and the risk to develop asthma in children with AD. *Abbreviations*: FLG, filaggrin; SPINK5, LEKTI; KLK7, stratum corneum tryptic enzyme.

well as by underlying inflammatory events driven by actors of the adaptive immune system such as T cells (32). This is best illustrated by the downregulation of the secretion of distinct antimicrobial peptides by T-cells derived cytokines in AD (33,34), favoring the strong colonization of *Staphylococcus aureus*. It is also of importance to note that with this respect both AD and eczema forms display a strong colonization with *S. aureus* and that the mechanisms of suppression of AMP secretion are similar in both the forms (35). Similarly, the role of dendritic cells (DC) linking innate and adaptive immunity in this context has been largely documented (36). The behavior of DC and the outcome of the T-cell response are finely tuned by the nature of the innate signals received by DC via TLRs as well as the local inflammatory micromilieu. Moreover, the strong colonization with *S. aureus* and the complex spectrum of the biologic activity of their products, such as exotoxins, are further factors that substantially influence the biology of DC. As shown in murine models, IgE sensitization to high-molecular-weight allergens may occur through the epidermal compartment, particularly when the barrier function is impaired as in the case for AD (37). Thus, it is likely that at least a part of the IgE sensitization emerging in infants during the initial course of AD is mediated by actors of the innate and adaptive immune system in the skin. Indeed, at the same time (*i*) the increased permeability facilitates the penetration of environmental allergens, (*ii*) local innate signals from bacterial colonization, and (*iii*) keratinocyte-derived mediators (such as TSLP) as well as (*iv*) allergen-derived mediators on DC are shaping their behavior. Moreover, it is assumed that (*v*) the "unspecific" local inflammation has a dramatic impact on the overall systemic immune response, favoring the sensitization mechanisms. Thus, the skin should be considered as a point of entry for IgE sensitization in the early phase of AD.

An important issue to address in future investigations will be the identification of the mechanisms underlying the very initial phase of the disease in infants as well as in patients suffering from eczema. Indeed, since IgE sensitization is not detectable, it is expected that other mechanisms are operative in this condition. As the role of food staff as a provocation factor has been documented in such patients, it is likely that IgE-independent allergic mechanisms, presumably related to allergen-specific T-cell reactivity, may explain this paradoxical situation.

Although their pathophysiologic role in AD had not yet been formally proven, the presence of IgE antibodies directed against self-proteins such as Hom S 1–4 has introduced another level of complexity in the issue of the natural history and the pathophysiology of AD (38,39). Because patients affected by eczema do not display such autoantibodies, their presence could be attributed to an overall predisposition to develop IgE antibodies without any further pathophysiologic significance. In this case, this would potentially question the overall significance of other allergen-specific IgE in this disease as well as all the proposed allergen avoidance strategies. However, the presence of such antibodies in a high proportion (up to 80%) of children before the age of six years (and before the putative spontaneous remission) (40) is in strong contrast to only 25% of adults with IgE-associated form who usually have a persistent and mostly therapeutically resistant disease. This peculiar observation opens the door for speculations about their putative role in the natural course of the disease.

Therefore, the investigation of the postnatal maturation phenomenon of the innate and adaptive immune systems in the skin is fascinating new field of research which should provide us better insights into the mechanisms driving the initial, eczema phase of AD and its role in the course of sensitization.

ATOPIC DERMATITIS: ONE OR SEVERAL DISEASES?

The above-exposed scientific evidence delivers a number of clues to the natural history of the disease, that is, the transition of a nonatopic eczema to an AD due to a facilitated penetration and sensitization to aeroallergens during chronic skin inflammation; the inflamed epidermis and dermis being the "entry point" for subsequent allergic diseases, that is, the atopic march. This scenario is further confirmed by our understanding of the genetic origin of the epidermal barrier dysfunction, for example, the filaggrin mutations/variants. However, because the FLG story may explain only 30% of the AD and the overall xerosis issue, further genetic variations in genes encoding for epidermal structures involved in the barrier function are still to be identified. On the other hand, as exposed above, the disease emerges on the background of at least two distinct sets of genes, that is, the skin-related genes (e. g., FLG) and the allergy/atopy-related genes (e. g., IL-4R). Therefore, an important question to address in the future would be whether AD and eczema differ genetically at the level of the skin-related and/or the allergy-related genes. Clearly, a dichotomic classification such as AD and eczema/atopiform dermatitis based only on the presence or the absence of one or a few distinct gene defects is theoretically possible but, in contrast to monogenic diseases, rather questionable because to the expected high degree of genetic complexity.

Therefore, our current knowledge of the genetics, epidemiology, and immunology of AD rather favors the classical concept of AD as a continuum where eczema is at one end and IgE-associated form with significant risk to develop an atopic march is on the other end of the spectrum. The degree of sensitization and the natural history of the disease are dictated by the individual genetic constellation and the environmental factors (Fig. 2).

Environment

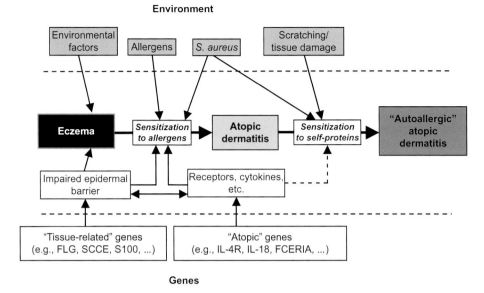

Genes

FIGURE 2 Gene–gene and gene–environment interactions in the natural history of atopic dermatitis. *Source*: Adapted from Ref. 2.

REFERENCES

1. Nestle FO. Psoriasis. Curr Dir Autoimmun 2008; 10:65–75.
2. Bieber T. Atopic dermatitis. N Engl J Med 2008; 358(14):1483–1494.
3. Williams HC, Johansson SG. Two types of eczema—Or are there? J Allergy Clin Immunol 2005; 116(5):1064–1066.
4. Flohr C, Johansson SG, Wahlgren CF, et al. How atopic is atopic dermatitis? J Allergy Clin Immunol 2004; 114(1):150–158.
5. Hanifin JM. Atopiform dermatitis: Do we need another confusing name for atopic dermatitis? Br J Dermatol 2002; 147(3):430–432.
6. Wüthrich B. Serum IgE in atopic dermatitis: Relationship to severity of cutaneous involvement and course of disease as well as coexistence of atopic respiratory diseases. Clin Allergy 1978; 8(3):241–248.
7. Wüthrich B, Schmid-Grendelmeier P. The atopic eczema/dermatitis syndrome. Epidemiology, natural course, and immunology of the IgE-associated ("extrinsic") and the nonallergic ("intrinsic") AEDS. J Investig Allergol Clin Immunol 2003; 13(1):1–5.
8. Bos JD. Atopiform dermatitis. Br J Dermatol 2002; 147(3):426–429.
9. Johansson SG, Bieber T, Dahl R, et al. Revised nomenclature for allergy for global use: Report of the Nomenclature Review Committee of the World Allergy Organization, October 2003. J Allergy Clin Immunol 2004; 113(5):832–836.
10. Brenninkmeijer EE, Spuls PI, Legierse CM, et al. Clinical differences between atopic and atopiform dermatitis. J Am Acad Dermatol 2008; 58(3):407–414.
11. Novak N, Allam JP, Bieber T. Allergic hyperreactivity to microbial components: A trigger factor of "intrinsic" atopic dermatitis? J Allergy Clin Immunol 2003; 112(1):215–216.
12. Illi S, von Mutius E, Lau S, et al. The natural course of atopic dermatitis from birth to age 7 years and the association with asthma. J Allergy Clin Immunol 2004; 113(5): 925–931.
13. Host A, Halken S, Muraro A, et al. Dietary prevention of allergic diseases in infants and small children. Pediatr Allergy Immunol 2008; 19(1):1–4.

14. Sampson HA. The evaluation and management of food allergy in atopic dermatitis. Clin Dermatol 2003; 21(3):183–192.
15. Novak N, Bieber T. Allergic and nonallergic forms of atopic diseases. J Allergy Clin Immunol 2003; 112(2):252–262.
16. Spergel JM, Paller AS. Atopic dermatitis and the atopic march. J Allergy Clin Immunol 2003; 112(6 suppl.):S118–S127.
17. Lowe AJ, Carlin JB, Bennett CM, et al. Do boys do the atopic march while girls dawdle? J Allergy Clin Immunol 2008; 121(5):1190–1195.
18. Palmer CN, Irvine AD, Terron-Kwiatkowski A, et al. Common loss-of-function variants of the epidermal barrier protein filaggrin are a major predisposing factor for atopic dermatitis. Nat Genet 2006; 38(4):441–446.
19. Sandilands A, O'Regan GM, Liao H, et al. Prevalent and rare mutations in the gene encoding filaggrin cause ichthyosis vulgaris and predispose individuals to atopic dermatitis. J Invest Dermatol 2006; 126(8):1770–1775.
20. Seguchi T, Cui CY, Kusuda S, et al. Decreased expression of filaggrin in atopic skin. Arch Dermatol Res 1996; 288(8):442–446.
21. Weidinger S, Illig T, Baurecht H, et al. Loss-of-function variations within the filaggrin gene predispose for atopic dermatitis with allergic sensitizations. J Allergy Clin Immunol 2006; 118(1):214–219.
22. Nomura T, Sandilands A, Akiyama M, et al. Unique mutations in the filaggrin gene in Japanese patients with ichthyosis vulgaris and atopic dermatitis. J Allergy Clin Immunol 2007; 119(2):434–440.
23. Weidinger S, O'Sullivan M, Illig T, et al. Filaggrin mutations, atopic eczema, hay fever, and asthma in children. J Allergy Clin Immunol 2008; 121(5):1203–1209.e1.
24. McGrath JA, Uitto J. The filaggrin story: Novel insights into skin-barrier function and disease. Trends Mol Med 2008; 14(1):20–27.
25. Vasilopoulos Y, Cork MJ, Murphy R, et al. Genetic association between an AACC insertion in the 3'UTR of the stratum corneum chymotryptic enzyme gene and atopic dermatitis. J Invest Dermatol 2004; 123(1):62–66.
26. Morar N, Willis-Owen SA, Moffatt MF, et al. The genetics of atopic dermatitis. J Allergy Clin Immunol 2006; 118(1):24–34 [quiz 5–6].
27. Nickel RG, Casolaro V, Wahn U, et al. Atopic dermatitis is associated with a functional mutation in the promoter of the C-C chemokine RANTES. J Immunol 2000; 164(3):1612–1616.
28. Hershey GK, Friedrich MF, Esswein LA, et al. The association of atopy with a gain-of-function mutation in the alpha subunit of the interleukin-4 receptor. N Engl J Med 1997; 337(24):1720–1725.
29. Novak N, Kruse S, Kraft S, et al. Dichotomic nature of atopic dermatitis reflected by combined analysis of monocyte immunophenotyping and single nucleotide polymorphisms of the interleukin-4/interleukin-13 receptor gene: The dichotomy of extrinsic and intrinsic atopic dermatitis. J Invest Dermatol 2002; 119(4):870–875.
30. Novak N, Kruse S, Potreck J, et al. Single nucleotide polymorphisms of the IL18 gene are associated with atopic eczema. J Allergy Clin Immunol 2005; 115(4):828–833.
31. Elias PM. Skin barrier function. Curr Allergy Asthma Rep 2008; 8(4):299–305.
32. Howell MD, Kim BE, Gao P, et al. Cytokine modulation of atopic dermatitis filaggrin skin expression. J Allergy Clin Immunol 2007; 120(1):150–155.
33. Ong PY, Ohtake T, Brandt C, et al. Endogenous antimicrobial peptides and skin infections in atopic dermatitis. N Engl J Med 2002; 347(15):1151–1160.
34. Hata TR, Gallo RL. Antimicrobial peptides, skin infections, and atopic dermatitis. Semin Cutan Med Surg 2008; 27(2):144–150.
35. Howell MD, Boguniewicz M, Pastore S, et al. Mechanism of HBD-3 deficiency in atopic dermatitis. Clin Immunol 2006; 121(3):332–338.
36. Steinman RM, Hemmi H. Dendritic cells: Translating innate to adaptive immunity. Curr Top Microbiol Immunol 2006; 311:17–58.
37. Spergel JM, Mizoguchi E, Brewer JP, et al. Epicutaneous sensitization with protein antigen induces localized allergic dermatitis and hyperresponsiveness to methacholine after single exposure to aerosolized antigen in mice. J Clin Invest 1998; 101(8):1614–1622.

38. Valenta R, Maurer D, Steiner R, et al. Immunoglobulin E response to human proteins in atopic patients. J Invest Dermatol 1996; 107(2):203–208.
39. Altrichter S, Kriehuber E, Moser J, et al. Serum IgE autoantibodies target keratinocytes in patients with atopic dermatitis. J Invest Dermatol 2008; 128(9):2232–2239.
40. Mothes N, Niggemann B, Jenneck C, et al. The cradle of IgE autoreactivity in atopic eczema lies in early infancy. J Allergy Clin Immunol 2005; 116(3):706–709.

2 Epidemiology

Carsten Flohr and Hywel C. Williams

Centre of Evidence Based Dermatology, University of Nottingham, Nottingham, U.K.

INTRODUCTION: WHAT IS EPIDEMIOLOGY?

The aim of this chapter is to review the way in which the concepts and methods of epidemiology have been applied to the study of atopic dermatitis (syn. atopic eczema, childhood eczema) in order to advance our knowledge and understanding of the disease. Epidemiology involves the study of the distribution and determinants of disease in specified populations and the application of such knowledge to the control of diseases (1). It involves a study of patterns of disease in whole populations to allow a broad understanding of etiology and natural history that cannot be gained from the study of sick individuals alone. The basic principles of epidemiology are to describe the distribution (where it occurs—geographically and in which social groups) and burden of disease (how common it is and how much morbidity it causes), to identify etiologic factors of the disease by measuring putative risk factors in sick and healthy populations, and to provide data essential for the evaluation and planning of services for prevention, control, and treatment of the disease. The findings of such research are not only essential for population-based public health planning, but they can also contribute greatly to the scientific basis of routine clinical practice and individual patient care.

Epidemiologic research can provide a natural foundation for the study of chronic diseases such as atopic dermatitis. In the past, much research into atopic dermatitis has been directed around the cellular and immunologic mechanisms of the disease. It is only over the last 15 years that epidemiologic studies of atopic dermatitis have started to flourish. Recent research has generated important information on disease frequency and has provided clues about genetic and environmental risk factors, as well as highlighted associated morbidity and costs to patients and health providers.

This chapter will describe our current knowledge of the distribution and frequency of atopic dermatitis worldwide and review recent advances in our understanding of the natural history of the disease. Epidemiologic studies that explore etiology and risk factors for disease are not covered in this chapter.

In order to ensure that information covered in this chapter is up-to-date, the authors carried out an electronic literature search of Medline (1966–June 2008) and Embase (1977–June 2008), using the key search terms "atopic dermatitis," "atopic eczema," "eczema," "prevalence," "incidence," and "epidemiology." Articles for which an English translation was not available were not considered, which inevitably leads to a potential English language bias; although based on the extensive body of literature identified, it is hoped that the chapter provides a general overview of past and recent epidemiologic research into atopic dermatitis. Much of the global data have been obtained from the International Study of Asthma and Allergies in Childhood (ISAAC), which now includes around 100 countries (http://isaac.auckland.ac.nz).

PREVALENCE AND INCIDENCE

There are many difficulties in providing an overall estimate of atopic dermatitis frequency, as studies have differed greatly in methodology, measuring disease frequency over different time periods, in different age groups, by using different techniques of data collection, and different diagnostic criteria. The effects of such methodological variations on the measurement of disease frequency are discussed below.

Defining Atopic Dermatitis

Variations in disease definition have made epidemiologic studies of atopic dermatitis difficult to interpret and compare. Patients seen in a clinic setting typically present with a spectrum of disease distribution, morphology, and severity, along with a variable time course of disease activity. This means that it is not always easy to say whether patients definitely have atopic dermatitis at a single time point, particularly those at the mild end of the spectrum. Researchers have used various methods to define the presence of disease. Some questionnaire-based surveys have relied on maternal reporting of "eczema" (although the accuracy of parental diagnosis remains unclear), while others have measured those with a history of doctor-diagnosed atopic dermatitis (which may depend on the knowledge and experience of the physician and also on diagnostic trends). Other questionnaires have recorded patient symptoms to establish the diagnosis. Even those studies based on examination by a dermatologist have used various combinations of signs and symptoms to aid diagnosis, reflecting different ideas about what constitutes a typical case of atopic dermatitis.

Although there is no definitive gold standard disease definition, various well-established diagnostic criteria have been developed, both to improve diagnostic accuracy in population studies and to aid in the comparison of results from different studies (2,3). The development of Hanifin and Rajka's diagnostic criteria in 1980 (2) represented an important milestone for atopic dermatitis research, but their complexity has limited their use in large-scale epidemiologic studies. Furthermore, they were derived largely from experience with the more severe subset of patients attending hospitals, whereas epidemiologic studies are often carried out in the community among patients with less severe disease. The U.K. Working Party's diagnostic criteria were developed in 1990 and have provided a shortened list of reliable disease criteria based on the original proposal by Hanifin and Rajka (3). The six diagnostic criteria have been independently validated and tested for repeatability (4,5). In order to capture the episodic nature of atopic dermatitis and minimize the effect of possible seasonal variations, the criteria have been developed as a 12-month period prevalence measure.

An important recent systematic review of diagnostic criteria for atopic dermatitis has identified 27 validation studies of diagnostic criteria (6). Two studies evaluated the Hanifin and Rajka diagnostic criteria and found a sensitivity and specificity ranging from 87.9% to 96.0% and from 77.6% to 93.8%, respectively. Nineteen validation studies of the U.K. refinement of Hanifin and Rajka's criteria showed a sensitivity ranging from 10% to 100% and specificity ranging from 89.3% to 99.1%.

Three studies referring to criteria proposed by Schultz-Larsen criteria showed sensitivity from 88% to 94.4% and specificity from 77.6% to 95.9%. One study evaluated Diepgen et al.'s criteria and found a sensitivity of 87.7% and specificity of 87.0%. The Kang and Tian criteria reported 95.5% sensitivity and 100% specificity. Only one fully published article validated the ISAAC questionnaire criteria, which showed a positive and negative predictive value of 48.8% and 91.1%, respectively. While the U.K. criteria are certainly the most validated and widely used criteria worldwide, like any other criteria they may be susceptible to translational and cultural problems (7). Ideally, any criteria employed in an epidemiologic study should first be validated in the country and setting in which it is to be used, and should also be accompanied by a separate analysis of how many in the survey population demonstrate physical signs of flexural dermatitis, which is less prone to cultural/language bias, especially when fieldworkers are trained and quality assessed using an online manual (8).

Measuring Disease Frequency

The most common measure of disease frequency in epidemiologic research is disease prevalence, defined as the total number of cases in the population under study. Disease prevalence can be measured at any one point in time (point prevalence) or over a defined period (period prevalence). Prevalence estimates provide useful information about the *burden* of disease in a population. The majority of epidemiologic studies have examined disease prevalence in the community because surveys of disease prevalence in hospital clinics or private practices are subject to referral bias, that is, referral may favor more severe cases which are also more likely to be atopic and have associated asthma and hay fever. Hospital-based studies also lack an appropriate population-based denominator. Population-based prevalence measurements usually involve a cross-sectional study design, and much of the data on atopic dermatitis have arisen from questionnaire surveys in schools. Point prevalence measurements using clinical examination are potentially more accurate but rely on subjects having active eczema at the time examination. One-year period prevalence measurements are probably the most useful for comparative purposes, as they take into account the relapsing and remitting nature of the disease, while minimizing the recall bias of lifetime prevalence estimates.

Much harder to obtain are incidence figures that provide information on the number of new cases developing over a period of time (usually one year). Incidence data provide a more precise insight into changes in disease frequency over time and minimize the risk of recall bias. However, measuring atopic dermatitis incidence usually requires a cohort study design, and such longitudinal studies are costly and time-consuming to perform. Furthermore, measuring new cases may be difficult because disease chronicity is often regarded as a major diagnostic feature of atopic dermatitis, and it is sometimes difficult to decide whether a child developing eczematous inflammation for the first time will go on to develop the more typical atopic dermatitis. Rather than describing the number of new cases per year, some studies have reported cumulative incidence, defined as the number of new cases developing since birth over a defined period. However, such studies have often relied on patients' recall of ever having had eczema at a certain age rather than being based on a prospective study design. A commonly used measure is cumulative lifetime incidence, which is synonymous with lifetime prevalence, although the latter term is preferable when data have been collected retrospectively.

HOW COMMON IS ATOPIC DERMATITIS?

Taking into account these difficulties, prevalence estimates from studies of varying methodology over the last 20 years are shown in Table 1 (7,9–50). The table is by no means exhaustive as many prevalence estimates have been buried within other studies, and other single country estimates of prevalence based on the ISAAC study have been omitted as they are discussed collectively under the topic of international variation in Section VII. The majority of prevalence studies have been carried out in children with lifetime prevalence figures in temperate developed countries ranging from 13% to 37% up until early adolescence. Point prevalence figures are lower, partly reflecting the fluctuating nature of the disease. The few studies of adults have shown lower prevalence rates in temperate developed countries such as the United Kingdom (26).

DISEASE SEVERITY

Overall population-based prevalence data may include many mild or asymptomatic cases. In public health terms the severity distribution of atopic dermatitis is of greater importance than total prevalence because this is more likely to closely reflect the need for health services. As with the diagnosis of atopic dermatitis, there are numerous methods of measuring disease severity. Population-based studies that have included a measurement of disease severity have generally used simple scales such as Rajka and Langeland's scoring system (51) or global severity estimates undertaken by the assessor. Some studies have graded severity according to the percentage of body surface area involved, although this may not provide an accurate reflection of patient morbidity, because involvement of small but functionally or cosmetically important sites such as the hands and face can be extremely disabling. More complex measures such as Costa et al.'s scoring system (52) and the well-validated SCORAD, EASI, and SASSAD indexes (53) are more complex and time-consuming and therefore are less suitable for large epidemiologic studies. However, some have successfully used the SCORAD index in population-based settings (20). Other well-tested and simple patient-orientated severity scores, such as the Patient Oriented Eczema Measure (POEM) (54,55) may prove to be useful for population-based severity scores because they do not depend on a physical examination.

Atopic dermatitis tends to be more severe in hospital compared to community settings, where 65% to 90% of cases are mild and only 1% to 2% are classified as severe (28). For instance, a survey of Australian school students aged 4 to 18 years found 86% of detected eczema cases to be "minimal to mild" on clinical examination (31), and this is in keeping with a U.K. survey among preschool children in which 84% of cases were classified as mild by a dermatologist (28). A study among Romanian school children showed that 93% of cases were very mild or mild (32), and in Japanese kindergarten and school children between 81% and 87% of cases were classified as mild (23). In a further study of Norwegian school children, two-thirds showed mild and one-third moderate symptoms, with less than 0.01% having severe disease confirmed by clinical examination (16). In contrast, the 40% of children, who continue to have atopic dermatitis as adults, are likely to have persistent and moderate-to-severe disease (56). In addition, atopic dermatitis can start in adult life, but very little prevalence data exists (56). A questionnaire-based study among Swedish adult patients with atopic dermatitis suggests that in this subgroup of patients, head and neck distribution as well as allergic sensitization are significant risk factors for disease chronicity and morbidity (56).

TABLE 1 Summary of Studies Measuring Prevalence of Atopic Dermatitis from 1990 to 2008

Country (Ref.)	Prevalence (%)	No. in study	Measurements and definitions	Age group (yr)	Year
Finland (9)	9.7	1712	12-Month period prevalence (questionnaire–symptoms)	15–16	1990
Germany (10)	12.9	1273	Point prevalence (dermatologist's examination)	5–7	1991
Norway (11)	23.6	551	Lifetime prevalence (questionnaire–symptoms)	7–12	1991
UK (12)	14.0	322	Point prevalence (history/examination by trained observer)	1–4	1992
Denmark (13)	22.9	437	Lifetime prevalence (questionnaire)	7	1992
Germany (13)	13.1	1164	Lifetime prevalence (questionnaire)	7	1992
Sweden (13)	15.5	1054	Lifetime prevalence (questionnaire)	7	1992
Germany (14)	14.9	2402	Lifetime prevalence (questionnaire–symptoms)	5–14	1992
	2.6	2200	Point prevalence (dermatologist's examination)		
Hong Kong (15)	20.1	1062	Lifetime prevalence (questionnaire–symptoms)	11–20	1992
Malaysia (15)	7.6	409	Lifetime prevalence (questionnaire–symptoms)		
China (15)	7.2	737	Lifetime prevalence (questionnaire–symptoms)		
Norway (16)	23	424	Point prevalence (dermatologist's examination)	7–12	1992
	37	424	Lifetime prevalence (interview)		
UK (17)	10.7	413	Point prevalence (dermatologist's examination)	1	1993
	15.5	413	12-Month period prevalence (interview–symptoms)		
Turkey (18)	5.0	1334	Lifetime prevalence (questionnaire–doctor diagnosis)	6–14	1993
UK (19)	11.7	693	Point prevalence (dermatologist's examination)	3–11	1994
Germany (20)	11.3	1511	Point prevalence (dermatologist's examination)	5–6	1994
Russia (21)	5.9	3368	Lifetime prevalence (questionnaire–symptoms)	Adults	1994
Turkey (22)	2.2	5412	Lifetime prevalence (questionnaire–doctor diagnosis)	7–12	1994

(Continued)

TABLE 1   Summary of Studies Measuring Prevalence of Atopic Dermatitis from 1990 to 2008
(*Continued*)

Country (Ref.)	Prevalence (%)	No. in study	Measurements and definitions	Age group (yr)	Year
	0.9	5412	12-Month period prevalence (questionnaire–doctor diagnosis)		
Japan (23)	24	994	Point prevalence (dermatologist's examination)	5–6	1994
	19	1240	Point prevalence (dermatologist's examination)	7–9	1994
	15	1152	Point prevalence (dermatologist's examination)	10–12	1995
	14	1670	Point prevalence (dermatologist's examination)	13–15	1995
Japan (24)	14.2	1378	Point prevalence (Japanese Dermatological Association Diagnostic Criteria)	Elementary schools	1995
Norway (25)	19.6	8676	Lifetime prevalence (questionnaire)	7–13	1995
	5.2	8676	12-Month period prevalence (questionnaire)		
UK (26)	2.3	9786	12-Month period prevalence (medical records and examination)	All ages	1995
UK (27)	8.5	695	Point prevalence (dermatologist's examination)	3–11	1995
	5.9	695	Point prevalence (UK Working Party Diagnostic Criteria)		
Japan (23)	11	2159	Point prevalence (dermatologist's examination)	16–18	1996
UK (28)	16.5	1523	12-Month period prevalence (history/dermatologist's examination)	1–5	1996
UK (29)	14.2	260	Point prevalence (dermatologist's examination)	4	1996
	12.3	260	UK Working Party Diagnostic Criteria (dermatologist's examination)		
Turkey (30)	4.3	738	12-Month prevalence (questionnaire–doctor diagnosis)	6–13	1997
	6.5	738	Lifetime prevalence (questionnaire–doctor diagnosis)		
Australia (31)	16.3	2491	Point prevalence (dermatologist's examination)	4–18	1997
	10.8	2491	UK Working Party's Diagnostic Criteria (dermatologist's examination)		
Romania (32)	2.4	1114	Point prevalence (dermatologist's examination)	6–12	1997
	1.8	1114	UK Working Party Diagnostic Criteria (dermatologist's examination)		

Country (Ref.)	Prevalence (%)	No. in study	Measurements and definitions	Age group (yr)	Year
USA (33)	17.2	1465	Lifetime prevalence (questionnaire–symptoms)	5–9	2000
Sweden (34)	11.5	742	Questionnaire and UK Working Party Diagnostic Criteria (dermatologist's examination)	5.5	2000
Denmark (35)	6.7	1340	12 months period prevalence (questionnaire and dermatologist's examination)	12–16	2001
Finland (36)	16.0	320	Cumulative prevalence (retrospective cohort study of well-baby clinic case records)	0–5	2003
Ethiopia (37)	1.8	7915	12 months period prevalence UK Working Party Diagnostic Criteria (questionnaire)	1–5	2005
New Zealand (38)	15.8	550	Point prevalence (questionnaire and physical examination) as part of a birth cohort study	At 3.5	2005
Germany (39)	8.4	1739	Self reported eczema verified by telephone interview	18–65	2006
Denmark (40)	44.0	356	Cumulative incidence (Hanifin & Rajka Criteria; 6-monthly physical examination) in birth cohort born to mothers with asthma	By age 3 years	2007
South Africa (7)	1.0	3067	Point prevalence in a rural setting (dermatologist's examination)	3–11	2007
UK (41)	25.3	593	Cumulative incidence UK Working Party Diagnostic Criteria (questionnaire and physical examination)	By age 8 years	2007
25 European countries and USA (42)	7.1 (2.2–17.6)	8206	Lifetime prevalence (questionnaire European Community Respiratory Health Survey)	27–56	2007
USA (43)	6.0	116202	Empirically defined eczema (self-administered questionnaire)	All ages	2007
Japan (44)	6.8	23044	12 months period prevalence (International Study of Asthma and Allergies in Childhood Phase One questionnaire)	6–15	2007

(Continued)

TABLE 1   Summary of Studies Measuring Prevalence of Atopic Dermatitis from 1990 to 2008 (*Continued*)

Country (Ref.)	Prevalence (%)	No. in study	Measurements and definitions	Age group (yr)	Year
Australia (45)	28.7	443	Cumulative prevalence (parental recall of doctor diagnosis of eczema in children who also had at least one positive skin prick test; birth cohort of high risk children)	By age 2 years	2007
Taiwan (46)	6.1 boys, 4.9 girls	23980	12 months period prevalence of flexural eczema (International Study of Asthma and Allergies in Childhood Phase One questionnaire)	6–12	2007
Thailand (47)	7.4	4021	Cumulative prevalence (questionnaire; population-based birth cohort study)	By age 1 year	2007
Norway (48)	15.9	390	UK Working Party Criteria (questionnaire and dermatologist's examination) in a random subsample from a larger cross-sectional study (n=4784)	2	2008
Taiwan (49)	1.7	317926	12 months period prevalence of flexural eczema (International Study of Asthma and Allergies in Childhood Phase One questionnaire)	13–15	2008
Denmark (50)	14.4	404	12 months period prevalence (Hanifin & Rajka Criteria questionnaire and clinical examination) in a birth cohort study	6	2008

MORBIDITY

The physical impact of atopic dermatitis depends on the severity of the disease and can range from annoying dryness to severely itchy skin with painful cracking, weeping, and secondary infection. Studies suggest that 60%–90% of children suffer from sleep disturbance, secondary to the severe pruritus, usually associated with the disease (57,58). Sleep disturbance and constant scratching may trigger other psychologic and social problems, especially in children. Irritability and lack of concentration can lead to detrimental effects on schooling, educational development, and social interactions. Furthermore, the stigmata of a visible skin disease can lead to teasing and bullying (59,60). Higher levels of dependency and clinginess have been found in children attending hospital outpatient clinics for their atopic dermatitis (61). The stress of caring for a child with eczema can have profound effects on all family members, especially for mothers of severely affected children, who have been shown to have higher stress levels than mothers of healthy control children (57,61).

Compared to other skin diseases atopic dermatitis rates highly on morbidity scores designed to capture the impact of disease on aspects of everyday life (62). In the past much of the emphasis in atopic dermatitis research has been on the measurement of physical signs, although the concept of measuring disease-related disability and quality of life is being increasingly recognized.

WHO GETS IT?

Age
Atopic dermatitis is predominantly a disease of childhood, as reflected in the prevalence data in Table 1. Prevalence estimates show a continuous reduction with increasing age (23,26). A Norwegian study based on review of medical records found a prevalence of atopic dermatitis of 13% in patients younger than 20 years compared to 2% for those older than 20 years (63). In the United Kingdom, 2% of adults aged 16 to 40 years and less than 0.2% of adults older than 40 years are affected (26). Adult atopic dermatitis has been relatively ignored in epidemiologic research. However, in developed countries adults make up approximately 80% of the population, meaning that up to a third of all subjects with the disease are adults (26). Furthermore, there is evidence that the number of adults presenting to hospital with the disease is increasing in some countries (64).

Sex
Although overall no strong relationship with sex has been demonstrated, a slight female preponderance has been demonstrated in some studies (10,11,16, 26,31,33,65), but not in others (14,17,22,63). A small female preponderance was also noted in the ISAAC study with an overall female:male ratio of 1.3:1, being higher in countries with the highest prevalence of atopic dermatitis symptoms. Interestingly, in children younger than two years this difference is not observed and the ratio may even be reversed (16,26), suggesting that increased disease chronicity in females may be partly responsible.

Ethnicity
Various studies have examined the effect of ethnic group on the prevalence of atopic dermatitis. It is difficult to draw conclusions about ethnic differences in prevalences by examining results from different countries because environmental factors may contribute to any differences seen. Therefore, studies of different ethnic groups in the same environment are particularly helpful to assess the contribution of genetic factors. In the United Kingdom, atopic dermatitis prevalence is similar in Asian schoolchildren compared to nonAsian schoolchildren (mainly European Caucasian), although Asian patients are three times more likely to be referred to the local dermatology department, perhaps due to less familiarity with the disease (12,17). However, atopic dermatitis is almost twice as common in black Caribbean schoolchildren born in the United Kingdom than their white counterparts (19). Similarly, the disease is more prevalent among Chinese infants born in the United States compared to local Caucasians (66). In Australia the 12-month cumulative incidence of atopic dermatitis is much higher in Chinese babies (44%) compared to that of Caucasians living under similar environmental conditions (21%) (67). Although this data suggests that genetic factors predispose to atopic dermatitis, migrant

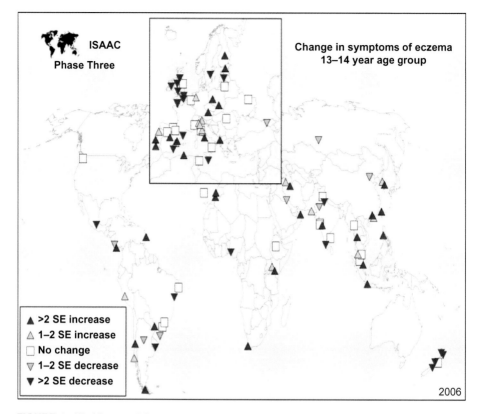

FIGURE 1 World map of flexural eczema symptoms in the last year showing changes in the prevalence of eczema symptoms for 13- to 14-year olds in consecutive International Study of Asthma and Allergies in Childhood prevalence surveys conducted 5 to 10 years apart (Phase One vs. Phase Three).

studies clearly demonstrate that environmental exposure must be equally involved (see below). Gene–environment interaction is likely and a currently unexplored area of research.

Socioeconomic Status

Atopic dermatitis shows a strong relationship to social class, but in contrast to many diseases it is significantly more common in higher social class groups (67–70). The disease is also more frequent in children from smaller families (71) and in those from privately owned properties rather than council rented properties (72). Various factors relating to education, lifestyle, type of home furnishing, and microbial exposure (the so-called (73) "hygiene hypothesis") could be contributing to this effect.

The socioeconomic gradient can also be seen on a wider scale, with disease prevalence being generally higher in more affluent countries with a westernized lifestyle and market economy (15,74). A comparison of disease prevalence in northern and eastern Europe (Fig. 1) shows a higher prevalence of atopic dermatitis in industrialized countries such as Scandinavia, compared to the western part of the formerly disadvantaged socialist region, for example, Estonia, Latvia, and Poland, with the lowest frequency in former socialist countries with a lifestyle even more different from that in western Europe, such as Albania.

Eczema and Allergic Sensitization

Although the name of "atopic dermatitis" suggests an atopic component to the disease, it is interesting to note that a previous systematic review as well as a recent population-based study among almost 30,000 schoolchildren in 20 affluent and non-affluent countries have shown that the strength of the association between allergic sensitization (skin prick test positivity and raised specific IgE levels to environmental allergens) and atopic dermatitis was positively related to gross national per capita income (75,76), with weak and often nonsignificant associations seen in low income countries (Table 2). This suggests that allergic sensitization is not a universal cause of atopic dermatitis. One explanation would be that there are two distinct phenotypes of atopic dermatitis, an atopic and a nonatopic one and that the prevalence of the nonatopic phenotype is higher in developing countries. However, given the universal clinical picture of atopic dermatitis across populations and the fact that allergic sensitization per se is at least as prevalent in developing country settings as in industrialized nations (76), it appears more likely that allergic sensitization is associated with childhood eczema in affluent countries due to shared causes linked with a "western" lifestyle rather than direct causality. The term "atopic" dermatitis or eczema in this context is misleading, certainly in children without proven allergic sensitization, and this has been highlighted in the recent nomenclature update of the World Allergy Organization (77). This is not to say that allergic sensitization cannot worsen existing eczema in some cases, and it may even be an etiologic factor in some affluent settings (78). Indeed, the discovery of the filaggrin and other skin barrier dysfunction genes may provide the missing link between atopic dermatitis risk, environmental exposures associated with westernization, such as increased use of detergents and reduced microbial exposure, and genetic predisposition to an impaired skin barrier. In this explanatory model, allergic sensitization is a secondary phenomenon in individuals who carry skin barrier gene mutations. Though not formally proven, environmental allergens are thought to be able to penetrate the impaired epidermal barrier, making contact with antigen-presenting cells and, as a consequence, amplifying the well-known immunologic processes seen in atopic dermatitis (Chapter 1). This may also be the reason why children with more severe disease have a higher risk of allergic sensitization (75).

Eczema and Other Specific Risk Factors

The role of genetic and other risk factors in disease expression will be discussed fully in other chapters of this book.

WHERE DOES IT OCCUR?

International Variation

Describing the geographical occurrence of disease comprises a basic component of epidemiologic research and can lead to the identification of important risk factors. Although the lack of standardized methodology has been a significant obstacle in

TABLE 2 Association Between Atopy and Flexural Eczema: Odds Ratios, Population Attributable Risk Fractions (PAF), and the Relationship Between the Number of Positive SPT Responses and Flexural Eczema Probability

Country, center	Study center characteristics	Children without flexural eczema		Children with flexural eczema		Age- and sex-adjusted OR (95% CI)	PAF (%)	Test for linear trend between FE probability and SPT positivity (P value)
		Number	% With atopy	Number	% With atopy			
Affluent								
China, Hong Kong[a]	Urban	1277	44.3	46	73.9	3.66[b] (1.88–7.12)	53.2	<0.001[b]
Germany, Dresden	Urban	2128	24.6	131	44.3	2.65[b] (1.83–3.82)	26.2	<0.001[b]
Germany, Munich	Urban	2225	21.6	92	40.2	2.55[b] (1.65–3.93)	23.8	<0.001[b]
Greece, Athens[a]	Urban	972	14.3	13	23.1	1.79 (0.49–6.52)	10.2	0.16
Greece, Thessaloniki[a]	Urban	1004	26.8	14	28.6	1.14 (0.34–3.77)	2.4	0.27
Iceland, Reykjavik	Urban	577	22.2	56	37.5	2.41[b] (1.33–4.37)	19.6	0.01[b]
Italy, Rome[a]	Urban	1285	28.6	22	45.5	2.43[b] (1.03–5.75)	23.6	0.11
Netherlands, Utrecht[a]	Urban	1000	28.9	63	54.0	3.13[b] (1.86–5.27)	35.2	<0.001[b]
New Zealand, Hawkes Bay	Urban/rural	1182	32.4	106	58.5	3.00[b] (1.99–4.53)	38.6	<0.001[b]
Norway, Tromso	Urban/rural	598	27.9	71	45.1	2.32[b] (1.39–3.88)	23.8	<0.001[b]
Spain, Almeria	Urban	1041	42.9	20	60.0	2.04 (0.81–5.13)	29.8	0.68
Spain, Cartagena[a]	Urban	1004	23.5	7	42.9	2.44 (0.64–9.32)	25.2	0.24
Spain, Madrid[a]	Urban	613	33.1	19	68.4	4.53[b] (1.72–11.93)	52.8	0.001[b]
Spain, Valencia[a]	Urban	951	13.7	37	27.0	2.32[b] (1.09–4.91)	15.4	0.008[b]
Sweden, Linkoeping[a]	Urban	150	20.6	18	46.2	3.72[b] (1.19–11.64)	40.2	0.005[b]

						OR (95% CI)	PAF	
Sweden, Östersund[a]	Urban/rural	200	29.8	43	48.9	2.67[b] (1.13–6.30)	33.2	0.005[b]
U.K., West Sussex	Urban/rural	835	16.3	61	34.4	2.89[b] (1.65–5.08)	21.6	<0.001[b]
Pooled adjusted OR						2.69[b] (2.31–3.13)	27.9[c]	
Nonaffluent								
Albania. Tirana[a]	Urban	879	15.1	23	13.0	0.85 (0.25–2.91)	−2.4	0.74
China, Beijing[a]	Urban	1034	23.9	10	20.0	0.77 (0.16–3.76)	−5.0	0.72
China, Guangzhou[a]	Urban	1070	32.0	8	37.5	1.24 (0.31–5.01)	8.2	0.22
Ecuador, Pichincha[a]	Rural	854	19.9	40	15.0	0.74 (0.31–1.81)	−6.2	0.92
Estonia, Tallinn[a]	Urban	612	14.1	30	26.7	2.32[b] (1.01–5.34)	14.6	0.02[b]
Georgia, Tbilisi[a]	Urban	148	33.9	25	26.8	0.75 (0.28–2.03)	−11.8	0.63
Ghana, Kintampo	Rural	1317	1.7	5	0.0	–	–	–
India, Mumbai	Urban	1537	6.3	15	20.0	3.65 (0.98–13.60)	14.6	0.05
Latvia, Riga	Urban	184	17.4	12	16.7	1.00 (0.25–4.10)	−0.8	0.80
Palestine, Ramallah[a]	Urban/rural	215	10.6	6	0.0	–	–	–
Turkey, Ankara[a]	Urban	2669	24.4	37	24.3	1.06 (0.50–2.26)	0	0.76
Pooled adjusted OR						1.17 (0.81–1.70)	1.2[c]	

[a] Local allergens were added to the six standard aeroallergens.
[b] Statistically significant at 5% level.
[c] Mean PAF.

Abbreviations: OR, odds ratio; PAF, population attributable fraction; FE, flexural eczema.

comparing international data, research suggests large geographical variations in atopic dermatitis prevalence both within and between countries (Table 1). The most comprehensive and standardized comparisons can be made from the ISAAC Phase One study (Fig. 2), which found a 60-fold variation in prevalence between the 56 countries studied, with 12-month prevalences ranging from 0.3% to 20.5% (74). The questions used in the ISAAC study are shown in Table 3. The study revealed some interesting patterns of disease frequency, such as a band of low prevalence running from China through central Asia to Eastern Europe, and low prevalences throughout the former socialist Eastern Europe. In contrast, very high prevalences were observed in developed countries such as Scandinavia, the United Kingdom, Japan, Australia, and New Zealand. The study also revealed that atopic dermatitis is a major problem in African cities such as Addis Ababa and Ibadan. Prior to this study there had been few epidemiologic studies of atopic dermatitis in developing countries. Some caution must be taken in the interpretation of results in countries such as India and Nigeria where the sensitivity of the ISAAC questionnaire may have been reduced due to the high prevalence of other itchy dermatoses in childhood such as scabies and onchocerciasis. Interestingly, the prevalence of eczema diagnosed by a doctor was also high in Nigeria (38.3%) (79). Interpretation of the ISAAC results also needs to take into account cultural factors such as differing thresholds for complaining about skin symptoms or an association of skin disease with stigmata of uncleanliness in some countries, which may have affected responses. Point prevalence estimates of flexural eczema based on physical examination using the validated U.K. visible flexural dermatitis protocol (80) undertaken in 28,951 children aged 8 to 12 years in 20 countries taking part in ISAAC Phase Two vary from 0.4% in Ghana to 14.2% in Sweden (76).

Another international study using standardized methodology has also found large variations in atopic dermatitis prevalence between genetically similar secondary school students in three different countries—Malaysia, China, and Hong Kong (Table 1) (15). As with the results of the ISAAC study, both genetic and environmental factors such as climate and air pollution may all contribute to these differences in disease prevalence.

Regional Variation
Wide regional variations in atopic dermatitis prevalence have been demonstrated across the United Kingdom, with higher prevalences in the southern and eastern areas of the country after adjustment for confounders such as social class (68,81). Several studies found a higher prevalence of atopic dermatitis in eastern Germany compared to western Germany (82–84). Higher prevalences of atopic dermatitis have also been noted in urban versus rural areas in the United States (33), Southeast Asia (15), Sweden (85), Finland (86), and Germany (10). On a smaller geographical scale the disease has also been associated with water hardness in a U.K. study (87), a finding that has been replicated in Japan (88) and Spain (89). These regional differences highlight the potential role of a variety of environmental exposures that may be amenable to public health manipulation, and a randomized controlled trial of water softeners for treating atopic dermatitis is currently underway (90). The role of airborne pollutants, climatic factors, and water quality are all possible risk factors that may contribute to such regional variation.

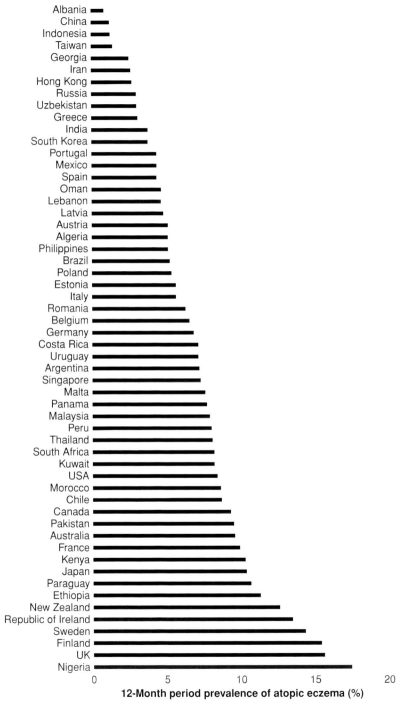

FIGURE 2 Summary of 12-month period prevalences for atopic dermatitis from the International Study of Asthma and Allergies in Childhood (ISAAC) Phase One.

TABLE 3 Questions Relating to Eczema Symptoms Used in International Study of Asthma and Allergies in Childhood (ISAAC) Phase One

1	Have you (has your child) ever had an itchy rash that was coming and going for at least 6 months?
2	Have you (has your child) had this itchy rash at any time in the last 12 months?
3	Has this itchy rash at any time affected any of the following places: the folds of the elbows, behind the knees, in front of the ankles, under the buttocks, or around the neck, ears, or eyes?

Migrant Studies

The study of disease in migrant groups compared to genetically similar groups in their country of origin allows insight into the role of environmental factors in disease expression (123). Children from Tokelau who migrated to New Zealand have higher prevalences of atopic dermatitis compared to genetically similar children who remained in Tokelau (91). The risk of atopic dermatitis in Asian migrants is significantly larger for those born in Australia compared to those of the same age who have recently immigrated to Australia (92). There is some evidence that people from less developed countries who move to industrialized countries may become more vulnerable than the local population. For example, IgE levels are significantly higher in migrant Turks residing in Sweden than among similar Swedish residents, with levels declining with increasing periods of residence in the country (93). These studies suggest that environmental factors associated with urbanization and development may be important in the etiology of atopic dermatitis in genetically susceptible individuals. Furthermore, the timing of migration may play a critical role in the expression of the disease.

TIME TRENDS

Seasonal Trends

Many studies have focused attention on the importance of month of birth on subsequent development of atopic dermatitis. These studies have arisen from the hypothesis that exposure to seasonal allergens during the initial few months of life, when the immune response is maturing, may result in sensitization and subsequent disease. Some studies have suggested that infants born in the autumn have higher prevalences of atopic dermatitis compared to those born in the spring (94). However, other studies have found no significant association with month of birth (95,96).

The effect of seasonality on the expression of established atopic dermatitis has also been studied. Atopic dermatitis characteristically runs a relapsing and remitting course, and point prevalence measurements can be used to compare the prevalence of active disease in different seasons. A study in Japan found no significant difference in disease prevalence in schoolchildren examined in the spring and autumn, although half of the children showed symptoms in only one season (24). However, a questionnaire study of teenagers in Finland found distinct seasonal variation, with atopic dermatitis occurring most commonly in the winter and least commonly in the summer (6). The majority of patients with established eczema report deterioration in winter months and improvement in the summer. The extent to which these changes are related to the effects of centrally heated houses or to the immuno-modulatory effect of sunlight remains to be fully established.

Trends

Epidemiologic research suggests that the prevalence of atopic dermatitis has increased two- to threefold over the last 30 to 50 years (97,98). It is important to separate out real changes in disease frequency from secular changes in diagnosis or reporting over time. Changes in the acceptability of eczema as a diagnosis or changes in the medical use of the word eczema, along with improved diagnostic methods and higher parental awareness and expectations, may all have exaggerated the trends seen in recent years. However, the increased prevalence has been consistently observed in different studies, suggesting that at least some of the observed changes are due to a true change in disease frequency.

The increasing prevalence of atopic dermatitis has been reported mainly in developed countries. One of the most widely quoted epidemiologic studies supporting an increasing prevalence have been the study of three British cohorts of children born in 1946, 1958, and 1970. The prevalence of a history of eczema determined when the children were aged between five and seven years increased from 5.1% to 7.3% to 12.2% in children born in the three successive cohorts, respectively, although the results of the three cohorts were drawn from three separate studies using slightly different methodologies (70). A further study of atopic twins in Denmark has shown that the percentage of at-risk individuals who developed atopic dermatitis between zero and seven years rose from 3% for the 1960–1964 birth cohort to 10% for the 1970–1974 birth cohort (99). Another study from Sweden has shown that the prevalence of atopic dermatitis had increased from 7% to 18% in schoolchildren between 1979 and 1991 (100). In Japan there is evidence that the prevalence of atopic dermatitis has doubled in 9- to 12-year olds and increased five times in 18-year olds over the last 20 years (23).

The largest and the most standardized comparison of changes in disease prevalences in atopic dermatitis has come from the ISAAC [Fig. 1; (101)]. In that comparison, children ($n = 302{,}159$) aged 13 to 14 years in 105 centers from 55 countries and children aged 6 to 7 years ($n = 187{,}943$) in 64 centers from 35 countries were surveyed from the same study centers taking part in Phase One and Three of ISAAC, using the same validated and translated questionnaires 5 to 10 years apart. Atopic dermatitis was defined as an itchy, relapsing, flexural skin rash in the last 12 months. Among the 13- to 14-year olds, atopic dermatitis symptoms decreased in some previously high-prevalence centers from the developed world, such as the United Kingdom, whereas centers with previously high prevalence rates from developing countries saw further increases. In the younger age group (6–7 years), most centers showed an increase in eczema symptoms, and similar patterns were observed for children with severe eczema across the two time periods.

The increasing disease prevalence reported over the last three to five decades cannot be explained by genetic factors alone because the time span is too short to allow specific genetic selection. It may be that environmental changes have led to a shift in the distribution of latent atopic disease, with more genetically predisposed individuals progressing to clinical disease. Changes in environmental exposure to irritants, decreased exposure to infectious agents, changes in domestic house dust mite levels with increased indoor humidity, carpets, and soft furnishing, and increasing exposure to allergens in childhood and pregnancy have all been

investigated as potential contributing factors. These risk factors will be discussed
further in later chapters.

NATURAL HISTORY

Much of the data on the natural history of atopic dermatitis have been generated
from the hospital patients, with a paucity of long-term follow-up studies of community cases. Summaries of the percentage of cases of atopic dermatitis developing
with age are clearly dependent on the age group studied, as surveys of very young
children may include many who will later go on to develop the disease. Atopic
dermatitis usually begins in infancy when it may be confused with seborrhoeic dermatitis (102). However, the former usually clears in the first year of life, whereas
atopic dermatitis is characterized by a more chronic relapsing and remitting course.
The distribution of atopic dermatitis may change early in life, from involvement
of the scalp and face to involvement of the neck and flexures between one and two
years of age (103). Age of onset in community cases of atopic dermatitis may be later
than that reported in hospital-based studies. From the available epidemiologic data
approximately 70% of cases begin before the age of five years, suggesting that factors in early life may be crucial in determining disease expression (104). In one U.K.
study, the disease developed within the first six months of life in 47.5% of cases and
within the first year of life in 60% of cases (105). The National Child Development
Study (NCDS) is a U.K. birth cohort study of children born in March 1958 with cases
of atopic dermatitis based on examination by a medical officer. Of the 870 cases with
examined or reported eczema by the age of 16 years, 43% had onset before the age
of one year and 66% had onset before the age of seven years (106). In a study of 551
Norwegian children, the onset of eczema occurred before one year of age in 25%
of children and before five years of age in 75% (11). A prospective study including a large number of high-risk infants (family history of atopic dermatitis and elevated IgE) showed a lifetime prevalence of 4.8%, 8.7%, 13%, and 18% at 3, 6, 12, and
24 months of age, respectively (107,108).

Because there is currently no cure for atopic dermatitis, epidemiologic data
on clearance rates can be extremely helpful when it comes to making predictions
about patients' long-term prognosis. It is generally agreed that a number of mild-to-
moderate cases clear spontaneously in early life, although good prospective studies
are lacking. Given the limitations of comparing research of varying methodology,
examination of studies including representative cases (milder community cases as
well as hospital patients) suggests clearance rates of approximately 60% by early
adolescence (104,109). Data from the NCDS have shown that at the age 11 and 16
years, 65% and 74% of children, respectively, are clear of their disease in terms of
examined eczema or a history of eczema in the previous year (106). In a study of
260 children in the United Kingdom, of those who had atopic dermatitis at age
one year, almost 50% no longer had the disease by age four years (29). Cessation
of atopic dermatitis occurred in 13% before the age of five years and 17% before
the age of seven years in an interview study of 156 Norwegian children (16). However, it is not always easy to say whether the disease has resolved permanently
because atopic dermatitis is characterized by a relapsing and remitting course,
and recurrences in adult life are not uncommon (106,110). Such recurrences often
occur on the hands and may be triggered by occupations such as food preparation,
housework, or hairdressing. In the hospital setting approximately 10% of patients
still suffer from eczema in adult life (111). The strongest and the most consistent

factors that appear to predict more persistent atopic dermatitis are early onset, severe widespread disease in early infancy, concomitant asthma or hay fever, and a family history of atopic dermatitis (104,109,112). There is also evidence to suggest that allergic sensitization-associated atopic dermatitis has a worse long-term prognosis than atopic dermatitis that is not associated with atopy (75).

PRIMARY, SECONDARY, AND TERTIARY PREVENTION

One of the major goals of epidemiologic research is to identify groups who are at high risk for the disease with the hope of modifying potential risk factors to prevent the disease. In this respect it is important to distinguish between primary, secondary, and tertiary prevention. Primary prevention refers to action taken to prevent the development of the disease in individuals who are free from the disease. Because atopic dermatitis usually begins in the first five years of life, there is potential for epidemiologic research to identify prenatal or early life factors that may be involved in sensitization and development of the disease. This raises the real possibility of primary prevention, either by altering exposures during pregnancy or by the prevention of sensitization in early infancy. Much interest has been focused on the role of dietary factors, breast-feeding, the timing of introduction of potentially allergenic solid foods, and the reduction of house dust mite levels around the home. Several cohort studies are currently evaluating manipulation of such factors, especially in individuals at a genetically high risk of developing atopic disease. If simple manipulation of these factors can be shown to be important in the development of the disease, this would have huge health implications. A Cochrane review of four trials involving 334 families concluded that the evidence did not suggest that maternal allergen avoidance *during pregnancy* reduced the incidence of atopic dermatitis, and such restrictive diets during pregnancy were associated with lower birth weights (113). Although some interventions such as delayed introduction of solids and administration of probiotics to pregnant mothers and their newborns may have a role in disease prevention (114–116), more studies are needed before primary prevention becomes a reality (117).

Secondary prevention refers to the identification of those who have already developed the disease at an early stage in its natural history, with the implication of intervention measures to reduce the associated morbidity and complications. Epidemiologic research can help identify key genetic and environmental factors involved in disease expression, and manipulation of these factors may help to diminish the progression of established atopic dermatitis (118). It is possible, for example, that early enhancement of the skin barrier may reduce the occurrence of atopic dermatitis, especially in those with filaggrin gene mutations that result in defective skin barrier function (119).

Tertiary prevention involves the treatment of established disease, which will be covered in detail in later chapters. One systematic review has summarized all the published data available from randomized controlled clinical trials of treatments for atopic dermatitis, covering more than 284 different studies (120). That systematic review is now out of date, as over 100 randomized controlled trials in atopic dermatitis have been published since. The review will be updated in 2009 at the Centre of Evidence-Based Dermatology, and the results will be freely available in the public domain (www.nottingham.ac.uk/dermatology). Unfortunately, prospective studies evaluating the effect of common treatments such as topical steroids on long-term disease progression or those that evaluate systemic consequences of long-term therapy are few. Most trials have been of less than six-week duration, and while they may show beneficial effects in controlling the acute phase of the disease, they do not capture the chronic relapsing course or the long-term effects of treatment such as the number of disease-free periods per year (121). For many other commonly employed therapies such as emollients and wet wrap bandaging, there are as yet no truly informative randomized controlled trials.

FUTURE RESEARCH AGENDA

The epidemiologic developments in the last 25 years have provided a strong foundation on which to build our knowledge and understanding of this common and distressing skin condition. These advances have included the development of valid and reliable disease definitions, the production of a worldwide map of the disease in the ISAAC study, tracking time trends of disease prevalence in many countries worldwide, and developments in the understanding of the mechanisms of allergic inflammation and the genetics of skin barrier defects (122). Yet, a number of important questions remain unanswered, and future research is desperately needed to fill the gaps of knowledge identified by recent studies. In particular, further investigation is needed into the factors associated with the "western" lifestyle that seems so strongly associated with atopic dermatitis expression, as we are still unable to adequately explain the global distribution of disease as documented by the ISAAC study. Prospective cohort studies are required to examine how the incidence and natural history of the disease is changing with time. The challenge remains to identify, refine, and evaluate those factors that can be easily manipulated at a population level in order to prevent the inexorable increase in disease prevalence.

REFERENCES

1. Last JM. A Dictionary of Epidemiology, 2nd ed. New York, NY: Oxford University Press, 1988.
2. Hanifin JM, Rajka G. Diagnostic features of atopic dermatitis. Acta Derm Venereol Suppl (Stockh) 1980; 92:44–47.
3. Williams HC, Burney PGJ, Hay RJ, et al. The UK working party's diagnostic criteria for atopic dermatitis I. Derivation of a minimum set of discriminators for atopic dermatitis. Br J Dermatol 1994; 131:383–396.
4. Williams HC, Burney PGJ, Strachan D, et al. The UK working party's diagnostic criteria for atopic dermatitis II: Observer variation of clinical diagnosis and signs of atopic dermatitis. Br J Dermatol 1994; 131:397–405.
5. Williams HC, Burney PGJ, Pembroke AC, et al. The UK working party's diagnostic criteria for atopic dermatitis III: Independent hospital validation. Br J Dermatol 1994; 131:406–416.
6. Brenninkmeijer EE, Schram ME, Leeflang MM, et al. Diagnostic criteria for atopic dermatitis: A systematic review. Br J Dermatol 2008; 158:754–765.
7. Chalmers DA, Todd G, Saxe N, et al. Validation of the U.K. working party diagnostic criteria for atopic eczema in a Xhosa-speaking African population. Br J Dermatol 2007; 156:111–116.
8. Williams HC, Flohr C. So how do I define atopic eczema? A practical manual for researchers wishing to define atopic eczema. http://www.nottingham.ac.uk/dermatology/eczema/index.html (last accessed 18th August 2008).
9. Varjonen E, Kalimo K, Lammintausta K, et al. Prevalence of atopic disorders among adolescents in Turku, Finland. Allergy 1992; 47:243–248.
10. Schäfer T, Vieluf D, Behrendt H, et al. Atopic eczema and other manifestations of atopy: Results of a study in East and West Germany. Allergy 1996; 51:532–539.

11. Dotterud LK, Kvammen B, Bolle R, et al. A survey of atopic disease among school children in Sør-Varanger community. Acta Derm Venereol (Stockh) 1994; 74:124–128.
12. Neame RL, Berth-Jones J, Kurinczuk JJ, et al. Prevalence of atopic dermatitis in Leicester: A study of methodology and examination of possible ethnic variation. Br J Dermatol 1995; 132:772–777.
13. Schultz Larsen F, Diepgen T, Svensson A. The occurrence of atopic dermatitis in northern Europe: An international questionnaire study. J Am Acad Dermatol 1996; 34:760–764.
14. Schäfer T, Heinrich J, Wjst M, et al. Indoor risk factors for atopic eczema in school children from East Germany. Environ Res Sect A 1999; 81:151–158.
15. Leung R, Ho P. Asthma, allergy and atopy in three south-east Asian populations. Thorax 1994; 49:1205–1210.
16. Dotterud LK, Kvammen B, Lund E, et al. Prevalence and some clinical aspects of atopic dermatitis in the community of Sør-Varanger. Acta Derm Venereol (Stockh) 1995; 75: 50–53.
17. Berth-Jones J, George S, Graham-Brown RAC. Predictors of atopic dermatitis in Leicester children. Br J Dermatol 1997; 136:498–501.
18. Kendirli GS, Altinta DU, Alparslan N, et al. Prevalence of childhood allergic diseases in Adana, Southern Turkey. Eur J Epidemiol 1998; 14:347–350.
19. Williams HC, Pembroke AC, Forsdyke H, et al. London-born black Caribbean children are at increased risk of atopic dermatitis. J Am Acad Dermatol 1995; 32:212–217.
20. Schäfer T, Dockery D, Krämer U, et al. Experiences with the severity scoring of atopic dermatitis in a population of German pre-school children. Br J Dermatol 1997; 137: 558–562.
21. Dotterud LK, Falk ES. Atopic disease among adults in northern Russia, an area with heavy air pollution. Acta Derm Venereol 1999; 79:448–450.
22. Selçuk ZT, Caglar T, Enunlu T, et al. The prevalence of allergic diseases in primary school children in Edirne, Turkey. Clin Exp Allergy 1997; 27:262–269.
23. Sugiura H, Umemoto N, Deguchi H, et al. Prevalence of childhood and adolescent atopic dermatitis in a Japanese population: Comparison with the disease frequency examined 20 years ago. Acta Derm Venereol (Stockh) 1998; 78:293–294.
24. Kimura Y, Kanazawa Y, Kida K, et al. A study of atopic dermatitis in elementary school children in Hirosaki City, Aomori Prefecture, Japan. Environ Health Prev Med 1998; 3:141–145.
25. Selnes A, Bolle R, Holt J, et al. Atopic diseases in Sami and Norse schoolchildren living in northern Norway. Pediatr Allergy Immunol 1999; 10:216–220.
26. Herd RM, Tidman MJ, Prescott RJ, et al. Prevalence of atopic eczema in the community: The Lothian atopic dermatitis study. Br J Dermatol 1996; 135:18–19.
27. Williams HC, Burney PGJ, Pembroke AC, et al. Validation of the UK diagnostic criteria for atopic dermatitis in a population setting. Br J Dermatol 1996; 135:12–17.
28. Emerson RM, Williams HC, Allen BR. Severity distribution of atopic dermatitis in the community and its relationship to secondary referral. Br J Dermatol 1998; 139: 73–76.
29. Bleiker TO, Shahidullah H, Dutton E, et al. The prevalence and incidence of atopic dermatitis in a birth cohort: The importance of a family history of atopy. Arch Dermatol 2000; 136:274.
30. Kalyoncu AF, Selçuk ZT, Enünlü T, et al. Prevalence of asthma and allergic diseases in primary school children in Ankara, Turkey: Two cross-sectional studies, five years apart. Pediatr Allergy Immunol 1999; 10:261–265.
31. Marks M, Kilkenny M, Plunkett A, et al. The prevalence of common skin conditions in Australian school students: 2. Atopic dermatitis. Br J Dermatol 1999; 140:468–473.
32. Popescu CM, Popescu R, Williams H, et al. Community validation of the United Kingdom diagnostic criteria for atopic dermatitis in Romanian schoolchildren. Br J Dermatol 1998; 138:436–442.
33. Laughter D, Istvan JA, Tofte SJ, et al. The prevalence of atopic dermatitis in Oregon schoolchildren. J Am Acad Dermatol 2000; 43:649–655.

34. Broberg A, Svensson A, Borres MP, et al. Atopic dermatitis in 5–6-year-old Swedish children: Cumulative incidence, point prevalence, and severity scoring. Allergy 2000; 55:1025–1029.
35. Mortz CG, Lauritsen JM, Bindslev-Jensen C, et al. Prevalence of atopic dermatitis, asthma, allergic rhinitis, and hand and contact dermatitis in adolescents. The Odense Adolescence Cohort Study on Atopic Diseases and Dermatitis. Br J Dermatol 2001; 144:523–532.
36. Lehtonen EP, Holmberg-Marttila D, Kaila M. Cumulative prevalence of atopic eczema and related skin symptoms in a well-baby clinic: A retrospective cohort study. Pediatr Allergy Immunol 2003; 14:405–408.
37. Haileamlak A, Lewis SA, Britton J, et al. Validation of the International Study of Asthma and Allergies in Children (ISAAC) and U.K. criteria for atopic eczema in Ethiopian children. Br J Dermatol 2005; 152:735–741.
38. Purvis DJ, Thompson JM, Clark PM, et al. Risk factors for atopic dermatitis in New Zealand children at 3.5 years of age. Br J Dermatol 2005; 152:742–749.
39. Worm M, Forschner K, Lee HH, et al. Frequency of atopic dermatitis and relevance of food allergy in adults in Germany. Acta Derm Venereol 2006; 86:119–122.
40. Halkjaer LB, Loland L, Buchvald FF, et al. Development of atopic dermatitis during the first 3 years of life: The Copenhagen prospective study on asthma in childhood cohort study in high-risk children. Arch Dermatol 2006; 142:561–566.
41. Harris JM, Williams HC, White C, et al. Early allergen exposure and atopic eczema. Br J Dermatol 2007; 156:698–704.
42. Harrop J, Chinn S, Verlato G, et al. Eczema, atopy and allergen exposure in adults: A population-based study. Clin Exp Allergy 2007; 37:526–535.
43. Hanifin JM, Reed ML; Eczema Prevalence and Impact Working Group. A population-based survey of eczema prevalence in the United States. Dermatitis 2007; 18:82–91.
44. Tanaka K, Miyake Y, Arakawa M, et al. Prevalence of asthma and wheeze in relation to passive smoking in Japanese children. Ann Epidemiol 2007; 17:1004–1010.
45. Lowe AJ, Hosking CS, Bennett CM, et al. Skin prick test can identify eczematous infants at risk of asthma and allergic rhinitis. Clin Exp Allergy 2007; 37:1624–1631.
46. Lee YL, Li CW, Sung FC, et al. Environmental factors, parental atopy and atopic eczema in primary-school children: A cross-sectional study in Taiwan. Br J Dermatol 2007; 157:1217–1224.
47. Sangsupawanich P, Chongsuvivatwong V, Mo-Suwan L, et al. Relationship between atopic dermatitis and wheeze in the first year of life: Analysis of a prospective cohort of Thai children. J Invest Allergol Clin Immunol 2007; 17:292–296.
48. Smidesang I, Saunes M, Storrø O. et al. Atopic dermatitis among 2-year olds; high prevalence, but predominantly mild disease—The PACT study, Norway. Pediatr Dermatol 2008; 25:13–18.
49. Lee YL, Su HJ, Sheu HM, et al. Traffic-related air pollution, climate, and prevalence of eczema in Taiwanese school children. J Invest Dermatol 2008; 128:2412–2420.
50. Kjaer HF, Eller E, Høst A, et al. The prevalence of allergic diseases in an unselected group of 6-year-old children. The DARC birth cohort study. Pediatr Allergy Immunol 2008 [Epub ahead of print].
51. Rajka G, Langeland T. Grading of the severity of atopic dermatitis. Acta Derm Venereol (Stockh) 1989; 144(suppl.):13–14.
52. Costa C, Rilliet A, Nicolet M, et al. Scoring atopic dermatitis: The simpler the better? Acta Derm Venereol (Stockh) 1989; 69:41–45.
53. European Task Force on Atopic Dermatitis. Severity scoring of atopic dermatitis: The SCORAD index. Dermatology 1993; 186:23–31.
54. Schmitt J, Langan S, Williams HC. What are the best outcome measurements for atopic eczema? J Allergy Clin Immunol 2007; 120:1389–1398.
55. Charman C, Venn A, Williams HC. The patient-oriented eczema measure. Development and initial validation of a new tool for measuring atopic eczema severity from the patients' perspective. Arch Dermatol 2004; 140:1513–1519.

56. Sandström MH, Faergemann J. Prognosis and prognostic factors in adult patients with atopic dermatitis: A long-term follow-up questionnaire study. Brit J Dermatol 2004; 150:103–110.
57. Lawson V, Lewis-Jones MS, Finlay AY, et al. The family impact of atopic dermatitis: The dermatitis family impact questionnaire. Br J Dermatol 1998; 138:107–113.
58. Reid P, Lewis-Jones M. Sleep difficulties and their management in preschoolers with atopic eczema. Clin Exp Dermatol 1995; 20:38–41.
59. Fennessy M, Coupland S, Popay J, et al. The epidemiology and experience of atopic eczema during childhood: A discussion paper on the implications of current knowledge for health care, public health policy and research. J Epidemiol Community Health 2000; 54:581–589.
60. Jowett S, Ryan T. Skin disease and handicap: An analysis of the impact of skin conditions. Soc Sci Med 1985; 20:425–429.
61. Daud LR, Garralda ME, David TJ. Psychosocial adjustment in preschool children with atopic eczema. Arch Dis Childhood 1993; 69:670–676.
62. Finlay AY, Khan GK. The Dermatology Life Quality Index. A simple practical measure for routine clinical use. Clin Exp Dermatol 1994; 19:210–216.
63. Falk E. Atopic diseases in Norwegian Lapps. Acta Derm Venereol Suppl (Stockh) 1993; 182:10–14.
64. Nishioka K. Atopic eczema of the adult type in Japan. Australas J Dermatol 1996; 37:S7–S9.
65. Saval P, Fuglsang G, Østerballe O. Prevalence of atopic disease among Danish school children. Pediatr Allergy Immunol 1993; 4:117–122.
66. Worth RM. Atopic dermatitis among Chinese infants in Honolulu and San Francisco. Hawaii Med J 1962; 22:31–34.
67. Mar A, Tam M, Jolley D, et al. The cumulative incidence of atopic dermatitis in the first 12 months among Chinese, Vietnamese, and Caucasian infants born in Melbourne, Australia. J Am Acad Dermatol 1999; 40:597–602.
68. Golding J, Peters TJ. The epidemiology of childhood eczema. Pediatr Perinat Epidemiol 1987; 1:67–79.
69. Wüthrich B. Epidemiology and natural history of atopic dermatitis. Allergy Clin Immunol Int 1996; 8(3):77–82.
70. Taylor B, Wadsworth J, Wadsworth M, et al. Changes in the reported prevalence of childhood eczema since the 1938–45 war. Lancet 1984; 2:1255–1257.
71. Strachan DP. Hay fever, hygiene, and household size. Br Med J 1989; 299:1259–1260.
72. Williams HC, Strachan DP, Hay RJ. Childhood eczema: Disease of the advantaged? Br Med J 1994; 308:1132–1135.
73. Flohr C, Pascoe D, Williams HC. Atopic dermatitis and the 'hygiene hypothesis': too clean to be true? British Journal of Dermatology 2005; 152:202–216.
74. Williams HC, Robertson C, Stewart A, et al. Worldwide variations in the prevalence of symptoms of atopic eczema in the International Study of Asthma and Allergies in Childhood. J Allergy Clin Immunol 1999; 103:125–138.
75. Flohr C, Johansson SGO, Wahlgren CF, et al. How atopic is atopic dermatitis? J Allergy Clin Immunol 2004; 114:150–158.
76. Flohr C, Weiland SK, Weinmayr G, et al. The role of atopic sensitization in flexural eczema: Findings from the International Study of Asthma and Allergies in Childhood Phase Two. J Allergy Clin Immunol 2008; 121:141–147.
77. Johansson SGO, Bieber T, Dahl R, et al. Revised nomenclature for allergy for global use. Report of the nomenclature review committee of the world allergy organization, October 2003. J Allergy Clin Immunol 2004; 113:832–836.
78. Williams H, Flohr C. How epidemiology has challenged 3 prevailing concepts about atopic dermatitis. J Allergy Clin Immunol 2006; 118:209–213.
79. Falade AG, Olawuyi F, Osinusi K, et al. Prevalence and severity of symptoms of asthma, allergic rhino-conjunctivitis and atopic eczema in secondary school children in Ibadan, Nigeria. East Afr Med J 1998; 75(12):695–698.

80. Williams HC, Forsdyke H, Boodoo G, et al. A protocol for recording the sign of visible flexural dermatitis. Br J Dermatol 1995; 133:941–949.
81. Strachan DP, Golding J, Anderson HR. Regional variations in wheezing illness in British children: Effect of migration during early childhood. J Epidemiol Community Health 1990; 44:231–236.
82. Weiland SK, von Mutius E, Hirsch T, et al. Prevalence of respiratory and atopic disorders among children in the east and west of Germany five years after unification. Eur Respir J 1999; 14:862–870.
83. Behrendt H, Krämer U, Dolgner R, et al. Elevated levels of total serum IgE in East German children: Atopy, parasites or pollutants? Allergy J 1993; 2:31–40.
84. Schäfer T, Ring J. Epidemiology of allergic diseases. Allergy 1997; 52(suppl. 38):14–22.
85. Kjellman B, Petterson R, Hyensjö B. Allergy among school children in a Swedish country. Allergy 1982; 37(suppl. 1):5.
86. Pösä I, Korppi M, Pietikäinen M, et al. Asthma, allergic rhinitis and atopioc eczema in Finnish children and adolescents. Allergy 1991; 46:161–165.
87. McNally NJ, Williams HC, Phillips DR, et al. Water hardness and atopic eczema. Lancet 1998; 352:527–553.
88. Miyake Y, Yokoyama T, Yura A, et al. Ecological association of water hardness with prevalence of childhood atopic dermatitis in a Japanese urban area. Environ Res 2004; 94:33–37.
89. Arnedo-Pena A, Bellido-Blasco J, Puig-Barbera J, et al. Domestic water hardness and prevalence of atopic eczema in Castellon (Spain) school children. Salud Publica Mex 2007; 49:295–301.
90. Thomas KS, Sach TH; on behalf of the SWET Trial Investigators. A multicentre randomized controlled trial of ion-exchange water softeners for the treatment of eczema in children: Protocol for the Softened Water Eczema Trial (SWET) (ISRCTN: 71423189). Br J Dermatol 2008 Jun 26 [Epub ahead of print].
91. Waite DA, Eyles EF, Tonkin SL, et al. Asthma prevalence in Tokelauan children in two environments. Clin Allergy 1980; 10:71–75.
92. Leung R. Asthma, allergy and atopy in south-east Asian immigrants in Australia. Aust N Z J Med 1994; 24:255.
93. Kalyoncu AF, Selcuk ZT, Karakoca Y, et al. Prevalence of childhood asthma and allergic diseases in Ankara, Turkey. Allergy 1994; 49:485–488.
94. Kusunoki T, Kouichi A, Harazaki M, et al. Month of birth and prevalence of atopic dermatitis in schoolchildren: Dry skin in early infancy as a possible etiological factor. J Allergy Clin Immunol 1999; 103(6):1148–1152.
95. Anderson HR, Bailey PA, Bland JM. The effect of birth month on asthma, eczema, hay fever, respiratory symptoms, lung function, and hospital admissions for asthma. Int J Epidemiol 1981; 10:45–51.
96. Schäfer T, Przybilla B, Ring J, et al. Manifestation of atopy is not related to patient's month of birth. Allergy 1993; 48:291–294.
97. Schultz-Larsen F, Hanifin JM. Secular changes in the occurrence of atopic dermatitis. Acta Derm Venereol Suppl (Stockh) 1992; 176:7–12.
98. Williams HC. Is the prevalence of atopic dermatitis increasing? Clin Exp Derm 1992; 17:385–391.
99. Schultz Larson F, Holm NV, Henningsen K. Atopic dermatitis. A genetic-epidemiological study in a population-based twin sample. J Am Acad Dermatol 1986; 15:487–494.
100. Åberg N, Hesselmar B, Åberg B, et al. Increase of asthma, allergic rhinitis and eczema in Swedish schoolchildren between 1979 and 1991. Clin Exp Allergy 1995; 25:815–819.
101. Williams H, Stewart A, von Mutius E, et al.; the International Study of Asthma and Allergies in Childhood (ISAAC) Phase One and Three Study groups. Is eczema really on the increase worldwide? J Allergy Clin Immunol 2008; 121:947–954.
102. Yates VM, Kerr REI, MacKie RM. Early diagnosis of infantile seborrhoeic dermatitis and atopic dermatitis—Clinical features. Br J Dermatol 1983; 108:633–638.
103. Aoki T, Fukuzumi T, Adachi J, et al. Re-evaluation of skin lesion distribution in atopic dermatitis. Acta Derm Venereol Suppl (Stockh) 1992; 176:19–23.

104. Williams HC, Wüthrich B. The natural history of atopic dermatitis. In: Williams HC, ed. Atopic Dermatitis: The Epidemiology, Causes and Prevention of Atopic Eczema. Cambridge, MA: Cambridge University Press, 2000:41–59.
105. Kay J, Gawkrodger DJ, Mortimer MJ, et al. The prevalence of childhood atopic eczema in a general population. J Am Acad Dermatol 1994; 30:35–39.
106. Williams HC, Strachan DP. The natural history of childhood eczema: Observations from the 1958 British cohort study. Br J Dermatol 1998; 139:834–839.
107. Bergmann RL, Bergmann KE, Lau-Schadensdorf S, et al. Atopic diseases in infancy. The German multicenter atopy study (MAS-90). Pediatr Allergy Immunol 1994; 5(suppl. 1):19–25.
108. Bergmann RL, Edenharter G, Bergmann KE, et al. Predictability of early atopy by cord blood-IgE and parental history. Clin Exp Allergy 1997; 27:752–760.
109. Rystedt I. Long term follow-up in atopic dermatitis. Acta Dermatol Venereol Suppl (Stockh) 1986; 114:117–120.
110. Vickers CFH. The natural history of atopic eczema. Acta Dermatol Venereol Suppl (Stockh) 1980; 92:113–115.
111. Schultz Larsen F. The epidemiology of atopic dermatitis. In: Burr ML, ed. Epidemiology of Clinical Allergy. Monogr Allergy, vol. 31. Basel, Switzerland: Karger, 1993:9–28.
112. Musgrove K, Morgan JK. Infantile eczema. A long-term follow-up study. Br J Dermatol 1976; 95:365–372.
113. Kramer MS, Kakuma R. Maternal dietary antigen avoidance during pregnancy or lactation, or both, for preventing or treating atopic disease in the child. Cochrane Database Syst Rev 2003; (4):CD000133.
114. Lee J, Seto D, Bielory L. Meta-analysis of clinical trials of probiotics for prevention and treatment of pediatric atopic dermatitis. J Allergy Clin Immunol 2008; 121:116–121.
115. Osborn DA, Sinn JK. Probiotics in infants for prevention of allergic disease and food hypersensitivity. Cochrane Database Syst Rev 2007; (4):CD006475.
116. Høst A, Halken S, Muraro A, et al. Dietary prevention of allergic diseases in infants and small children. Pediatr Allergy Immunol 2008; 19:1–4.
117. Mar A, Marks R. Prevention of atopic dermatitis. In: Williams HC, ed. Atopic Dermatitis: The Epidemiology, Causes and Prevention of Atopic Eczema. Cambridge, MA: Cambridge University Press, 2000:205–218.
118. Anonymous. Allergic factors associated with the development of asthma and the influence of cetirizine in a double-blind, randomised, placebo-controlled trial: First results of ETAC. Early treatment of the atopic child. Pediatr Allergy Immunol 1998; 9:116–124.
119. Baurecht H, Irvine AD, Novak N, et al. Toward a major risk factor for atopic eczema: Meta-analysis of filaggrin polymorphism data. J Allergy Clin Immunol 2007; 120:1406–1412.
120. Hoare C, Li A, Wan Po, et al. Systematic review of treatments for atopic eczema. Health Technol Assess 2000; 4(37).
121. Langan SM, Thomas KS, Williams HC. What is meant by a "flare" in atopic dermatitis? A systematic review and proposal. Arch Dermatol 2006; 142;1190–1196.
122. Bieber T. Atopic dermatitis. N Engl J Med 2008; 358:1483–1494.
123. Burrel-Morris C, Williams HC. Atopic dermatitis in migrant populations. In: Williams HC, ed. Atopic dermatitis. The epidemiology, causes and prevention of atopic eczema. Cambridge, MA: Cambridge University Press, 2000:169–182.

Genetics of Atopic Eczema

Stephan Weidinger

Department of Dermatology and Allergy Biederstein, Technische Universität München (TUM), Munich, Germany

Elke Rodriguez

Division of Environmental Dermatology and Allergy, Helmholtz Zentrum München and ZAUM-Center for Allergy and Environment, Technische Universität München (TUM), Munich, Germany

Alan D. Irvine

Paediatric Dermatology, Our Lady's Children's Hospital, Crumlin, and Trinity College Dublin, Dublin, Ireland

INTRODUCTION: DEFINITIONS, EMPIRICAL EVIDENCE FOR A GENETIC ROLE

Atopic Eczema: Defining a Phenotype for Molecular Investigation

Atopic eczema (AE) is a chronic and relapsing inflammatory skin disease, which is characterized by dry skin, intense pruritus, and a typical age-related distribution of inflammatory lesions. In the majority of cases the disease starts in early childhood and shows a spontaneous remission before adolescence (1). During the last three decades, there has been an increase in the prevalence of AE, especially in industrialized countries, where 15% to 30% of children and 2% to 10% of adults are affected (2). Due to its frequent co-occurrence with asthma and allergic rhinitis and since parental atopy is a strong risk factor, AE is considered to be part of a syndrome of "atopic diseases," which are characterized by the development of IgE antibodies to ubiquitous allergens (3). Many individuals with AE (especially those with moderate or severe disease in secondary care settings) exhibit increased total IgE levels and IgE-mediated sensitivity to food and environmental allergens. However, in many with features otherwise typical of AE, particularly children who are affected in the first two years of life and adult-onset AE, there are no signs of IgE-mediated sensitization (4,5). Consistent with these observations, recent epidemiologic research questions a primary, causative role for allergic sensitization in AE (2,6). The role and temporal significance of elevated IgE in AE are, at present, unresolved but currently the balance of evidence weighs in favor of elevated serum IgE being a secondary phenomenon that may well amplify existing inflammatory lesions either directly or through mediation of autoimmune processes (1). In this regard, as increasingly sophisticated genetic linkage and association studies dissect out the pathways associated with AE and with other atopic diseases, the precise role of IgE in AE versus atopy *sensu latu* will become clearer.

The study of complex genetic illnesses demands accurate definitions of the phenotypes being investigated in order to detect causal associations and to reduce the likelihood of detecting confounding associations (7). Phenotype standardization and nomenclature have been a central activity of committees and organizations for years (8–10). However, standardization often results in a less specific phenotype in order to gain maximum consensus. Reconciling the tension between quality of phenotyping and standardization of methodology is a great challenge for the constitution of phenotype databases and has presented severe problems for the study of atopic illnesses.

The term "atopy" (Greek: atopos) was first introduced by Coca and Cooke in 1923 to describe some phenomena of hypersensitivity in man (11). They considered "atopy" as a hereditary disorder clinically characterized by asthma or hay fever, which is associated with immediate-type skin reactions and which is different from "anaphylaxis," as a lack of protection, and "allergy," as altered reactivity. Since Prausnitz and Küstner had already demonstrated the passive transfer of immediate hypersensitivity in man by serum (12), Coca and Grove later designated the causative serum factor as ""atopic reagins" (13). In 1933, Wise and Sulzberger included "AE" into the group of atopic diseases proposing the term "atopic dermatitis" to denote confusing types of localized and generalized lichenification, generalized neurodermatitis, or a manifestation of atopy (14). After the identification of reagins as IgE (15), Pepys defined atopy as inherited tendency to produce increased amounts of IgE against low doses of environmental allergens (16). Since then, the definition of "atopy" has been a matter of controversy, as, for example, this concept of "atopy" does not explain IgE-negative disease manifestations, nonfamilial IgE-responses, or parenterally induced IgE reactions. Thus, it is unclear whether AE is a single disorder with variable clinical manifestations or a group of syndromes, each with a unique or overlapping pathophysiology. Thus, the extant terminology for atopic diseases remains confusing and terms such as AE, atopic dermatitis, childhood eczema, atopiform dermatitis, and flexural dermatitis are frequently used synonymously in the literature. Recently, in an attempt to standardize the nosology for allergic diseases, the task force on nomenclature of the European Academy of Allergy and Clinical Immunology (EAACI) (9) and the nomenclature committee of the World Allergy Organisation (WAO) (8) defined atopy as a "personal or familial tendency to become sensitized and produce IgE antibodies in response to low doses of allergens, usually proteins" and to "develop typical symptoms such as asthma, rhinoconjunctivitis, or eczema/dermatitis. Following this definition, the term "eczema" designates the disease formerly called "AE" or "atopic dermatitis". The term "AE" is reserved for those patients with eczema and showing evidence for IgE involvement, while the others (formerly called "intrinsic") will be classified as non-AE. However, as pointed out in a recent review, this division might not adequately reflect the natural history of this disease (1), and it has to be considered that so far most, if not all, studies on the genetics of AE were performed prior to these definitional suggestions. Also, most existing DNA collections will have been assembled using older definitions; given the time, money, and effort that these collections demand, it is likely that this will remain the case for future genetic studies.

In AE, a clear-cut definition and diagnosis are further hampered by the wide spectrum of clinical presentations, such as presentation, severity and distribution, and course of the disease. Furthermore, different combinations of symptoms exist in different individuals. Thus, there might be subtypes in which the genetic determinants are distinct from those relevant to the condition suggested by wider, more inclusive definitions. Furthermore, although a diagnosis made by a dermatological examination might be looked upon as a gold standard, clinical examinations by experts are not practicable in large epidemiologic studies. In the absence of a single diagnostic parameter, numerous lists of diagnostic criteria have been developed to establish a definition for AE with known validity and reproducibility by using reliable discriminators. At present, the U.K. diagnostic criteria have been the most widely validated and appear to be applicable and repeatable across all ages and many ethinicities. However, as shown in a recent review, the ideal set of diagnostic criteria still has to be established (10).

Thus, accurate phenotyping and a clear-cut definition of the phenotype are crucial when studying the genetics of AE and judging observations made by genetic association studies in different patient collections and in different ethnic populations.

Atopic Eczema As Complex Genetic Trait

A strong genetic component in atopic diseases was recognized almost a century ago, when Cooke and van der Veer were the first to report a strong familial clustering of allergic diseases (17). Since then, a genetic predisposition to the development of asthma, allergic rhinitis, and AE has been confirmed by numerous epidemiological studies with the strongest evidence delivered by twin studies, which show a distinctly higher concordance rate among monozygotic twins as compared to dizygotic twin pairs (for AE: 0.72–0.77 vs. 0.15–0.23), and segregation analyses, which suggest that genetic factors account for more than 80% of the variance in the susceptibility to AE (18–21). However, unlike monogenic disorders, which are caused by mutations in a single gene, AE and atopic disorders do not follow a Mendelian mode of inheritance, but are complex multifactorial traits, which are thought to arise from a complex interaction of genetic and environmental factors (7). The importance of environmental factors in genetically susceptible individuals is indicated by the incomplete concordance among monozygotic twins and the rapid rise in prevalence, which cannot be explained in genetic terms. In addition, single genetic factors are likely to exert additive or synergistic effects known as epistatic interactions (7). The dissection of these traits is further hampered by phenocopy, incomplete penetrance, and genetic heterogeneity (7).

Nevertheless, significant progress has been made in the field of AE genetics with the identification of numerous loci and potential candidate genes linked and associated.

This chapter will provide a structured overview on the current knowledge of genetic susceptibility to AE and will briefly discuss future developments in this fast-moving field.

METHODOLOGIES USED IN THE GENETIC ANALYSIS OF ATOPIC ECZEMA

It is clear from genetic epidemiology that despite familial aggregation in AE, there is no clear Mendelian single gene inheritance pattern, and that the mode of transmission is complex (22). Hallmarks of complex diseases include variable disease onset, expression and progression, incomplete penetrance, confounding by other genes (allelic or locus heterogeneity, multigene inheritance, copy number variation, epistasis, modifier genes, sex influence, parental effects), and nonclassical genetic phenomena (imprinting—parent of origin effect, mitochondrial inheritance) (23). In general there are two major methodological approaches to identify gene variants associated with susceptibility to common diseases: pedigree and affected sib-pair linkage studies (studies using related subjects) and association studies (where unrelated cases are compared with population controls).

Genome Screens: Linkage Studies

Initially, whole-genome searches for disease loci in complex diseases were based on linkage approaches. Linkage between a genetic marker and a disease means that the disease and marker transmissions in families are not independent, implying the presence of a susceptibility gene in the marker region. Linkage can be used to map disease genes by genotyping polymorphic DNA markers (short tandem repeats or microsatellites) and evaluating if their alleles co-segregate with the disease within families. In general, there are two approaches: parametric analysis [reviewed in (24)], also known as logarithm of the odds (LOD) score analysis, and nonparametric methods, which evaluate allele sharing by affected relatives. Parametric analysis is also termed "model-based," whereas nonparametric analysis is named "model-free" [reviewed in (25)].

For LOD score analysis, the parameters of the disease model, for example, mode of inheritance, penetrance, and allele frequencies need to be specified prior to analysis. The LOD score is a likelihood ratio testing the hypothesis of linkage (against the hypothesis of no linkage) for different genetic distances (or recombination fractions) between the phenotype locus and the marker locus. A LOD of 3 or more is generally taken as "significant" evidence for linkage (equivalent to a 1 in 1000 chance of nonlinkage or roughly equivalent to a P value of 0.0001), whereas a LOD score less than -2 proves nonlinkage (26). Nonparametric methods, which do not need specification of a genetic model, are often preferred for complex traits, but are poor at providing a precise location of the disease gene compared to the LOD score method. Most nonparametric linkage methods are based on the proportion of marker alleles identical by descent (i.e., the same allele inherited from the same parent) in sets of relatives (usually pairs of siblings) compared with the phenotypic similarity between the relatives. The strength of evidence in favor of linkage can be given by a chi-squared statistic or by a maximum likelihood score (MLS), the latter being similar to a LOD score [reviewed in (27)].

Linkage studies are capable of detecting a disease gene over a relatively large range, so that genome screens typically use only 400 polymorphic markers spread evenly over the chromosomes. However, linkage regions identified in this way usually extend over large distances (>10 cm) that might contain hundreds of genes. Thus, intensive follow-up fine mapping analyses are needed to narrow down the region of interest and to further refine the localization of disease genes, by applying a directed genomic screening or utilizing a candidate gene approach.

Genome Screens: Association Studies

Although the traditional approach for mapping disease genes by linkage mapping followed by progressive fine-mapping of candidate linkage peaks has been extremely successful at identifying genes that predispose carriers to rare Mendelian disorders, for example, cystic fibrosis (28), it has met only limited success when applied to complex traits such as AE (29,30). Therefore molecular epidemiologists increasingly have utilized genome-wide association studies (GWAS), which use dense maps of single nucleotide polymorphisms (SNPs) that cover the human genome to look for allele-frequency differences between cases and controls (31). GWAS have become commercially viable through recent developments in ultra-high-volume genotyping chip technology. Currently available commercial SNP-typing products deploy up to 1,000,000 SNPs, and are designed by using two different SNP selection approaches, the direct gene-centric approach focusing on genetic variants in genic regions, and the indirect approach using either random/anonymous SNPs that are spread across the genome, or sets of linkage-disequilibrium (LD)–based tag SNPs that are specifically chosen to saturate the genome (32). Assuming that genotyping technologies continue to develop at the current pace, in the near future, assays that capture all common SNPs and population-specific chips as well as disease- or pathway-specific chips and copy number variation analyses should become available soon.

Candidate Gene Approach

In contrast to the "hypothesis-free" approach of whole genome mapping studies, an alternative (or at times complementary) approach is to select biologically plausible candidate genes and to test polymorphisms within these genes for either linkage (family based studies) or association (case:control studies) with eczema. Both the choice of a suitable and plausible candidate gene and the particular polymorphisms to be analyzed are of crucial importance. Candidate genes can be chosen for their position, if they are located in a region showing linkage or association in prior genomic screening studies or if they may be chosen based on a biological model because of their function and expression patterns. Combined strategies appear to be the most successful method of identifying disease genes (33). Examples of biologically plausible candidate genes, derived from Mendelian disorders, include *filaggrin* (FLG) (the causative gene for ichthyosis vulgaris (IV)) and *SPINK5* (the causative gene in Netherton syndrome). In principle, candidate gene studies aim at identifying interindividual genetic variants, mostly SNPs, which are associated with the phenotype of interest, either because they are causal or, more likely, statistically correlated or in linkage disequilibrium (LD) with (an) unobserved causal variant(s).

Although candidate gene studies are an essential and powerful tool for studying the genetic architecture of complex traits (29), there are multiple potential pitfalls in both the design and interpretation of such studies that have led to some inconsistency of both linkage and association data and ambiguous results (34). Potential reasons for conflicting findings include small sample sizes and low statistical power, inadequate assessment of the trait of interest and inappropriate controls, inappropriate statistical modeling and failure to correct for multiple comparisons, genetic and environmental heterogeneity, publication bias (more positive reports are submitted to and accepted by journals), and lack of independent replication (35).

What is the Optimal Approach to Elucidate the Genetic Basis of Atopic Eczema?

Currently, the most widely used strategy of association studies is the case-control design; this will continue to be the dominant methodology, as larger cases collections are assembled and marker panels with increasing density of markers become available. Family-based procedures such as the transmission disequilibrium test (TDT), a method which identifies markers preferentially transmitted to affected individuals and tests for both linkage and association, are robust to population stratification, migration, and admixture, but have several disadvantages, such as the need to collect DNA samples from parents of affected individuals, which are not easily accessible, especially for late-onset disorders, and the limited use of infor-mation due to its reliance on heterozygous parents. A population-based case-control or cohort designs permits valid extrapolation to larger groups within the popula-tion, but might have limited power due to their being few affected individuals (36).

Alternative Approaches to Gene Identification

The use of animal models and quantitative trait locus (QTL) mapping has aided in the identification of genes that affect multifactorial traits (37). Advantages of animal models include a reduced genetic heterogeneity in inbred strains, the possibility to generate large numbers of offspring in short generation times, and the opportunity to investigate gene–environment interactions in controlled settings. A number of different murine models of AE have been reported, but so far there is no repro-ducible and accessible animal model which combines all of the different aspects of AE (38). Due to the complexity and variability of this disease it is anticipated that, given the lack of a single comprehensive animal model, many of the disease components will have to be modeled initially as isolated traits and subsequently in combination to explore pathophysiological mechanisms and to provide models for testing new treatments.

Microarray technology now allows monitoring of messenger RNA abundance for thousands of genes simultaneously. Synergistic analysis of gene expression data in tandem with genetic locus data from association or linkage studies can advance the gene discovery process, for example by reducing the number of candidate genes in QTL regions and by validating genes found to be associated in genome-wide scans, as has been recently shown for asthma and diabetes (39). In AE, expression-array studies are still in their infancy. So far, most reported studies were performed in small samples only and have methodological weaknesses such as inappropriate controls and the use of full thickness skin biopsy specimens with heterogeneous cellular populations (40–42). However, well-designed single cell and population cell profiling in large cohorts using whole-genome microarray platforms together with improved proteomic and metabolomic technologies have the potential to greatly enhance the identification of candidate disease genes.

WHOLE GENOME LINKAGE STUDIES IN ATOPIC ECZEMA

At least 15 whole-genome screens have been reported for asthma and associated phenotypes such as bronchial hyper-responsiveness, elevated IgE levels, and atopy, with numerous suggestive linkage findings in different chromosomal regions, but limited validity due to low statistical power and the potential for type I and type II errors as discussed above (43,44). In contrast, very few whole-genome linkage screens for AE have been carried out, all of which have been of modest size (45–48). The first screen was carried out in 199 nuclear families of mainly German origin using 380 microsatellite markers and found linkage for AE and suggestive link-age for total IgE on chromosome 3q21. The second screen was performed with 385 microsatellite markers in 148 nuclear British families and found suggestive evidence for linkage of AE to 1q21 and 17q25, as well as total IgE to chromosomes 5q31 and 16qtel (46). The candidate region on chromosome 1q21 overlies the epidermal dif-ferentiation complex (EDC) and that on chromosome 17q contains the keratin type I gene cluster. Mutations in several genes located in these regions have been shown to cause different monogenic disorders of epidermal differentiation and function (49). A third genome screen was carried out in Swedish adults with AE by means of 367 microsatellite marker in 109 families, with less conclusive results suggesting linkage to chromosome region 3p24–22 (45). More recently, an SNP-based linkage approach in 77 Japanese families with 111 affected sib-pairs suggested linkage to 15q21 (48).

Additional loci have been mapped by using composite phenotypes, such as AE and asthma (20p) (46), AE with increased allergen-specific IgE levels (3p, 4p, and 18q) (50), and total serum IgE level (16q) (46). In addition, some candidate loci originally identified in analyses of AE or other atopic phenotypes have been examined for replication by means of region-specific linkage mapping. Thereby additional evidence of linkage has been obtained on chromosomes 5q (51), 13q (51) and 14q (52) for AE, and on chromosome 5q (52) for severity of AE.

In general, there is no substantial overlap between the results of these linkage studies, this might be explained by differences in sample sizes, marker panels, statistical methods, phenotype definitions, and different populations, but perhaps the most likely explanation for these inconsistencies is that they are largely due to the limitations of linkage studies for the dissection of complex traits, especially when utilized on small samples sizes. Apart from *FLG*, which accounts for a large part of the significant linkage signal on 1q21 (53), the underlying disease genes remain elusive. Interestingly, as shown in Table 1, the regions linked to AE do not overlap with those known for asthma, suggesting that susceptibility to asthma and AE is mediated through different genes rather than through a shared susceptibility to a common atopic background. The AE loci identified thus far are, however, closely coincident with psoriasis susceptibility regions, for example 1q21, suggesting that these conditions share susceptibility loci in genomic regions encoding tissue-specific genes, perhaps with general effects on dermal inflammation, immunity, and structure, and an important role for proteins expressed by epithelial cells (54).

CANDIDATE GENE STUDIES IN ATOPIC ECZEMA

In the past two decades, numerous candidate gene studies have been conducted for AE, often yielding inconsistent results as discussed above (Table 2). In addition, the specific phenotypes found to be associated with many candidate genes vary, possibly indicating a role for the atopic state rather than eczema *per se*. Very few genes have been associated consistently with AE. These are presented and discussed in more detail below. These genes can be considered as falling into two major functional groups: genes encoding epidermal or other epithelial structural proteins, and genes encoding major elements of the immune system.

Genes Associated with Epithelial Barrier Function

Filaggrin (FLG)

Hallmark features of AE are dry, itchy skin, a marked permeability barrier abnormality, and stratum corneum abnormalities (55,56). Among the loci linked to AE is the susceptibility region for psoriasis and IV, a common monogenic disorder of keratinization, on chromosome 1q21 (57), which contains the epidermal differentiation complex (EDC)(58). The EDC is a dense cluster of approximately 50 genes encoding proteins involved in the terminal differentiation of the epidermis (59). The EDC gene *FLG* is a key protein in the formation of the outermost keratin layer of the skin (60). Profilaggrin is expressed as large (300 kD) insoluble and highly phosphorylated protein in the keratohyalin granules in the stratum granulosum and consists of a unique N-terminal Ca-binding S-100 domain, followed by a downstream B-domain comprising a putative bipartite nuclear localization sequence, 10 to 12 tandem filaggrin monomer repeats, and the C-terminal end containing a

TABLE 1 Genome Screens for AE

Ref.	Study population	Individuals/affected sib-pairs/families	Microsatellite marker sets	Phenotypes	Region of highest linkage	P-value	Additional traits linked to these regions
(47)	European	839/199/199	380	AE	3q21	8.4×10^{-6}	Psoriasis, SLE, asthma, AR
				Allergic sensitization		6.7×10^{-4}	
(46)	British	383/213/148	385	AE	1q21	5.0×10^{-4}	Psoriasis, SLE, IV, asthma, RA
					17q25	4.0×10^{-4}	Psoriasis, EV, SLD
				AE plus asthma	20p	5.0×10^{-4}	Psoriasis
				Total serum	5q31	0.004	
				IgE	16q	7.0×10^{-4}	
(45)	Swedish	470/197(9)[b]/109	367	AE	3p24–22	<0.001	
					5p13	<0.005	
					6q16	<0.01	
					10p13–12	<0.01	
				Severity score of AE	3q14	$<7.4 \times 10^{-4}$	
					13q14	$<7.4 \times 10^{-4}$	Asthma
					15q14–15	$<7.4 \times 10^{-4}$	
					17q21	$<7.4 \times 10^{-4}$	
		144/100(2)[b]/62		AE with elevated specific IgE	1p32	<0.01	
					4q24–26	<0.005	
					6p	<0.005	
					18q21	<0.001	
		74/53/32		Extreme severe AE	7p14	<0.005	
					18p	<0.005	
					21q21	<0.005	
(50)	Danish	103/28/23	446	AE with elevated specific IgE	3p26–24	≤ 0.001[a]	
					4p15–14	≤ 0.0126[a]	
					18q11–12	≤ 0.004[a]	
(48)	Japanese	287/111/77	5861 SNPs	AE	1q24	0.008	Asthma, RA, GD
					15q21	0.0012	

[a] Studies with a maximum likelihood score >2.
[b] Affected half-sib pairs.

Abbreviations: AD, atopic dermatitis; AR, allergic rhinitis; EV, epidermodysplasia verruciformis; GD, Graves' disease; IgE, immunoglobulin E; IV, ichthyosis vulgaris; RA, rheumatoid arthritis; SLE, systemic lupus erythematosus; SLD, seborrhea-like dermatitis.

TABLE 2 Genes That Have Been Associated with AE Ordered by Their Chromosomal Position

Gene symbol	Gene name	Location	Phenotype(s)	AE cases	Marker(s)	Ass.	Ref.
IL10	Interleukin 10	1q31–32	AE	94 Germans	−1082A/G	No	(194)
			Childhood AE	185 Japanese	−627C/A	Yes	(195)
			AE, nonatopic eczema	358 Koreans	−819T/C,−592A/C	Yes	(196)
IL1RL1	Interleukin 1 receptor-like 1	2q11.2	AE	452 Japanese	−26999G/A	Yes	(197)
CTLA4	Cytotoxic T-lymphocyte-associated protein 4	2q33	Early onset AE	112 Australian families	49A/G, haplotypes	Yes	(198)
TLR9	Toll-like receptor 9	3p21.3	AE, Intrinsic AE	483 German families	rs5743836, haplotype	Yes	(199)
				274 Germans		No	
IL5RA	Interleukin 5 receptor alpha	3p26-p24	AE	646 Koreans	rs334809	Yes	(200)
IL5	Interleukin-5	5q31	Extrinsic AE	646 Koreans	rs2522411 (−4597T/A), haplotype	Yes	(200)
IL4	Interleukin-4	5q31	Childhood AE	88 Japanese families	−590C/T	Yes	(139)
			Childhood AE	101 Australian families	−590C/T, −34C/T, haplotypes	No	(142)
			Intrinsic AE	190 Japanese	−590C/T	No	(140)
			Extrinsic AE	60 Germans	−590C/T	Yes	(148)
			AE severity	406 Swedish families	−590C/T	Yes	(141)
			Infantile AE (<2 years)	28 Canadians	−590C/T	No	(133)
			AE	94 Chinese	−590T/C, 33T/C	No	(201)
SPINK5	Serine protease inhibitor, Kazal type 5	5q32	AE	148 British families	rs2303067 (Glu420Lys)	Yes	(57)

(Continued)

TABLE 2 Genes That Have Been Associated with AE Ordered by Their Chromosomal Position (*Continued*)

Gene symbol	Gene name	Location	Phenotype(s)	AE cases	Marker(s)	Ass.	Ref.
			AE severity	55 Japanese	rs2303067	Yes	(136)
			Childhood AE	41 Japanese families	rs2303067	Yes	(100)
			AE	124 Japanese	rs2303067	Yes	(99)
			AE	274 german	rs2303067	No	(202)
			Childhood AE	200 Dutch families	rs2303067	No	(103)
			Childhood AE	308 German families	rs2303067	No	(102)
			AE	99 French	rs2303067	No	(101)
			AE	2774 Germans, Irish, English	rs2303067	No	(104)
CARD4 (NOD1)	Caspase recruitment domain-containing protein 4	7p14–15	AE	189 German families	rs2975632, rs2075822, rs2907749, rs2907748	Yes	(185)
				227 Germans	Haplotype	Yes	(185)
				1417[a]/28 Germans	rs2736726, rs2075817, haplotype	Yes	
			AE	392 Germans	Haplotypes, SNP-SNP interaction	Yes	(180)
FCER1B	High affinity IgE receptor beta chain	11q13	AE	148 British families	RsaI in2, RsaI ex7	Yes	(125)
IL18	Interleukin-18	11q22	Adult AE	225 Germans	113T/G, 127C/T, −137G/C, −133C/G	Yes	(203)
			Extrinsic AE	646 Koreans	rs795467, haplotype	Yes	(204)
IL31	Interleukin 31	12q24.31	Nonatopic eczema	690 European families	Haplotype	Yes	(205)
PHF11	Plant homeodomain Zink finger protein 11	13q14	Childhood AE	111 Australian families	T/C intron 3, G/A 3′ UTR	Yes	(206)

TABLE 2   Genes That Have Been Associated with AE Ordered by Their Chromosomal Position (*Continued*)

Gene		Position	Phenotype	Cases	SNP	Population-based[a]	Ref.
CMA1	Mast cell chymase	14q11.2	Adult AE	100 Japanese	−1903A/G	Yes	(113)
			Childhood AE	145 Japanese	−1903A/G	Yes	(167)
			Childhood and young Adult AE	100 Japanese	−1903A/G	No	(171)
			AE	70 Italians	−1903A/G	No	(172)
			AE	242 Germans	−1903A/G	Yes	(169)
CARD15 (NOD2)	Caspase recruitment domain-containing protein 15	16q12	Childhood AE	330 Germans	2722G/C (G881R)	Yes	(179)
			AE	242 Germans	Multiple SNPs	No	(181)
			AE	392 Germans	rs2066844 (R702W)	No	(180)
RANTES	Regulated on activation, normally T-cell expressed and secreted	17q11.2	Childhood AE	188 Germans	−403A/G	Yes	(156)
			Childhood AE	128 Hungarian	−403A/G, −28C/G	No	(158)
			AE	389 Japanese	−403A/G	No	(130)
					−28C/G	Yes	
IL12RB1	Interleukin 12 receptor, beta-1	19p13.1	AE	382 Japanese	rs393548, rs436857	Yes	(207)
GSTT1	Glutathion S-transferase, Theta 1	22q11.2	AE	325 Russians	Haplotypes	Yes	(208)

Published candidate genes for which association with AE has been reported in at least one study population of sufficient size (total cases studied, $n > 200$).

a Population-based cross-sectional

TABLE 3 Overview on Association Studies on *FLG* Mutations and AE

Ref.	Study population and size (cases/controls or families)	Variants	Ass.
(74)	Irish (52/189)	R501X, 2282del4	Y
	Danish (142/190)		
(89)	German (476)	R501X, 2282del4	Y
(209)	European (490)	R501X, 2282del4	Y
	German (189/314)		
(210)	German (338)	R501X	Y
	German (272/276)		
(211)	British (163/1463)	R501X, 2282del4	Y
(92)	German (274/252)	R501X, 2282del4	Y
(53)	Mixed (657)	R501X, 2282del4	Y
(212)	German (378/433)	R501X, 2282del4	Y
(84)	Irish (188/736)	R501X, 2282del4, R2247X, S3247X, 3702delG	Y
(79)	Japanese (143/156)	S2554X, 3321delA	Y
(213)	North American (646, case only cohort for asthma)	R501X, 2282del4	Y
(101)	French (99/102)	R501X, 2282del4	Y
(214)	Italian (178/210)	R501X, 2282del4	N
(215)	Japanese (102/133)	S2554X, 3321delA, S2889X, S3269X	Y
(216)	Swedish (406)	R501X, 2282del4	Y
(217)	German (540/2994)	R501X, 2282del4, R2247X, S3247X	Y
(218)	British (190/599)	R501X, 2282del4, R2247X, S3247X, 3702delG	Y
(85)	British (1445/5255)	R501X, 2282del4	Y
(104)	Germans, Irish, English (2774/10607)	R501X, 2282del4	Y

truncated filaggrin unit and a unique peptide of 23 amino acids (61–64) (Fig. 1). During cornification of the keratinocytes, profilaggrin is dephosphorylated and proteolytically cleaved into the N-terminal S-100 protein, which translocates to the nucleus where it is believed to function as a calcium-dependent transcriptional regulator of genes associated with late stratum corneum differentiation (63,64), and individual 37 kDa filaggrin repeats (65,66). These filaggrin monomers aid in packing keratin intermediate filaments into macrofibril bundles leading to compaction of the keratinocytes into corneocytes (67). Thereafter they are released from the filaments and progressively degraded into hygroscopic amino acids and derivatives of amino acids which are believed to function as "natural moisturizers" of the skin (68,69) (Fig. 2).

Based on immunohistochemical and immunoblotting studies showing a diminished or absent filaggrin expression in IV patients (70–73), as well as linkage findings between IV and markers in the EDC region, a genetically determined filaggrin deficiency was first considered and confirmed to be involved in IV. In 2006, two null mutations in the *filaggrin* (FLG) gene with an estimated combined population allele frequency of approximately 6% (74,75) were identified in IV patients from Irish, Scottish, and European-American populations (75). In the meantime a total of 32 *FLG* mutations have been reported (76), seven of them are common in at least

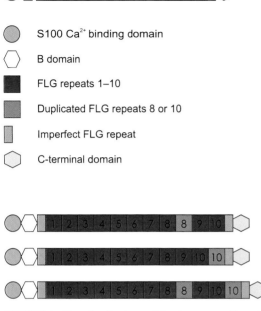

FIGURE 1 Domain structure of the human profilaggrin protein. [(78) with permission of Future Medicine Ltd.]. The N-terminus consists of two distinct domains: a conserved S100-like domain and a less-conserved cationic B domain, followed by an imperfect filaggrin unit and 10 to 12 almost identical filaggrin monomers. The C-terminus contains a truncated filaggrin unit and a unique peptide of 23 amino acids. There are distinct size variants of the *FLG* gene in the human population, which have resulted from duplication of repeat 8 and/or repeat 10. It is likely that size variants involving other repeats also exist. A fewer number of repeats has been reported to be associated with dry skin (219).

one population studied thus far (77,78). Interestingly, most of the mutations appear to be population-specific, with most so far identified in those of European ancestry, with other *FLG* gene mutations apparently restricted to Asian populations (77,79) (Fig. 3). All these variants lead to frameshifts, premature stop codons, or nonsense mutations and prevent the production of free filaggrin in the epidermis. Carriers of one *FLG* mutation immunohistochemically show marked reduction of *FLG* expression, whereas processed filaggrin is virtually completely absent in homozygotes and compound heterozygotes (75,77).

The well-known clinical association between IV and AE, coupled with the prior observation of decreased expression of *FLG* in AE (40,80) suggested that *FLG* loss-of-function mutations might also be of relevance for AE. Subsequently, Palmer et al. showed that both the R501X and 2282del4 alleles are strong predisposing factors for AE (74); over the past two years an impressive series of independent replication studies [for review see (78,81)] has provided unequivocal evidence that *FLG* null alleles are major risk factors for AE (Table 3). Many studies have now shown that *FLG* null alleles predispose particularly to an early-onset, severe, and persistent course of eczema [for review see (78,82)]. Remarkably, *FLG* null alleles are rather

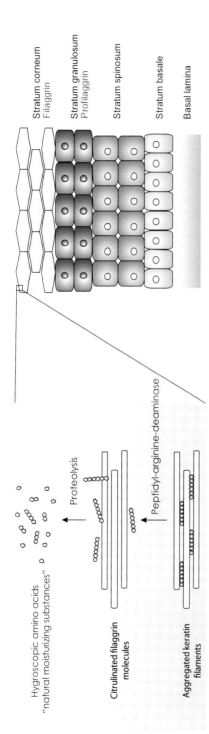

FIGURE 2 Epidermal differentiation and filaggrin [(78) with permission of Future Medicine Ltd.]. The epidermis is mainly composed of keratinocytes proliferating out of the basal layer. These multipotent cells undergo various phases of differentiation before they transform into corneocytes, which are dead flattened squames consisting of a keratin filament matrix encased within the so-called cornified cell envelope and embedded in a lamellar lipid matrix. The precursor of filaggrin, profilaggrin, is expressed as large (435 kD) insoluble and highly phosphorylated protein in the keratohyalin granules in the stratum granulosum. During cornification of the keratinocytes, profilaggrin is proteolytically cleaved into individual 37 kDa filaggrin repeats, which aid in packing keratin intermediate filaments into macrofibril bundles leading to a compaction of the keratinocytes. In the squamous cells, the arginines in filaggrin are converted to citrulline, which dissociates from the keratin filaments. The filaggrin is then broken down to a pool of hygroscopic amino acids and derivatives of amino acids in the outermost layers of the stratum corneum where they are believed to function as "natural moisturizers" of the skin.

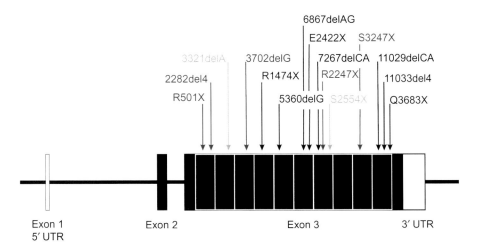

FIGURE 3 Diagram of the human profilaggrin gene [(78) with permission of Future Medicine Ltd.]. Like other members of the S-100 "fused-type" gene family, *FLG* shares a conserved gene structure consisting of three exons and two introns. Exon 1 encodes untranslated sequence only, exon 2 contains the start codon, and the unusually large (12,753 bp) exon 3 encodes most of the N-terminal domain and 10 to 12 filaggrin monomers. The position of reported loss-of-function mutations is indicated by arrows. The null alleles shown in red have been reported to be present in up to 8% of the population (83); those in black are either very rare or family-specific (77). Blue arrows indicate variants identified in Asian populations.

common with carrier frequencies of ~8% in the general population and up to 48% in AE cases (83,84). In two recent large population-based studies (85,86), it was demonstrated that, assuming causality, *FLG* mutations account for up to 15% of the total causality of all AE in these populations. Thus, *FLG* mutations are the strongest and best replicated genetic risk for AE to date.

Until recently, studies on *FLG* mutations were primarily performed in AE cohorts while their role in atopic diseases independently from AE has not been fully determined. Several studies have shown that *FLG*-deficient eczema is characterized by an increased risk for allergic sensitization, elevated IgE levels, and concomitant asthma and/or allergic rhinitis [for review see (78,82)]. However, filaggrin is not expressed in the human bronchial mucosa (87), and so far only associations with asthma in the presence of AE and with asthma severity, but not with asthma per se, have been observed (74,88,89). This has led to the hypothesis that reduction or loss of filaggrin expression primarily leads to a dry, disturbed skin barrier, which allows an increased passage of antigens, allergens, and chemicals through the epidermis, leading to inflammation and—depending on the host's immunological properties—facilitating allergic sensitization (90,91). Thus, it has been suggested that asthma in individuals with AE could be secondary to sensitization through a primarily defective epidermal barrier. This hypothesis is supported by a recent population-based study on adults which demonstrated associations of *FLG* mutations with "dry skin" independent from the presence of AE, whereas associations with elevated IgE levels were only observed in atopic individuals (92).

However, the functional consequences and exact phenotypic characteristics caused by *FLG* mutations remain incompletely understood and the hypothesis of a "dry or defective barrier" in *FLG*-mutation carriers remains to be proven (82).

The findings on *FLG* are a milestone in molecular genetic research in atopic disorders, and the knowledge gained on the disturbance of barrier function is expected to lead to the development of more rational and more effective treatments.

SPINK5 and KLK7

As outlined above, the key barrier protein filaggrin is initially synthesized as biologically inactive profilaggrin which, during the transition from granular cells to flattened squames, is processed to biologically active filaggrin monomers by several dephosphorylation and proteolytic steps (66,93). Thus, dysregulation of filaggrin processing might also impair skin barrier function. One of the proteases that has been suggested to be implicated in profilaggrin processing is the stratum corneum chymotryptic enzyme (SCCE) (94,95). Interestingly, an insertion in the 3′ untranslated region of the *kallikrein 7* gene (*KLK7*) that encodes SCCE (96) has been reported to be associated with eczema in a small cohort of 103 British children, but has not been replicated so far. SCCE is putatively regulated by the serine protease inhibitor LETKI, encoded by *SPINK5* (95,97,98), the gene underlying Netherton syndrome, a rare autosomal-recessive disease characterized by congenital erythroderma and ichthyosis, bamboo hair (trichorrhexis invaginata), and atopic manifestations, including AE. Early genome-wide linkage analysis of eczema family studies suggested a potential locus on 5q31 and, after identification of six common polymorphisms in *SPINK5*, the variant Glu420Lys (rs2303067), was associated with eczema in a cohort of British children (57) with significant maternal effects. The association of *SPINK5* variants was replicated in two small Japanese studies (99,100), whereas other studies failed to replicate this association (101–103). Very recently, in a large-scale study on several cohorts, which involved more than 2700 AE cases and more than 10,000 controls, the *SPINK5* Glu420Lys mutation conferred a risk of eczema only when maternally inherited, but did not appear to be a major eczema risk factor (104). The balance of evidence on the larger studies conducted to date thus supports minor susceptibility to AE from the maternally inherited Lys420Ser polymorphism. The *KLK7* insertion was not associated with eczema in this large study and in a smaller French study (95), and no evidence was found for significant interaction effects between *KLK7* or *SPINK5* variants and *FLG* mutations (104).

Genes Associated with Immunoregulation
The High Affinity IgE Receptor (FcεRI)

The high affinity receptor for IgE represents not only the central receptor of IgE-induced type I hypersensitivity reactions such as the liberation of vasoactive mediators including serotonin and histamine, but also induces of profound immune responses through the activation of NFkappaB and downstream genes (105). It is usually expressed as an $\alpha\beta\gamma_2$ complex on mast cells and basophils, but additionally as an $\alpha\beta_2$ complex on antigen-presenting cells (APCs) (105). The β subunit functions act as amplifier of FcεRI surface expression and signaling. The gene encoding FcεRIβ is located on chromosome 11q13, a region that was originally linked to atopy (106,107) and for which a maternal pattern of inheritance was reported (108). The *FcεRIβ* coding variant Glu237Gly was associated with a range of atopy-related traits such as bronchial hyperresponsiveness (109–111), atopic asthma (112,113), and allergic sensitization (110,114), but several studies have failed to replicate these associations (115–117). Results for total IgE are also inconsistent (112,113,118–124). A British study reported significant association of two noncoding *FcεRIβ* polymorphisms with AE in two panels of 60 and 88 families (125). However, the association was only present with maternally derived alleles, and so far lacks robust replication.

FcεRI expression is substantially influenced by the binding of IgE to either form of the receptor, as bound IgE apparently protects the receptor from degradation and thus enhances surface expression without de novo protein synthesis. Of note, binding of IgE in the two different complexes only uses the α-subunit of the receptor, lacking contact sites with the β- or γ-subunits. Consequently, the expression level of the α-subunit is crucial for IgE levels on immune cells (105).

Very recently, in a population-based genome-wide association scan, the gene encoding the α-chain of the high affinity receptor for IgE (*FcεRIα*) on chromosome 1q23 was identified as quantitative trait locus strongly associated with total IgE levels, but no association with AE was detected (126). On balance of evidence to date mutations in the FcεRI genes are unlikely to be major players in AE susceptibility.

The Cytokine Gene Cluster and Cytokine Receptors

The cytokine gene cluster is located on chromosome 5q31–33, a region which was originally linked to total IgE (127) and subsequently to asthma and a range of atopy-related traits in multiple linkage studies [for review see (128)]. In addition, there is a weaker evidence for linkage to AE (51) and AE severity (52,129). The cytokine cluster contains a tightly linked group of immunoregulatory genes such as *IL4*, *IL5*, *IL9*, *IL13*, and *CD14*, which are plausible candidates for atopy-related phenotypes. However, association studies have shown conflicting and inconsistent results. Assuming that at least some of the reported genetic effects are real, it appears that they might be more relevant for the atopic state *sensu latu* than for any individual distinct atopic disease. In addition, due to the high level of linkage disequilibrium across this genomic region and the potential for gene–gene interactions through overlapping functional pathways, it is difficult to reliably differentiate the specific sources of signals and to identify causal variants.

The gene most consistently associated with allergic phenotypes is *IL13*. Notably, two functional *IL13* polymorphisms, *IL13*–1112CT (rs1800925) in the promoter region and *IL13* +2044GA (*IL13* Arg130Gln, rs20541) in exon 4, have been shown to be associated with a range of atopy-related disorders, including asthma, bronchial hyper-responsiveness, total IgE levels, and "atopy" [reviewed in: (128,130)]. IL13 has been reported to be over-expressed in both subacute and lichenified AE lesions (131), particularly in extrinsic forms of AE (132). Association of the Arg130Gln variation with AE was reported in Canadian (133), Japanese (134), and German cohorts (135). The promoter polymorphism was associated with AE in a Dutch cohort (136), a finding that could not be replicated in the aforementioned Japanese cohort (134).

In a recent genome-wide scan, several variants within the *RAD50* gene, which is located between the *IL5* and the *IL13* gene, were found to be associated with total IgE, some of which in addition showed associations with AE and with asthma in independent cohorts (126). Since RAD50 is hypothesized to play an important role in the regulation of Th2 cytokine gene transcription, this finding is biologically compelling. However, due to the strong linkage disequilibrium in this region the authors could not reliably differentiate the specific source of the signal between *RAD50* and *IL13*. Clearly, further studies are needed to assess whether *RAD50* is a true causal gene.

IL13 and *IL4* share overlapping biological functions, and both signal via a complex network of receptors (137). A functional SNP in the promoter of *IL4* (589C/T) has been associated with total serum IgE level, asthma, and asthma-related phenotypes [reviewed in (44,138)]. Concerning AE, in a Japanese study on 377 individuals from 88 nuclear families, markers flanking the *IL4* gene showed evidence for linkage, and significant transmission distortion was observed for the 589C/T variant (139). This association, however, could not be confirmed in a larger Japanese study (140). In another study investigating 406 affected sibling families from Sweden neither linkage nor association of AE to the *IL-4* promoter region was observed, but there was association of 589C/T with AE severity (141). Likewise, in an Australian cohort of 76 small nuclear families and 25 triads neither the −589C/T variant nor a newly identified *IL4* promoter polymorphism was associated with childhood AE (142).

The effects of IL4 are mediated by the IL4 receptor, a heterodimer consisting of an α-subunit (αIL4R) and either a γc-subunit (type 1 receptor) or an IL-13Ra1 unit (type 2 receptor). The common α-chain is encoded by the *IL4RA* gene on chromosome 16p12. *IL4RA* polymorphisms may significantly influence the outcome of IL-4 receptor signaling and consequently IgE secretion (143). Several *IL4RA* polymorphisms have been explored for associations with total serum IgE levels with conflicting results [reviewed in (144)]. Association of the coding variant Gln551Arg has been reported for severe AE in a small American cohort (145) and with adult AE in a Japanese population (146), but was not confirmed in a larger Japanese sample (140). A promoter SNP associated with decreased levels of soluble IL-4 receptor protein (147) was found to be associated with extrinsic AD in Germans (148) as well as with AE in a Japanese sample (149).

Within the gene encoding CD14, an innate immunity receptor for endotoxin, a promoter polymorphism (rs2569190) has been reported to be associated with elevated soluble CD14 levels (150,151). Analysis for association of this variant with various atopic traits yielded inconsistent results [reviewed in (152)]. Association with AE was observed in a single study on 344 white children from the US (153), but has not been replicated so far. Interestingly, recent data indicates that the effect of *CD14* variants might depend upon the level of endotoxin exposure (152).

Thus although some interesting and biologically plausible genetic associations have been demonstrated with the cytokine cluster on 5q31–33, these results remain inconclusive and require further investigation to confirm or refute whether there is a true genetic role for this genomic region and if so which specific genes are implicated. This will require more definitive studies in much larger cohorts, including very high SNP density whole-genome association studies.

RANTES

Chemotactic cytokines or C-C chemokines are small signaling proteins that mainly regulate trafficking of leukocytes through interaction with a subset of transmembrane G protein–coupled receptors (154). *RANTES* (regulated on activation of normal T cell expressed and secreted), mainly produced in dermal fibroblasts, is a potent eosinophil, monocyte, basophil, and lymphocyte chemoattractant at the site of inflammation, and has been reported to be overexpressed in lesional AE skin

(155). The *RANTES* gene is located within the C-C chemokine cluster on 17q11–12, but is some distance from the region of linkage to AE and psoriasis described above. Association of a functional mutation in the proximal promoter of the *RANTES* gene with AE has been reported in 188 children with AE and 98 controls from the German multicenter study (MAS-90) (156) and in a small Japanese cohort of 62 AE patients and 14 controls (157), but could not be replicated in other cohorts (158,159).

Mast Cell Chymase

Mast cells represent key effector cells of IgE-dependent immediate reactions, and also contribute significantly to certain features of IgE-associated late-phase reactions and chronic allergic inflammation [reviewed in (160)]. Mast cell chymase is a proinflammatory serine protease that is present in large quantities in the secretory granules. A variety of features have rendered the gene encoding chymase, *CMA1*, a premier candidate gene for atopy and AE, viz, together with tryptase and histamine it appears to exert a plethora of actions consistent with key roles in inflammation, tissue remodeling, and bronchial hyperresponsiveness [reviewed in (161)]. Enhanced expression has been observed in lesional as well as nonlesional AE skin (162,163). Finally, *CMA1* maps to chromosome 14q11, which has been linked with specific allergic reactions, asthma, total IgE, and AE (52,64–166). Several studies have reported a significant association between variants within the *CMA1* promoter and AE. Initially, an association of the promoter polymorphism rs1800875 was observed in a cohort of Japanese adults (113). In two subsequent studies on individuals with the same ethnic background, this observation was confirmed, with the strongest effect on AE with low total serum IgE levels (167,168), indicating that the effect might be independent of IgE. Interestingly, in a more recent large-scale association study we found a significant association of this polymorphism with AE, but no effects on serum IgE levels or other atopic phenotypes (169). In contrast, in a U.K. Caucasian family cohort for asthma, associations with total IgE levels were found (170). Although these data appear convincing, it has to be noted that two smaller studies on Japanese (171) and Italian (172) individuals failed to replicate the associations, possibly due to low statistical power and limited comparability of Asian and Caucasian populations. On the balance of date to date, *CMA1* remains an interesting player in susceptibility to AE, but further replication would be helpful in clarifying the precise role for this candidate gene.

Innate Immunity Receptors

Innate immunity represents the first line of host defence recognizing a few highly conserved structures present in many different microorganisms. These pathogen-associated molecular patterns (PAMPs) are recognized through a set of germ-line–encoded pattern recognition receptors (PRRs). PRRs located in the cell membrane such as Toll-like-receptors (TLRs) or CD14 respond to extracellular PAMPs. Cytosolic PPRs such as NOD1 (nucleotide-binding oligomerization domain protein 1, also designated as CARD4) and NOD2 (also designated as CARD15) recognize PAMPs that cross the plasma membrane [reviewed in (173,174)]. Genetic variations in innate immunity genes have been reported to be associated with a range of inflammatory disorders including both Th2-driven atopic and Th1-dominated autoimmune diseases [reviewed in (175)].

Polymorphisms in the *NOD2* gene have been identified at the *IBD1* locus. These DNA variants have been found to be associated with Crohn's disease and are considered causative for the etiology of the disease, in a percentage of patients (176–178). Evaluation of three functionally relevant *NOD2* polymorphisms related to Crohn's disease (3020insC, C2104T, G2722C) in two cross-sectional populations from Germany (total $N = 1872$) also indicated a role of *NOD2* variation in atopic diseases: strong associations with allergic rhinitis were observed for C2104T and G2722C, whereas 3020insC increased the risk of atopy and elevated serum IgE levels. In addition, for G2772C a significant effect on AE was observed (179). In a more recent study on 392 AE patients and 297 controls, the *NOD2* variant R702W showed association with AE, but significance was lost after Bonferroni correction for multiple testing (180). In a population-based study on German adults, we found an association of G2772C with total IgE levels, as well as associations of noncoding polymorphisms and a *NOD2* haplotype with asthma (181).

NOD1 shares many structural and functional similarities with *NOD2* and is located on chromosome 7p14–p15, a region which was reported to contain an atopy susceptibility locus (182). *NOD1* polymorphisms showed effects on increased IgE levels and asthma in British and Australian cohorts (183), with a complex indel polymorphism displaying the strongest associations. This variant was associated with IBD in a subsequent study performed by the same group (184). We observed associations of several *NOD1* variants with increased IgE levels and/or AE in three large and independent study samples: a cross-sectional study, a case-control cohort, and a family collection from Germany (185). In contrast, no association of *NOD1* SNPs with AE could be detected in another smaller study from Germany (180). Thus, despite some promising results for *NOD1* and *NOD2*, further clarification is needed.

Further innate immune receptor genes that have been investigated for association with atopic traits are *TLR2*, *TLR4*, and *TLR9*. TLR2 recognizes peptidoglycan, a predomiant component of the cell wall of *Staphylococcus aureus* (174), a pathogen with important implications for AE. TLR4 is the principal receptor for bacterial endotoxin, exposure to which has been suggested to protect from the development of asthma and atopy. TLR9 ligands are immunostimulatory sequence oligodeoxynucleotides (ISS-ODN) containing unmethylated CpG dinucleotides (also known as CpG-ODN) [reviewed in (186)]. Associations between the *TLR2* polymorphism rs4696480 (187) as well as the *TLR4* polymorphism rs4986790 (188) with asthma, and of the *TLR4* variant rs4986791 with a modified response to endotoxin (189) have been reported.

In a study on 78 AE patients and 39 controls (120) and in a subsequent extension of the case series to 175 patients (no controls), an overrepresentation of the heterozygous genotype of the TLR2 variant R753Q (rs5743708) in AE cases (frequency 11%) was reported. However, this finding appears to be false-positive due to a number of methodological issues. Notably, the 39 controls displayed a frequency of 2.5% for the heterozygous genotype, which is in contrast to several other studies as well as public databases, which report frequencies of 8% to 10%. Supportive of this assumption is the lack of association of rs5743708 and *TLR2* tagSNPs in our large-scale study on 275 AE families (190). Concerning *TLR4* variation, so far no evidence for a specific effect on AE has been reported.

In another large-scale study on two independent panels of AE families as well as a case-control sample analyzing four common *TLR9* SNPs, a significant overtransmission of the common T-allele of a functional *TLR9* promoter polymorphism was observed in both family panels, but not in the case-control cohort. As one possible explanation for this lack of replication the higher age of cases in the case-control sample was assumed. Interestingly, in a recent study involving 210 asthmatic children, 224 controls and 80 asthma families from Tunisia, the −1237C allele in *TLR9* gene polymorphisms was associated with increased risk of asthma (191), supporting a potential role for *TLR9* variation in atopy. Overall the case for a strong role for genetic susceptibility to AE conferred by polymorphisms in the innate immune system, while an intriguing possibility, remains to be proven.

CONCLUSIONS AND FUTURE DIRECTIONS

Despite much effort and progress over the past two decades, our understanding of the complex genetic susceptibility to AE remains in the early stages, compared to psoriasis, the most closely analogous complex inflammatory skin disease and more especially to other complex diseases such as diabetes. One main barrier to progress is the lack or really large collections of cases or families in contrast to other complex traits such as multiple sclerosis (192) and diabetes (193), where association studies are now being reported with meta-analysis available on greater than 10,000 subjects.

Based on reported data, only *FLG* appears to clearly convey a strong and consistent AE risk across all collections in all populations and in multiple large independent studies. Good data now exist in two large family collections to support a minor role for maternally inherited *SPINK5* polymorphisms and, on the balance of evidence to date, *CMA1* also appears to have a minor role. As has been demonstrated earlier, initial reports of intriguing and biologically plausible linkages to candidate genes more often than not fail to replicate. Therefore there is a need for large scale and detailed whole-genome studies both to clarify the roles of these currently suggested candidate genes and, more hopefully, to identify additional novel susceptibility loci. Recent results in a large asthma study that resulted in the identification of *ORMDL3* by positional cloning offer a glimpse of these possibilities. That said, even very large studies occasionally fail to reveal significant additional loci and may merely confirm that the major proportion of genetic risk to a complex trait rests within a previously identified single gene or genomic region, with smaller effects seem for a small number of additional alleles as was recently seen with multiple sclerosis (192). In addition, copy number variation, a heretofore unexamined aspect of AE genetics, may have a role to play. The future for AE genetics looks to be very exciting and full of promise.

REFERENCES

1. Bieber T. Atopic dermatitis. N Engl J Med 2008; 358(14):1483–1494.
2. Williams H, Flohr C. How epidemiology has challenged 3 prevailing concepts about atopic dermatitis. J Allergy Clin Immunol 2006; 118(1):209–213.
3. Wuthrich B, Schmid-Grendelmeier P. The atopic eczema/dermatitis syndrome. Epidemiology, natural course, and immunology of the IgE-associated ("extrinsic") and the nonallergic ("intrinsic") AEDS. J Invest Allergol Clin Immunol 2003; 13(1):1–5.
4. Illi S, von Mutius E, Lau S, et al. The natural course of atopic dermatitis from birth to age 7 years and the association with asthma. J Allergy Clin Immunol 2004; 113(5):925–931.
5. Novak N, Bieber T. Allergic and nonallergic forms of atopic diseases. J Allergy Clin Immunol 2003; 112(2):252–262.

6. Flohr C, Weiland SK, Weinmayr G, et al. The role of atopic sensitization in flexural eczema: Findings from the International Study of Asthma and Allergies in Childhood Phase Two. J Allergy Clin Immunol 2008; 121(1):141–147.e4.
7. Glazier AM, Nadeau JH, Aitman TJ. Finding genes that underlie complex traits. Science 2002; 298(5602):2345–2349.
8. Johansson SG, Bieber T, Dahl R, et al. Revised nomenclature for allergy for global use: Report of the Nomenclature Review Committee of the World Allergy Organization, October 2003. J Allergy Clin Immunol 2004; 113(5):832–836.
9. Johansson SG, Hourihane JO, Bousquet J, et al. A revised nomenclature for allergy. An EAACI position statement from the EAACI nomenclature task force. Allergy 2001; 56(9):813–824.
10. Brenninkmeijer EE, Schram ME, Leeflang MM, et al. Diagnostic criteria for atopic dermatitis: A systematic review. Br J Dermatol 2008; 158(4):754–765.
11. Coca AF, Cooke RA. On the classification of the phenonema of hypersensitiveness. J Immunol 1923; (10):163–182.
12. Prausnitz C, Küstner H. Studien über die Überempfiindlichkeit. Zentralbl Bakteriol Parasit Infect 1921; (86):160–169.
13. Coca AF, Grove EF. Study in hypersensitiveness. XIII. Study of atopic reagins. J Immunol 1925; (10):445–464.
14. Wise F, Sulzberger MB. Footnote on problem of eczema, neurodermitis and lichenification. In: Wise F, Sulzberger MB, eds. The 1933 Year Book of Dermatology and Syphilology. Chicago, IL: Year Book Publishers, 1993:38–39.
15. Ishizaka K, Ishizaka T, Hornbrook MM. Physicochemical properties of reaginic antibody. V. Correlation of reaginic activity wth gamma-E-globulin antibody. J Immunol 1966; 97(6):840–853.
16. Pepys J. Atopy: A study in definition. Allergy 1994; 49(6):397–399.
17. Cooke R, Van Der Veer A. Human sensitization. J Immunol 1916; (1):201–305.
18. Schultz Larsen F. Atopic dermatitis: A genetic-epidemiologic study in a population-based twin sample. J Am Acad Dermatol 1993; 28(5 Pt 1):719–723.
19. Larsen FS, Holm NV, Henningsen K. Atopic dermatitis. A genetic-epidemiologic study in a population-based twin sample. J Am Acad Dermatol 1986; 15(3):487–494.
20. Thomsen SF, Ulrik CS, Kyvik KO, et al. Findings on the atopic triad from a Danish twin registry. Int J Tuberc Lung Dis 2006; 10(11):1268–1272.
21. van Beijsterveldt CE, Boomsma DI. Genetics of parentally reported asthma, eczema and rhinitis in 5-yr-old twins. Eur Respir J 2007; 29(3):516–521.
22. Morar N, Willis-Owen SA, Moffatt MF, et al. The genetics of atopic dermatitis. J Allergy Clin Immunol 2006; 118(1):24–34 [quiz 5–6].
23. Hirschhorn JN. Genetic approaches to studying common diseases and complex traits. Pediatr Res 2005; 57(5 Pt 2):74R–77R.
24. Rice JP, Saccone NL, Corbett J. Model-based methods for linkage analysis. Adv Genet 2008; 60:155–173.
25. Almasy L, Blangero J. Contemporary model-free methods for linkage analysis. Adv Genet 2008; 60:175–193.
26. Wilkinson J, Grimley S, Collins A, et al. Linkage of asthma to markers on chromosome 12 in a sample of 240 families using quantitative phenotype scores. Genomics 1998; 53(3):251–259.
27. Strauch K, Bogdanow M, Fimmers R, et al. Linkage analysis of asthma and atopy including models with genomic imprinting. Genet Epidemiol 2001; 21(suppl. 1):S204–S209.
28. McKusick VA. Mendelian Inheritance in Man and its online version, OMIM. Am J Hum Genet 2007; 80(4):588–604.
29. Botstein D, Risch N. Discovering genotypes underlying human phenotypes: Past successes for Mendelian disease, future approaches for complex disease. Nat Genet 2003; 33(suppl.):228–237.
30. Altmuller J, Palmer LJ, Fischer G, et al. Genomewide scans of complex human diseases: True linkage is hard to find. Am J Hum Genet 2001; 69(5):936–950.

31. Markianos K, Carlson S, Gibbs M, et al. A joint analysis of asthma affection status and IgE levels in multiple data sets collected for asthma. Genet Epidemiol 2001; 21(suppl 1):S148–S153.

32. Grant SF, Hakonarson H. Microarray technology and applications in the arena of genome-wide association. Clin Chem 2008; 54(7):1116–1124.

33. Tabor HK, Risch NJ, Myers RM. Candidate–gene approaches for studying complex genetic traits: Practical considerations. Nat Rev Genet 2002; 3(5):391–397.

34. Cardon LR, Bell JI. Association study designs for complex diseases. Nat Rev Genet 2001; 2(2):91–99.

35. Risch NJ. Searching for genetic determinants in the new millennium. Nature 2000; 405(6788):847–856.

36. Cordell HJ, Clayton DG. Genetic association studies. Lancet 2005; 366(9491):1121–1131.

37. Korstanje R, Paigen B. From QTL to gene: The harvest begins. Nat Genet 2002; 31(3):235–236.

38. Gutermuth J, Ollert M, Ring J, et al. Mouse models of atopic eczema critically evaluated. Int Arch Allergy Immunol 2004; 135(3):262–276.

39. Dixon AL, Liang L, Moffatt MF, et al. A genome-wide association study of global gene expression. Nat Genet 2007; 39(10):1202–1207.

40. Sugiura H, Ebise H, Tazawa T, et al. Large-scale DNA microarray analysis of atopic skin lesions shows overexpression of an epidermal differentiation gene cluster in the alternative pathway and lack of protective gene expression in the cornified envelope. Br J Dermatol 2005; 152(1):146–149.

41. Nomura I, Gao B, Boguniewicz M, et al. Distinct patterns of gene expression in the skin lesions of atopic dermatitis and psoriasis: A gene microarray analysis. J Allergy Clin Immunol 2003; 112(6):1195–1202.

42. Ogawa K, Ito M, Takeuchi K, et al. Tenascin-C is upregulated in the skin lesions of patients with atopic dermatitis. J Dermatol Sci 2005; 40(1):35–41.

43. Denham S, Koppelman GH, Blakey J, et al. Meta-analysis of genome-wide linkage studies of asthma and related traits. Respir Res 2008; 9:38.

44. Scirica CV, Celedon JC. Genetics of asthma: Potential implications for reducing asthma disparities. Chest 2007; 132(5 suppl.):770S–781S.

45. Bradley M, Soderhall C, Luthman H, et al. Susceptibility loci for atopic dermatitis on chromosomes 3, 13, 15, 17 and 18 in a Swedish population. Hum Mol Genet 2002; 11(13):1539–1548.

46. Cookson WO, Ubhi B, Lawrence R, et al. Genetic linkage of childhood atopic dermatitis to psoriasis susceptibility loci. Nat Genet 2001; 27(4):372–373.

47. Lee YA, Wahn U, Kehrt R, et al. A major susceptibility locus for atopic dermatitis maps to chromosome 3q21. Nat Genet 2000; 26(4):470–473.

48. Enomoto H, Noguchi E, Iijima S, et al. Single nucleotide polymorphism-based genome-wide linkage analysis in Japanese atopic dermatitis families. BMC Dermatol 2007; 7:5.

49. Irvine AD, McLean WH. The molecular genetics of the genodermatoses: Progress to date and future directions. Br J Dermatol 2003; 148(1):1–13.

50. Haagerup A, Bjerke T, Schiotz PO, et al. Atopic dermatitis—A total genome-scan for susceptibility genes. Acta Derm Venereol 2004; 84(5):346–352.

51. Beyer K, Nickel R, Freidhoff L, et al. Association and linkage of atopic dermatitis with chromosome 13q12–14 and 5q31–33 markers. J Invest Dermatol 2000; 115(5):906–908.

52. Soderhall C, Bradley M, Kockum I, et al. Linkage and association to candidate regions in Swedish atopic dermatitis families. Hum Genet 2001; 109(2):129–135.

53. Morar N, Cookson WO, Harper JI, et al. Filaggrin mutations in children with severe atopic dermatitis. J Invest Dermatol 2007; 127(7):1667–1672.

54. Cookson W. The immunogenetics of asthma and eczema: A new focus on the epithelium. Nat Rev Immunol 2004; 4(12):978–988.

55. Linde YW. Dry skin in atopic dermatitis. Acta Derm Venereol Suppl (Stockh) 1992; 177:9–13.

56. Tabata N, Tagami H, Kligman AM. A twenty-four-hour occlusive exposure to 1% sodium lauryl sulfate induces a unique histopathologic inflammatory response in the xerotic skin of atopic dermatitis patients. Acta Derm Venereol 1998; 78(4):244–247.

57. Walley AJ, Chavanas S, Moffatt MF, et al. Gene polymorphism in Netherton and common atopic disease. Nat Genet 2001; 29(2):175–178.

58. Mischke D, Korge BP, Marenholz I, et al. Genes encoding structural proteins of epidermal cornification and S100 calcium-binding proteins form a gene complex ("epidermal differentiation complex") on human chromosome 1q21. J Invest Dermatol 1996; (106):989–992.

59. Toulza E, Mattiuzzo NR, Galliano MF, et al. Large-scale identification of human genes implicated in epidermal barrier function. Genome Biol 2007; 8(6):R107.

60. Candi E, Schmidt R, Melino G. The cornified envelope: A model of cell death in the skin. Nat Rev Mol Cell Biol 2005; 6(4):328–340.

61. Rothnagel JA, Steinert PM. The structure of the gene for mouse filaggrin and a comparison of the repeating units. J Biol Chem 1990; 265(4):1862–1865.

62. Presland RB, Haydock PV, Fleckman P, et al. Characterization of the human epidermal profilaggrin gene. Genomic organization and identification of an S-100-like calcium binding domain at the amino terminus. J Biol Chem 1992; 267(33):23772–23781.

63. Zhang D, Karunaratne S, Kessler M, et al. Characterization of mouse profilaggrin: Evidence for nuclear engulfment and translocation of the profilaggrin B-domain during epidermal differentiation. J Invest Dermatol 2002; 119(4):905–912.

64. Pearton DJ, Dale BA, Presland RB. Functional analysis of the profilaggrin N-terminal peptide: Identification of domains that regulate nuclear and cytoplasmic distribution. J Invest Dermatol 2002; 119(3):661–669.

65. Presland RB, Kimball JR, Kautsky MB, et al. Evidence for specific proteolytic cleavage of the N-terminal domain of human profilaggrin during epidermal differentiation. J Invest Dermatol 1997; 108(2):170–178.

66. Resing KA, Walsh KA, Dale BA. Identification of two intermediates during processing of profilaggrin to filaggrin in neonatal mouse epidermis. J Cell Biol 1984; 99(4 Pt 1):1372–1378.

67. Dale BA, Holbrook KA, Steinert PM. Assembly of stratum corneum basic protein and keratin filaments in macrofibrils. Nature 1978; 276(5689):729–731.

68. Scott IR, Harding CR, Barrett JG. Histidine-rich protein of the keratohyalin granules. Source of the free amino acids, urocanic acid and pyrrolidone carboxylic acid in the stratum corneum. Biochim Biophys Acta 1982; 719(1):110–117.

69. Rawlings AV, Harding CR. Moisturization and skin barrier function. Dermatol Ther 2004; 17(suppl. 1):43–48.

70. Fleckman P, Holbrook KA, Dale BA, et al. Keratinocytes cultured from subjects with ichthyosis vulgaris are phenotypically abnormal. J Invest Dermatol 1987; 88(5):640–645.

71. Sybert VP, Dale BA, Holbrook KA. Ichthyosis vulgaris: Identification of a defect in synthesis of filaggrin correlated with an absence of keratohyaline granules. J Invest Dermatol 1985; 84(3):191–194.

72. Nirunsuksiri W, Presland RB, Brumbaugh SG, et al. Decreased profilaggrin expression in ichthyosis vulgaris is a result of selectively impaired posttranscriptional control. J Biol Chem 1995; 270(2):871–876.

73. Fleckman P, Brumbaugh S. Absence of the granular layer and keratohyalin define a morphologically distinct subset of individuals with ichthyosis vulgaris. Exp Dermatol 2002; 11(4):327–336.

74. Palmer CN, Irvine AD, Terron-Kwiatkowski A, et al. Common loss-of-function variants of the epidermal barrier protein filaggrin are a major predisposing factor for atopic dermatitis. Nat Genet 2006; 38(4):441–446.

75. Smith FJ, Irvine AD, Terron-Kwiatkowski A, et al. Loss-of-function mutations in the gene encoding filaggrin cause ichthyosis vulgaris. Nat Genet 2006; 38(3):337–342.

76. O'Regan G, Irvine AD, Chen H, et al. The genetic architecture and population genetics of filaggrin-related atopic dermatitis. International Investigative Dermatology Meeting, Kyoto. J Invest Dermatol 2008; 128.

77. Sandilands A, Terron-Kwiatkowski A, Hull PR, et al. Comprehensive analysis of the gene encoding filaggrin uncovers prevalent and rare mutations in ichthyosis vulgaris and atopic eczema. Nat Genet 2007; 39(5):650–654.
78. Rodriguez E, Illig T, Weidinger S. Filaggrin loss-of-function mutations and association with allergic diseases. Pharmacogenomics 2008; 9(4):399–413.
79. Nomura T, Sandilands A, Akiyama M, et al. Unique mutations in the filaggrin gene in Japanese patients with ichthyosis vulgaris and atopic dermatitis. J Allergy Clin Immunol 2007; 119(2):434–440.
80. Seguchi T, Cui CY, Kusuda S, et al. Decreased expression of filaggrin in atopic skin. Arch Dermatol Res 1996; 288(8):442–446.
81. Baurecht H, Irvine AD, Novak N, et al. Toward a major risk factor for atopic eczema: Meta-analysis of filaggrin polymorphism data. J Allergy Clin Immunol 2007; 120(6):1406–1412.
82. Irvine AD. Fleshing out filaggrin phenotypes. J Invest Dermatol 2007; 127(3):504–507.
83. Baurecht H, Irvine AD, Novak N, et al. Towards a major risk factor for atopic eczema: Meta-analysis of filaggrin mutation data. J Allergy Clin Immunol 2007; 120(6):1406–1412.
84. Sandilands A, Smith FJ, Irvine AD, et al. Filaggrin's fuller figure: A glimpse into the genetic architecture of atopic dermatitis. J Invest Dermatol 2007; 127(6):1282–1284.
85. Henderson J, Northstone K, Lee SP, et al. The burden of disease associated with filaggrin mutations: A population-based, longitudinal birth cohort study. J Allergy Clin Immunol 2008; 121(4):872–877.e9.
86. Weidinger S, O'Sullivan M, Illig T, et al. Filaggrin mutations, atopic eczema, hay fever, and asthma in children. J Allergy Clin Immunol 2008; 121(5):1203—1209.e1.
87. Ying S, Meng Q, Corrigan CJ, et al. Lack of filaggrin expression in the human bronchial mucosa. J Allergy Clin Immunol 2006; 118(6):1386–1388.
88. Palmer CN, Ismail T, Lee SP, et al. Filaggrin null mutations are associated with increased asthma severity in children and young adults. J Allergy Clin Immunol 2007; 120(1):64–68.
89. Weidinger S, Illig T, Baurecht H, et al. Loss-of-function variations within the filaggrin gene predispose for atopic dermatitis with allergic sensitizations. J Allergy Clin Immunol 2006; 118(1):214–219.
90. McLean WH, Hull PR. Breach delivery: Increased solute uptake points to a defective skin barrier in atopic dermatitis. J Invest Dermatol 2007; 127(1):8–10.
91. Hudson TJ. Skin barrier function and allergic risk. Nat Genet 2006; 38(4):399–400.
92. Weidinger S, Rodriguez E, Stahl C, et al. Filaggrin mutations strongly predispose to early-onset and extrinsic atopic dermatitis. J Invest Dermatol 2007; 127(3):724–726.
93. Resing KA, Walsh KA, Haugen-Scofield J, et al. Identification of proteolytic cleavage sites in the conversion of profilaggrin to filaggrin in mammalian epidermis. J Biol Chem 1989; 264(3):1837–1845.
94. Resing KA, Thulin C, Whiting K, et al. Characterization of profilaggrin endoproteinase 1. A regulated cytoplasmic endoproteinase of epidermis. J Biol Chem 1995; 270(47):28193–28198.
95. Descargues P, Deraison C, Bonnart C, et al. Spink5-deficient mice mimic Netherton syndrome through degradation of desmoglein 1 by epidermal protease hyperactivity. Nat Genet 2005; 37(1):56–65.
96. Vasilopoulos Y, Cork MJ, Murphy R, et al. Genetic association between an AACC insertion in the 3'UTR of the stratum corneum chymotryptic enzyme gene and atopic dermatitis. J Invest Dermatol 2004; 123(1):62–66.
97. Komatsu N, Takata M, Otsuki N, et al. Elevated stratum corneum hydrolytic activity in Netherton syndrome suggests an inhibitory regulation of desquamation by SPINK5-derived peptides. J Invest Dermatol 2002; 118(3):436–443.
98. Bitoun E, Micheloni A, Lamant L, et al. LEKTI proteolytic processing in human primary keratinocytes, tissue distribution and defective expression in Netherton syndrome. Hum Mol Genet 2003; 12(19):2417–2430.
99. Kato A, Fukai K, Oiso N, et al. Association of SPINK5 gene polymorphisms with atopic dermatitis in the Japanese population. Br J Dermatol 2003; 148(4):665–669.

100. Nishio Y, Noguchi E, Shibasaki M, et al. Association between polymorphisms in the SPINK5 gene and atopic dermatitis in the Japanese. Genes Immun 2003; 4(7):515–517.

101. Hubiche T, Ged C, Benard A, et al. Analysis of SPINK 5, KLK 7 and FLG genotypes in a French atopic dermatitis cohort. Acta Derm Venereol 2007; 87(6):499–505.

102. Folster-Holst R, Stoll M, Koch WA, et al. Lack of association of SPINK5 polymorphisms with nonsyndromic atopic dermatitis in the population of Northern Germany. Br J Dermatol 2005; 152(6):1365–1367.

103. Jongepier H, Koppelman GH, Nolte IM, et al. Polymorphisms in SPINK5 are not associated with asthma in a Dutch population. J Allergy Clin Immunol 2005; 115(3):486–492.

104. Weidinger S, Baurecht H, Wagenpfeil S, et al. Analysis of the individual and aggregate genetic contributions of previously identified SPINK5, KLK7 and FLG polymorphisms to eczema risk. J Allergy Clin Immunol 2008; 122(3):560–8.e4.

105. Kraft S, Kinet JP. New developments in FcepsilonRI regulation, function and inhibition. Nat Rev Immunol 2007; 7(5):365–378.

106. Cookson WO, Sharp PA, Faux JA, et al. Linkage between immunoglobulin E responses underlying asthma and rhinitis and chromosome 11q. Lancet 1989; 1(8650):1292–1295.

107. Sandford AJ, Shirakawa T, Moffatt MF, et al. Localisation of atopy and beta subunit of high-affinity IgE receptor (Fc epsilon RI) on chromosome 11q. Lancet 1993; 341(8841):332–334.

108. Cookson WO, Young RP, Sandford AJ, et al. Maternal inheritance of atopic IgE responsiveness on chromosome 11q. Lancet 1992; 340(8816):381–384.

109. van Herwerden L, Harrap SB, Wong ZY, et al. Linkage of high-affinity IgE receptor gene with bronchial hyperreactivity, even in absence of atopy. Lancet 1995; 346(8985):1262–1265.

110. Hill MR, Cookson WO. A new variant of the beta subunit of the high-affinity receptor for immunoglobulin E (Fc epsilon RI-beta E237G): Associations with measures of atopy and bronchial hyper-responsiveness. Hum Mol Genet 1996; 5(7):959–962.

111. Kim YK, Park HW, Yang JS, et al. Association and functional relevance of E237G, a polymorphism of the high-affinity immunoglobulin E-receptor beta chain gene, to airway hyper-responsiveness. Clin Exp Allergy 2007; 37(4):592–598.

112. Shirakawa T, Li A, Dubowitz M, et al. Association between atopy and variants of the beta subunit of the high-affinity immunoglobulin E receptor. Nat Genet 1994; 7(2):125–129.

113. Mao XQ, Shirakawa T, Yoshikawa T, et al. Association between genetic variants of mast-cell chymase and eczema. Lancet 1996; 348(9027):581–583.

114. Laprise C, Boulet LP, Morissette J, et al. Evidence for association and linkage between atopy, airway hyper-responsiveness, and the beta subunit Glu237Gly variant of the high-affinity receptor for immunoglobulin E in the French-Canadian population. Immunogenetics 2000; 51(8–9):695–702.

115. Sandford AJ, Chagani T, Zhu S, et al. Polymorphisms in the IL4, IL4RA, and FCERIB genes and asthma severity. J Allergy Clin Immunol 2000; 106(1 Pt 1):135–140.

116. Takabayashi A, Ihara K, Sasaki Y, et al. Childhood atopic asthma: Positive association with a polymorphism of IL-4 receptor alpha gene but not with that of IL-4 promoter or Fc epsilon receptor I beta gene. Exp Clin Immunogenet 2000; 17(2):63–70.

117. Zhu S, Chan-Yeung M, Becker AB, et al. Polymorphisms of the IL-4, TNF-alpha, and Fcepsilon RIbeta genes and the risk of allergic disorders in at-risk infants. Am J Respir Crit Care Med 2000; 161(5):1655–1659.

118. Hizawa N, Yamaguchi E, Jinushi E, et al. A common FCER1B gene promoter polymorphism influences total serum IgE levels in a Japanese population. Am J Respir Crit Care Med 2000; 161(3 Pt 1):906–909.

119. Hizawa N, Yamaguchi E, Jinushi E, et al. Increased total serum IgE levels in patients with asthma and promoter polymorphisms at CTLA4 and FCER1B. J Allergy Clin Immunol 2001; 108(1):74–79.

120. Ahmad-Nejad P, Mrabet-Dahbi S, Breuer K, et al. The toll-like receptor 2 R753Q polymorphism defines a subgroup of patients with atopic dermatitis having severe phenotype. J Allergy Clin Immunol 2004; 113(3):565–567.

121. Traherne JA, Hill MR, Hysi P, et al. LD mapping of maternally and non-maternally derived alleles and atopy in FcepsilonRI-beta. Hum Mol Genet 2003; 12(20):2577–2585.

122. Wjst M, Fischer G, Immervoll T, et al. A genome-wide search for linkage to asthma. German Asthma Genetics Group. Genomics 1999; 58(1):1–8.

123. Hoffjan S, Ostrovnaja I, Nicolae D, et al. Genetic variation in immunoregulatory pathways and atopic phenotypes in infancy. J Allergy Clin Immunol 2004; 113(3):511–518.

124. Palmer LJ, Rye PJ, Gibson NA, et al. Association of FcepsilonR1-beta polymorphisms with asthma and associated traits in Australian asthmatic families. Clin Exp Allergy 1999; 29(11):1555–1562.

125. Cox HE, Moffatt MF, Faux JA, et al. Association of atopic dermatitis to the beta subunit of the high affinity immunoglobulin E receptor. Br J Dermatol 1998; 138(1):182–187.

126. Weidinger S, Gieger C, Rodriguez E, et al. Genome-wide scan on total serum IgE levels identifies FCER1A as novel susceptibility locus PLOS. Genet 2008; 4(8):e1000166.

127. Marsh DG, Neely JD, Breazeale DR, et al. Linkage analysis of IL4 and other chromosome 5q31.1 markers and total serum immunoglobulin E concentrations. Science 1994; 264(5162):1152–1156.

128. Vercelli D. Discovering susceptibility genes for asthma and allergy. Nat Rev Immunol 2008; 8(3):169–182.

129. Forrest S, Dunn K, Elliott K, et al. Identifying genes predisposing to atopic eczema. J Allergy Clin Immunol 1999; 104(5):1066–1070.

130. Tanaka K, Roberts MH, Yamamoto N, et al. Upregulating promoter polymorphisms of RANTES relate to atopic dermatitis. Int J Immunogenet 2006; 33(6):423–428.

131. Tazawa T, Sugiura H, Sugiura Y, et al. Relative importance of IL-4 and IL-13 in lesional skin of atopic dermatitis. Arch Dermatol Res 2004; 295(11):459–464.

132. Jeong CW, Ahn KS, Rho NK, et al. Differential in vivo cytokine mRNA expression in lesional skin of intrinsic vs. extrinsic atopic dermatitis patients using semiquantitative RT-PCR. Clin Exp Allergy 2003; 33(12):1717–1724.

133. He JQ, Chan-Yeung M, Becker AB, et al. Genetic variants of the IL13 and IL4 genes and atopic diseases in at-risk children. Genes Immun 2003; 4(5):385–389.

134. Tsunemi Y, Saeki H, Nakamura K, et al. Interleukin-13 gene polymorphism G4257A is associated with atopic dermatitis in Japanese patients. J Dermatol Sci 2002; 30(2):100–107.

135. Liu X, Nickel R, Beyer K, et al. An IL13 coding region variant is associated with a high total serum IgE level and atopic dermatitis in the German multicenter atopy study (MAS-90). J Allergy Clin Immunol 2000; 106(1 Pt 1):167–170.

136. Hummelshoj T, Bodtger U, Datta P, et al. Association between an interleukin-13 promoter polymorphism and atopy. Eur J Immunogenet 2003; 30(5):355–359.

137. Munitz A, Brandt EB, Mingler M, et al. Distinct roles for IL-13 and IL-4 via IL-13 receptor alpha1 and the type II IL-4 receptor in asthma pathogenesis. Proc Natl Acad Sci U S A 2008; 105(20):7240–7245.

138. Hoffjan S, Nicolae D, Ober C. Association studies for asthma and atopic diseases: A comprehensive review of the literature. Respir Res 2003; 4:14.

139. Kawashima T, Noguchi E, Arinami T, et al. Linkage and association of an interleukin 4 gene polymorphism with atopic dermatitis in Japanese families. J Med Genet 1998; 35(6):502–504.

140. Tanaka K, Sugiura H, Uehara M, et al. Lack of association between atopic eczema and the genetic variants of interleukin-4 and the interleukin-4 receptor alpha chain gene: Heterogeneity of genetic backgrounds on immunoglobulin E production in atopic eczema patients. Clin Exp Allergy 2001; 31(10):1522–1527.

141. Soderhall C, Bradley M, Kockum I, et al. Analysis of association and linkage for the interleukin-4 and interleukin-4 receptor b;alpha; regions in Swedish atopic dermatitis families. Clin Exp Allergy 2002; 32(8):1199–1202.

142. Elliott K, Fitzpatrick E, Hill D, et al. The −590C/T and −34C/T interleukin-4 promoter polymorphisms are not associated with atopic eczema in childhood. J Allergy Clin Immunol 2001; 108(2):285–287.

143. Kruse S, Japha T, Tedner M, et al. The polymorphisms S503P and Q576R in the interleukin-4 receptor alpha gene are associated with atopy and influence the signal transduction. Immunology 1999; 96(3):365–371.
144. Franjkovic I, Gessner A, König I, et al. Effects of common atopy-associated amino acid substitutions in the IL-4 receptor alpha chain on IL-4 induced phenotypes. Immunogenetics 2005; 56(11):808–817.
145. Hershey GK, Friedrich MF, Esswein LA, et al. The association of atopy with a gain-of-function mutation in the alpha subunit of the interleukin-4 receptor. N Engl J Med 1997; 337(24):1720–1725.
146. Oiso N, Fukai K, Ishii M. Interleukin 4 receptor alpha chain polymorphism Gln551Arg is associated with adult atopic dermatitis in Japan. Br J Dermatol 2000; 142(5):1003–1006.
147. Hackstein H, Hecker M, Kruse S, et al. A novel polymorphism in the 5′ promoter region of the human interleukin-4 receptor alpha-chain gene is associated with decreased soluble interleukin-4 receptor protein levels. Immunogenetics 2001; 53(4):264–269.
148. Novak N, Kruse S, Kraft S, et al. Dichotomic nature of atopic dermatitis reflected by combined analysis of monocyte immunophenotyping and single nucleotide polymorphisms of the interleukin-4/interleukin-13 receptor gene: The dichotomy of extrinsic and intrinsic atopic dermatitis. J Invest Dermatol 2002; 119(4):870–875.
149. Hosomi N, Fukai K, Oiso N, et al. Polymorphisms in the promoter of the interleukin-4 receptor alpha chain gene are associated with atopic dermatitis in Japan. J Invest Dermatol 2004; 122(3):843–845.
150. Kabesch M, Hasemann K, Schickinger V, et al. A promoter polymorphism in the CD14 gene is associated with elevated levels of soluble CD14 but not with IgE or atopic diseases. Allergy 2004; 59(5):520–525.
151. Baldini M, Lohman IC, Halonen M, et al. A Polymorphism* in the 5′ flanking region of the CD14 gene is associated with circulating soluble CD14 levels and with total serum immunoglobulin E. Am J Respir Cell Mol Biol 1999; 20(5):976–983.
152. Simpson A, John SL, Jury F, et al. Endotoxin exposure, CD14, and allergic disease: An interaction between genes and the environment. Am J Respir Crit Care Med 2006; 174(4):386–392.
153. Litonjua AA, Belanger K, Celedon JC, et al. Polymorphisms in the 5′ region of the CD14 gene are associated with eczema in young children. J Allergy Clin Immunol 2005; 115(5):1056–1062.
154. Pease JE, Williams TJ. Chemokines and their receptors in allergic disease. J Allergy Clin Immunol 2006; 118(2):305–318 [quiz 19–20].
155. Kato Y, Pawankar R, Kimura Y, et al. Increased expression of RANTES, CCR3 and CCR5 in the lesional skin of patients with atopic eczema. Int Arch Allergy Immunol 2006; 139(3):245–257.
156. Nickel RG, Casolaro V, Wahn U, et al. Atopic dermatitis is associated with a functional mutation in the promoter of the C-C chemokine RANTES. J Immunol 2000; 164(3):1612–1616.
157. Bai B, Tanaka K, Tazawa T, et al. Association between RANTES promoter polymorphism −401A and enhanced RANTES production in atopic dermatitis patients. J Dermatol Sci 2005; 39(3):189–191.
158. Kozma GT, Falus A, Bojszko A, et al. Lack of association between atopic eczema/dermatitis syndrome and polymorphisms in the promoter region of RANTES and regulatory region of MCP-1. Allergy 2002; 57(2):160–163.
159. Muro M, Marin L, Torio A, et al. CCL5/RANTES chemokine gene promoter polymorphisms are not associated with atopic and nonatopic asthma in a Spanish population. Int J Immunogenet 2008; 35(1):19–23.
160. Williams CM, Galli SJ. The diverse potential effector and immunoregulatory roles of mast cells in allergic disease. J Allergy Clin Immunol 2000; 105(5):847–859.
161. Caughey GH. Mast cell tryptases and chymases in inflammation and host defense. Immunol Rev 2007; 217:141–154.
162. Badertscher K, Bronnimann M, Karlen S, et al. Mast cell chymase is increased in chronic atopic dermatitis but not in psoriasis. Arch Dermatol Res 2005; 296(10):503–506.

163. Jarvikallio A, Naukkarinen A, Harvima IT, et al. Quantitative analysis of tryptase- and chymase-containing mast cells in atopic dermatitis and nummular eczema. Br J Dermatol 1997; 136(6):871–877.
164. Moffatt MF, Hill MR, Cornelis F, et al. Genetic linkage of T-cell receptor alpha/delta complex to specific IgE responses. Lancet 1994; 343(8913):1597–1600.
165. A genome-wide search for asthma susceptibility loci in ethnically diverse populations. The Collaborative Study on the Genetics of Asthma (CSGA). Nat Genet 1997; 15(4):389–392.
166. Deichmann KA, Heinzmann A, Forster J, et al. Linkage and allelic association of atopy and markers flanking the IL4-receptor gene. Clin Exp Allergy 1998; 28(2):151–155.
167. Mao XQ, Shirakawa T, Enomoto T, et al. Association between variants of mast cell chymase gene and serum IgE levels in eczema. Hum Hered 1998; 48(1):38–41.
168. Tanaka K, Sugiura H, Uehara M, et al. Association between mast cell chymase genotype and atopic eczema: Comparison between patients with atopic eczema alone and those with atopic eczema and atopic respiratory disease. Clin Exp Allergy 1999; 29(6):800–803.
169. Weidinger S, Rummler L, Klopp N, et al. Association study of mast cell chymase polymorphisms with atopy. Allergy 2005; 60(10):1256–1261.
170. Iwanaga T, McEuen A, Walls AF, et al. Polymorphism of the mast cell chymase gene (CMA1) promoter region: Lack of association with asthma but association with serum total immunoglobulin E levels in adult atopic dermatitis. Clin Exp Allergy 2004; 34(7):1037–1042.
171. Kawashima T, Noguchi E, Arinami T, et al. No evidence for an association between a variant of the mast cell chymase gene and atopic dermatitis based on case-control and haplotype-relative-risk analyses. Hum Hered 1998; 48(5):271–274.
172. Pascale E, Tarani L, Meglio P, et al. Absence of association between a variant of the mast cell chymase gene and atopic dermatitis in an Italian population. Hum Hered 2001; 51(3):177–179.
173. Inohara N, Nunez G. NODs: Intracellular proteins involved in inflammation and apoptosis. Nat Rev Immunol 2003; 3(5):371–382.
174. Athman R, Philpott D. Innate immunity via Toll-like receptors and Nod proteins. Curr Opin Microbiol 2004; 7(1):25–32.
175. Lazarus R, Vercelli D, Palmer LJ, et al. Single nucleotide polymorphisms in innate immunity genes: Abundant variation and potential role in complex human disease. Immunol Rev 2002; 190:9–25.
176. Hugot JP, Chamaillard M, Zouali H, et al. Association of NOD2 leucine-rich repeat variants with susceptibility to Crohn's disease. Nature 2001; 411(6837):599–603.
177. Hampe J, Frenzel H, Mirza MM, et al. Evidence for a NOD2-independent susceptibility locus for inflammatory bowel disease on chromosome 16p. Proc Natl Acad Sci U S A 2002; 99(1):321–326.
178. Ogura Y, Bonen DK, Inohara N, et al. A frameshift mutation in NOD2 associated with susceptibility to Crohn's disease. Nature 2001; 411(6837):603–606.
179. Kabesch M, Peters W, Carr D, et al. Association between polymorphisms in caspase recruitment domain containing protein 15 and allergy in two German populations. J Allergy Clin Immunol 2003; 111(4):813–817.
180. Macaluso F, Nothnagel M, Parwez Q, et al. Polymorphisms in NACHT-LRR (NLR) genes in atopic dermatitis. Exp Dermatol 2007; 16(8):692–698.
181. Weidinger S, Klopp N, Rummler L, et al. Association of CARD15 polymorphisms with atopy-related traits in a population-based cohort of Caucasian adults. Clin Exp Allergy 2005; 35(7):866–872.
182. Laitinen T, Daly MJ, Rioux JD, et al. A susceptibility locus for asthma-related traits on chromosome 7 revealed by genome-wide scan in a founder population. Nat Genet 2001; 28(1):87–91.
183. Hysi P, Kabesch M, Moffatt MF, et al. NOD1 variation, immunoglobulin E and asthma. Hum Mol Genet 2005; 14(7):935–941.

184. McGovern DP, Hysi P, Ahmad T, et al. Association between a complex insertion/deletion polymorphism in NOD1 (CARD4) and susceptibility to inflammatory bowel disease. Hum Mol Genet 2005; 14(10):1245–1250.
185. Weidinger S, Klopp N, Rummler L, et al. Association of NOD1 polymorphisms with atopic eczema and related phenotypes. J Allergy Clin Immunol 2005; 116(1):177–184.
186. Upham JW, Holt PG. Environment and development of atopy. Curr Opin Allergy Clin Immunol 2005; 5(2):167–172.
187. Eder W, Klimecki W, Yu L, et al. Toll-like receptor 2 as a major gene for asthma in children of European farmers. J Allergy Clin Immunol 2004; 113(3):482–488.
188. Fageras Bottcher M, Hmani-Aifa M, Lindstrom A, et al. A TLR4 polymorphism is associated with asthma and reduced lipopolysaccharide-induced interleukin-12(p70) responses in Swedish children. J Allergy Clin Immunol 2004; 114(3):561–567.
189. Werner M, Topp R, Wimmer K, et al. TLR4 gene variants modify endotoxin effects on asthma. J Allergy Clin Immunol 2003; 112(2):323–330.
190. Weidinger S, Novak N, Klopp N, et al. Lack of association between Toll-like receptor 2 and Toll-like receptor 4 polymorphisms and atopic eczema. J Allergy Clin Immunol 2006; 118(1):277–279.
191. Lachheb J, Dhifallah IB, Chelbi H, et al. Toll-like receptors and CD14 genes polymorphisms and susceptibility to asthma in Tunisian children. Tissue Antigens 2008; 71(5):417–425.
192. Hafler DA, Compston A, Sawcer S, et al. Risk alleles for multiple sclerosis identified by a genomewide study. N Engl J Med 2007; 357(9):851–862.
193. Zeggini E, Scott LJ, Saxena R, et al. Meta-analysis of genome-wide association data and large-scale replication identifies additional susceptibility loci for type 2 diabetes. Nat Genet 2008; 40(5):638–645.
194. Reich K, Westphal G, Konig IR, et al. Cytokine gene polymorphisms in atopic dermatitis. Br J Dermatol 2003; 148(6):1237–1241.
195. Negoro T, Orihara K, Irahara T, et al. Influence of SNPs in cytokine-related genes on the severity of food allergy and atopic eczema in children. Pediatr Allergy Immunol 2006; 17(8):583–590.
196. Sohn MH, Song JS, Kim KW, et al. Association of interleukin-10 gene promoter polymorphism in children with atopic dermatitis. J Pediatr 2007; 150(1):106–108.
197. Shimizu M, Matsuda A, Yanagisawa K, et al. Functional SNPs in the distal promoter of the ST2 gene are associated with atopic dermatitis. Hum Mol Genet 2005; 14(19):2919–2927.
198. Jones G, Wu S, Jang N, et al. Polymorphisms within the CTLA4 gene are associated with infant atopic dermatitis. Br J Dermatol 2006; 154(3):467–471.
199. Novak N, Yu CF, Bussmann C, et al. Putative association of a TLR9 promoter polymorphism with atopic eczema. Allergy 2007; 62(7):766–772.
200. Namkung JH, Lee JE, Kim E, et al. IL-5 and IL-5 receptor alpha polymorphisms are associated with atopic dermatitis in Koreans. Allergy 2007; 62(8):934–942.
201. Chang YT, Lee WR, Yu CW, et al. No association of cytokine gene polymorphisms in Chinese patients with atopic dermatitis. Clin Exp Dermatol 2006; 31(3):419–423.
202. Kabesch M, Carr D, Weiland SK, et al. Association between polymorphisms in serine protease inhibitor, kazal type 5 and asthma phenotypes in a large German population sample. Clin Exp Allergy 2004; 34(3):340–345.
203. Novak N, Kruse S, Potreck J, et al. Single nucleotide polymorphisms of the IL18 gene are associated with atopic eczema. J Allergy Clin Immunol 2005; 115(4):828–833.
204. Kim E, Lee JE, Namkung JH, et al. Association of the single-nucleotide polymorphism and haplotype of the interleukin 18 gene with atopic dermatitis in Koreans. Clin Exp Allergy 2007; 37(6):865–871.
205. Schulz F, Marenholz I, Folster-Holst R, et al. A common haplotype of the IL-31 gene influencing gene expression is associated with nonatopic eczema. J Allergy Clin Immunol 2007; 120(5):1097–1102.
206. Jang N, Stewart G, Jones G. Polymorphisms within the PHF11 gene at chromosome 13q14 are associated with childhood atopic dermatitis. Genes Immun 2005; 6(3):262–264.

207. Takahashi N, Akahoshi M, Matsuda A, et al. Association of the IL12RB1 promoter poly-morphisms with increased risk of atopic dermatitis and other allergic phenotypes. Hum Mol Genet 2005; 14(21):3149–3159.
208. Vavilin VA, Safronova OG, Lyapunova AA, et al. Interaction of GSTM1, GSTT1, and GSTP1 genotypes in determination of predisposition to atopic dermatitis. Bull Exp Biol Med 2003; 136(4):388–391.
209. Marenholz I, Nickel R, Ruschendorf F, et al. Filaggrin loss-of-function mutations pre-dispose to phenotypes involved in the atopic march. J Allergy Clin Immunol 2006; 118(4):866–871.
210. Ruether A, Stoll M, Schwarz T, et al. Filaggrin loss-of-function variant contributes to atopic dermatitis risk in the population of Northern Germany. Br J Dermatol 2006; 155(5):1093–1094.
211. Barker JN, Palmer CN, Zhao Y, et al. Null mutations in the filaggrin gene (FLG) deter-mine major susceptibility to early-onset atopic dermatitis that persists into adulthood. J Invest Dermatol 2007; 127(3):564–567.
212. Stemmler S, Parwez Q, Petrasch-Parwez E, et al. Two common loss-of-function muta-tions within the filaggrin gene predispose for early onset of atopic dermatitis. J Invest Dermatol 2006; 127(3):722–724.
213. Rogers AJ, Celedon JC, Lasky-Su JA, et al. Filaggrin mutations confer susceptibility to atopic dermatitis but not to asthma. J Allergy Clin Immunol 2007; 120(6):1332–1337.
214. Giardina E, Paolillo N, Sinibaldi C, et al. R501X and 2282del4 filaggrin mutations do not confer susceptibility to psoriasis and atopic dermatitis in Italian patients. Dermatology 2008; 216(1):83–84.
215. Nomura T, Akiyama M, Sandilands A, et al. Specific filaggrin mutations cause ichthyosis vulgaris and are significantly associated with atopic dermatitis in Japan. J Invest Dermatol 2008; 128(6):1436–1441.
216. Ekelund E, Lieden A, Link J, et al. Loss-of-function variants of the filaggrin gene are associated with atopic eczema and associated phenotypes in Swedish families. Acta Derm Venereol 2008; 88(1):15–19.
217. Weidinger S, O'Sullivan M, Illig T, et al. Filaggrin mutations, atopic eczema, hay fever, and asthma in children. J Allergy Clin Immunol 2008; 121(5):1203–1209.e1.
218. Brown SJ, Relton CL, Liao H, et al. Filaggrin null mutations and childhood atopic eczema: A population-based case-control study. J Allergy Clin Immunol 2008; 121(4):940–946.e3.
219. Ginger RS, Blachford S, Rowland J, et al. Filaggrin repeat number polymorphism is associated with a dry skin phenotype. Arch Dermatol Res 2005; 297(6):235–241.

4 | Epidermal Barrier in Atopic Dermatitis

Ehrhardt Proksch, Regina Fölster-Holst, and Jens-Michael Jensen

Department of Dermatology, University of Kiel, Kiel, Germany

INTRODUCTION

A defect in skin permeability barrier function is a well-accepted component of atopic dermatitis (AD). The physical barrier, located in the outermost part of the epidermis, the stratum corneum, is one instrument in a concert of different skin barriers including the chemical/biochemical or antimicrobial barrier of the innate immune system. Although epidermal changes in atopic skin are often viewed as a secondary consequence of the inflammatory process, there is overwhelming evidence that impaired skin barrier function is centrally involved in the pathogenesis of AD (1,2). This chapter focuses on the role of the physical barrier and its interactions with the immune barrier in AD.

THE SKIN'S PERMEABILITY BARRIER

The permeability barrier is formed during epidermal proliferation and differentiation, which begins in the basal layer (Fig. 1). The stratum corneum, composed of protein-enriched cells, the corneocytes, and lipid-enriched intercellular domains, is particularly important in the formation of the physical barrier. During transition from the basal layer to the stratum corneum, a variety of biochemical reactions occur in the keratinocytes, including the synthesis of specific basal (K5 and K14) and suprabasal (K1 and K10) keratins and cornified envelope-associated proteins. Cornified envelopes are formed in the upper spinous and granular cell layers of the epidermis through the cross-linking of involucrin and envoplakin on the intracellular surface of the plasma membrane. This process begins at the sides of the desmosomes and is followed by the addition of elafin, small proline-rich proteins, and loricrin. The phospholipid-enriched plasma membrane is replaced by a ceramide-containing layer, which is then covalently attached to involucrin, envoplakin, and periplakin by ω-hydroxyester bonds (3).

The synthesis of lipids necessary for barrier function occurs within keratinocytes in all nucleated epidermal layers. Lipid storage occurs within the epidermal lamellar bodies, which are ultrastructurally visible in the upper spinous and granular layers. In the outermost granular layer, the contents of lamellar bodies are secreted into the intercellular domains of the stratum granulosom–stratum corneum interface (Fig. 2). Lamellar bodies contain phospholipids, glucosylceramides, and cholesterol as well as hydrolytic enzymes, which are necessary for the conversion of phospholipids, glucosylceramides, and sphingomyelinase to free fatty acids and ceramides. In addition, the antimicrobial peptide β-defensin 2, a component of the skin's innate immunity, has been found in lamellar bodies (4). Several proteases essential for desquamation including the aspartate protease cathepsin D (5) are also delivered to the stratum granulosom–stratum corneum interface during this

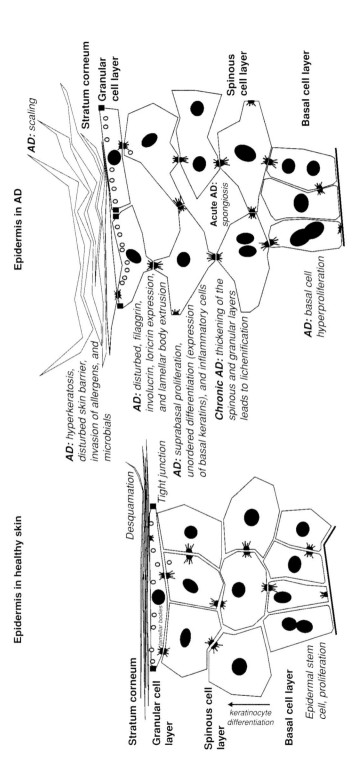

FIGURE 1 Epidermal changes in atopic dermatitis.

Stratum granulosum/stratum corneum interface in healthy skin

Corneocyte

Extracellular
lipid bilayer

Granular cell

*Fusion of a lamellar body with
the cell membrane, extruding
lipids, and enzymes into the
transition zone, and generating
ordered extracellular lipid
bilayers in the SC*

*lamellar body containing lipids and
hydrolytic enzymes transported
from the Golgi apparatus toward
the granular cell/horny layer interface*

Stratum granulosum/stratum corneum interface in AD

*AD: lipid bilayers lack proper anchoring to
involucrin and barely develop even bilayer
architecture*

Transition desmosome

*AD: lamellar body
containing mostly
unordered lipid
structures and
hydrolytic enzymes;
prevalently unextruded
lamellar bodies*

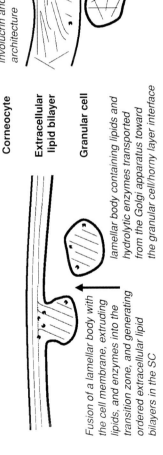

FIGURE 2 Lamellar body exocytosis into the transition zone SG/SC.

transition. In response to certain signals such as calcium concentration and cytokine release, the lamellar bodies begin to fuse with the plasma membrane and exocytotically secrete their lipid and enzyme content into the intercellular space (6).

Stratum corneum lipids contain approximately equal quantities of ceramides, cholesterol, and free fatty acids. Ceramides are considered essential for barrier function, not only because of their quantitative significance, but also because of their amphiphilic structure and long-chain, constituent N-acyl fatty acids (7). It has been classified that the stratum corneum contains nine major free ceramides (8). Three of them are ω-hydroxyceramide linked to polyunsaturated fatty acids, prevalently linoleic acid. In addition, the stratum corneum contains two ω-hydroxyceramides A and B, which are covalently bound to cornified envelope proteins, most importantly to involucrin (9,10). It was recently shown that the stratum corneum of forearm skin contains 342 ceramides (11). In AD, total ceramides, as well as ceramide 1 (according to the Robson classification) individually, were found to be reduced in the stratum corneum (12). Reduced ceramide content might be a result of reduced acid sphingomyelinase activity in atopic skin (1). Reduced amounts of ω-hydroxyceramide in nonlesional and lesional atopic skin were recently reported (13), suggesting that a reduction in covalently bound ceramides could contribute to barrier function disturbance in AD. Because ceramides are the backbone of the lipid envelope, with subsequent addition of cholesterol and free fatty acids, a reduced amount of ceramides in the stratum corneum results in disturbed skin barrier function.

SKIN BARRIER FUNCTION AND STRATUM CORNEUM HYDRATION IN AD

We determined skin barrier function and stratum corneum hydration in atopic skin using biophysical methods. We found a twofold increase in transepidermal water loss (TEWL) in nonlesional skin and a fourfold increase in lesional skin, as compared to normal controls (1). This demonstrates that the inside–out barrier is already impaired in nonlesional skin and is more significantly impaired in lesional atopic skin. The outside–in barrier is also disturbed in lesional and nonlesional AD, which has been shown by an increased penetration of theophylline, an asthma medication with structural and pharmacological similarity to caffeine (14), polyethylene glycol, and sodium lauryl sulfate (15,16). The disturbed outside–inside barrier in AD may allow the penetration of harmful substances into the skin, particularly allergens like house dust mites, pollen, and cat dander, which initiate immune response and inflammation. Interestingly, there is a correlation between TEWL and the prevalence of sensitization to aeroallergens. In 59 children with AD, it was shown that the higher the TEWL, the higher the prevalence of sensitization to aeroallergens (17).

From this and other studies there is evidence that immunodysregulation in AD results from inherited impaired barrier function alleviating the penetration of aeroallergens into the skin ("outside–inside" hypothesis).

An inverse relationship between TEWL and stratum corneum hydration is well known. High TEWL values are frequently correlated with low hydration of the stratum corneum; this has been shown in experimental settings after skin cleansing with soaps and detergents (18) and in lesional AD (2), where the skin barrier defect is also shown with electron microscopy and penetration studies (16,19). Although it is also well known that moisturizers often improve skin barrier function (20), the mechanisms involved have not yet been studied systematically. We as well as other authors think that disturbed skin barrier function leads to changes in epidermal differentiation, particularly in filaggrin expression, which, in turn, influences water-binding filaggrin break down products (2,21,22).

CUTANEOUS AND MUCOCUTANEOUS BARRIER DYSFUNCTION IN THE ATOPIC SYNDROME

As AD, allergic rhinitis/conjunctivitis and allergic bronchial asthma belong to the atopic syndrome, Ogawa and Yoshiike have suggested that the atopic syndrome represents a mucocutaneous barrier dysfunction (14). A defect in mucocutaneous barrier function allows the penetration of multiple antigens and irritants. Increased response to irritants has been widely observed in atopic skin. Disturbances in skin barrier function not only allow enhanced penetration of irritants, resulting in inflammation, but also enable allergens to reach the lower epidermal layers more easily. Positive patch test reactions for type I allergens are regularly seen in atopic patients but not in normal controls. Penetration of type I allergens into the mucous membranes and their contact with the immune cells, only possible due to a disturbed barrier, lead to irritant rhinitis and clinically more significant allergic rhinitis in patients with AD. There is additional evidence that patients with the atopic syndrome exhibit disturbed bronchial mucous membranes and increased irritant response in the lungs, which may lead to bronchial asthma (23–25). Although immunologic tolerance normally develops, repeated allergen exposure can cause hypersensitivity, which initiates allergic inflammatory responses. Nishijima et al. have suggested that the interaction between immunologically induced inflammation and the resulting disruptions in barrier function is an essential dynamic in the manifestation of atopic conditions (26). After challenging with milk, higher levels of protein antigen immune complex in IgA, IgG, and IgE are found in the serum of AD patients than in control subjects. This finding was attributed to deficient intestinal permeability and possibly to maldigestion (27–31). Overall, there is significant evidence that disturbed cutaneous and mucocutaneous barrier dysfunction is involved in the atopic syndrome.

SKIN LIPIDS IN AD

Disturbed skin barrier function in AD is at least partly related to the disturbed composition of lipids in the stratum corneum. Skin surface lipids have been examined first and found to be significantly lower than that in normal controls or in patients with ichthyosis vulgaris, suggesting an overall decrease in total stratum corneum lipids (32,33). The reduced skin surface lipids correlate with the reduced hydration in AD (34). Skin surface lipids are sebaceously derived, whereas lipids for skin barrier function are derived from epidermal keratinocytes (35). Epidermal lipids in AD have been extensively studied. AD displays a decrease in total lipids, phospholipids, and sterol esters as well as an increase in free fatty acids and sterols in contrast to normal controls. It is likely that the decrease in phospholipids reflects a decrease in sphingolipid content, specifically sphingomyelin.

Special attention has been given to the role of ceramides in barrier abnormalities in AD. Decreased stratum corneum ceramides have also been observed in the back skin and toenails of AD patients (36,37); a significant reduction in ceramides is observed in lesional forearm skin (38). A significant decrease in the ceramide fraction, expressed as percentage of total lipids, was found in the nonlesional plantar skin of AD patients (12). Reduced ceramide 1 in the stratum corneum of clinically dry, noneczematous skin has also been described (39). In contrast, the relative amounts of all other stratum corneum lipid classes in AD, including squalene, cholesterol esters, triglycerides, free fatty acids, cholesterol, cholesterol sulfate, and phospholipids were not significantly different from amounts present in controls (12).

Ceramides are synthesized by serine-palmitoyl transferase as rate-limiting enzyme and by hydrolysis of glucosylceramide (by β-glucocerebrosidase) and sphingomyeline (by acid sphingomyelinase) (40,41). Ceramide synthesis rates and serine-palmitoyl transferase activity have not yet been measured in AD. Differences in the activity of hydrolytic enzymes, β-glucocerebrosidase, and ceramidase activities in uninvolved stratum corneum of AD could not be observed. The ceramide decrease in AD could not be attributed to the enhanced degradation of ceramides. Unchanged β-glucocerebrosidase activity in atopic stratum corneum was also found (42). We found decreased epidermal acid sphingomyelinase activity in lesional and nonlesional skin, which correlates with reduced stratum corneum ceramide content and disturbed barrier function in AD (1).

Prosaposins, the precursor proteins that stimulate enzymatic hydrolysis of sphingolipids, including glucosylceramide and sphingomyelin, are also reduced in AD. These findings suggest that reduced activation of β-glucocerebrosidase, acid sphingomyelinase, and reduced prosaposin levels in AD may cause ceramide content to decrease in atopic skin. An alternative explanation for reduced ceramide content in AD has also been forwarded. A novel enzyme called glucosylceramide/sphingomyelin deacylase, which cleaves the N-acyl linkage of both sphingomyelin and glucosylceramide, has been described in atopic skin (43). Extremely elevated sphingomyelin hydrolysis in the stratum corneum of uninvolved and involved skin has been described (44), suggesting that sphingomyelin metabolism is altered in AD, resulting in decreased levels of ceramides.

The importance of lipids for the pathogenesis of AD has been recently shown in a mouse model. Mice with transgenic expression of human apolipoprotein C1 (APOC1) in liver and skin have strongly increased serum levels of cholesterol, triglycerides, and free fatty acids. These mice displayed a disturbed skin barrier function, increased TEWL, and spontaneously developed symptoms of dermatitis including scaling, lichenification, excoriations, and pruritus. Histology revealed increased epidermal thickening and spongiosis in conjunction with elevated numbers of inflammatory cells (eosinophils, neutrophils, mast cells, macrophages, and CD4+ T cells). Affected mice have increased serum levels of IgE and show abundant IgE(+) mast cells. Partial inhibition of disease could be achieved by restoration of the skin barrier function with topical application of a lipophilic ointment. The development of AD in these mice was suppressed by corticosteroid treatment (45).

METABOLISM OF ESSENTIAL FREE FATTY ACIDS IN AD

It is well established that n-6 essential fatty acid (EFA) deficiency causes inflammatory skin conditions in both animals and humans. EFA deficiency in mice causes red scaly skin and an up to 10-fold increase in transepidermal water loss, which can easily be reversed with systemic or topical application of n-6 EFAs (linoleic acid, γ-linolenic acid, and columbinic acid) (46). Although no linoleic acid deficiency has been observed in AD, it has been proposed that linoleic to γ-linolenic acid conversion might be impaired. The effects of systemic and topical administration of γ-linolenic acid in AD have been studied with controversial findings. While some studies report an improvement of AD after γ-linolenic acid treatment, other trials show no significant effects from either n-6 or n-3 EFA supplementation (47). Own clinical experience has shown that only a subgroup of patients experienced an improvement in atopic symptoms after EFA supplementation.

New evidence for a role of unsaturated fatty acids derives from studies in mice. It has been shown that 12R-lipoxygenase deficiency in mice resulted in a severe degree of skin barrier impairment, associated with disturbance of the assembly/extrusion of lamellar bodies. Lipid analysis demonstrates a disordered composition of ceramides, in particular a decrease of ester-bound ceramide species. Moreover, processing of profilaggrin to monomeric filaggrin was impaired (48).

Skin surface lipids increased and skin and hair coat condition improved in dogs fed increased total fat diets containing polyunsaturated fatty acids (49).

GENETICS AND DISTURBED BARRIER FUNCTION

Genetic impairment of the epidermal barrier has been proposed as a cause of AD and respiratory atopy for several years. Increased postnatal exposure to irritants and allergens that disrupts the permeability barrier in predisposed individuals may cause a subset of specific Th2 cell activation favoring the development of IgE response (50). Ichthyosis vulgaris, an autosomal dominant disorder causing defective epidermal filaggrin expression, occurs in 20% to 37% of atopic patients (51). Concomitant AD in patients with ichthyosis vulgaris was found in 30% of patients (52). Wiscott–Aldrich syndrome, linked to the X-chromosome, involves immunologic deficiencies, low platelet counts, and a comorbid eczema (29,53) clinically resembling AD. A genetic defect associated with AD can lead to decreased serine protease inhibitor activity, such as that occurring in Netherton's syndrome, which is caused by mutations in the *SPINK5* gene encoding the serine-protease inhibitor co-protein lymphoepithelial Kazal-type inhibitor 1 (LEKTI 1) (54,55). However, we did not find the SPINK5 polymorphism in patients with AD (56).

The central role of the terminally differentiating epithelium was recently observed in the genetic mapping in asthma and AD (57). Genetic linkage studies of AD and psoriasis have highlighted the importance of the chromosomal region 1q21, known as the epidermal differentiation complex. Many of these genes have shown increased expression in atopic and psoriatic skin. Two independent loss-of-function genetic variants in the gene encoding filaggrin (R510X and 2282del4) were identified, which are associated with a high degree of significance with AD-associated asthma (58). These genetic variants were found in 9% of people of European origin. Factors compromising the function of the various barrier layers increase opportunities for allergens to penetrate into the living epidermal and dermal layers and induce response by antigen-presenting cells, possibly representing the pathologic mechanism for the development of asthma in AD (58,59). Several other gene families are present within this complex, which encodes small proline-rich region proteins (SPRRs), S100 A calcium-binding proteins, and late enveloped proteins. Expression of epidermal differentiation proteins occurs at a late stage in keratinocyte maturation, primarily just beneath the cornified envelope. Some of the S100 A calcium-binding proteins are often secreted in response to inflammation and have a wide range of immunologic actions including chemotactic activity for eosinophiles or CD4+ T-cells and neutrophils and also have antimicrobial activity, in particular S100A7 (psoriasin). An understanding of the innate mechanisms of epithelial defense is essential for the treatment of asthma and AD (57).

It has been shown that E-cadherin expression and cellular distribution are reduced in keratinocyte membranes in areas of spongiosis in acute eczematous dermatitis (60). The gene for a rare autosomal dominant form of pompholyx was also very recently mapped to chromosome 18q22.1–18q22.3. Two genes part of the cadherin superfamily are also located in these regions (61). This indicates that the blister formations on palmar and plantar skin often seen in AD rely on the biochemical changes in the epidermis. We recently found that ADAM10 is the shedding protease for E-cadherin and that this process is active in eczema (62). It has also been proposed that T-cells migrating into the epidermis mediate apoptosis in keratinocytes via the release of IFN-γ or TNF-α, which upregulate Fas molecules on the surface of keratinocytes and contribute to spongiosis (63). Spongiosis is an important component of impaired epithelial homeostasis in eczema, irrespective of the sequence of events.

EPIDERMAL PROLIFERATION AND DIFFERENTIATION IN AD

AD is a scaling dermatitis in which epidermal changes are clinically and histologically visible (2). Changes in the stratum corneum have been described in AD, which correspond with disturbed epidermal differentiation. A thinner stratum corneum cell layer has been observed in asymptomatic atopic skin (64). Although the number of stratum corneum cell layers was substantially larger in atopic xerosis than in controls, their turnover time was shorter. Superficial corneocytes are significantly smaller in atopic, xerotic skin, and in skin displaying disturbed epidermal differentiation than in control samples (65).

Using the Ki-67 marker, we found increased epidermal proliferation in nonlesional skin and more pronouncedly in lesional skin. Increased proliferation is often accompanied by disturbed differentiation. Extended expression of basal keratin K5, paralleled by a reduced expression of suprabasal/differentiation-related K 10 was found in lesional AD (1). We have also noted K10 reduction in dry skin in previous studies (66,67). Proliferation-associated cytokeratin K6 and inflammation-associated K17 were expressed in AD, correlating with an increase in their proliferation rates and inflammation (1).

Involucrin is the most important substrate for covalent attachment of ceramides to the cornified envelope. In AD we found premature involucrin expression. Involucrin expression is normally seen in the upper spinous and granular layers, already in the mid-spinous layer. However, the staining intensity for involucrin was reduced, which explains the decreased amount of ω-hydroxyceramides bound to the cornified envelope (13). Loricrin staining was increased. Although the filaggrin, involucrin, and loricrin genes are all localized in the epidermal differentiation complex 1q21, the loricrin gene does not necessarily share the filaggrin and involucrin genes' regulatory elements (68).

FILAGGRIN, DRY SKIN, AND SKIN BARRIER FUNCTION IN AD

Both our group and Tezuka's group found reduced filaggrin expression in nonlesional skin and particularly in lesional skin of AD (1,69). This was one reason why the group of McLean et al. searched for filaggrin mutations in AD. In a landmark paper extremely high significant mutations in the filaggrin gene were reported in ichthyosis vulgaris and in AD (58). The results were immediately confirmed independently by several other groups (70–73). Mutations in the filaggrin gene are present in 9% of people of European origin. The rate of filaggrin mutations is increased to about 20% in general and to about 50% in severe cases of AD (see Chapter 3 Genetics of Atopic Eczema).

As filaggrin is an important component of the skin's water binding capacity, the loss of function mutations may explain the well-established dryness of ichthyosis vulgaris and AD (1,74,75). Filaggrin breakdown products, different amino acids, in particular histidine, which is transformed to urocanic acid and pyrrolidone carboxylic acid, have been considered important for water binding for years (21). Shortly before the McLean findings, polymorphisms in the filaggrin gene, in association with dry skin, have been described as an important cause of dry skin (76). Recently, it has been shown that loss-of-function mutations in the filaggrin gene lead to a reduced level of natural moisturizing factor in the stratum corneum of AD (77). Therefore, the connection between filaggrin mutations and dry skin in AD is well established.

The connection between disturbed skin barrier function and mutations in the filaggrin gene is not easily explained, although numerous studies have shown that there is a relationship between the two, and examination of filaggrin mutation has finally brought significant attention to the role of the skin barrier in AD. Filaggrin is encoded as part of the epidermal differentiation complex 1q21, as are involucrin and loricrin. We as well as other authors have shown that epidermal differentiation is centrally involved in skin barrier homeostasis (1,69,78).

Although filaggrin's role in skin barrier homeostasis is only partly understood, it is known that filaggrin aggregates keratin filaments into tight bundles, which promotes the collapse of the cell into the flattened shape characteristic of corneocytes in the cornified layer (58). Together, keratins and filaggrin constitute 80% to 90% of the protein mass of mammalian epidermis (79,80). Mouse models, ichthyosis vulgaris, and AD involving aberrant filaggrin expression clearly demonstrate the importance of filaggrin for epidermal barrier homeostasis (58,70,73,81). Filaggrin overexpression in murine suprabasal epidermis has been shown to cause a delay in barrier repair (82). Loss of normal profilaggrin and filaggrin has been found in flaky tail (ft/ft) mice, which characteristically display dry, flaky skin, and annular tail, and paw constrictions in the neonatal period (83).

A few functional studies on the role of the disrupted skin barrier in patients with filaggrin mutations have been performed. Loss-of-function polymorphisms in the filaggrin gene have been found to be associated with an increased susceptibility to chronic irritant contact dermatitis (84). This is in accordance with the well-known clinical finding that people with dry skin and AD are prone to irritant contact dermatitis. The role of filaggrin mutations for allergic contact sensitization (type IV) is not as clear. It is widely accepted that the rate of type IV sensitization in AD (regardless of filaggrin mutations) is not increased in general (85), with the possible exception of nickel sensitization. Recently, filaggrin loss of function mutation was accounted for allowing easier hapten intrusion into the skin, which might explain the possibly increased rate of contact sensitization to nickel (86). However, no correlation between filaggrin mutations and hand eczema or contact allergy in general has been found (87), although hand eczema is often regarded as being caused by an atopic predisposition. However, an increased rate of type I allergies has been found in AD patients with filaggrin mutations. It has been shown that patients with filaggrin mutations had a higher risk for developing sensitization against cats but not against dogs, when exposed in early life (88).

Filaggrin mutations are certainly very important for skin barrier dysfunction in AD. However, filaggrin mutation accounted for only 20% to 50% of the patients. The remaining patients without filaggrin mutations also have a defect in skin barrier function. In recent, yet unpublished, studies a tendency toward increased TEWL has been found in patients without filaggrin mutations as compared to patients with these mutations (89). Therefore, it is still an open question whether filaggrin mutations are the most important cause for skin barrier impairment in AD.

The role of filaggrin in allergic rhinitis and bronchial asthma remains unclear. It has been shown that patients with filaggrin mutations are at higher risk of developing bronchial asthma and allergic rhinitis. Nasal biopsies demonstrated strong filaggrin expression in the cornified epithelium of the nasal vestibular lining, but not the transitional and respiratory nasal epithelia (90). The bronchial system does not contain filaggrin. Therefore, it was proposed that the sensitization for asthma develops by skin penetration.

EPIDERMAL BARRIER AND INFLAMMATION IN AD

Inflammatory skin diseases can be induced by either exogenous or endogenous causes. In several diseases it is obvious that the disturbed skin barrier is the first event followed by inflammation. In irritant and allergic contact dermatitis or skin infection, a disruption of the stratum corneum permeability barrier leads to invasion of the noxious agents, which is followed by injury to living epidermal layers, immunologic reactions, and inflammation. Mild skin barrier impairment is found in monogenetic diseases expressing impaired epidermal differentiation or lipid composition without inflammation, for example, ichthyosis vulgaris (filaggrin mutations) (58,81,90) and x-linked recessive ichthyosis (steroid sulfatase deficiency) (91). This means that a certain degree of skin barrier disruption may be necessary for substantial invasion of harmful substances into the skin. Only substantial invasion of irritants or allergens may lead to inflammation. Additional factors, which may be genetically determined, may also be necessary to develop an inflammatory skin disease. An unsolved question is why patients with the same filaggrin mutations develop ichthyosis vulgaris or AD, although there is a considerable overlap between both diseases.

There are skin diseases in which barrier abnormality is triggered by abnormalities of the living epidermal layers or the inflammatory cells, such as autoimmune bullous diseases or T-cell lymphoma (mycosis fungoides). In T-cell lymphoma an endogenous cause of expansion of clonal malignant CD4+ T-cells leads to changes in epidermal proliferation, differentiation, and skin barrier disruption (92).

AD may show integrating elements of both primary barrier abnormality, which may trigger immunologic reactions, and primary immunologic reactions, which may trigger barrier abnormalities. Barrier disruption and immunologic mechanisms may mutually enhance the initiation and sustaining of skin lesions. With the discovery of the filaggrin mutations in about 20% of the patients with AD it is very likely that barrier abnormalities are the first event in that group. For the remaining about 80% it is unclear whether further genetic defects exist that lead to skin barrier disruption first or whether there are genetic defects that primarily lead to inflammation followed by barrier disruption.

The vast majority of reports on the pathogenesis of AD have focused on the primary role of immune abnormalities [reviewed in (93,94)]. However, an "outside–inside" pathogenesis for AD and other inflammatory dermatoses involving barrier abnormalities has been proposed (1,95). Data primarily obtained during the last 10 years favor the barrier hypothesis (1,58). Exogenous factors that disturb the permeability barrier surely aggravates AD (Fig. 3). Water containing solvents or detergents may impair skin barrier function by removing lipids or disturbing lipid organization in the extracellular lipid bilayers (96). Penetration of irritants or allergens induces keratinocyte proliferation for the removal of the invading pathogen and may activate T-cells (26). Barrier disruption alone leads to increased Langerhans cell density in the skin (97). Also, proteases from house dust mites disturb the epidermal permeability barrier (98).

CLIMATE AND ENVIRONMENTAL ASPECTS IN THE PATHOGENESIS OF AD
Changes in lifestyle or climate may cause barrier dysfunction, which may, in turn, explain the increased incidence of AD. Physiologic stress associated with demanding modern lifestyles appears to enhance skin irritability (99–102). Excessive use of soaps, detergents, and shampoos may also irritate the skin and disturb the skin barrier, while air conditioning and inadequate ventilation may increase exposure to environmental antigens such as house dust mites and pollens. Antigens may also penetrate the intestinal barriers of babies prematurely fed animal protein (27).

Climate may also influence AD. Although a large number of Asians have the atopic syndrome, they do not develop AD as long as they live in humid, tropical climates. Upon moving to different climate zones, individuals with previously subclinical disease often develop cutaneous symptoms. Patients of Southeast Asian and Chinese origin living in the northern areas of the United States and Europe often develop dry skin and eczema in the winter.

It has also been proposed that exposure to atmospheric indoor pollution and the presence of low-grade irritant cause children's skin to become more vulnerable to sensitization (103). Outdoor industrial pollution does not seem to be of equal importance, because in the heavily polluted industrial areas of the former East Germany the rate of AD and bronchial asthma was not increased (in contrast to the increased rate of unspecific bronchitis). Central heating, improved insulation, and other changes in residential environments may increase potential exposure to allergens, particularly dust mites, causing children with already disturbed barrier function to be more vulnerable when exposed to allergens. Global warming and the increased use of fertilizer may enhance the density and the allergenic potency of pollen from trees and grains.

THERAPEUTIC IMPLICATIONS
Treatment strategies in eczema often address immunogenic abnormalities and barrier function. Treatments involving corticosteroids, tacrolimus, pimecrolimus, cyclosporin, and UV light have been shown to improve barrier function and reduce cell inflammation.

Low dose UVB exposed mice showed accelerated permeability barrier repair after artificial barrier disruption, which can be explained by an increase of mRNA levels of rate-limiting enzymes of the lipid synthesis such as FAS, serine palmitoyl transferase, and HMG-CoA (104).

Topical treatment with hydrocortisone ointments may promote barrier restoration in atopic skin (105). However, we recently showed that treatment with the potent corticosteroid betamethasone does not lead to proper permeability barrier repair and restoration of skin barrier structure. In contrast, pimecrolimus led

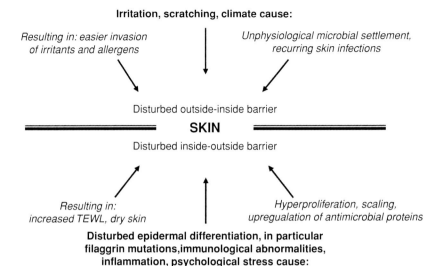

FIGURE 3 Causes and consequences of skin barrier disruption.

to more pronounced repair of skin barrier function and in particular skin barrier structure (106).

The application of creams and ointments containing lipids and lipid-like substances, fatty acids, cholesterol esters, triglycerides, and hydrocarbons, increases stratum corneum hydration and stimulates barrier repair. Petrolatum, the most commonly applied hydrocarbon, has been shown to enhance permeability barrier repair after artificial disruption (107). Topical application of lipids, glycerol, and hydrocarbons may partially correct the permeability barrier defects associated with reduced lipid composition commonly present in AD (108). Improved barrier function has also been described after treatment with moisturizers (20,109). It has been proposed that application of a lipid mixture containing ceramides, cholesterol, and free fatty acids, the three key lipid groups, improves skin barrier function and stratum corneum hydration in AD (110). The efficacy of a nanoparticle cream containing ceramide 3 for restoring barrier function in AD has also been described (111). Nonetheless, several research groups and companies report that creams containing ceramides and key lipids are no more effective than traditional creams and ointments. As these preparations have not yet been widely used, more research and clinical experience are necessary to determine the role of ceramides and the treatment composition with the most therapeutic benefit.

During acute exacerbation of AD the treatment with cream and moisturizers alone does not seem to be sufficient for the treatment. However, these treatments are of invaluable importance for the interval and long-term treatment of patients with AD.

It has been shown that emollients improve treatment results with topical corticosteroids in childhood AD (112). Therefore, future development of treatment remedies should focus on how we can develop pharmaceuticals, which improve epidermal function in AD.

CONCLUSION

The physical barrier of the skin in AD is a very complex system, formed by a tremendous number of interrelated components and embedded in many other physiologic and immunologic processes. Epidermal lipids, proliferation, and differentiation play central roles in the regulation of skin barrier function. The disturbed skin barrier in AD is caused by disturbed lipid content, increased epidermal proliferation, and changes in epidermal differentiation. The skin barrier regulates the entry of type I and IV allergens into the skin. The genetically impaired skin barrier function, which, in particular, is caused by filaggrin mutations, points to the central role of epithelial defense in the pathogenesis of AD. Whether there are inherited abnormalities in neurotropic or immunologic factors that lead to inflammation and to a disruption of the skin barrier in AD remains unknown. Also, mutations in lipid metabolism have not yet been found. However, lipid and lipid-based creams and ointments are most often used for the treatment of eczema, as they are able to remedy reduced lipid content and restore skin barrier function. Drugs like calcineurin inhibitors, which have previously been regarded as influencing the immune system, may primarily influence skin barrier function and structure in AD. Therefore, altered skin barrier function is of central importance in the pathogenesis of AD and treatments should seek to correct the barrier dysfunction.

REFERENCES

1. Jensen JM, Fölster-Holst R, Baranowsky A, et al. Impaired sphingomyelinase activity and epidermal differentiation in atopic dermatitis. J Invest Dermatol 2004; 122:1423–1431.
2. Proksch E, Fölster-Holst R, Jensen JM. Skin barrier function, epidermal proliferation and differentiation in eczema. J Dermatol Sci 2006; 43:159–169.
3. Marekov LN, Steinert PM. Ceramides are bound to structural proteins of the human foreskin epidermal cornified cell envelope. J Biol Chem 1998; 273:17763–17770.
4. Oren A, Ganz T, Liu L, et al. In human epidermis, beta-defensin 2 is packaged in lamellar bodies. Exp Mol Pathol 2003; 74:180–182.
5. Egberts F, Heinrich M, Jensen JM, et al. Cathepsin D is involved in the regulation of transglutaminase 1 and epidermal differentiation. J Cell Sci 2004; 117:2295–2307.
6. Menon GK, Feingold KR, Elias PM. Lamellar body secretory response to barrier disruption. J Invest Dermatol 1992; 98(3):279–289.
7. Holleran WM, Man MQ, Gao WN, et al. Sphingolipids are required for mammalian epidermal barrier function. Inhibition of sphingolipid synthesis delays barrier recovery after acute perturbation. J Clin Invest 1991; 88:1338–1345.
8. Uchida Y, Hamanaka S. Stratum corneum ceramides: Function, origins, and therapeutic implications. In: Elias PM, Feingold KR, eds. Skin Barrier. New York, NY: Taylor & Francis, 2006:43–64.
9. Robson KJ, Stewart ME, Michelsen S, et al. 6-Hydroxy-4-sphingenine in human epidermal ceramides. J Lipid Res 1994; 35:2060–2068.
10. Bouwstra JA, Pilgrim K, Ponec M. Structure of the skin barrier. In: Elias PM and Feingold KR, eds. Skin Barrier. New York, NY: Taylor & Francis, 2006:65–95.
11. Masukawa Y, Narita H, Shimizu E, et al. Characterization of overall ceramide species in human stratum corneum. J Lipid Res 2008; 49(7):1466–1476.
12. Di Nardo A, Wertz P, Giannetti A, et al. Ceramide and cholesterol composition of the skin of patients with atopic dermatitis. Acta Derm Venereol 1998; 78:27–30.
13. Macheleidt O, Kaiser HW, Sandhoff K. Deficiency of epidermal protein-bound ω-hydroxyceramides in atopic dermatitis. J Invest Dermatol 2002; 119(1):166–173.

14. Ogawa H, Yoshiike TJ. A speculative view of atopic dermatitis: Barrier dysfunction in pathogenesis. Dermatol Sci 1993; 5:197–204.
15. Jakasa I, de Jongh CM, Verberk MM, et al. Percutaneous penetration of sodium lauryl sulphate is increased in uninvolved skin of patients with atopic dermatitis compared with control subjects. Br J Dermatol 2006; 155(1):104–109.
16. Jakasa I, Verberk MM, Esposito M, et al. Altered penetration of polyethylene glycols into uninvolved skin of atopic dermatitis patients. J Invest Dermatol 2007; 127(1): 129–134.
17. Boralevi F, Hubiche T, Léauté-Labrèze C, et al. Epicutaneous aeroallergen sensitization in atopic dermatitis infants—Determining the role of epidermal barrier impairment. Allergy 2008; 63(2):205–210.
18. Thune P, Nilsen T, Hanstad IK, et al. The water barrier function of the skin in relation to the water content of stratum corneum, pH and skin lipids. The effect of alkaline soap and syndet on dry skin in elderly, non-atopic patients. Acta Derm Venereol 1988; 68: 277–283.
19. Segre JA. Epidermal barrier formation and recovery in skin disorders. J Clin Invest 2006; 116:1150–1158.
20. Lodén M, Andersson AC, Lindberg M. Improvement in skin barrier function in patients with atopic dermatitis after treatment with a moisturizing cream (Canoderm). Br J Dermatol 1999; 140:264–267.
21. Scott IR, Harding CR. Filaggrin breakdown to water binding compounds during development of the rat stratum corneum is controlled by the water activity of the environment. Dev Biol 1986; 115:84–92.
22. Djian P, Easley K, Green H. Targeted ablation of the murine involucrin gene. J Cell Biol 2000; 151:381–388.
23. Mitchell EB, Crow J, Chapman MD, et al. Basophils in allergen-induced patch test sites in atopic dermatitis. Lancet 1982; 16:127–130.
24. Conti A, Di Nardo A, Seidenari S. No alteration of biophysical parameters in the skin of subjects with respiratory atopy. Dermatology 1996; 192:317–320.
25. Conti A, Seidenari S. No increased skin reactivity in subjects with allergic rhinitis during the active phase of the disease. Acta Derm Venereol 2000; 80:192–195.
26. Nishijima T, Tokura Y, Imokawa G, et al. Altered permeability and disordered cutaneous immunoregulatory function in mice with acute barrier disruption. J Invest Dermatol 1997; 109:175–182.
27. Paganelli R, Atherton DJ, Levinski RI. Differences between normal and milk allergic subjects in their immune response after milk ingestion. Arch Dis Child 1983; 58: 201–206.
28. Barba A, Schena D, Andreaus MC, et al. Intestinal permeability in patients with atopic eczema. Br J Dermatol 1989; 120:71–75.
29. Ochs HD. The Wiskott–Aldrich syndrome. Clin Rev Allergy Immunol 2001; 20:61–86.
30. Ukabam SO, Mann RJ, Cooper BT. Small intestinal permeability to sugars in patients with atopic eczema. Br J Dermatol 1984; 110:649–652.
31. Pike MG, Heddle RJ, Boulton P, et al. Increased intestinal permeability in atopic eczema. J Invest Dermatol 1986; 86:101–104.
32. Jakobza D, Reichmann G, Langnick W, et al. Surface skin lipids in atopic dermatitis (author's transl) [Article in German]. Dermatol Monatsschr 1981; 167:26–29.
33. Barth J, Gatti S, Jatzke M. Skin surface lipids in atopic eczema and ichthyosis. Chron Derm 1989; 10:609–612.
34. Sator PG, Schmidt JB, Hönigsmann H. Comparison of epidermal hydration and skin surface lipids in healthy individuals and in patients with atopic dermatitis. J Am Acad Dermatol 2003; 48(3):352–358.
35. Elias PM, Friend DS. The permeability barrier in mammalian epidermis. J Cell Biol 1975; 65(1):180–191.
36. Melnik BC, Hollmann J, Erler E, et al. Microanalytical screening of all major stratum corneum lipids by sequential high-performance thin-layer chromatography. J Invest Dermatol 1989; 92:231–234.

37. Melnik BC, Plewig G. Is the origin of atopy linked to deficient conversion of omega-6-fatty acids to prostaglandin E1? J Am Acad Dermatol 1989; 21:557–563.
38. Imokawa G, Abe A, Jin Y, et al. Decreased level of ceramides in stratum corneum of atopic dermatitis: An etiologic factor in atopic dry skin? J Invest Dermatol 1991; 96: 523–526.
39. Yamamoto A, Serizawa S, Ito M, et al. Stratum corneum lipid abnormalities in atopic dermatitis. Arch Dermatol Res 1991; 283:219–223.
40. Holleran WM, Gao WN, Feingold KR, et al. Localization of epidermal sphingolipid synthesis and serine palmitoyl transferase activity: Alterations imposed by permeability barrier requirements. Arch Dermatol Res 1995; 287(3–4):254–258.
41. Jensen JM, Schütze S, Förl M, et al. Roles for tumor necrosis factor receptor p55 and sphingomyelinase in repairing the cutaneous permeability barrier. J Clin Invest 1999; 104:1761–1770.
42. Jin K, Higaki Y, Takagi Y, et al. Analysis of beta-glucocerebrosidase and ceramidase activities in atopic and aged dry skin. Acta Derm Venereol 1994; 74(5):337–340.
43. Higuchi K, Hara J, Okamoto R, et al. The skin of atopic dermatitis patients contains a novel enzyme, glucosylceramide sphingomyelin deacylase, which cleaves the N-acyl linkage of sphingomyelin and glucosylceramide. Biochem J 2000; 15(350 Pt 3):747–756.
44. Hara J, Higuchi K, Okamoto R, et al. High-expression of sphingomyelin deacylase is an important determinant of ceramide deficiency leading to barrier disruption in atopic dermatitis. J Invest Dermatol 2000; 115:406–413.
45. Nagelkerken L, Verzaal P, Lagerweij T, et al. Development of atopic dermatitis in mice transgenic for human apolipoprotein C1. J Invest Dermatol 2008; 128(5):1165–1172.
46. Proksch E, Feingold KR, Elias PM. Epidermal HMG CoA reductase activity in essential fatty acid deficiency: Barrier requirements rather than eicosanoid generation regulate cholesterol synthesis. J Invest Dermatol 1992; 99:216–220.
47. van Gool CJ, Zeegers MP, Thijs C. Oral essential fatty acid supplementation in atopic dermatitis—A meta-analysis of placebo-controlled trials. Br J Dermatol 2004; 150(4):728–740.
48. Epp N, Fürstenberger G, Müller K, et al. 12R-lipoxygenase deficiency disrupts epidermal barrier function. J Cell Biol 2007; 177(1):173–182.
49. Kirby NA, Hester SL, Rees CA, et al. Skin surface lipids and skin and hair coat condition in dogs fed increased total fat diets containing polyunsaturated fatty acids. J Anim Physiol Anim Nutr (Berl). In press.
50. Taieb A. Hypothesis: From barrier dysfunction to atopic disorders. Contact Dern 1999; 41:177–180.
51. Uehara M, Hayashi S. Hyperlinear palms: Association with ichthyosis and atopic dermatitis. Arch Dermatol 1981; 117(8):490–491.
52. Mevorah B, Marazzi A, Frenk E. The prevalence of accentuated palmoplantar markings and keratosis pilaris in atopic dermatitis, autosomal dominant ichthyosis and control dermatological patients. Br J Dermatol 1985; 112(6):679–685.
53. Spitz JL. Genodermatosis. Baltimore, MD: Williams & Wilkins, 1996:214–215.
54. Hachem JP, Wagberg F, Schmuth M, et al. Serine protease activity and residual LEKTI expression determine phenotype in netherton syndrome. J Invest Dermatol 2006; 126(7):1609–1621.
55. Descargues P, Deraison C, Bonnart C, et al. SPINK5-deficient mice mimic Netherton syndrome through degradation of desmoglein 1 by epidermal protease hyperactivity. Nat Genet 2005; 37:56–65.
56. Fölster-Holst R, Stoll M, Koch WA, et al. Lack of association of SPINK5 polymorphisms with nonsyndromic atopic dermatitis in the population of Northern Germany. Br J Dermatol 2005; 152:1365–1367.
57. Cookson W. The immunogenetics of asthma and eczema: A new focus on the epithelium. Nat Rev Immunol 2004; 4(12):978–988.
58. Palmer CN, Irvine AD, Terron-Kwiatkowski A, et al. Common loss-of-function variants of the epidermal barrier protein filaggrin are a major predisposing factor for atopic dermatitis. Nat Genet 2006; 38(4):441–446.

59. Hudson TJ. Skin barrier function and allergic risk. Nat Genet 2006; 38(4):399–400.
60. Trautmann A, Altznauer F, Akdis M, et al. The differential fate of cadherins during T-cell-induced keratinocyte apoptosis leads to spongiosis in eczematous dermatitis. J Invest Dermatol 2001; 117:927–934.
61. Chen JJ, Liang YH, Zhou FS, et al. The gene for a rare autosomal dominant form of pompholyx maps to chromosome 18q22.1–18q22.3. J Invest Dermatol 2006; 126(2): 300–304.
62. Maretzky T, Reiss K, Ludwig A, et al. ADAM10 mediates E-cadherin shedding and regulates epithelial cell–cell adhesion, migration, and beta-catenin translocation. Proc Natl Acad Sci U S A 2005; 102:9182–9187.
63. Trautmann A, Akdis M, Kleemann D, et al. T cell-mediated Fas-induced keratinocyte apoptosis plays a key pathogenetic role in eczematous dermatitis. J Clin Invest 2000; 106(1):25–35.
64. Al-Jaberi H, Marks R. Studies of the clinically uninvolved skin in patients with dermatitis. Br J Dermatol 1984; 111:437–443.
65. Watanabe M, Tagami H, Horii I, et al. Functional analyses of the superficial stratum corneum in atopic xerosis. Arch Dermatol 1991; 127:1689–1692.
66. Engelke M, Jensen J-M, Ekanayake-Mudiyanselage S, et al. Effects of xerosis and aging in epidermal proliferation and differentiation. Br J Dermatol 1997; 137:219–225.
67. Proksch E. The role of emollients in the management of diseases with chronic dry skin. Skin Pharmacol Physiol 2008; 21(2):75–80.
68. Yoneda K, McBride OW, Korge BP, et al. The cornified cell envelope: Loricrin and transglutaminases. J Dermatol 1992; 19(11):761–764.
69. Seguchi T, Cui CY, Kusuda S, et al. Decreased expression of filaggrin in atopic skin. Arch Dermatol Res 1996; 288(8):442–446.
70. Smith FJ, Irvine AD, Terron-Kwiatkowski A, et al. Loss-of-function mutations in the gene encoding filaggrin cause ichthyosis vulgaris. Nat Genet 2006; 38:337–342.
71. Sandilands A, O'Regan GM, Liao H, et al. Prevalent and rare mutations in the gene encoding filaggrin cause ichthyosis vulgaris and predispose individuals to atopic dermatitis. J Invest Dermatol 2006; 126(8):1770–1775.
72. Weidinger S, Illig T, Baurecht H, et al. Loss-of-function variations within the filaggrin gene predispose for atopic dermatitis with allergic sensitizations. J Allergy Clin Immunol 2006; 118(1):214–219.
73. Ruether A, Stoll M, Schwarz T, et al. Filaggrin loss-of-function variant contributes to atopic dermatitis risk in the population of Northern Germany. Br J Dermatol 2006; 155(5):1093–1094.
74. Linde YW. Dry skin in atopic dermatitis. Acta Derm Venereol Suppl (Stockh) 1992; 177:9–13.
75. Proksch E, Nissen HP, Bremgartner M, et al. Bathing in a magnesium-rich dead sea salt solution improves skin barrier function, enhances skin hydration, and reduces inflammation in atopic dry skin. Int J Dermatol 2005; 44(2):151–157.
76. Ginger RS, Blachford S, Rowland J, et al. Filaggrin repeat number polymorphism is associated with a dry skin phenotype. Arch Dermatol Res 2005; 297(6):235–241.
77. Kezic S, Kemperman PM, Koster ES, et al. Loss-of-function mutations in the filaggrin gene lead to reduced level of natural moisturizing factor in the stratum corneum. J Invest Dermatol 2008; 128(8):2117–2119.
78. Ekanayake-Mudiyanselage S, Aschauer H, Schmook FP, et al. Expression of epidermal keratins and the cornified envelope protein involucrin is influenced by permeability barrier disruption. J Invest Dermatol 1998; 111:517–523.
79. Roop D. Defects in the barrier. Science 1995; 267:474–475.
80. Nemes Z, Steinert PM. Bricks and mortar of the epidermal barrier. Exp Mol Med 1999; 31:5–19.
81. Irvine AD, McLean WH. Breaking the (un)sound barrier: Filaggrin is a major gene for atopic dermatitis. J Invest Dermatol 2006; 126:1200–1202.
82. Presland RB, Coulombe PA, Eckert RL, et al. Barrier function in transgenic mice overexpressing K16, involucrin, and filaggrin in the suprabasal epidermis. J Invest Dermatol 2004; 123:603–606.

83. Presland RB, Boggess D, Lewis SP, et al. Loss of normal profilaggrin and filaggrin in flaky tail (ft/ft) mice: An animal model for the filaggrin-deficient skin disease ichthyosis vulgaris. J Invest Dermatol 2000; 115:1072–1081.

84. de Jongh CM, Khrenova L, Verberk MM, et al. Loss-of-function polymorphisms in the filaggrin gene are associated with an increased susceptibility to chronic irritant contact dermatitis: A case-control study. Br J Dermatol 2008; 159(3):621–627.

85. Heine G, Schnuch A, Uter W, et al. Information Network of Departments of Dermatology (IVDK); German Contact Dermatitis Research Group (DKG). Type-IV sensitization profile of individuals with atopic eczema: Results from the Information Network of Departments of Dermatology (IVDK) and the German Contact Dermatitis Research Group (DKG). Allergy 2006; 61(5):611–616.

86. Novak N, Baurecht H, Schäfer T, et al. Loss-of-function mutations in the filaggrin gene and allergic contact sensitization to nickel. J Invest Dermatol 2008; 128(6):1430–1435.

87. Lerbaek A, Kyvik KO, Ravn H, et al. Incidence of hand eczema in a population-based twin cohort: Genetic and environmental risk factors. Br J Dermatol 2007; 157(3):552–557.

88. Bisgaard H, Simpson A, Palmer CN, et al. Gene–environment interaction in the onset of eczema in infancy: Filaggrin loss-of-function mutations enhanced by neonatal cat exposure. PLoS Med 2008; 5(6):e131.

89. Nemoto-Hasebe I, Akiyama M, Nomura T, et al. Clinical severity is correlated with barrier defect in atopic dermatitis associated with filaggrin mutations. J Invest Dermatol 2008; 128:S94.

90. Weidinger S, O'Sullivan M, Illig T, et al. Filaggrin mutations, atopic eczema, hay fever, and asthma in children. J Allergy Clin Immunol 2008; 121(5):1203–1209.

91. Thauvin-Robinet C, Mugneret F, Callier P, et al. Unique survival in chrondrodysplasia-hermaphrodism syndrome. Am J Med Genet A 2005; 132:335–337.

92. Berger CL, Edelson R. The life cycle of cutaneous T cell lymphoma reveals opportunities for targeted drug therapy. Curr Cancer Drug Targets 2004; 4:609–619.

93. Leung DY. New insights into the complex gene–environment interactions evolving into atopic dermatitis. J Allergy Clin Immunol 2006; 118:37–45.

94. Ong PY, Leung DY. Immune dysregulation in atopic dermatitis. Curr Allergy Asthma Rep 2006; 6:384–389.

95. Elias PM, Feingold KR. Does the tail wag the dog? Role of the barrier in the pathogenesis of inflammatory dermatoses and therapeutic implications. Arch Dermatol 2001; 137:1079–1081.

96. Fartasch M. Epidermal barrier in disorders of the skin. Microsc Res Tech 1997; 38:361–372.

97. Proksch E, Brasch J, Sterry W. Integrity of the permeability barrier regulates epidermal Langerhans cell density. Br J Dermatol 1996; 134(4):630–638.

98. Jeong SK, Kim HJ, Youm JK, et al. Mite and cockroach allergens activate protease-activated receptor 2 and delay epidermal permeability barrier recovery. J Invest Dermatol 2008; 128(8):1930–1939.

99. Elias PM, Wood LC, Feingold KR. Epidermal pathogenesis of inflammatory dermatoses. Am J Contact Derm 1999; 10:119–126.

100. Garg A, Chren MM, Sands LP, et al. Psychological stress perturbs epidermal permeability barrier homeostasis: Implications for the pathogenesis and treatment of stress-associated skin disorders. Arch Dermatol 2001; 137:53–59.

101. Altemus M, Rao B, Dhabhar FS, et al. Stress-induced changes in skin barrier function in healthy women. J Invest Dermatol 2001; 117:309–317.

102. Choi EH, Brown BE, Crumrine D, et al. Mechanisms by which psychologic stress alters cutaneous permeability barrier homeostasis and stratum corneum integrity. J Invest Dermatol 2005; 124(3):587–595.

103. Huss-Marp J, Eberlein-König B, Breuer K, et al. Influence of short-term exposure to airborne Der p 1 and volatile organic compounds on skin barrier function and dermal blood flow in patients with atopic eczema and healthy individuals. Clin Exp Allergy 2006; 36(3):338–345.

104. Hong SP, Kim MJ, Jung MY, et al. Biopositive effects of low-dose UVB on epidermis: Coordinate upregulation of antimicrobial peptides and permeability barrier reinforcement. J Invest Dermatol 2008; 128(12):2880–2887.
105. Aalto-Korte K. Improvement of skin barrier function during treatment of atopic dermatitis. J Am Acad Dermatol 1995; 33(6):969–972.
106. Proksch E, Jensen JM, Bräutigam M, et al. Pimecrolimus but not corticosteroid improves the skin barrier in atopic dermatitis. J Invest Dermatol 2008; 128:S104.
107. Ghadially R, Halkier-Sörensen L, Elias PM. Effects of petrolatum on stratum corneum structure and function. J Am Acad Dermatol 1992; 26:387–396.
108. Fluhr JW, Darlenski R, Surber C. Glycerol and the skin: Holistic approach to its origin and functions. Br J Dermatol 2008; 159(1):23–34.
109. Tabata N, O'Goshi K, Zhen YX, et al. Biophysical assessment of persistent effects of moisturizers after their daily applications: Evaluation of corneotherapy. Dermatology 2000; 200:308–313.
110. Chamlin SL, Frieden IJ, Fowler A, et al. Ceramide-dominant, barrier repair lipids improve childhood atopic dermatitis. Arch Dermatol 2001; 137:1110–1112.
111. Berardesca E, Barbareschi M, Veraldi S, et al. Evaluation of efficacy of a skin lipid mixture in patients with irritant contact dermatitis, allergic contact dermatitis or atopic dermatitis: A multicenter study. Contact Dermatitis 2001; 45:280–285.
112. Szczepanowska J, Reich A, Szepietowski JC. Emollients improve treatment results with topical corticosteroids in childhood atopic dermatitis: A randomized comparative study. Pediatr Allergy Immunol 2008; 19(7):614–618.

5 Keratinocytes and the Cytokine/Chemokine Orchestra

Bernhard Homey

Department of Dermatology, Heinrich-Heine-University, Düsseldorf, Germany

INTRODUCTION

Keratinocytes are gatekeepers at the interface between the host and the environment. Taking into account that environmental factors play a critical role in the initiation and maintenance of atopic dermatitis (AD), the aim of this review is to unravel the role of keratinocytes in orchestrating the complex immunologic events underlying this chronically relapsing inflammatory skin disease.

Keratinocytes take on a leading role in a cycle of events that will finally lead to the development of an AD phenotype (Fig. 1). The breakdown of the epidermal barrier is a hallmark of AD. Disruption of the epidermal barrier may lead, on the one hand, to increased transepidermal water loss, resulting in dryness of the skin, which is associated with the development of pruritus. In turn, atopic patients may scratch and induce mechanical trauma leading to the production of proinflammatory cytokines and chemokines. On the other hand, skin barrier defects facilitate the transepidermal penetration of allergens and irritants, which in turn will sustain the production of proinflammatory cytokines and chemokines by keratinocytes and other resident cells of the skin. Subsequently, chemokines in concert with different adhesion molecules direct the recruitment of pathogenic leukocytes to the skin (1–4). Within the skin, distinct leukocyte subsets are activated via different pathways: (a) The keratinocyte-derived cytokine thymic stromal lymphopoietin (TSLP) instructs dendritic cells to induce T_H2 cell differentiation (5–9); (b) Memory T cells encounter their specific antigen/allergen (e.g., Bet v1 from birch pollen or Der p2 from house dust mites) or bacterial superantigens (e.g., staphylococcal enterotoxins) (2); (c) Dendritic cells bind allergen-specific IgE-complexes, capture antigen, and show enhanced antigen presentation capabilities (2); and (d) Allergen-specific IgE-complexes induce Fcε receptor aggregation and activate mast cells (2). Viruses, fungi, and bacteria take advantage of a reduced level of antimicrobial peptides present in AD skin, colonize inflamed skin, and release proinflammatory products resulting in the modulation and amplification of leukocyte activation (10,11). As a common feature, leukocyte activation results in the release of inflammatory mediators including effector cytokines (e.g., IL-31), which perpetuate pruritic signals (12–15). Taken together, these amplifying processes sustain inflammatory responses within the skin and lead to the development of an AD phenotype (Fig. 1).

KERATINOCYTES AND THE PRODUCTION OF PROINFLAMMATORY CYTOKINES

The very early events, which initiate atopic skin inflammation remain largely elusive, however, the production of primary proinflammatory cytokines following mechanical trauma and skin barrier disruption is a well-accepted scenario. Several

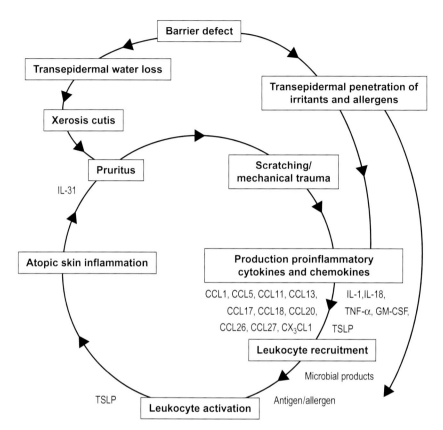

FIGURE 1 Keratinocytes and the cycle of events leading to an atopic dermatitis phenotype.

studies showed that mechanical trauma and skin barrier disruption following tape stripping of the skin result in the rapid and marked upregulation of IL-1α, IL-1β, TNF-α, and GM-CSF (16,17). These primary proinflammatory cytokines in turn induce the production of chemoattractants and adhesion molecules supporting the recruitment, proliferation, and survival of leukocytes within the skin. Besides mechanical trauma, the staphylococcal product, peptidoglycan as well as histamine have been suggested to contribute to the elevated expression of GM-CSF in keratinocytes within lesional skin of AD patients (18,19). Hence, GM-CSF is regulated under the control of innate and adaptive immune pathways and may support the survival and retention of dendritic cell subsets at sites of atopic skin inflammation.

Recently, a member of the rapidly expanding IL-1 superfamily, IL-18, has been shown to participate in the development of a relapsing dermatitis with mastocytosis, T_H2 cytokine accumulation, and systemic elevation of IgE and histamine (20). Macrophages as well as keratinocytes store IL-18 as a biologically inactive precursor. After stimulation by danger signals, caspase-1 or caspase-like enzymes cleave pro–IL-18 and release the active form. Moreover, skin-specific expression of IL-18 and caspase-1 leads to this atopy-like dermatitis (20). Notably, the dermatitis phenotype is independent of Stat6 signaling pathways but critically dependent on the presence of active IL-18 (20). Therefore, Konishi and colleagues suggest that IL-18 induces IgE-independent allergic disorders and mediates an innate-type of allergic response (20). In contrast to these findings, Higa et al. could not demonstrate a role for IL-18 in the development of AD-like skin lesions in NC/Nga mice (21). Although IL-18 serum levels were significantly increased prior to and during the development in NC/Nga mice, administration of a neutralizing antibody failed to inhibit the onset and development of dermatitis and IgE elevation. The treatment, rather, tended to lead to an exacerbation of dermatitis and scratching behavior (21). Although genetic approaches as well as intervention studies using neutralizing antibodies in murine models for human diseases have their own limitations, findings of a recent study by Novak and colleagues support a role for IL-18 in the pathogenesis of AD (22). Single nucleotide polymorphisms (SNPs) in exon 1 and the promoter region of the *IL18* gene were significantly associated with an AD phenotype. These associations were independent of the concomitant manifestation of allergic rhinitis or asthma. Furthermore, the amount of IL-18 in the supernatants of PBMCs of patients with AD stimulated with staphylococcal enterotoxin B (SEB) was significantly higher than that in healthy control subjects. In parallel, the amount of active IL-18 in the sera of patients with AD was enhanced at the exacerbation of their disease. These observations suggest that SNPs in the *IL18* gene might be involved in the development of AD by contributing to a functional dysregulation of the IL-18 production in vivo (22).

Taken together, mechanical trauma and skin barrier disruption induce a set of primary proinflammatory cytokines that initiate inflammation in atopic individuals. Moreover, staphylococcal as well as mast cell products may sustain the release of these mediators and support the cycle of inflammation.

KERATINOCYTES AND CHEMOKINE-INDUCED RECRUITMENT OF PATHOGENIC LEUKOCYTE SUBSETS

Chemokines are small (8–12 kD), cytokine-like chemotactic peptides that critically regulate leukocyte trafficking and organize innate as well as adaptive immune responses (23). To date, 46 human chemokine ligands have been identified and this superfamily is thought to be among the first functional protein families completely characterized at the molecular level. This offers the opportunity to identify all relevant members of a particular protein family in physiologic and pathophysiologic processes. On the basis of the arrangement of the amino terminal cysteine residues, chemokines are classified into: (*i*) CXC-chemokines (termed as CXC ligands, CXCL), (*ii*) CC-chemokines (CCL), (*iii*) C-chemokines (XCL), and (*iv*) CX_3C-chemokine (CX_3CL) (24).

Chemokines bind pertussis toxin-sensitive, seven-transmembrane-spanning G-protein coupled receptors (GPCRs), and to date 10 CC-chemokine, 7 CXC-chemokine, 1 CX_3C, and 1 XCR receptors have been characterized (23,25). During the multistep process of leukocyte trafficking, chemokine ligand–receptor interactions initiate the firm adhesion of leukocytes to the endothelium and mediate transendothelial migration from the blood vessel into perivascular pockets (26). From perivascular spaces matrix-bound sustained chemokine gradients direct skin-infiltrating leukocyte subsets to subepidermal or intraepidermal locations.

Recent studies have identified several homeostatic and inflammatory chemokines including CCL1, CCL2, CCL3, CCL4, CCL5, CCL11, CCL13, CCL17, CCL18, CCL20, CCL22, CCL26, and CCL27 to be associated with an ΛD phenotype

(1,27–53). Moreover, serum levels of the following chemokines including CCL11, CCL17, CCL22, CCL26, CCL27, and CX₃CL1 directly correlated with disease severity, suggesting an important role in the pathogenesis of AD. Recent studies support that keratinocytes serve as a cellular source for a distinct set of AD-associated chemokines such as CCL5, CCL17, CCL20, CCL26, CCL27, and CX₃CL1.

The inflammatory infiltrate of AD mainly consists of CD4$^+$ memory T cells located in perivascular, subepidermal as well as intraepidermal spaces (2). Besides T cells, distinct dendritic cell subsets, mast cells, and eosinophils constitute the inflammatory infiltrate (2).

Recruitment of Skin-Homing Memory T Cells

Over the last decade, findings of numerous clinical and experimental studies indicate that T cells play a crucial role in the immunopathogenesis of atopic skin inflammation (2,54,55).

The cutaneous lymphocyte–associated antigen (CLA) identifies a subset of skin-homing memory T cells (4,26). CLA interacts with its vascular ligand E-selectin and mediates the rolling of distinct leukocyte subsets along the vascular endothelium (4,26). E-selectin is not skin-specific but is expressed on inflamed endothelium of various tissues (4,26). Hence, other skin-specific cues must regulate the tissue-specific homing capacity of CLA$^+$ memory T cells.

CCL27 represents a skin-specific chemokine exclusively produced by epidermal keratinocytes (1,56). This novel chemokine is abundantly expressed under homeostatic conditions and is inducible by proinflammatory mediators such as TNF-α and IL-1β (1,56). It binds with high affinity to extracellular matrix proteins and is displayed on cutaneous vascular endothelium (1,56). CCL27 binds the formerly orphan G-protein coupled receptor GPR-2 (CCR10) (57). In vivo, the CCL27–CCR10 interaction regulates memory T cell recruitment to the skin as well as allergen-specific skin inflammation (1). Neutralization of CCL27 significantly impairs cutaneous inflammation in mouse models of allergic contact dermatitis and AD (1). Besides CCR10, skin-homing CLA$^+$ memory T cells abundantly express CCR4 on their cell surface.

A recent study by Reiss et al. suggests that CCR4 and CCR10 ligands cooperate in the recruitment of memory T cells to inflamed skin (3). The endothelium of cutaneous venules expresses the CCR4 ligand CCL17. Its expression is not exclusive to the skin but widely detected at various noncutaneous sites (3). Hence, endothelial cell–derived CCL17 may cooperate with CCL27 in mediating leukocyte arrest and diapedesis. Sustained gradients of matrix-bound CCL27 may subsequently direct lymphocytes from perivascular pockets to subepidermal or intraepidermal locations.

Next to the keratinocyte-specific chemokine CCL27, a comprehensive analysis of the expression of all known chemokines in chronic inflammatory skin diseases identified the chemokines CCL18 and CCL1 to be specifically associated with an AD phenotype but absent in other chronic inflammatory or autoimmune skin diseases such as psoriasis or cutaneous lupus erythematosus (27,43).

CCL18 represented the most highly expressed ligand in AD, and the absolute amount of CCL18 mRNA in lesional atopic skin was more than 100-fold higher than those seen for CCL17 (43). In good accordance with this finding, DNA microarray analyses by Nomura and coworkers also identified CCL18 as one of the genes showing the strongest association with AD compared to psoriatic or normal skin specimens (10). Notably, trigger factors of atopic skin inflammation such as allergen exposure and staphylococcal superantigens markedly induced this chemokine in vitro and in vivo, suggesting important CCL18-driven processes during the initiation and amplification of atopic skin inflammation (43). CCL18 binds to CLA$^+$ memory T cells in peripheral blood of AD patients, in vitro and induces the recruitment of memory T cells into human skin, in vivo (44). Hence, CCL18 may play a role in the organization of T cell responses (44). This hypothesis is supported by a study demonstrating that human CCL18 enhanced Ag-specific primary CD8$^+$ T cell responses when co-administered with malaria vaccines in mice (58). Dermal dendritic cells produce CCL18 and are in a close proximity to infiltrating T cells suggesting the involvement of this chemokine during the formation of T cell–dendritic cell clusters (43). Taken together, CCL18, produced by antigen presenting cells after contact with specific allergens or microbial products may support the recruitment of T cells into the skin and ensure their encounter with allergen- or superantigen-loaded dendritic cells.

Recently, Gombert et al. demonstrated that the expression of the CC chemokine CCL1 is also significantly and selectively upregulated in AD in comparison to psoriasis, cutaneous lupus erythematosus, or normal skin (27). CCL1 serum levels of AD patients were significantly higher than those of healthy individuals (27). Dendritic cells, mast cells, and dermal endothelial cells were abundant sources of CCL1 during atopic skin inflammation and allergen challenge as well as *Staphylococcus aureus*–derived products induced its production (27). In vitro, binding and cross-linking of IgE on mast cells resulted in a significant upregulation of this inflammatory chemokine. A small subset of circulating T cells, interstitial dendritic cells, Langerhans cells as well as their monocytic precursors expressed CCR8 (27). Moreover, the inflammatory and atopy-associated chemokine CCL1 synergized with the homeostatic chemokine CXCL12, resulting in the recruitment of T cell (CD8 > CD4) and Langerhans cell-like dendritic cells (27).

Interestingly, CCL1 has also been described as a potent antiapoptotic factor for thymocytes suggesting that CCL1–CCR8 interactions may provide survival signals for T cells and dendritic cells at sites of atopic skin inflammation. These findings suggest that allergen or microbial products (*S. aureus*) may trigger CCL1 and CCL18 production in atopic individuals which in turn recruit memory T cells and in particular Langerhans cells into the skin and lead to their accumulation in subepidermal and intraepidermal locations. Because activated dendritic cells secrete large amounts of CCL1, CCL1–CCR8 driven recruitment pathways may facilitate dendritic cell–T cell interactions at sites of atopic skin inflammation. Moreover, CCR8 signaling may enhance cell survival providing a potential mechanism that sustains atopic inflammation and prevents activation-induced apoptosis of skin-infiltrating leukocytes. Thus, CCL1 and CCL18 together may provide pathways linking adaptive and innate immune functions, leading to the accumulation of relevant leukocyte subsets at sites of atopic skin inflammation and supporting the initiation and amplification of AD.

Dendritic Cell Trafficking

Dendritic cell precursors migrate from postcapillary venules into peripheral tissues, differentiate, and capture, while in an immature state, antigens or allergens. Following stimulation with proinflammatory mediators, dendritic cells mature and leave peripheral sites, enter afferent lymphatics, and migrate to local draining lymph nodes, where they prime naïve T cells and initiate immune responses (59,60). During their activation and differentiation, T cells critically depend on the stimulation of antigen, presenting cells to differentiate into effector cells. In AD, an increased number of epidermal Langerhans cells , inflammatory dendritic epidermal cells (IDEC) as well as tissue macrophages, and interstitial/dermal dendritic cells is present in the epidermal and dermal compartment (2,60).

Extensive analyses of the chemokine receptor repertoire and chemokine responsiveness of dendritic cell populations during their development and maturation have been performed during recent years. Overall, immature dendritic cells respond to many CC and CXC chemokines including CCL3, CCL4, CCL13, CCL5, CCL20, CCL25, and CXCL12, but each immature dendritic cell subpopulation shows a unique spectrum of chemokine responsiveness (59).

On broad terms, immature dendritic cells can be classified into four distinct groups of related cells: epithelial dendritic cells (LC), intersitial/dermal dendritic cell, monocyte-derived dendritic cell, and CD11 c$^-$ dendritic cell precursors. Peripheral blood dendritic cell and monocytes display many chemokine receptors including CCR1, CCR2, CCR5, CXCR4, and CX$_3$CR1 on their cell surface but primarily respond towards CCR2 ligands (59). In contrast, ex vivo–derived LC or in vitro–generated Langerhans-type dendritic cells demonstrate a restricted chemokine receptor repertoire with CCR6 being the only abundantly expressed receptor on this dendritic cell subset (59,61). Since no CCR6$^+$ populations are detected among putative dendritic cell precursors within the peripheral blood, a model of sequential chemokine responsiveness has been suggested (62). Blood dendritic cells or dendritic cell precursors are recruited into peripheral tissues via CCR2 ligands expressed in the context of endothelial cells and blood vessels. Within perivascular spaces, dendritic cell precursors differentiate through the influence of the tissue microenvironment and gain CCR6 expression (62). Subsequently, CCL20 production by keratinocytes at sites of injury or allergen exposure may direct Langerhans cell precursors into the epidermis and lead to their accumulation in AD (62). Nakayama et al. demonstrated that CCL20 is weakly expressed in normal skin but markedly produced by keratinocytes in lesional skin of AD patients and associated CCL20–CCR6-driven pathways with the accumulation of immature dendritic cells and memory T cells within atopic skin (45).

Hence, the chemokine ligands CCL1, CCL2, CCL5, CCL13, CCL20, and CX$_3$CL1 have been shown to be induced and are likely candidates to recruit dendritic cell precursors from the circulation to sites of atopic skin inflammation.

Once entering peripheral tissues, immature dendritic cell serves as sentinels of the immune system. Upon stimulation with inflammatory mediators such as IL-1, TNF-α, CD40 L, virus or bacterial products dendritic cells mature and undergo phenotypic changes. Uniformly, mature dendritic cell subpopulations loose their ability to capture antigen and chemotactic responsiveness toward inflammatory chemokines but upregulate the chemokine receptor CCR7 (59). In turn, CCR7 ligands, for example, CCL19, CCL21 are abundantly expressed in afferent lymphatics and with secondary lymphoid tissues directing dendritic cell migration to local draining lymph nodes (59).

Taken together, dendritic cells and their precursors perform tightly controlled migration processes, and the temporal–spatial expression pattern of chemokines decides the composition and anatomical distribution of dendritic cells in the different phases of atopic skin inflammation.

Recruitment of Eosinophils

Elevated numbers of circulating eosinophils are frequently observed in patients with AD (2). Although controversial data on the chemokine receptor repertoire of human peripheral blood eosinophils has been published, there is increasing evidence that CCR2, CCR3, and CXCR4 are expressed on the cell surface of human eosinophils and induce significant chemotactic responses. Among all chemokine receptors associated with eosinophils, CCR3 represents the most extensively studied member of this protein family. CCR3 represents a highly promiscuous receptor binding at least nine different human chemokine ligands. Among those CCL5, CCL11, CCL13, and CCL26 have been reported in AD.

Yawalkar et al. showed the expression of CCL11 and CCR3 in AD. CCL11 and CCR3 were significantly increased in lesional skin from AD patients but not in nonatopic controls (33). Predominantly, mononuclear cells of the dermis expressed CCL11 and CCR3 (33). Analysis of serial sections suggested that $CD3^+$ lymphocytes were major sources of these proteins. Besides mononuclear cells, fibroblasts and eosinophils were identified as producers of CCL11 in lesional atopic skin (33). Thus, the authors suggested a positive feedback loop that may preferentially amplify the chemotactic response of T lymphocytes and eosinophils.

Moreover, Gluck and Rogala demonstrated that CCL5 serum levels were significantly increased in AD patients compared to healthy nonatopic control subjects (29). However, serum levels did not correlate with clinical scores of patients. In contrast, serum levels of CCL11, CCL13, and CCL26 were significantly upregulated in AD patients and directly correlated with disease activity.

Findings in CCR3-deficient mice recently showed that this chemokine receptor is essential for skin eosinophilia and airway hyperresponsiveness in a murine model of AD and asthma (63). Although eosinophils and the eosinophil-produced major basic protein were absent from the skin of sham and ovalbumin-sensitized CCR3$-/-$ mice, mast cell numbers and the expression of IL-4 mRNA were normal within the skin suggesting that CCR3 is not essential for the infiltration of mast cells and T_H2 cells into the skin (63). Furthermore, CCR3$-/-$ mice produced normal levels of OVA-specific IgE and their splenocytes secreted normal amounts of IL-4 and IL-5 following in vitro stimulation with OVA indicating effective generation of systemic T_H2 responses (63). Hence findings of this study suggest that CCR3 ligands are critical for eosinophil recruitment during atopic skin inflammation but may not play a dominant role in T cell differentiation and recruitment.

Taken together, CCR3-driven pathways are essential for the recruitment of eosinophils to sites of atopic skin inflammation. In lesional skin of AD patients, keratinocyte-derived CCR3 ligands including CCL5 and CCL26 may be candidates to mediate the influx of eosinophils into the skin. Within the complex puzzle of mediators regulating leukocyte trafficking under homeostatic and inflammatory conditions, a picture emerges suggesting that an orchestrated process of temporal–spatial expression of adhesion molecules and chemokines is responsible for the recruitment and accumulation of distinct leukocyte subsets during atopic skin inflammation.

KERATINOCYTES DIRECT T-CELL DIFFERENTIATION TOWARD A PROATOPIC/ALLERGIC PHENOTYPE

For decades, the role of keratinocytes during the initiation of allergic responses remained an enigma. Recently, Soumelis et al. demonstrated that keratinocytes trigger dendritic cell–mediated allergic inflammation by producing the novel IL-7–like hematopoietic cytokine thymic stromal lymphopoietin (TSLP) (9). Keratinocytes in lesional skin of AD patients abundantly produced TSLP. Keratinocyte-derived TSLP instructed human CD11 c$^+$ dendritic cells to prime T cells into the direction of a proallergic T$_H$2 phenotype with the production of IL-4, IL-5, and IL-13 but no IL-10 or IFN-γ (9). Moreover, stimulation of human CD11 c$^+$ dendritic cells with this novel hematopoietic cytokine resulted in the release of CCL17 and CCL22, two atopy-associated chemokines which preferentially attract CCR4$^+$ T$_H$2 cells (9). Besides CD4$^+$ T cell responses, TSLP-activated human CD11 c$^+$ dendritic cells potently activated naïve CD8$^+$ T cells to expand and differentiate into IL-5- and IL-13-producing effector cells (5). Simultaneous CD40 L triggering of TSLP-activated dendritic cells induced CD8$^+$ T cells with potent cytolytic activity, producing large amounts of IFN-γ, while retaining their capacity to produce IL-5 and IL-13 (5). Hence, TSLP may represent an early keratinocyte-derived trigger of atopic T cell responses and suggest that in concert with CD40L expressing cells, TSLP may amplify and sustain proallergic responses as well as cause tissue damage by promoting the generation of IFN-γ–producing cytotoxic effectors.

These findings contradict the perception of epithelial cells as pure lining cells and include effector functions determining the direction and type of immune responses.

Indeed, two independent in vivo studies underscored the important role of TSLP in the development of AD-like skin inflammation (6,8). Inducible skin-specific overexpression of TSLP resulted in an AD-like phenotype (8). Histopathologic examinations of eczematous lesions demonstrated acanthosis, spongiosis, hyperkeratosis, and a dermal mononuclear infiltrate containing increased numbers of lymphocytes, macrophages, eosinophils, and mast cells (8). In addition to the skin phenotype, mice showed increased IgG1 and IgE immunoglobulins within the serum (8). In addition, a striking increase of the skin-homing receptors such as P- and E-selectin ligands on T$_H$2 cells was observed in K5-TSLP-transgenic mice (8). In skin lesions, the expression of the atopy-associated chemokine CCL17 and its receptor CCR4 were markedly increased (8). In addition to Yoo et al., findings of Li and coworkers further supported the important role of TSLP in the development of atopic skin inflammation (6). Overexpression of TSLP under the regulation of the keratin-14 promoter (K14-TSLP mice) resulted in the development of pruritic eczematous lesions on the ears, face, and neck region of mice (6). Skin lesions showed numerous CD4$^+$ T cells, CD11 c$^+$ dendritic cells and eosinophils, and a molecular signature with increased levels of IL-4, IL-5, IL-13, IL-10, and IL-31 transcripts (6). Moreover, serum IgE levels were elevated (6).

Taken together, transgenic mice overexpressing TSLP within the skin demonstrated that TSLP can initiate a cascade of inflammation that leads to the development of AD-like skin lesions. Notably, TSLP is also increased in asthmatic airway epithelial cells and TSLP expression correlates with disease severity in asthma patients, while lung-specific overexpression of TSLP leads to airway inflammation in mice (7,64,65).

KERATINOCYTES AND THE PERPETUATION OF PRURITUS SIGNALS

Until recently, the contribution of T cells to the development of pruritus remained an enigma. Dillon et al. recently showed that transgenic overexpression of the novel four helix bundle cytokine interleukin (IL)-31 in lymphocytes induces severe pruritus and subsequently a dermatitis phenotype in mice (12). T$_H$2 cells preferentially expressed IL-31 which signals through a heterodimeric receptor composed of IL-31 receptor A (IL-31RA) and oncostatin M receptor (OSMR) (12,66). Sonkoly et al. as well as Bilsborough et al. extended these findings and showed that human IL-31 is significantly upregulated in "pruritic" (AD, prurigo nodularis) but not in "non-pruritic" (psoriasis) forms of chronic skin inflammation (67,68). Within the inflammatory infiltrate of AD patients, inflammatory cells of the lymphocytic lineage, with the majority staining for CLA and CD3 overexpressed IL-31 mRNA (67). In vivo, exposure to staphylococcal superantigen rapidly induced IL-31 expression in atopic individuals. In vitro, IL-31 was induced by staphylococcal superantigens but not by T_H1- or T_H2-type cytokines or viruses in leukocytes (68). In atopic individuals, activated leukocytes expressed higher levels of IL-31 transcripts compared to healthy, nonatopic subjects (68). These observations were in line with findings of Bilsborough showing that circulating CLA^+ memory T cells of AD patients were capable of producing elevated levels of IL-31 protein when compared with T cells of psoriatic donors (67).

Monocytes, dendritic cells and epithelial cells including keratinocytes are likely candidates to express heterodimeric IL-31 receptor (IL-31RA/OSMR) (12,67,68). In cultured human keratinocytes, IL-31 activates Stat3 and induces among other genes the expression of a distinct set of atopy-associated chemokines such as CCL1, CCL17, and CCL22 (12). Notably, Sonkoly and coworkers reported that OSMR and IL-31RA transcripts are also abundantly expressed in dorsal root ganglia, the anatomical location where the cell bodies of the primary sensory and itch-mediating neurons reside (68). Hence, keratinocytes initiate the recruitment of skin-homing CLA^+ T cells through the release of CCL27, in turn skin-infiltrating T cells produce the effector cytokine IL-31 in response to the stimulation with bacterial superantigens or allergen. Subsequently, peripheral sensory neurons as well as keratinocytes are a target of IL-31 resulting in the transmission of pruritus signals to the CNS and sustaining the recruitment of IL-31–producing effector memory T cell recruitment through the induction of CCL1, CCL17, and CCL22.

Taken together, IL-31 may provide the missing link between increased *S. aureus* colonization, subsequent T cell recruitment/activation, and the induction of pruritus to close the amplification cycle in atopic skin inflammation.

CONCLUSIONS AND PERSPECTIVE

Insights into the immunopathogenesis of AD provide numerous interesting therapeutic targets. We are currently witnessing an interesting development integrating structural cells, in particular the keratinocyte, into the complex puzzle of AD. Although findings of recent studies substantially enhanced our understanding of the molecular and cellular events leading to the development of AD, significant therapeutic challenges remain. In particular, the long-term management patients suffering from severe chronically relapsing inflammatory skin diseases still represents a significant unmet medical need. A large number of preclinical studies are currently targeting AD-associated cytokine- and chemokine-pathways and may provide interesting new therapeutic tools in the years to come.

REFERENCES

1. Homey B, Alenius H, Muller A, et al. CCL27–CCR10 interactions regulate T cell-mediated skin inflammation. Nat Med 2002; 8:157–165.

2. Leung DY, Bieber T. Atopic dermatitis. Lancet 2003; 361:151–160.
3. Reiss Y, Proudfoot AE, Power CA, et al. CC chemokine receptor (CCR)4 and the CCR10 ligand cutaneous T cell-attracting chemokine (CTACK) in lymphocyte trafficking to inflamed skin. J Exp Med 2001; 194:1541–1547.
4. Campbell JJ, Butcher EC. Chemokines in tissue-specific and microenvironment-specific lymphocyte homing. Curr Opin Immunol 2000; 12:336–341.
5. Gilliet M, Soumelis V, Watanabe N, et al. Human dendritic cells activated by TSLP and CD40 L induce proallergic cytotoxic T cells. J Exp Med 2003; 197:1059–1063.
6. Li M, Messaddeq N, Teletin M, et al. Retinoid X receptor ablation in adult mouse keratinocytes generates an atopic dermatitis triggered by thymic stromal lymphopoietin. Proc Natl Acad Sci U S A 2005; 102:14795–14800.
7. Liu YJ. Thymic stromal lymphopoietin: Master switch for allergic inflammation. J Exp Med 2006; 203:269–273.
8. Yoo J, Omori M, Gyarmati D, et al. Spontaneous atopic dermatitis in mice expressing an inducible thymic stromal lymphopoietin transgene specifically in the skin. J Exp Med 2005; 202:541–549.
9. Soumelis V, Reche PA, Kanzler H, et al. Human epithelial cells trigger dendritic cell mediated allergic inflammation by producing TSLP. Nat Immunol 2002; 3:673–680.
10. Nomura I, Gao B, Boguniewicz M, et al. Distinct patterns of gene expression in the skin lesions of atopic dermatitis and psoriasis: A gene microarray analysis. J Allergy Clin Immunol 2003; 112:1195–1202.
11. Ong PY, Ohtake T, Brandt C, et al. Endogenous antimicrobial peptides and skin infections in atopic dermatitis. N Engl J Med 2002; 347:1151–1160.
12. Dillon SR, Sprecher C, Hammond A, et al. Interleukin 31, a cytokine produced by activated T cells, induces dermatitis in mice. Nat Immunol 2004; 5:752–760.
13. Schmelz M. Itch—mediators and mechanisms. J Dermatol Sci 2002; 28:91–96.
14. Stander S, Steinhoff M. Pathophysiology of pruritus in atopic dermatitis: An overview. Exp Dermatol 2002; 11:12–24.
15. Steinhoff M, Neisius U, Ikoma A, et al. Proteinase-activated receptor-2 mediates itch: A novel pathway for pruritus in human skin. J Neurosci 2003; 23:6176–6180.
16. Wood LC, Jackson SM, Elias PM, et al. Cutaneous barrier perturbation stimulates cytokine production in the epidermis of mice. J Clin Invest 1992; 90:482–487.
17. Wood LC, Elias PM, Calhoun C, et al. Barrier disruption stimulates interleukin-1 alpha expression and release from a pre-formed pool in murine epidermis. J Invest Dermatol 1996; 106:397–403.
18. Matsubara M, Harada D, Manabe H, et al. *Staphylococcus aureus* peptidoglycan stimulates granulocyte macrophage colony-stimulating factor production from human epidermal keratinocytes via mitogen-activated protein kinases. FEBS Lett 2004; 566:195–200.
19. Kanda N, Watanabe S. Histamine enhances the production of granulocyte-macrophage colony-stimulating factor via protein kinase Calpha and extracellular signal-regulated kinase in human keratinocytes. J Invest Dermatol 2004; 122:863–872.
20. Konishi H, Tsutsui H, Murakami T, et al. IL-18 contributes to the spontaneous development of atopic dermatitis-like inflammatory skin lesion independently of IgE/stat6 under specific pathogen-free conditions. Proc Natl Acad Sci U S A 2002; 99:11340–11345.
21. Higa S, Kotani M, Matsumoto M, et al. Administration of anti-interleukin 18 antibody fails to inhibit development of dermatitis in atopic dermatitis-model mice NC/Nga. Br J Dermatol 2003; 149:39–45.
22. Novak N, Kruse S, Potreck J, et al. Single nucleotide polymorphisms of the IL18 gene are associated with atopic eczema. J Allergy Clin Immunol 2005; 115:828–833.
23. Zlotnik A, Yoshie O. Chemokines: A new classification system and their role in immunity. Immunity 2000; 12:121–127.
24. Rossi D, Zlotnik A. The biology of chemokines and their receptors. Annu Rev Immunol 2000; 18:217–242.
25. Balabanian K, Lagane B, Infantino S, et al. The chemokine SDF-1/CXCL12 binds to and signals through the orphan receptor RDC1 in T lymphocytes. J Biol Chem 2005; 280:35760–35766.

26. Butcher EC, Picker LJ. Lymphocyte homing and homeostasis. Science 1996; 272:60–66.
27. Gombert M, Dieu-Nosjean MC, Winterberg F, et al. CCL1–CCR8 interactions: An axis mediating the recruitment of T cells and Langerhans-type dendritic cells to sites of atopic skin inflammation. J Immunol 2005; 174:5082–5091.
28. Kaburagi Y, Shimada Y, Nagaoka T, et al. Enhanced production of CC-chemokines (RANTES, MCP-1, MIP-1alpha, MIP-1beta, and eotaxin) in patients with atopic dermatitis. Arch Dermatol Res 2001; 293:350–355.
29. Gluck J, Rogala B. Chemokine RANTES in atopic dermatitis. Arch Immunol Ther Exp (Warsz) 1999; 47:367–372.
30. Niwa Y. Elevated RANTES levels in plasma or skin and decreased plasma IL-10 levels in subsets of patients with severe atopic dermatitis. Arch Dermatol 2000; 136:125–126.
31. Park CW, Lee BH, Han HJ, et al. Tacrolimus decreases the expression of eotaxin, CCR3, RANTES and interleukin-5 in atopic dermatitis. Br J Dermatol 2005; 152:1173–1181.
32. Yamada H, Chihara J, Matsukura M, et al. Elevated plasma RANTES levels in patients with atopic dermatitis. J Clin Lab Immunol 1996; 48:87–91.
33. Yawalkar N, Uguccioni M, Scharer J, et al. Enhanced expression of eotaxin and CCR3 in atopic dermatitis. J Invest Dermatol 1999; 113:43–48.
34. Leung TF, Wong CK, Chan IH, et al. Plasma concentration of thymus and activation-regulated chemokine is elevated in childhood asthma. J Allergy Clin Immunol 2002; 110:404–409.
35. Jahnz-Rozyk K, Targowski T, Paluchowska E, et al. Serum thymus and activation-regulated chemokine, macrophage-derived chemokine and eotaxin as markers of severity of atopic dermatitis. Allergy 2005; 60:685–688.
36. Hossny E, Aboul-Magd M, Bakr S. Increased plasma eotaxin in atopic dermatitis and acute urticaria in infants and children. Allergy 2001; 56:996–1002.
37. Taha RA, Minshall EM, Leung DY, et al. Evidence for increased expression of eotaxin and monocyte chemotactic protein-4 in atopic dermatitis. J Allergy Clin Immunol 2000; 105:1002–1007.
38. Hijnen D, De Bruin-Weller M, Oosting B, et al. Serum thymus and activation-regulated chemokine (TARC) and cutaneous T cell-attracting chemokine (CTACK) levels in allergic diseases: TARC and CTACK are disease-specific markers for atopic dermatitis. J Allergy Clin Immunol 2004; 113:334–340.
39. Kakinuma T, Nakamura K, Wakugawa M, et al. Thymus and activation-regulated chemokine in atopic dermatitis: Serum thymus and activation-regulated chemokine level is closely related with disease activity. J Allergy Clin Immunol 2001; 107:535–541.
40. Lin L, Nonoyama S, Oshiba A, et al. TARC and MDC are produced by CD40 activated human B cells and are elevated in the sera of infantile atopic dermatitis patients. J Med Dent Sci 2003; 50:27–33.
41. Morita E, Hiragun T, Mihara S, et al. Determination of thymus and activation-regulated chemokine (TARC)-contents in scales of atopic dermatitis. J Dermatol Sci 2004; 34:237–240.
42. Uchida T, Suto H, Ra C, et al. Preferential expression of T(h)2-type chemokine and its receptor in atopic dermatitis. Int Immunol 2002; 14:1431–1438.
43. Pivarcsi A, Gombert M, Dieu-Nosjean MC, et al. CC chemokine ligand 18, an atopic dermatitis-associated and dendritic cell-derived chemokine, is regulated by staphylococcal products and allergen exposure. J Immunol 2004; 173:5810–5817.
44. Gunther C, Bello-Fernandez C, Kopp T, et al. CCL18 is expressed in atopic dermatitis and mediates skin homing of human memory T cells. J Immunol 2005; 174:1723–1728.
45. Nakayama T, Fujisawa R, Yamada H, et al. Inducible expression of a CC chemokine liver- and activation-regulated chemokine (LARC)/macrophage inflammatory protein (MIP)-3 alpha/CCL20 by epidermal keratinocytes and its role in atopic dermatitis. Int Immunol 2001; 13:95–103.
46. Horikawa T, Nakayama T, Hikita I, et al. IFN-gamma-inducible expression of thymus and activation-regulated chemokine/CCL17 and macrophage-derived chemokine/CCL22 in epidermal keratinocytes and their roles in atopic dermatitis. Int Immunol 2002; 14:767–773.

47. Leung TF, Ma KC, Hon KL, et al. Serum concentration of macrophage-derived chemokine may be a useful inflammatory marker for assessing severity of atopic dermatitis in infants and young children. Pediatr Allergy Immunol 2003; 14:296–301.
48. Kagami S, Kakinuma T, Saeki H, et al. Significant elevation of serum levels of eotaxin-3/CCL26, but not of eotaxin-2/CCL24, in patients with atopic dermatitis: Serum eotaxin-3/CCL26 levels reflect the disease activity of atopic dermatitis. Clin Exp Immunol 2003; 134:309–313.
49. Shimada Y, Takehara K, Sato S. Both Th2 and Th1 chemokines (TARC/CCL17, MDC/CCL22, and Mig/CXCL9) are elevated in sera from patients with atopic dermatitis. J Dermatol Sci 2004; 34:201–208.
50. Hon KL, Leung TF, Ma KC, et al. Serum levels of cutaneous T-cell attracting chemokine (CTACK) as a laboratory marker of the severity of atopic dermatitis in children. Clin Exp Dermatol 2004; 29:293–296.
51. Kakinuma T, Nakamura K, Wakugawa M, et al. Serum macrophage-derived chemokine (MDC) levels are closely related with the disease activity of atopic dermatitis. Clin Exp Immunol 2002; 127:270–273.
52. Kakinuma T, Saeki H, Tsunemi Y, et al. Increased serum cutaneous T cell-attracting chemokine (CCL27) levels in patients with atopic dermatitis and psoriasis vulgaris. J Allergy Clin Immunol 2003; 111:592–597.
53. Echigo T, Hasegawa M, Shimada Y, et al. Expression of fractalkine and its receptor, CX3CR1, in atopic dermatitis: Possible contribution to skin inflammation. J Allergy Clin Immunol 2004; 113:940–948.
54. Ruzicka T, Bieber T, Schopf E, et al. A short-term trial of tacrolimus ointment for atopic dermatitis. European Tacrolimus Multicenter Atopic Dermatitis Study Group. N Engl J Med 1997; 337:816–821.
55. Woodward AL, Spergel JM, Alenius H, et al. An obligate role for T-cell receptor alphabeta + T cells but not T-cell receptor gammadelta + T cells, B cells, or CD40/CD40 L interactions in a mouse model of atopic dermatitis. J Allergy Clin Immunol 2001; 107:359–366.
56. Morales J, Homey B, Vicari AP, et al. CTACK, a skin-associated chemokine that preferentially attracts skin-homing memory T cells. Proc Natl Acad Sci U S A 1999; 96:14470–14475.
57. Homey B, Wang W, Soto H, et al. Cutting edge: The orphan chemokine receptor G protein-coupled receptor-2 (GPR-2, CCR10) binds the skin-associated chemokine CCL27 (CTACK/ALP/ILC). J Immunol 2000; 164:3465–3470.
58. Bruna-Romero O, Schmieg J, Del Val M, et al. The dendritic cell-specific chemokine, dendritic cell-derived CC chemokine 1, enhances protective cell-mediated immunity to murine malaria. J Immunol 2003; 170:3195–3203.
59. Caux C, Ait-Yahia S, Chemin K, et al. Dendritic cell biology and regulation of dendritic cell trafficking by chemokines. Springer Semin Immunopathol 2000; 22:345–369.
60. Koch S, Kohl K, Klein E, et al. Skin homing of Langerhans cell precursors: Adhesion, chemotaxis, and migration. J Allergy Clin Immunol 2006; 117:163–168.
61. Dieu MC, Vanbervliet B, Vicari A, et al. Selective recruitment of immature and mature dendritic cells by distinct chemokines expressed in different anatomic sites. J Exp Med 1998; 188:373–386.
62. Vanbervliet B, Homey B, Durand I, et al. Sequential involvement of CCR2 and CCR6 ligands for immature dendritic cell recruitment: Possible role at inflamed epithelial surfaces. Eur J Immunol 2002; 32:231–242.
63. Ma W, Bryce PJ, Humbles AA, et al. CCR3 is essential for skin eosinophilia and airway hyperresponsiveness in a murine model of allergic skin inflammation. J Clin Invest 2002; 109:621–628.
64. Ying S, O'Connor B, Ratoff J, et al. Thymic stromal lymphopoietin expression is increased in asthmatic airways and correlates with expression of Th2-attracting chemokines and disease severity. J Immunol 2005; 174:8183–8190.
65. Al-Shami A, Spolski R, Kelly J, et al. A role for TSLP in the development of inflammation in an asthma model. J Exp Med 2005; 202:829–839.

66. Diveu C, Lak-Hal AH, Froger J, et al. Predominant expression of the long isoform of GP130-like (GPL) receptor is required for interleukin-31 signaling. Eur Cytokine Netw 2004; 15:291–302.

67. Bilsborough J, Leung DY, Maurer M, et al. IL-31 is associated with cutaneous lymphocyte antigen-positive skin homing T cells in patients with atopic dermatitis. J Allergy Clin Immunol 2006; 117:418–425.

68. Sonkoly E, Muller A, Lauerma AI, et al. IL-31: A new link between T cells and pruritus in atopic skin inflammation. J Allergy Clin Immunol 2006; 117:411–417.

6 Innate Immunity in Atopic Dermatitis

Tissa R. Hata and Richard L. Gallo

Division of Dermatology, University of California, San Diego, California, U.S.A.

The innate immune system evolved more than two billion years ago as a first line, immediate, nonspecific, but efficient mechanism for an organism to fight pathogens. It is found among plants and animals, vertebrate and invertebrates. Although adaptive immunity exists only in vertebrates, and provides immunologic memory, innate immune systems shape the adaptive response. In humans, when a pathogen first encounters the host, the innate immune system is there to recognize and respond by a process that inhibits microbial proliferation as well as triggers events that later control the inflammatory and adaptive response. Unfortunately, this fine orchestration of systems to recognize microbes and resist infection is defective in atopic dermatitis (AD). Several distinct defects in innate and adaptive immunity account for the decreased ability of the atopic patient to fight infections and may result in the abnormal inflammatory infiltrate that characterizes this disorder. This chapter will focus on defects in the innate immune system of AD.

THE DEFECTIVE BARRIER

The first element of the innate immune defense system is the physical barrier presented by the epidermis. Not surprisingly, a significant proportion of patients with AD have an abnormality in this barrier. This may be partially explained by observations of altered or absent production of the structural protein filaggrin. Filaggrin is essential for epidermal barrier formation and hydration (1). To date, 17 loss-of-function nonsense or frameshift mutations in filaggrin have been identified (2–4). These filaggrin mutations have been shown to be a major predisposing factor to the development of AD (5), asthma, and allergic rhinitis (6,7). Furthermore, null mutations in the filaggrin gene seem to be indicative of a more severe, persistent phenotype, as they are associated with an early onset AD phenotype that persists into adulthood (8,9), as well as increased asthma severity (10).

These mutations in filaggrin on a molecular level support the clinical observation of improvement in AD with daily emollient use, use of mild soaps, and reduction in exposure to water. An intact epidermal barrier is an important first-line component of the ability of atopics to fight infections.

Although the defects in filaggrin in the epidermal barrier play an important role in the development of cutaneous infections in AD, the immune barrier of AD patients is compromised at several levels. The combination of epidermal barrier defects and an impaired microbial recognition and response system all contribute to the increased incidence of skin infections in atopics.

PATTERN RECOGNITION RECEPTORS

The first job of the innate immune system is to recognize an invader. Is this organism a pathogen or nonpathogen, self or nonself? Secondly, the innate immune system must execute a coordinated physiologic response to the offenders, which results in the production of cytokines, chemokines, endogenous antimicrobial substances, transcription factors, and activation of immune cells.

The innate immune system recognizes invading pathogens through the imprecisely named pathogen-associated molecular patterns (PAMPs) via pattern recognition receptors (PRRs). PRRs are present both intracellularly, on cell membranes, and in circulating plasma and tissues (11–13). PAMPs are poorly named as these molecules are not unique to pathogens, but are found as part of all organisms and can include molecules released by host as well as nonself invading organisms. Once activated, the molecules that recognize the PAMPs participate in phagocytosis, opsinization, activation of complement and coagulation cascades, activation of proinflammatory signaling pathways, and induction of the antimicrobial response (14–16).

Best known of the PRRs are the toll receptors, which are structurally related to the *Drosophila* toll receptor and the interleukin-1 receptor, and are expressed in human keratinocytes and antigen-presenting cells (17,18). TLRs are transmembrane proteins with a leucine-rich extracellular domain, and a highly conserved intracellular domain (19). To date, 10 TLRs have been identified, with each receptor characterized by the microbial ligand it recognizes (11,20–22)(Fig. 1). The extracellular portion is responsible for specific ligand recognition, and the intracellular portion mediates signal transduction through coupling with different adaptor molecules. At least four different adaptor molecules are known: myeloid differentiation factor 88 (MyD88), TIR-domain containing adaptor, TIR-domain containing adaptor protein inducing IFN-β (TRIF), and the TRIF-related adaptor molecule (TRAM). Most TLRs utilize the adaptor molecule MyD88 which in turn activates the MAPK kinases and the transcription factor NF-κB leading to the expression of several proinflammatory and regulatory cytokines and chemokines, including IL-1β, TNF-α, IL-6, and IL-12 (21).

Examples of PAMPS include lipopolysaccharides (lps) from gram-negative bacteria, lipoteichoic acid (LTA), and peptidoglycan from gram-positive bacteria, and mannans of yeast/fungi. Each TLR has been found to recognize specific PRRs. TLR2 is a heterodimer that associates with TLR1 or TLR6 and CD14 to recognize lipopeptides from bacteria, peptidoglycan, and LTA. TLR3 recognizes double-stranded RNA produced during viral replication, and TLR4/CD14 recognizes lps from gram-negative bacteria. Flagellin is recognized by TLR5, and viral single-stranded RNA by TLR7 and TLR8. TLR9 recognizes unmethylated CpGDNA found primarily in bacteria. TLR11 recognizes uropathogenic *Escherichia coli* (23).

TLR stimulation by microbes results in activation of signaling pathways to not only produce antimicrobials, but to also trigger dendritic cell maturation, induce costimulatory molecules, and increase antigen presentation. This cascade of events helps to initiate and direct the adaptive immune response. The TLRs play an important role as a mediator between innate and adaptive immunity.

Polymorphisms of TLR2 (Arg753Gln), located within the intracellular part of the receptor, have been associated with *Staphylococcus aureus* infection, and present in higher frequency in AD patients compared to controls (24), although there have been conflicting reports (25). These patients also have increased disease severity

a

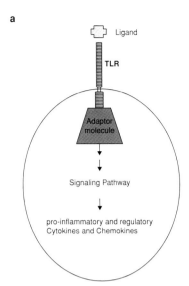

b

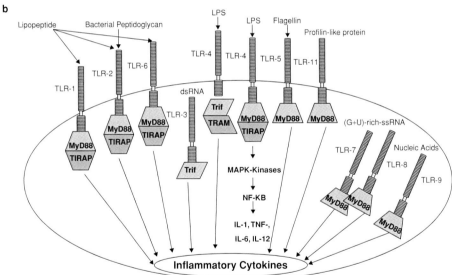

FIGURE 1   TLRs mediate innate immune responses in host defense. (**A**) After binding of a ligand, TLR couples with adaptor molecule(s) and initiate signaling pathways that lead to the production of inflammatory cytokines and chemokines. In addition, costimulatory molecules are induced that instruct the type of adaptive immune response. (**B**) A number of TLRs are expressed on the cell surface and recognize extracellular bacterial components; TLR4 binds LPS, TLR2 binds bacterial peptidoglycan, and TLR5 recognizes flagellin. Intracellular TLRs bind viral and bacterial components including nucleic acids (TLR9), ds RNA (TLR3) or (G + U)-rich-ss RNA (TLR7 and 8). At least four different adaptor molecules are known to associate with TLRs: MyD88, TIR-domain-containing adaptor (TIRAP), TRIF, and TRIF-related adaptor molecule (TRAM).

with high IgE antibodies to *S. aureus* superantigens and a more severe clinical phenotype. Further analysis of these subjects revealed that monocytes from AD subjects with the TLR-2 R753Q mutation produced significantly more IL-6 and IL-12 compared to wild-type AD subjects upon stimulation with TLR-2 agonists. The authors speculate that these proinflammatory cytokines may explain the enhanced skin inflammation in patients with the TLR-2 R753Q SNP because of "chronification" by IL-12 (26).

Intracellular PAMPs such as peptidoglycan are recognized by nucleotide-binding oligomerization domains (NOD) NOD 1 and NOD 2 (27). NOD1 senses diaminopimelic acid–type PGN produced by gram-negative bacteria, and NOD2 senses muramyl dipeptide found in PGNs from all bacteria including *S. aureus* (27). Polymorphisms in the NOD1/caspase recruitment domain containing protein (CARD) 4 have been associated with AD. Interestingly, these polymorphisms were also associated with asthma and total serum IgE levels, but not with allergic rhinoconjunctivitis (28).

CD14 is a multifunctional receptor for LPS and other bacterial wall components (28). CD14 binds LPS and LPS-binding protein and is required for LPS-induced macrophage activation via TLR4. It has also been found to induce cellular activation in response to LTA through a TLR2-dependent pathway (29) and has binding activity for peptidoglycans (30). Reduced levels of CD14 have been observed in atopic children (31). In breast-fed children, low levels of soluble CD14 in breast milk had been associated with an increased risk for AD and asthma (32,33).

These defects in the PRRs, which are one of the first lines of defense in the innate immune system reduce the ability of AD patients to recognize cutaneous microbial pathogens resulting in an increase in their incidence of bacterial and viral infections.

ANTIMICROBIAL PEPTIDES

In the 1980s, Steiner et al. identified a 37-amino-acid cationic peptide from hemolymph of the cecropia moth after injection of bacteria (34). The peptide was devoid of disulfide bonds, had a linear α-helical structure, and exhibited antimicrobial activity against gram-negative bacteria. This family was classified under the cecropin family of AMPs. Since this time, other AMPs have been identified with variable activity against bacteria, fungi, and viruses. We now understand that the AMPs represent an essential system that the skin uses to respond and prevent the uncontrolled growth of microbes and trigger and coordinate multiple components of the innate and adaptive immune system (35). Many different cell types that reside in the skin produce AMPs, including keratinocytes, sebocytes, eccrine glands, and mast cells, thus giving the host ample ammunition against invading organisms (36–39). Circulating cells such as neutrophils and natural killer cells are also able to contribute to the total amount of AMPs present (40). Although cathelicidin and β-defensins are the most well characterized, there are actually more than 20 individual proteins that have shown antimicrobial activity(Table 1) (41). Unfortunately for the patient with AD, multiple AMPs, including defensins, cathelicidins, and dermcidin, have all been shown to have diminished expression and function compared to that expected when normal skin is injured. Better understanding of these molecules sheds further light on the mechanisms responsible for infections in AD.

TABLE 1 Mammalian Peptides with Antimicrobial Activity in Skin (AMPs)

AMP	Reference
AMPs identified in resident cells	
Cathelicidins	70
	76
β-Defensins	51
	134
Bactericidal/permeability-increasing protein (BPI)	135
Lactoferrin	136
Lysozyme	76
Dermcidin	27
	39
Histones	137
S100A15	138
RNase 7	139
Cathelicidins	140
	76
α-Defensins	141
Lactoferrin	142
Granulysin	143
Perforin	143
Eosinophil cationic protein (ECP)/RNase 3	144
Eosinophil-derived neurotoxin (EDN)/RNase 2	145
RANTES	146
AMPs identified as proteinase inhibitors	
hCAP18/LL-37 prosequence (cathelin-like domain)	147
Secretory leukocyte proteinase inhibitor (SLPI)/antileukoprotease	148
Elafin/skin-derived antileukoprotease (SKALP)	149
	150
P-cystatin A	135
Cystatin C	151
AMPs identified as chemokines	
Psoriasin	152
Monokine induced by IFN-γ (MIG/CXCL9)	153
IFN-γ–inducible protein of 10 kD (IP-10/CXCL10)	153
IFN-γ–inducible T cell α-chemoattractant (ITAC/CXCL11)	153
AMPs identified as neuropeptides	
α-Melanocyte–stimulating hormone	154
Substance P	155
Bradykinin	155
Neurotensin	155
Vasostatin-1 and chromofungin (chromogranin A)	156
Secretolytin (chromogranin B)	156
Enkelytin and peptide B (proenkephalin A)	156
Ubiquitin	157
Neuropeptide Y	158
Polypeptide YY/skin-polypeptide Y	158
Catestatin	159
Adrenomedullin	160

Defensins

Originally identified in human and rabbit neutrophils (42), defensins are cationic peptides containing cysteine-rich conserved motifs. There are three subfamilies of defensins, which include alpha, beta, and circular theta defensins. Alpha and beta defensins are distinguished by the position of three disulfide bridges. Alpha defensins have been identified in neutrophils and in the Paneth cells of the small intestine (43). Human beta defensins 1–4 are expressed in keratinocytes. The theta defensin pseudogene has been found in human bone marrow, but the peptide has not been identified in humans (44). Of the four best-known human beta defensins, only HBD-1 is constitutively expressed in the human epidermis and sweat gland ducts (45–47). HBD 2–3 are inducible by bacterial infection, cytokines IL-1α, IL-1β, TNF-α, and differentiation (48,49). HBD2–4 can be induced by calcium and phorbol 12 myristate 13 acetate (PMA) and can be inhibited by retinoic acid pretreatment (50). HBD-2 is highly sensitive to the physiologic environment, and shows preferential antimicrobial activity toward gram-negative bacteria such as *E. coli* and *Pseudomonas* (51). Because of HBD-2's high sensitivity, high salt concentrations such as that found in sweat can substantially reduce the antimicrobial capacity of HBD-2.

Alpha and beta defensins show a broad antibacterial activity against gram-positive and gram-negative bacteria (42,52), fungi (53,54), and viruses, including adenovirus (55), papilloma virus (56), human immunodeficiency virus (HIV) (57,58), and the human herpes simplex virus (HSV) (59). Binding of the positively charged defensin with the negatively charged bacterial membrane precedes membrane permeabilization and is thought to be the mechanism of bacterial killing by the defensins.

Defensins also induce cytokines. Alpha defensins upregulate the expression of TNF-α and IL-1β in monocytes activated with *S. aureus* (60). Defensins induce IL-8 and proinflammatory cytokines in lung epithelial cells (61,62) and IL-18 in primary keratinocytes (63).

Cathelicidins

Cathelicidins were originally named for a diverse group of peptides based upon their evolutionarily conserved cathelin-like-N-terminal domain and their structurally variable cationic antimicrobial C terminal domain (64). The cathelin-like domain is similar to the 12-kD protein, cathelin, which was originally isolated as a cathepsin L inhibitor (65). Most cathelicidins are amphipathic cationic peptides, which are α-helical in some buffer conditions (66). The amphipathic structure and cationic charge allow the cathelicidin peptides to interact in the aqueous environment, the lipid-rich membrane, and bind to the negatively charged bacterial membranes.

There are two major steps to cathelicidin expression and function: transcription to mRNA and posttranslational processing to active peptides. In the human genome, cathelicidin exons 1–4 are on chromosome 3p21. They are transcribed as a single gene called cathelicidin antimicrobial peptide (CAMP), which translated to the proprotein termed human cationic antimicrobial protein 18 kDa or hCAP 18, which is inactive as an antimicrobial peptide.

In the skin, hCAP 18 is stored in the lamellar bodies in keratinocytes and secreted in the granular and spinous layer of the epidermis (67) . After secretion SCTE (stratum corneum tryptic enzyme, kallikrein 5/hK5) first process hCAP 18 to LL-37, and a combination of SCTE and SCCE (stratum corneum chymotryptic enzyme, kallikrein 7/hK7) further process the smaller peptides to RK-31 and

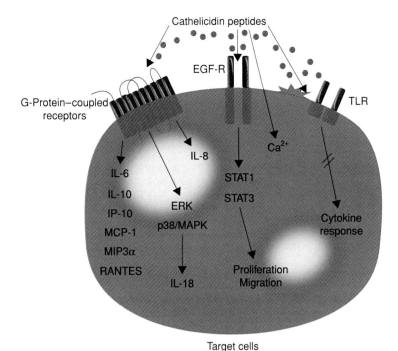

Target cells

FIGURE 2 Models for cell activation by cathelicidins. Multiple mechanisms have been proposed for cathelicidins to stimulate a cellular response. Responses are dependent on activation of G protein–coupled receptors and transactivation of the epidermal growth factor receptor or secondary to intracellular Ca^{2+} mobilization or a change in cell membrane function, leading to alterations in receptor responses. Finally, cathelicidins can influence the function of TLRs through both direct and indirect pathways. *Abbreviations*: EGF-R, epidermal growth factor receptor; IP-10, IFN-γ–inducible protein 10; MCP-1, monocyte chemoattractant protein 1; MIP3α, macrophage inflammatory protein 3α; ERK, extracellular signal-regulated kinase; MAPK, mitogen-activated protein kinase; STAT, signal transducer and activator of transcription.

KS-30 (68,69). In human keratinocytes, cathelicidin is inducible with wounding, infection, and skin inflammation from basal expression levels that are low and barely detectible (70).

LL-37 consists of 37 amino acids starting with two leucines and is expressed in various cells, tissues, and body fluids, including epidermal keratinocytes and intestinal cells (71), T cells (40), mast cells (36), neutrophils (72), wound fluids (73), bronchoalveolar lavage fluids (74), sweat (39), saliva (75), and vernix caseaosa of newborns (76). Cathelicidins are cationic, and thought to directly bind to the anionic cell wall and membrane of the microbe, increasing permeability of the microbe's cell wall (77,78). Through this method of killing they have a broad antimicrobial activity against gram-positive and gram-negative bacteria (79–81), vaccinia virus (82), and fungi (83,84).

Cathelicidins also act as alarmins, through a multitude of mechanisms. Alarmin functions include direct interactions of LL-37 with cell-surface receptors, such as the formyl-peptide receptor-like-1 or G-protein-coupled receptors, resulting in direct effects on intracellular signaling pathways(Fig. 2) (41,85–87). Cathelicidins

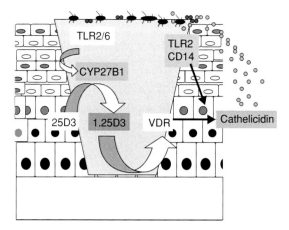

FIGURE 3 Injury or infection enhances TLR2 function and cathelicidin antimicrobial peptide expression through a vitamin D3 dependent mechanism.

also induce proinflammatory cytokine secretion. They stimulate IL-8 secretion from human epidermal keratinocytes via direct or indirect activation of the epidermal growth factor receptor (88,89). Both beta defensins and LL-37 induce production of IL-6, IL-10, and the chemokines (interferon inducible protein 10, monocyte chemoattractant protein 1, macrophage inflammatory protein 3α, RANTES), in keratinocytes, allowing them to work in both innate and adaptive immunity (86).

As mentioned earlier, cathelicidin expression is high in bacterial skin infection or cutaneous barrier disruption, however, the regulation of cathelicidin transcription remained a mystery, because classic mediators of inflammation or infection did not influence expression (71). Identification of the vitamin D responsive element in the cathelicidin promoter and identification of cathelicidin as the direct target of vitamin D3 in keratinocytes were significant breakthroughs in the understanding of cathelicidin expression in the skin (90–92). Additional elements of vitamin D3 signaling cascade have been identified that lead to increased cathelicidin expression, such as recruitment of coactivators or epigenetic changes (93). However, even with these findings it still remained a question as to how cathelicidin would be induced in bacterial infections or in wounds, because situations in which a sudden change in vitamin D3 levels would be unlikely. The answer came with the realization that CYP27B1 (which is present in skin) and TLR2 are under similar control by inflammatory stimuli (94). CYP27B1 executes a hydroxylation step in the skin and activates vitamin D3 to its most active form, 1,25-dihydroxy vitamin D3. With skin injury or bacterial infection, there is a local increase in expression of CYP27B1 and as a direct consequence more vitamin D3 is activated to induce cathelicidin expression (94,95)(Fig. 3). Interestingly, in mice that are typically nocturnal and would not be exposed to sunlight to generate vitamin D precursors, the cathelicidin gene for mCRAMP (Cnlp) derived from phagocytes is regulated in part by hypoxia inducible factor 1 alpha (HIF-alpha) (96,97), and not directly by vitamin D.

Dermcidin

The dermcidin gene and mature peptide have been identified only in humans to date. They are constitutively secreted in human sweat and are not inducible by skin injury or inflammation (98). Dermcidin is secreted as a proprotein, and post-secretory processing by cathepsin D cleaves the peptide from the C terminus of the proprotein thus allowing for the dermcidin peptides to be distributed to the skin surface in sweat (99). Dermcidin is an anionic peptide whose specific method of killing of microbes is still unknown, however, they have been shown to have potent antimicrobial activity against *S. aureus*, *E. coli*, and *Candida* (100).

STAPHYLOCOCCUS AND THE ATOPIC INNATE IMMUNE SYSTEM

Healthy skin of normal individuals has shown colonization of a large number of microorganisms which include *Staphylococcus epidermidis*, *Staphylococcus hemolyticus*, and *Staphylococcus hominus* (101). Colonization by *S. aureus* occurs in approximately 5% of the healthy population (102). In contrast, more than 90% of atopics have *S. aureus* colonization on their lesional and to a lesser extent on their nonlesional skin (103). The impaired skin barrier function may partially explain *S. aureus* colonization in AD; however, psoriatics, which also have a disrupted skin barrier are in comparison much more resistant to skin infections (104). Differences in resistance to cutaneous infections may be partially explained by the disrupted barrier, and differences in the cytokine milieu resulting in differential antimicrobial expression between psoriatics and atopics.

Ong et al. were the first to identify a deficiency in LL-37 and HBD-2 in atopic lesional skin compared to those of psoriatic lesional skin (105). Because AMPs can be induced in wounding and inflammation, it was initially expected that both the psoriatic and atopic lesional skin would have an elevation in AMPs. Quantitative real-time reverse transcriptase polymerase chain reaction (PCR) assays examining the relative expression of HBD-2 and LL-37 mRNA found significantly decreased levels of both AMPs in acute and chronic lesions of AD. Subsequently, Nomura et al. found reduced expression of HBD-3 by real-time PCR and immunohistochemistry (106). Because LL-37, HBD-2, and HBD-3 all have anti-staphylococcal activity, this observed decrease in induction of AMPs is thought to be an important factor in staphylococcal colonization and infections of atopic subjects.

The cytokine milieu in atopics plays a significant role in the reduction of AMPs. AD exhibits a Th2-directed cytokine pattern with high IgE levels and eosinophilia. The Th2 cytokine pattern is characterized by overexpression of IL-4, IL-10, and IL-13 (107–109). High levels of IL-4 and IL-13 inhibit HBD-2 and HBD-3 (110,111). IL-4 and IL-13 act directly on keratinocytes to downregulate the expression of LL-37 through activation of STAT-6 which inhibits the TNF-α/NF-κB system (112,113). Downregulation of HBD-3 has recently shown to be influenced by a S-100 calcium-binding protein A11 (S100/A11) (114). S100/A11 is significantly downregulated in the presence of IL-4 and Il-13, and shows decreased expression in atopic subjects (114). Thus the reduction in AMP expression in atopic lesional skin is thought to be secondary to the inhibitory effects of IL-4 and IL-13 on TNF-α/NF-κB system and the indirect effect of the immunomodulatory cytokine IL-10 on proinflammatory cytokine production of TNF-α and IFN-γ (107,113).

High levels of IL-4 and IL-13 also inhibit IL-8 and iNOS gene expression (115,116). IL-8 is a chemokine that attracts PMNs into the skin where they phagocytose and kill bacteria, and iNos can kill viruses, bacteria, and fungi through production of nitric oxide; thus both are important mediators of innate immunity.

IFN-γ is considered a key cytokine of innate and adaptive immunity. Its role in host defense against microbial pathogens is through activation of monocytes, macrophages, NK cells, enhancing antigen processing, and presentation and modulation of the humoral response. Thus a deficiency may result in an hampered pathogen elimination and increased propensity to skin infections in AD (117). Clinically, increased *S. aureus* skin colonization in AD directly correlates with an increase in the AD clinical severity as measured by the Scoring Atopic Dermatitis (SCORAD) index, and is inversely correlated with a decreased IFN-γ production by peripheral blood CD4 and CD8+ T cells (118).

The antimicrobial peptide dermcidin has also been shown to be decreased in atopics (119). It is constitutively expressed in eccrine sweat glands and secreted into sweat. Several dermcidin-derived peptides are significantly reduced in AD compared to healthy subjects, and atopics with previous bacterial or viral infections show the lowest concentration (119).

Adherence of *S. aureus* to the skin surface are also increased in AD compared to healthy subjects (120,121). The adhesions of *S. aureus* take place primarily in the stratum corneum, and are mediated by fibronectin and fibrinogen. The fibronectin-binding protein of *Staphylococcus* is a bifunctional protein that binds to fibrinogen (122). IL-4 appears to play a role in the staphylococcal binding to the skin. IL-4 induces the synthesis of fibronectin by skin fibroblasts (116). Fibronectin in combination with plasma exudation of fibrinogen allows *Staphylococcus* to bind to the skin (120,121). In the murine model, binding of *Staphylococcus* did not occur in IL-4 gene knockout mice (116). These staphylococcal mutants that were deficient in fibronectin or fibrinogen-binding proteins decreased binding to the AD skin, but not psoriatic or healthy skin (120). Scratching by AD also enhances the binding of *Staphylococcus* to the skin by disrupting the skin barrier, and by exposing epidermal and dermal laminin and fibronectin allowing *Staphylococcus* to bind.

ATOPICS AND VIRAL INFECTIONS

The importance of viral infections in atopics has been highlighted recently because of concerns of bioterrorism. The last case of smallpox in the United States was in 1949, and the last naturally occurring case in the world was in Somalia in 1977. Routine vaccination of the American public against smallpox stopped in 1972 after the disease was eradicated in the United States (123). In 1980, the World Health Organization (WHO) announced that smallpox had been eradicated from the world, thus eliminating the need for smallpox vaccinations worldwide. It is currently estimated that approximately 119 million residents have been born in the United States since the smallpox vaccination has been discontinued (124). With the resurgence of bioterrorism, the issue of vaccination has resurfaced. Currently, any individual with a history of or current active AD as well as those who have close household contacts to an atopic individual are currently excluded from the smallpox vaccination, because of the risk of eczema vaccinatum, which is a serious, life-threatening infection (125). This complication was recently highlighted in the case of transmission from an active military recruit that had received the vaccine three weeks earlier, and transmitted eczema vaccinatum to his two-year-old son and wife (126). Conventional treatment with immune globulin and the antiviral drug cidofovir failed. Only through treatment with an investigative drug through SIGA Technologies, called ST-246, did the child survive, highlighting the seriousness of infection with eczema vaccinatum.

Eczema herpeticum is a disseminated herpes simplex virus infection with either HSV 1 or 2, most commonly in atopic individuals (127). Most infections in ADEH start with a simple labial infection, which then spreads to involve the facial area, and in severe cases spreads over the entire body (127). Risk factors for ADEH within the atopic population are, higher total serum IgE levels, early age of onset of AD, location of eczema on the head and neck area, and higher sensitization against aeroallergens, especially the yeast *Malassezia sympodialis* (128).

As mentioned earlier, cathelicidin exhibits antiviral activity against HSV and vaccinia virus, and cathelicidin expression is inversely correlated with serum IgE levels in eczema herpeticum patients (129). Skin from atopic patients with eczema herpeticum shows reduced expression of cathelicidin, and cathelicidin deficient mice show higher levels of HSV-2 replication (129). Human and mouse cathelicidin reduce vaccinia virus plaque formation in vitro, and CRAMP knockout mice show more vaccinia pox formation than in control mice (82,129). Vaccinia virus also replicates faster in AD skin explants than in normal or psoriatic skin explants (112) and these explants show a reduced ability to express cathelicidin following stimulation with the vaccinia virus. The mechanism of this inhibition is thought to be through IL-4 and IL-13 inhibiting vaccinia virus mediated induction of cathelicidin through STAT-6 (112).

Plasmacytoid dendritic cells are also thought to play a key role in the antiviral immune response because of their ability to produce high amounts of antiviral type 1 IFN-α and IFN-β upon viral infection. Although the peripheral blood PDC is increased in AD (130), they have been shown to be depleted in AD skin compared to other inflammatory skin diseases such as psoriasis, contact dermatitis, or lupus (131). The reason for this depletion is by dose-dependent plasmacytoid dendritic cell apoptosis induction caused by IL-4, and potentiated by IL-10 (132). Interestingly, it has been recently postulated that these plasmacytoid dendritic cells may be responsible for the autoimmunity in psoriasis through mediation by cathelicidin. In contrast to AD, psoriatics possess a very high level of cathelicidin in lesional skin. Cathelicidin binds to self-DNA, then promotes translocation of this DNA into the endocytic pathway of plasmacytoid dendritic cells to produce TLR-9 mediated type 1 interferon (133). Thus in the case of psoriasis, cathelicidin is interfering in the toll receptors ability to distinguish self from nonself, and is allowing self-DNA to elicit a rapid and robust induction of IFN which begins the cascade of innate and adaptive immunity.

CONCLUSION

Many defects in the innate immune system resulting in a disequilibrium between innate and acquired immunity account for the increase in skin infections in atopics. The defects begin in the physical epidermal barrier, and continue to defects in PRRs, currently identified as the toll receptors and the intracellular PAMP NOD. Low levels of the antimicrobial peptides cathelicidin, HBD-2, and HBD-3 have been observed in the lesional skin of atopics, and the peptide dermcidin is decreased in sweat. And finally, plasmacytoid dendritic cells are depleted in AD skin compared to other inflammatory diseases such as psoriasis, contact dermatitis or lupus. Defects in the innate immune system beginning with the barrier, followed by defects in the identification of pathogens and the agents employed to disarm them, account for the increase in infections in atopics. In the future, identification of these defects may allow therapeutic intervention to correct these deficiencies and reduce the incidence of infection in atopic individuals.

REFERENCES

1. Irvine AD, McLean WH. Breaking the (un)sound barrier: Filaggrin is a major gene for atopic dermatitis. J Invest Dermatol 2006; 126:1200–1202.
2. Nomura T, Sandilands A, Akiyama M, et al. Unique mutations in the filaggrin gene in Japanese patients with ichthyosis vulgaris and atopic dermatitis. J Allergy Clin Immunol 2007; 119:434–440.
3. Nomura T, Akiyama M, Sandilands A, et al. Specific filaggrin mutations cause ichthyosis vulgaris and are significantly associated with atopic dermatitis in Japan. J Invest Dermatol 2008; 128:1436–1441.
4. Sandilands A, Terron-Kwiatkowski A, Hull PR, et al. Comprehensive analysis of the gene encoding filaggrin uncovers prevalent and rare mutations in ichthyosis vulgaris and atopic eczema. Nat Genet 2007; 39:650–654.
5. Irvine AD. Fleshing out filaggrin phenotypes. J Invest Dermatol 2007; 127:504–507.
6. Marenholz I, Nickel R, Ruschendorf F, et al. Filaggrin loss-of-function mutations predispose to phenotypes involved in the atopic march. J Allergy Clin Immunol 2006; 118:866–871.
7. Weidinger S, Illig T, Baurecht H, et al. Loss-of-function variations within the filaggrin gene predispose for atopic dermatitis with allergic sensitizations. J Allergy Clin Immunol 2006; 118:214–219.
8. Barker JN, Palmer CN, Zhao Y, et al. Null mutations in the filaggrin gene (FLG) determine major susceptibility to early-onset atopic dermatitis that persists into adulthood. J Invest Dermatol 2007; 127:564–567.
9. Weidinger S, Rodriguez E, Stahl C, et al. Filaggrin mutations strongly predispose to early-onset and extrinsic atopic dermatitis. J Invest Dermatol 2007; 127:724–726.
10. Palmer CN, Ismail T, Lee SP, et al. Filaggrin null mutations are associated with increased asthma severity in children and young adults. J Allergy Clin Immunol 2007; 120:64–68.
11. Kang SS, Kauls LS, Gaspari AA. Toll-like receptors: Applications to dermatologic disease. J Am Acad Dermatol 2006; 54:951–983 [quiz 83–86].
12. Janeway CA Jr, Medzhitov R. Innate immune recognition. Annu Rev Immunol 2002; 20:197–216.
13. Medzhitov R, Janeway CA Jr. Innate immunity: Impact on the adaptive immune response. Curr Opin Immunol 1997; 9:4–9.
14. Kuhlman M, Joiner K, Ezekowitz RA. The human mannose-binding protein functions as an opsonin. J Exp Med 1989; 169:1733–1745.
15. Matsushita M, Fujita T. Activation of the classical complement pathway by mannose-binding protein in association with a novel C1 s-like serine protease. J Exp Med 1992; 176:1497–1502.
16. Schweinle JE, Ezekowitz RA, Tenner AJ, et al. Human mannose-binding protein activates the alternative complement pathway and enhances serum bactericidal activity on a mannose-rich isolate of *Salmonella*. J Clin Invest 1989; 84:1821–1829.
17. Mempel M, Voelcker V, Kollisch G, et al. Toll-like receptor expression in human keratinocytes: Nuclear factor kappaB controlled gene activation by *Staphylococcus aureus* is toll-like receptor 2 but not toll-like receptor 4 or platelet activating factor receptor dependent. J Invest Dermatol 2003; 121:1389–1396.
18. Kollisch G, Kalali BN, Voelcker V, et al. Various members of the Toll-like receptor family contribute to the innate immune response of human epidermal keratinocytes. Immunology 2005; 114:531–541.
19. Gay NJ, Keith FJ. Drosophila Toll and IL-1 receptor. Nature 1991; 351:355–356.
20. Leulier F, Lemaitre B. Toll-like receptors—Taking an evolutionary approach. Nat Rev Genet 2008; 9:165–178.

21. Hawlisch H, Kohl J. Complement and Toll-like receptors: Key regulators of adaptive immune responses. Mol Immunol 2006; 43:13–21.
22. Goodarzi H, Trowbridge J, Gallo RL. Innate immunity: A cutaneous perspective. Clin Rev Allergy Immunol 2007; 33:15–26.
23. Beutler B. Toll-like receptors and their place in immunology. Where does the immune response to infection begin? Nat Rev Immunol 2004; 4:498.
24. Ahmad-Nejad P, Mrabet-Dahbi S, Breuer K, et al. The toll-like receptor 2 R753Q polymorphism defines a subgroup of patients with atopic dermatitis having severe phenotype. J Allergy Clin Immunol 2004; 113:565–567.
25. Weidinger S, Novak N, Klopp N, et al. Lack of association between Toll-like receptor 2 and Toll-like receptor 4 polymorphisms and atopic eczema. J Allergy Clin Immunol 2006; 118:277–279.
26. Niebuhr M, Langnickel J, Draing C, et al. Dysregulation of toll-like receptor-2 (TLR-2)-induced effects in monocytes from patients with atopic dermatitis: Impact of the TLR-2 R753Q polymorphism. Allergy 2008; 63:728–734.
27. Schittek B, Hipfel R, Sauer B, et al. Dermcidin: A novel human antibiotic peptide secreted by sweat glands. Nat Immunol 2001; 2:1133–1137.
28. Weidinger S, Klopp N, Rummler L, et al. Association of NOD1 polymorphisms with atopic eczema and related phenotypes. J Allergy Clin Immunol 2005; 116:177–184.
29. Schroder NW, Morath S, Alexander C, et al. Lipoteichoic acid (LTA) of *Streptococcus pneumoniae* and *Staphylococcus aureus* activates immune cells via Toll-like receptor (TLR)-2, lipopolysaccharide-binding protein (LBP), and CD14, whereas TLR-4 and MD-2 are not involved. J Biol Chem 2003; 278:15587–15594.
30. Dziarski R. Recognition of bacterial peptidoglycan by the innate immune system. Cell Mol Life Sci 2003; 60:1793–1804.
31. Zdolsek HA, Jenmalm MC. Reduced levels of soluble CD14 in atopic children. Clin Exp Allergy 2004; 34:532–539.
32. Rothenbacher D, Weyermann M, Beermann C, et al. Breastfeeding, soluble CD14 concentration in breast milk and risk of atopic dermatitis and asthma in early childhood: Birth cohort study. Clin Exp Allergy 2005; 35:1014–1021.
33. Jones CA, Holloway JA, Popplewell EJ, et al. Reduced soluble CD14 levels in amniotic fluid and breast milk are associated with the subsequent development of atopy, eczema, or both. J Allergy Clin Immunol 2002; 109:858–866.
34. Steiner H, Hultmark D, Engstrom A, et al. Sequence and specificity of two antibacterial proteins involved in insect immunity. Nature 1981; 292:246–248.
35. Braff MH, Bardan A, Nizet V, et al. Cutaneous defense mechanisms by antimicrobial peptides. J Invest Dermatol 2005; 125:9–13.
36. Di Nardo A, Vitiello A, Gallo RL. Cutting edge: Mast cell antimicrobial activity is mediated by expression of cathelicidin antimicrobial peptide. J Immunol 2003; 170:2274–2278.
37. Braff MH, Zaiou M, Fierer J, et al. Keratinocyte production of cathelicidin provides direct activity against bacterial skin pathogens. Infect Immun 2005; 73:6771–6781.
38. Lee DY, Yamasaki K, Rudsil J, et al. Sebocytes express functional cathelicidin antimicrobial peptides and can act to kill propionibacterium acnes. J Invest Dermatol 2008; 128:1863–1866.
39. Murakami M, Ohtake T, Dorschner RA, et al. Cathelicidin anti-microbial peptide expression in sweat, an innate defense system for the skin. J Invest Dermatol 2002; 119:1090–1095.
40. Agerberth B, Charo J, Werr J, et al. The human antimicrobial and chemotactic peptides LL-37 and alpha-defensins are expressed by specific lymphocyte and monocyte populations. Blood 2000; 96:3086–3093.
41. Schauber J, Gallo RL. Antimicrobial peptides and the skin immune defense system. J Allergy Clin Immunol 2008; 122(2):261–266.
42. Ganz T, Selsted ME, Szklarek D, et al. Defensins. Natural peptide antibiotics of human neutrophils. J Clin Invest 1985; 76:1427–1435.

43. Mallow EB, Harris A, Salzman N, et al. Human enteric defensins. Gene structure and developmental expression. J Biol Chem 1996; 271:4038–4045.
44. Cole AM, Hong T, Boo LM, et al. Retrocyclin: A primate peptide that protects cells from infection by T- and M-tropic strains of HIV-1. Proc Natl Acad Sci U S A 2002; 99:1813–1818.
45. Fulton C, Anderson GM, Zasloff M, et al. Expression of natural peptide antibiotics in human skin. Lancet 1997; 350:1750–1751.
46. Ali RS, Falconer A, Ikram M, et al. Expression of the peptide antibiotics human beta defensin-1 and human beta defensin-2 in normal human skin. J Invest Dermatol 2001; 117:106–111.
47. Zhao C, Wang I, Lehrer RI. Widespread expression of beta-defensin hBD-1 in human secretory glands and epithelial cells. FEBS Lett 1996; 396:319–322.
48. Liu AY, Destoumieux D, Wong AV, et al. Human beta-defensin-2 production in keratinocytes is regulated by interleukin-1, bacteria, and the state of differentiation. J Invest Dermatol 2002; 118:275–281.
49. Harder J, Bartels J, Christophers E, et al. Isolation and characterization of human beta-defensin-3, a novel human inducible peptide antibiotic. J Biol Chem 2001; 276:5707–5713.
50. Harder J, Meyer-Hoffert U, Wehkamp K, et al. Differential gene induction of human beta-defensins (hBD-1, -2, -3, and -4) in keratinocytes is inhibited by retinoic acid. J Invest Dermatol 2004; 123:522–529.
51. Harder J, Bartels J, Christophers E, et al. A peptide antibiotic from human skin. Nature 1997; 387:861.
52. Ericksen B, Wu Z, Lu W, et al. Antibacterial activity and specificity of the six human {alpha}-defensins. Antimicrob Agents Chemother 2005; 49:269–275.
53. Wilde CG, Griffith JE, Marra MN, et al. Purification and characterization of human neutrophil peptide 4, a novel member of the defensin family. J Biol Chem 1989; 264:11200–11203.
54. Hoover DM, Wu Z, Tucker K, et al. Antimicrobial characterization of human beta-defensin 3 derivatives. Antimicrob Agents Chemother 2003; 47:2804–2809.
55. Bastian A, Schafer H. Human alpha-defensin 1 (HNP-1) inhibits adenoviral infection in vitro. Regul Pept 2001; 101:157–161.
56. Buck CB, Day PM, Thompson CD, et al. Human alpha-defensins block papillomavirus infection. Proc Natl Acad Sci U S A 2006; 103:1516–1521.
57. Sun L, Finnegan CM, Kish-Catalone T, et al. Human beta-defensins suppress human immunodeficiency virus infection: Potential role in mucosal protection. J Virol 2005; 79:14318–14329.
58. Chang TL, Vargas J Jr, DelPortillo A, et al. Dual role of alpha-defensin-1 in anti-HIV-1 innate immunity. J Clin Invest 2005; 115:765–773.
59. Hazrati E, Galen B, Lu W, et al. Human alpha- and beta-defensins block multiple steps in herpes simplex virus infection. J Immunol 2006; 177:8658–8666.
60. Chaly YV, Paleolog EM, Kolesnikova TS, et al. Neutrophil alpha-defensin human neutrophil peptide modulates cytokine production in human monocytes and adhesion molecule expression in endothelial cells. Eur Cytokine Netw 2000; 11:257–266.
61. van Wetering S, Mannesse-Lazeroms SP, van Sterkenburg MA, et al. Neutrophil defensins stimulate the release of cytokines by airway epithelial cells: Modulation by dexamethasone. Inflamm Res 2002; 51:8–15.
62. Van Wetering S, Mannesse-Lazeroms SP, Van Sterkenburg MA, et al. Effect of defensins on interleukin-8 synthesis in airway epithelial cells. Am J Physiol 1997; 272:L888–L896.
63. Niyonsaba F, Ushio H, Nagaoka I, et al. The human beta-defensins (-1, -2, -3, -4) and cathelicidin LL-37 induce IL-18 secretion through p38 and ERK MAPK activation in primary human keratinocytes. J Immunol 2005; 175:1776–1784.
64. Zanetti M, Gennaro R, Romeo D. Cathelicidins: A novel protein family with a common proregion and a variable C-terminal antimicrobial domain. FEBS Lett 1995; 374:1–5.
65. Ritonja A, Kopitar M, Jerala R, et al. Primary structure of a new cysteine proteinase inhibitor from pig leucocytes. FEBS Lett 1989; 255:211–214.

66. Zelezetsky I, Pontillo A, Puzzi L, et al. Evolution of the primate cathelicidin. Correlation between structural variations and antimicrobial activity. J Biol Chem 2006; 281:19861–19871.
67. Braff MH, Di Nardo A, Gallo RL. Keratinocytes store the antimicrobial peptide cathelicidin in lamellar bodies. J Invest Dermatol 2005; 124:394–400.
68. Yamasaki K, Schauber J, Coda A, et al. Kallikrein-mediated proteolysis regulates the antimicrobial effects of cathelicidins in skin. FASEB J 2006; 20:2068–2080.
69. Murakami M, Lopez-Garcia B, Braff M, et al. Postsecretory processing generates multiple cathelicidins for enhanced topical antimicrobial defense. J Immunol 2004; 172:3070–3077.
70. Frohm M, Agerberth B, Ahangari G, et al. The expression of the gene coding for the antibacterial peptide LL-37 is induced in human keratinocytes during inflammatory disorders. J Biol Chem 1997; 272:15258–15263.
71. Schauber J, Dorschner RA, Yamasaki K, et al. Control of the innate epithelial antimicrobial response is cell-type specific and dependent on relevant microenvironmental stimuli. Immunology 2006; 118:509–519.
72. Borregaard N, Cowland JB. Granules of the human neutrophilic polymorphonuclear leukocyte. Blood 1997; 89:3503–3521.
73. Frohm M, Gunne H, Bergman AC, et al. Biochemical and antibacterial analysis of human wound and blister fluid. Eur J Biochem 1996; 237:86–92.
74. Agerberth B, Grunewald J, Castanos-Velez E, et al. Antibacterial components in bronchoalveolar lavage fluid from healthy individuals and sarcoidosis patients. Am J Respir Crit Care Med 1999; 160:283–290.
75. Murakami M, Ohtake T, Dorschner RA, et al. Cathelicidin antimicrobial peptides are expressed in salivary glands and saliva. J Dent Res 2002; 81:845–850.
76. Marchini G, Lindow S, Brismar H, et al. The newborn infant is protected by an innate antimicrobial barrier: Peptide antibiotics are present in the skin and vernix caseosa. Br J Dermatol 2002; 147:1127–1134.
77. Henzler Wildman KA, Lee DK, Ramamoorthy A. Mechanism of lipid bilayer disruption by the human antimicrobial peptide, LL-37. Biochemistry 2003; 42:6545–6558.
78. Gutsmann T, Hagge SO, Larrick JW, et al. Interaction of CAP18-derived peptides with membranes made from endotoxins or phospholipids. Biophys J 2001; 80:2935–2945.
79. Nizet V, Ohtake T, Lauth X, et al. Innate antimicrobial peptide protects the skin from invasive bacterial infection. Nature 2001; 414:454–457.
80. Rosenberger CM, Gallo RL, Finlay BB. Interplay between antibacterial effectors: A macrophage antimicrobial peptide impairs intracellular *Salmonella* replication. Proc Natl Acad Sci U S A 2004; 101:2422–2427.
81. Iimura M, Gallo RL, Hase K, et al. Cathelicidin mediates innate intestinal defense against colonization with epithelial adherent bacterial pathogens. J Immunol 2005; 174:4901–4907.
82. Howell MD, Jones JF, Kisich KO, et al. Selective killing of vaccinia virus by LL-37: Implications for eczema vaccinatum. J Immunol 2004; 172:1763–1767.
83. Lopez-Garcia B, Lee PH, Yamasaki K, et al. Anti-fungal activity of cathelicidins and their potential role in *Candida albicans* skin infection. J Invest Dermatol 2005; 125:108–115.
84. Dorschner RA, Lopez-Garcia B, Massie J, et al. Innate immune defense of the nail unit by antimicrobial peptides. J Am Acad Dermatol 2004; 50:343–348.
85. Braff MH, Gallo RL. Antimicrobial peptides: An essential component of the skin defensive barrier. Curr Top Microbiol Immunol 2006; 306:91–110.
86. Niyonsaba F, Ushio H, Nakano N, et al. Antimicrobial peptides human beta-defensins stimulate epidermal keratinocyte migration, proliferation and production of proinflammatory cytokines and chemokines. J Invest Dermatol 2007; 127:594–604.
87. Yang D, Chertov O, Oppenheim JJ. Participation of mammalian defensins and cathelicidins in anti-microbial immunity: Receptors and activities of human defensins and cathelicidin (LL-37). J Leukoc Biol 2001; 69:691–697.
88. Braff MH, Hawkins MA, Di Nardo A, et al. Structure–function relationships among human cathelicidin peptides: Dissociation of antimicrobial properties from host immunostimulatory activities. J Immunol 2005; 174:4271–4278.

89. Tjabringa GS, Aarbiou J, Ninaber DK, et al. The antimicrobial peptide LL-37 activates innate immunity at the airway epithelial surface by transactivation of the epidermal growth factor receptor. J Immunol 2003; 171:6690–6696.
90. Wang TT, Nestel FP, Bourdeau V, et al. Cutting edge: 1,25-Dihydroxyvitamin D3 is a direct inducer of antimicrobial peptide gene expression. J Immunol 2004; 173:2909–2912.
91. Gombart AF, Borregaard N, Koeffler HP. Human cathelicidin antimicrobial peptide (CAMP) gene is a direct target of the vitamin D receptor and is strongly up-regulated in myeloid cells by 1,25-dihydroxyvitamin D3. FASEB J 2005; 19:1067–1077.
92. Weber G, Heilborn JD, Chamorro Jimenez CI, et al. Vitamin D induces the antimicrobial protein hCAP18 in human skin. J Invest Dermatol 2005; 124:1080–1082.
93. Schauber J, Oda Y, Buchau AS, et al. Histone acetylation in keratinocytes enables control of the expression of cathelicidin and CD14 by 1,25-dihydroxyvitamin D3. J Invest Dermatol 2008; 128:816–824.
94. Schauber J, Dorschner RA, Coda AB, et al. Injury enhances TLR2 function and antimicrobial peptide expression through a vitamin D-dependent mechanism. J Clin Invest 2007; 117:803–811.
95. Liu PT, Stenger S, Li H, et al. Toll-like receptor triggering of a vitamin D-mediated human antimicrobial response. Science 2006; 311:1770–1773.
96. Peyssonaux C, Johnson RS. An unexpected role for hypoxic response: Oxygenation and inflammation. Cell Cycle 2004; 3:168–171.
97. Gallo RL, Kim KJ, Bernfield M, et al. Identification of CRAMP, a cathelin-related antimicrobial peptide expressed in the embryonic and adult mouse. J Biol Chem 1997; 272:13088–13093.
98. Rieg S, Garbe C, Sauer B, et al. Dermcidin is constitutively produced by eccrine sweat glands and is not induced in epidermal cells under inflammatory skin conditions. Br J Dermatol 2004; 151:534–539.
99. Baechle D, Flad T, Cansier A, et al. Cathepsin D is present in human eccrine sweat and involved in the postsecretory processing of the antimicrobial peptide DCD-1 L. J Biol Chem 2006; 281:5406–5415.
100. Lai YP, Peng YF, Zuo Y, et al. Functional and structural characterization of recombinant dermcidin-1 L, a human antimicrobial peptide. Biochem Biophys Res Commun 2005; 328:243–250.
101. Lin YT, Wang CT, Chiang BL. Role of bacterial pathogens in atopic dermatitis. Clin Rev Allergy Immunol 2007; 33:167–177.
102. Williams RE, Gibson AG, Aitchison TC, et al. Assessment of a contact-plate sampling technique and subsequent quantitative bacterial studies in atopic dermatitis. Br J Dermatol 1990; 123:493–501.
103. Leung DY. Infection in atopic dermatitis. Curr Opin Pediatr 2003; 15:399–404.
104. Grice K, Sattar H, Baker H, et al. The relationship of transepidermal water loss to skin temperature in psoriasis and eczema. J Invest Dermatol 1975; 64:313–315.
105. Ong PY, Ohtake T, Brandt C, et al. Endogenous antimicrobial peptides and skin infections in atopic dermatitis. N Engl J Med 2002; 347:1151–1160.
106. Nomura I, Goleva E, Howell MD, et al. Cytokine milieu of atopic dermatitis, as compared to psoriasis, skin prevents induction of innate immune response genes. J Immunol 2003; 171:3262–3269.
107. Howell MD, Novak N, Bieber T, et al. Interleukin-10 downregulates anti-microbial peptide expression in atopic dermatitis. J Invest Dermatol 2005; 125:738–745.
108. Homey B, Steinhoff M, Ruzicka T, et al. Cytokines and chemokines orchestrate atopic skin inflammation. J Allergy Clin Immunol 2006; 118:178–189.
109. Jeong CW, Ahn KS, Rho NK, et al. Differential in vivo cytokine mRNA expression in lesional skin of intrinsic vs. extrinsic atopic dermatitis patients using semiquantitative RT-PCR. Clin Exp Allergy 2003; 33:1717–1724.
110. Kaburagi Y, Shimada Y, Nagaoka T, et al. Enhanced production of CC-chemokines (RANTES, MCP-1, MIP-1alpha, MIP-1beta, and eotaxin) in patients with atopic dermatitis. Arch Dermatol Res 2001; 293:350–355.

111. Campbell JJ, Butcher EC. Chemokines in tissue-specific and microenvironment-specific lymphocyte homing. Curr Opin Immunol 2000; 12:336–341.
112. Howell MD, Gallo RL, Boguniewicz M, et al. Cytokine milieu of atopic dermatitis skin subverts the innate immune response to vaccinia virus. Immunity 2006; 24:341–348.
113. Howell MD, Boguniewicz M, Pastore S, et al. Mechanism of HBD-3 deficiency in atopic dermatitis. Clin Immunol 2006; 121:332–338.
114. Howell MD, Fairchild HR, Kim BE, et al. Th2 Cytokines Act on S100/A11 to Downregulate keratinocyte differentiation. J Invest Dermatol 2008; 128(9):2248–2258.
115. Nishijima S, Namura S, Kawai S, et al. *Staphylococcus aureus* on hand surface and nasal carriage in patients with atopic dermatitis. J Am Acad Dermatol 1995; 32:677–679.
116. Postlethwaite AE, Holness MA, Katai H, et al. Human fibroblasts synthesize elevated levels of extracellular matrix proteins in response to interleukin 4. J Clin Invest 1992; 90:1479–1485.
117. Grassegger A, Hopfl R. Significance of the cytokine interferon gamma in clinical dermatology. Clin Exp Dermatol 2004; 29:584–588.
118. Machura E, Mazur B, Golemiec E, et al. *Staphylococcus aureus* skin colonization in atopic dermatitis children is associated with decreased IFN-gamma production by peripheral blood CD4+ and CD8+ T cells. Pediatr Allergy Immunol 2008; 19:37–45.
119. Rieg S, Steffen H, Seeber S, et al. Deficiency of dermcidin-derived antimicrobial peptides in sweat of patients with atopic dermatitis correlates with an impaired innate defense of human skin in vivo. J Immunol 2005; 174:8003–8010.
120. Cho SH, Strickland I, Boguniewicz M, et al. Fibronectin and fibrinogen contribute to the enhanced binding of *Staphylococcus aureus* to atopic skin. J Allergy Clin Immunol 2001; 108:269–274.
121. Cho SH, Strickland I, Tomkinson A, et al. Preferential binding of *Staphylococcus aureus* to skin sites of Th2-mediated inflammation in a murine model. J Invest Dermatol 2001; 116:658–663.
122. Wann ER, Gurusiddappa S, Hook M. The fibronectin-binding MSCRAMM FnbpA of *Staphylococcus aureus* is a bifunctional protein that also binds to fibrinogen. J Biol Chem 2000; 275:13863–13871.
123. Plaut M, Tinkle SS. Risks of smallpox vaccination: 200 years after Jenner. J Allergy Clin Immunol 2003; 112:683–685.
124. Bicknell WJ. The case for voluntary smallpox vaccination. N Engl J Med 2002; 346:1323–1325.
125. Wharton M, Strikas RA, Harpaz R, et al. Recommendations for using smallpox vaccine in a pre-event vaccination program. Supplemental recommendations of the Advisory Committee on Immunization Practices (ACIP) and the Healthcare Infection Control Practices Advisory Committee (HICPAC). MMWR Recomm Rep 2003; 52:1–16.
126. Marris E. Dramatic rescue relieves rare case of smallpox infection. Nat Med 2007; 13:517.
127. Wollenberg A, Wetzel S, Burgdorf WH, et al. Viral infections in atopic dermatitis: Pathogenic aspects and clinical management. J Allergy Clin Immunol 2003; 112:667–674.
128. Peng WM, Jenneck C, Bussmann C, et al. Risk factors of atopic dermatitis patients for eczema herpeticum. J Invest Dermatol 2007; 127:1261–1263.
129. Howell MD, Wollenberg A, Gallo RL, et al. Cathelicidin deficiency predisposes to eczema herpeticum. J Allergy Clin Immunol 2006; 117:836–841.
130. Uchida Y, Kurasawa K, Nakajima H, et al. Increase of dendritic cells of type 2 (DC2) by altered response to IL-4 in atopic patients. J Allergy Clin Immunol 2001; 108:1005–1011.
131. Wollenberg A, Wagner M, Gunther S, et al. Plasmacytoid dendritic cells: A new cutaneous dendritic cell subset with distinct role in inflammatory skin diseases. J Invest Dermatol 2002; 119:1096–1102.
132. Rissoan MC, Soumelis V, Kadowaki N, et al. Reciprocal control of T helper cell and dendritic cell differentiation. Science 1999; 283:1183–1186.
133. Lande R, Gregorio J, Facchinetti V, et al. Plasmacytoid dendritic cells sense self-DNA coupled with antimicrobial peptide. Nature 2007; 449:564–569.

134. Liu L, Wang L, Jia HP, et al. Structure and mapping of the human beta-defensin HBD-2 gene and its expression at sites of inflammation. Gene 1998; 222:237–244.
135. Takahashi M, Horiuchi Y, Tezuka T. Presence of bactericidal/permeability-increasing protein in human and rat skin. Exp Dermatol 2004; 13:55–60.
136. Cumberbatch M, Dearman RJ, Uribe-Luna S, et al. Regulation of epidermal Langerhans cell migration by lactoferrin. Immunology 2000; 100:21–28.
137. Rose FR, Bailey K, Keyte JW, et al. Potential role of epithelial cell-derived histone H1 proteins in innate antimicrobial defense in the human gastrointestinal tract. Infect Immun 1998; 66:3255–3263.
138. Buchau AS, Hassan M, Kukova G, et al. S100A15, an antimicrobial protein of the skin: Regulation by E. coli through Toll-like receptor 4. J Invest Dermatol 2007; 127:2596–2604.
139. Harder J, Schroder JM. RNase 7, a novel innate immune defense antimicrobial protein of healthy human skin. J Biol Chem 2002; 277:46779–46784.
140. Gallo RL, Ono M, Povsic T, et al. Syndecans, cell surface heparan sulfate proteoglycans, are induced by a proline-rich antimicrobial peptide from wounds. Proc Natl Acad Sci U S A 1994; 91:11035–11039.
141. Harwig SS, Chen NP, Park AS, et al. Purification of cysteine-rich bioactive peptides from leukocytes by continuous acid-urea-polyacrylamide gel electrophoresis. Anal Biochem 1993; 208:382–386.
142. Caccavo D, Pellegrino NM, Altamura M, et al. Antimicrobial and immunoregulatory functions of lactoferrin and its potential therapeutic application. J Endotoxin Res 2002; 8:403–417.
143. Stenger S, Hanson DA, Teitelbaum R, et al. An antimicrobial activity of cytolytic T cells mediated by granulysin. Science 1998; 282:121–125.
144. Domachowske JB, Dyer KD, Bonville CA, et al. Recombinant human eosinophil-derived neurotoxin/RNase 2 functions as an effective antiviral agent against respiratory syncytial virus. J Infect Dis 1998; 177:1458–1464.
145. Domachowske JB, Dyer KD, Adams AG, et al. Eosinophil cationic protein/RNase 3 is another RNase A-family ribonuclease with direct antiviral activity. Nucleic Acids Res 1998; 26:3358–3363.
146. Tang YQ, Yeaman MR, Selsted ME. Antimicrobial peptides from human platelets. Infect Immun 2002; 70:6524–6533.
147. Zaiou M, Nizet V, Gallo RL. Antimicrobial and protease inhibitory functions of the human cathelicidin (hCAP18/LL-37) prosequence. J Invest Dermatol 2003; 120:810–816.
148. Wingens M, van Bergen BH, Hiemstra PS, et al. Induction of SLPI (ALP/HUSI-I) in epidermal keratinocytes. J Invest Dermatol 1998; 111:996–1002.
149. Simpson AJ, Maxwell AI, Govan JR, et al. Elafin (elastase-specific inhibitor) has antimicrobial activity against gram-positive and gram-negative respiratory pathogens. FEBS Lett 1999; 452:309–313.
150. Meyer-Hoffert U, Wichmann N, Schwichtenberg L, et al. Supernatants of Pseudomonas aeruginosa induce the Pseudomonas-specific antibiotic elafin in human keratinocytes. Exp Dermatol 2003; 12:418–425.
151. Blankenvoorde MF, van't Hof W, Walgreen-Weterings E, et al. Cystatin and cystatin-derived peptides have antibacterial activity against the pathogen Porphyromonas gingivalis. Biol Chem 1998; 379:1371–1375.
152. Glaser R, Harder J, Lange H, et al. Antimicrobial psoriasin (S100A7) protects human skin from Escherichia coli infection. Nat Immunol 2005; 6:57–64.
153. Cole AM, Ganz T, Liese AM, et al. Cutting edge: IFN-inducible ELR-CXC chemokines display defensin-like antimicrobial activity. J Immunol 2001; 167:623–627.
154. Cutuli M, Cristiani S, Lipton JM, et al. Antimicrobial effects of alpha-MSH peptides. J Leukoc Biol 2000; 67:233–239.
155. Kowalska K, Carr DB, Lipkowski AW. Direct antimicrobial properties of substance P. Life Sci 2002; 71:747–750.
156. Tasiemski A, Hammad H, Vandenbulcke F, et al. Presence of chromogranin-derived antimicrobial peptides in plasma during coronary artery bypass surgery and evidence of an immune origin of these peptides. Blood 2002; 100:553–559.

157. Kieffer AE, Goumon Y, Ruh O, et al. The N- and C-terminal fragments of ubiquitin are important for the antimicrobial activities. FASEB J 2003; 17:776–778.
158. Lambert RW, Campton K, Ding W, et al. Langerhans cell expression of neuropeptide Y and peptide YY. Neuropeptides 2002; 36:246–251.
159. Radek KA, Lopez-Garcia B, Hupe M, et al. The neuroendocrine peptide catestatin is a cutaneous antimicrobial and induced in the skin after injury. J Invest Dermatol 2008; 128:1525–1534.
160. Allaker RP, Zihni C, Kapas S. An investigation into the antimicrobial effects of adrenomedullin on members of the skin, oral, respiratory tract and gut microflora. FEMS Immunol Med Microbiol 1999; 23:289–293.

7 Role of T cells

Cevdet Ozdemir

Swiss Institute of Allergy and Asthma Research (SIAF), Davos, Switzerland and Marmara University, Division of Pediatric Allergy and Immunology, Istanbul, Turkey

Mübeccel Akdis and Cezmi A. Akdis

Swiss Institute of Allergy and Asthma Research (SIAF), Davos, Switzerland

INTRODUCTION

Atopic dermatitis (AD) is a chronic relapsing skin disorder with an interplay of migrating lymphocytes, fibrocytes, Langerhans cells, mast cells, and epidermal keratinocytes (KC). Recent investigations have greatly increased our understanding of immunologic mechanisms involved in the pathogenesis of AD (Fig. 1). Activation of the immune system, particularly skin-homing T cells, transmigration to skin, and effector functions such as induction of keratinocyte apoptosis, IgE, and eosinophilia represents cardinal features of allergic inflammation in AD (1). The mononuclear cellular infiltrate in lesional skin of AD is mainly constituted of CD4$^+$ T cells and to a lesser extent CD8$^+$ T cells (2). Aeroallergens, food antigens, autoantigens, and bacterial superantigens activate T cells in AD. Activated T cells are under the influence of skin-related chemokine network and they show skin-selective homing. Migration of activated T helper (Th) 2 cells to the dermis is then followed by acquiring a Th0/Th1 phenotype under the influence of interleukin (IL)-12, produced mainly by antigen-presenting cells or activated keratinocytes. Epidermal Langerhans cells and inflammatory dendritic epidermal cells (IDEC) are able to activate allergen-specific T cells through allergen-specific IgE-antibodies bound to Fc receptors for IgE (FcεRI and FcεRII) (3). This leads to continuous stimulation and survival of T cells in the skin. Apoptosis (i.e., activation-induced cell death) of activated T cells is prevented in the dermis by cytokines, chemokines, and extracellular matrix components (4). The Th0/Th1 cells are characterized by secretion of significant amounts of the effector cytokines tumor necrosis factor (TNF)-α and interferon (IFN)-γ. IFN-γ induces apoptosis of keratinocytes, leading eventually to the eczematous lesions characteristic of AD (5). T cells play important roles in AD with induction of hyper IgE. However, diagnosis of AD can be made in the absence of elevated total IgE and specific IgE to food or environmental allergens. The subgroup of AD patients with normal IgE levels and without specific IgE sensitization has been termed non-atopic dermatitis (NAD) (6). They show similar mechanisms in the pathogenesis except the induction of hyper IgE (2,7). In addition, recent data suggest that filaggrin mutations are key organ specific factors

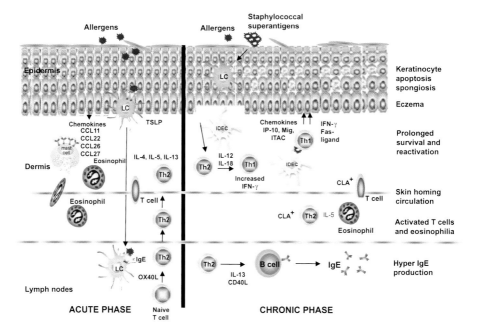

FIGURE 1 Mechanisms of T-cell–mediated allergic inflammation in atopic dermatitis. Aeroallergens, food antigens, autoantigens, and bacterial superantigens activate T cells. They are under the influence of skin-related chemokine network and they show skin-selective homing. In the skin they show increased survival and they are continuously stimulated. Activated T cells induce keratinocyte apoptosis as a key pathogenetic event in the formation of eczema. LCs and inflammatory dendritic epidermal cells (IDECs) are two different subtypes of dendritic cells in lesional skin of AD. LCs are also present in nonlesional skin. LCs induce Th2 immune responses, which predominate in the acute phase of the disease which also release chemotactic signals for the IDECs. IDECs produce proinflammatory cytokines and chemokines and play a role in the polarization of Th2 immune response into Th1 type. T-cells infiltrating the skin are CD45RO+, and use CLA and other receptors to recognize and cross the endothelium. In the peripheral blood of AD patients, both CD4+ and CD8+ subsets of CLA+ CD45RO+ T cells are in an activated state (CD25+, CD40L+, HLADR+). They express Fas and Fas-ligand and undergo activation-induced apoptosis. In contrast, T-cells infiltrating the skin of AD patients—despite expressing both Fas and Fas ligand—do not show any apoptosis, because they are protected from apoptosis by cytokines and ECM proteins. These T cells secrete IFN-γ, which upregulates Fas on keratinocytes, and render them susceptible to apoptosis in the skin. Fas ligand expressed on the surface of activated T cells or released to microenvironment induces keratinocyte apoptosis. Both CD4+ and CD8+ T cells isolated from skin or CLA+ CD45RO+ T cells from peripheral blood secrete high levels of IL-5 and IL-13 and therefore are capable of prolonging eosinophil life span and inducing IgE production.

predominantly affecting the development of eczema and confer significant risks of allergic sensitization and allergic rhinitis as well as asthma in the context of eczema (8). They are not included in this chapter, but discussed in detail elsewhere in other chapters.

T-CELL ACTIVATION IN AD

Mechanisms of T-Cell Activation

T cells constitute a large population of cellular infiltrate in AD, and a dysregulated, cytokine-mediated immune response appears to be an important pathogenetic factor (Fig. 1). Numerous studies have pointed to the role of activated $CD4^+$ T cells in AD and other allergic inflammatory diseases (9). Systemic activation of T cells in AD is supported by the observation that these patients possess increased numbers of activated cutaneous lymphocyte–associated antigen (CLA)-bearing T cells in the circulation and increased levels of serum L-selectin, a marker for leukocyte activation correlating with AD disease severity (10–12). CLA defines a subset of circulating memory T cells that selectively localizes to cutaneous sites. CLA^+ T cells constitute only 10% to 15% of the circulating T-cell pool and do not exceed 5% of lymphocytes within noncutaneous inflamed sites (13). CLA is expressed on Th1 cells during the differentiation process and can be induced on Th2 cells by stimulation with bacterial superantigen and/or IL-12 (14,15). Another supporting observation for the role of T cells in AD is the significant improvement seen in lesional rash with treatment models which specifically target activated T cells, as that with topical calcineurin inhibitor (TCI) therapies (16). Improvement in eczematous skin lesions seen in primary T-cell immunodeficiency disorders after successful bone marrow transplantation also remarks for the key role of immune effector T cells in AD. Dermal cellular infiltrate in AD mainly consists of $CD4^+$ and $CD8^+$ T cells with a CD4/CD8 ratio similar to peripheral blood levels (2,7). In studies, $CD8^+CLA^+$ T cells were demonstrated to be as potent as $CD4^+CLA^+$ T cells in the induction of IgE and inhibition of eosinophil survival (2,7).

A number of pathogenetic mechanisms leading to T-cell activation in AD including aeroallergens, food allergens, superantigens, and autoantigens have been emphasized. The role of aeroallergens in T-cell activation in AD has been extensively studied (17,18). Aeroallergens can induce both immediate type and delayed type responses in the skin (18). The frequency of aeroallergen-specific T cells was investigated in AD lesions and they were found to be less than 1% in nonchallenged AD lesions (19). Besides, such allergen-specific T cells can be detected in the skin of atopic patients after allergen administration, without any signs of AD lesions (20). The contribution of food allergens in the exacerbation of AD by T-cell activation was also demonstrated (21). Normally allergen-specific T cell responses in food and aeroallergen allergy are confined to $CD4^+$ T cells. This, however, may not explain the activation and recruitment of $CD8^+$ T cells in AD skin lesions. It has recently been demonstrated that allergens such as house dust mite (*Dermatophagoides pteronyssinus*) and birch pollen induce atopy patch test reactivity in NAD patients with the presence of specific IgG but not IgE antibodies (22). It is also known that bacterial superantigens can interact with certain Vβ elements of the T-cell receptor (TCR) leading to activation, expansion, anergy, or deletion of T cells. It is evident from mouse studies that superantigen response of T cells is not restricted to $CD4^+$ T cells. $CD8^+$ T cells (23) and even $CD4^-CD8^-$ T cells can respond to superantigenic stimuli (24). This may explain the existence and activation of $CD8^+$ T cells in eczema lesions and their contribution to IgE production and eosinophil survival and development, chronicity, and exacerbation of AD (2,7). One of the factors that may contribute to the pathophysiology of AD is autoreactivity to human proteins (25,26). IgE against autoantigens can stimulate type 1 hypersensitivity reactions as well as dendritic cells and induce the proliferation of autoreactive T cells (27). Another widely supported view is that dermal dendritic cells and epidermal Langerhans cells display an abnormal hyperstimulatory function for T cells, in addition to IL-12 and IL-18 production. IgE FcεRI and FcεRII (CD23) are upregulated in CD1a positive cells in AD. CD1a is a marker of dermal dendritic cells and Langerhans cells (28). Their role in IgE-facilitated antigen presentation and T-cell activation will be discussed below.

Role of Superantigens in T-Cell Activation in AD

In healthy skin, naturally occurring antimicrobial peptides including two major classes of peptides, β-defensins and cathelicidins (29,30), are critical components of innate immune system against bacterial, fungal, and viral pathogens (31). Among antimicrobial peptides, HBD-2 and LL-37 are produced by keratinocytes in response to inflammatory stimuli in normal skin (29). The importance of these peptides by reporting their deficiency in AD lesional skin both at the protein and mRNA level has been suggested (32). This defect may explain the exponential increase in *Staphylococcus aureus* (*S. aureus*) colony numbers in the upper layers of the epidermis between keratinocytes (33). It has also been stated that HBD-2 and LL-37 have activity not only against bacteria but also against fungi and viruses, which may explain the increased susceptibility of patients with AD to fungal and viral infections such as *Herpes simplex* and *Molluscum contagiosum* (32).

From a number of studies, it can be concluded that bacterial superantigens contribute to the pathogenesis and exacerbation of AD. Staphylococcal superantigens are frequent triggers of exacerbations in AD and are frequently isolated from skin of patients with AD (34). Superantigen patch test elicits skin inflammation in AD patients (35) and in human severe combined immunodeficiency mouse model (36). In addition, specific IgE antibodies to bacterial superantigens exist in AD (37). It was also demonstrated that $CD8^+$ T cells isolated from skin or CLA^+CD8^+ T cells isolated from peripheral blood efficiently proliferate by superantigenic stimulation (2). Furthermore, purified $CD4^+$ or $CD8^+$ T cells cultured from skin biopsies secrete high IL-5 and IL-13 by Staphylococcal enterotoxin B (SEB) stimulation (2). Induction of CLA expression by superantigens may play an important role in the pathogenesis of AD, which is associated with superantigen-producing staphylococci (15). Staphylococcal superantigens secreted at the skin surface may penetrate through the inflamed skin and stimulate epidermal macrophages or Langerhans cells to produce IL-1, TNF-α, and IL-12. SEB can induce the maturation of dendritic cells through activation of TLR2 leading to priming of naive allogenic T cells into Th2 (38). Superantigen-stimulated Langerhans cells may migrate to skin-associated lymph nodes and serve as antigen-presenting cells (APCs). They can upregulate the expression of CLA by IL-12 production (15,39) and alter the functional profile of virgin T cells. Moreover, superantigens presented by keratinocytes, Langerhans cells, and macrophages can stimulate T cells in the skin. This second round of stimulation is able to induce CLA expression (40). Local production of IL-1 and TNF-α may induce E-selectin on vascular endothelium allowing an initial migration of CLA^+ memory/effector cells (41). Effect of superantigens on regulatory T (Treg) cells has also been marked in patients with AD, who have significantly increased numbers of peripheral blood Treg cells with normal immunosuppressive activity, which then lose this after superantigen stimulation (42). Staphylococcal enterotoxin B upregulates GITR-L on monocytes and inhibits natural Treg ability to suppress effector T-cell proliferation via a cell contact interaction (43). Superantigens also induce corticosteroid resistance, thereby complicating the response to therapy (44). *S. aureus* isolates from patients with steroid-resistant AD appear to be selected on the basis of greater production of superantigens compared with that of isolates from control groups (45).

Role of Autoantigens in AD

It has been demonstrated that a considerable percentage of patients suffering from AD develop IgE autoantibodies against a broad variety of human proteins including endothelial cells and keratinocytes (26,46). Human antigens that cross-react with environmental allergens have been shown to induce basophil degranulation, autoreactive T-cell proliferation, dendritic cell stimulation, and immediate as well as late-phase skin reactions (46–48). Recently, it has been shown that IgE against manganese superoxide dismutase (MnSOD) from the skin-colonizing yeast *Malassezia sympodialis* cross-reacts with human MnSOD (46). In the Th2 environment of atopic patients, IgE antibodies against autoantigens due to their intracellular nature may have escaped tolerance induction. Role of autoimmunity and autoantibodies in AD has been considered, especially when exacerbations appeared without any exposure to environmental allergens (49). Also, several studies have shown that the severity of AD is closely related with IgE autoreactivity (25,26). Complementary DNAs (cDNAs) coding for IgE-reactive autoantigens have been isolated from human expression cDNA libraries using serum IgE autoantibodies from patients with AD (26,50). Hom s 4 represents a protein with an intrinsic property to induce Th1-mediated autoreactivity (50). On the other hand, it has recently been demonstrated that Hom s 2 has been shown to induce a strong IFN-γ response in both atopic and nonatopic individuals (51). The production of chemokines, which in turn promote the infiltration of IFN-γ-producing T cells into the epidermis, results with further damage to skin keratinocytes of AD patients [5,52].

Cytokine Profile of Activated T Cells in AD

Elevated IgE levels and eosinophilia in AD suggests increased expression of Th2-type cytokines (53). The majority of allergen-specific T cells derived from skin lesions that have been provoked in AD patients by epicutaneous allergen application or peripheral blood skin homing T cells produce predominantly Th2 cytokines such as IL-4, IL-5, and IL-13 (Fig. 1) (2,10,11,54). Previously, such polarized Th2 cytokine pattern was regarded as a specific feature reflecting immune dysregulation in AD. The inhibitory effect of IL-4 on the barrier recovery, especially in the early phase, in vivo supports the hypothesis that Th2 cytokines may impair the barrier recovery in inflammation (55). However, studies demonstrate that IFN-γ predominates over IL-4 in chronic skin lesions and older patch test reactions in AD, whereas IL-5 and IL-13 still remain at high levels (7,19,56,57). A number of factors may be involved in increased IFN-γ in older skin lesions. IL-12 produced by Langerhans cells, eosinophils, and keratinocytes appears to be a predominant mediator for the induction of IFN-γ in T cells after homing to skin (Fig. 1) (39,58,59). Furthermore, IL-18 produced in the microenvironment of skin may act in parallel to IL-12 (60). Characterization of the cells in the afferent skin-derived lymph from healthy individuals demonstrated the dominance of a type 1 cytokine profile with IFN-γ in

T cells and IL-12 in dendritic cells (61). Such studies performed in AD patients may further help to understand the immune regulation mechanisms. Another widely supported view is that dermal dendritic cells and epidermal Langerhans cells display an abnormal hyperstimulatory functions for T cells, in addition to their IL-12 and IL-18 production. IgE FcεRI and FcεRII (CD23) are upregulated in CD1a positive cells in AD (28).

The Role of IgE-Facilitated Antigen-Presentation in T-Cell Activation

The immune response to foreign proteins strongly depends on the efficiency and selectivity of antigen uptake by antigen-presenting cells. The two distinct dendritic cell populations that have been identified in inflamed epidermis of AD are the classical Langerhans cells and the IDEC (Fig. 1) (62). Langerhans cell population rather induces a Th2 type of T-cell response, while the IDEC population clearly induces a Th1 T-cell outcome (63). Concerning dendritic cells and Langerhans cells, the expression of IgE FcεRI and its increase on the surface of these cells is strongly related to distinct type of inflammatory status (64). IDEC express costimulatory molecules in situ, take up mannosylated antigens via mannose receptor-mediated endocytosis, and represent the relevant FcRI-expressing and IgE-binding epidermal dendritic cell population (65,66). It was shown that IgE bound to CD23 (FcεRII) on mouse B cells may be used to focus antigen to T cells (67). This finding initialized the understanding of focused antigen presentation via IgE receptors. Previously, the high affinity receptor for IgE has been believed to be present on mast cells and basophils. This was followed by the demonstration of IgE FcεRI on Langerhans cells, eosinophils, and epidermal cells (28,68,69). Low-affinity IgE receptor (CD23) has a widespread cellular distribution (70). Both types of IgE Fc receptors are thought to play a role in IgE-mediated antigen presentation (71–74). This mechanism operates selectively at low doses of allergens, and the presentation of extremely low doses of allergen to CD4$^+$ T lymphocytes is greatly enhanced by IgE-facilitated antigen presentation (73,75). Blocking IgG antibodies in IgG containing serum fractions induced by SIT of birch pollen allergy inhibits the IgE-facilitated antigen presentation at very low allergen concentrations (75). Accordingly, IgE acts as an immunoglobulin specialized in antigen capture or antigen focusing. Especially in extrinsic type of AD, the presence of high levels of specific IgE in serum and CD23 on APC (activated B cells) (7), together with FcεRI expressing APC (Langerhans cells in the skin) (28), may strongly contribute to the overstimulation of the allergen-specific immune responses. On the other hand, the role of FcεRI in the induction of allergen-specific tolerance has also been considered as the activation of monocytes and monocyte-derived dendritic cells, expressing that the FcεRI leads to the production of high amounts of IL-10 (76,77).

Capture of antigens via surface IgE and signal transduction through IgE cytoplasmic chain was shown as crucial events in specific IgE responses (78). Clinical trials with a neutralizing non-anaphylactogenic anti-IgE mAb treatment have demonstrated an inhibition in bronchial late-phase responses and decreased the number of eosinophils in sputum of allergic asthma patients (79). Correspondingly, the production of IL-4 and IL-5 and lung eosinophilia of house dust mite–sensitized mice is inhibited by anti-CD23 or anti-IgE mAb treatment (80). Moreover, studies performed using anti-CD23 mAb and CD23 deficient mice suggest that IgE-mediated antigen presentation plays a major role in Th2 cytokine production and lung eosinophilia (80). The development of humanized anti-IgE antibodies may also offer the possibility of reduced IgE-facilitated antigen presentation (81). Recently with low-dose anti-IgE therapy, successful preliminary experience has been reported in patients with generalized AD. The clinical improvement was paralleled by a decrease in the mRNA ratio for IgE/IgG in these patients' peripheral blood mononuclear cells (82). However, elimination of IgE may not be adequate in individuals with persisting T-cell–mediated inflammation, because in animal models of AD, allergic inflammation of the skin was elicited to the same extent in wild type and IgE knock-out mice (83).

HISTAMINE AND HISTAMINE RECEPTORS IN AD

Histamine is synthesized from L-histidine exclusively by histidine decarboxylase, an enzyme expressed in cells throughout the body, including central nervous system neurons, gastric mucosa parietal cells, mast cells, and basophils (84,85). Histamine exerts a range of effects on many physiologic and pathologic processes, and new roles are still being discovered. Histamine and the four histamine receptors constitute a multifaceted system, with distinct functions of receptor types due to their differential expression, which changes according to the stage of cell differentiation with the influence from the microenvironment (Fig. 2) (84,85).

Although contrasting findings have been reported, the histamine H_1-receptor (H_1R) stimulates cells of the immune system by enhancing proinflammatory activity through release of mediators and increase of cellular adhesion molecule expression and chemotaxis of eosinophils and neutrophils. H_1R also increase antigen-presenting cell capacity and costimulatory activity on B cells and exert a Th1-type immune response marked by increased IFN-γ production. The histamine H_2-receptor (H_2R), on the other hand, appears to be a potent suppressor of inflammatory and effector function. H_2R decreases eosinophil and neutrophil chemotaxis and decreases IL-12. H_2R increases IL-10 levels and induces the development of Th2 or tolerance inducing dendritic cells (84). Moreover, histamine modulates neurotransmitter release through presynaptic histamine H_3-receptors (H_3R) located on histaminergic and nonhistaminergic neurons in the central and peripheral nervous systems (86). The novel histamine receptor, H_4R facilitates several proinflammatory activities through increasing eosinophil chemotaxis and IL-16 production. H_4R plays role in chemotaxis of regulatory T cells (84,87).

Histamine contributes to the progression of allergic-inflammatory responses by enhancing the secretion of proinflammatory cytokines such as IL-1α, IL-1β, and IL-6, as well as chemokines such as RANTES and IL-8, by several cell types and in local tissues (88–91). Histamine possesses all the properties of a classic leukocyte chemoattractant, including agonist-induced actin polymerization, mobilization of intracellular calcium, alterations in cell shape, and upregulation of adhesion molecule expression (92). Histamine also plays role in skin defense. In addition to this, the role in skin defense in inducing the production of various cytokines and chemokines (93,94), histamine also enhances the production of TNF-α–induced or IFN-γ–induced human β-defensin-2 in human keratinocytes, which play pivotal roles in antimicrobial defense, hence preventing from effects of superantigens (95).

Histamine participates in activating dendritic cell precursors, as well as both immature and mature forms. Dendritic cells express all four histamine receptors (96–98). Although human monocyte-derived dendritic cells express both H_1R and H_2R and can induce CD86 expression by histamine, human epidermal Langerhans cells express neither H_1R nor H_2R, mainly because of the effect of transforming

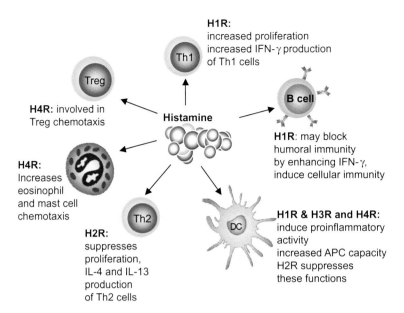

FIGURE 2 Role of histamine in immunoregulation. Histamine is synthesized and released by human basophils, mast cells, lymphocytes, dendritic cells, macrophages, neurons, and gastric enterochromaffin-like cells. Histamine regulates various cells of the immune system including monocytes, dendritic cells, T cells, and B cells in lymphatic organs and subepithelial tissues. Histamine H_1-receptor (H_1R) stimulates cells of the immune system by potentiating their proinflammatory activity through increased migration to areas of inflammation, as well as by increasing their effector function. The histamine H_2-receptor (H_2R) appears to be a potent suppressor of inflammatory and effector function. Histamine modulates neurotransmitter release through presynaptic histamine H_3-receptors (H_3R) located on histaminergic and nonhistaminergic neurons in the central and peripheral nervous systems, and it facilitates several proinflammatory activities through the novel histamine H_4-receptor (H_4R). Histamine H_1 receptor and histamine H_3 receptor induce proinflammatory activity and increased antigen-presenting cell capacity. Histamine induces increased proliferation and IFN-γ production in Th1 cells. Th2 cells express predominant histamine H_2 receptor, which acts as the negative regulator of proliferation, IL-4, and IL-13 production. Histamine enhances Th1-type responses by triggering the histamine H_1 receptor, whereas both Th1- and Th2-type responses are negatively regulated by histamine H_2 receptor. These distinct effects may suggest roles of histamine H_1 receptor and histamine H_2 receptor on T cells for autoimmunity and peripheral tolerance, respectively. Histamine directly effects B-cell antibody production as a costimulatory receptor on B cells. Histamine H_1 receptor predominantly expressed on Th1 cells may block humoral immune responses by enhancing Th1 type cytokine IFN-γ.

growth factor (TGF)-β (99). The possible interaction of histamine and previously mentioned IDECs in lesions of AD has been recently studied by investigating the expression and function of H_4R on IDECs (100). Skin IDECs express H_4R, which is upregulated by IFN-γ, but not by IL-4, TNF-α, poly I:C, or combinations of these, thus demonstrating that H_4R has a role in a Th1-related cytokine environment in the skin. It has been demonstrated that differential patterns of histamine receptor expression on Th1 and Th2 cells determine reciprocal T-cell responses following histamine stimulation (85). Th1 cells show predominant, but not exclusive, expression of H_1R, whereas Th2 cells show increased expression of H_2R. Histamine enhances Th1-type responses by triggering H_1R, whereas both Th1- and Th2-type responses are negatively regulated by H_2R (85). It has been suggested that downregulation of CCL2 and upregulation of IFN-γ by H_4R may contribute to the shift from a Th2 to a Th1 milieu, as seen in the transition from acute to chronic lesions of AD (100). It seems that H_1R and H_4R synergize in this process in which the upregulation of IFN-γ in T cells leads to keratinocyte apoptosis and eczema formation in AD (5).

SKIN-SELECTIVE T-CELL HOMING IN AD

Skin represents a functionally distinct immune compartment, and the location of the allergic/inflammatory disease in the skin is determined by tissue compartmentalization of the immune response. This is controlled by the expression of chemokines and chemokine receptors, the expression of skin-selective homing ligand, and the route of allergen/superantigen sensitization. The great majority of T-cells homing to the skin are of the CD45RO$^+$ memory/effector phenotype and express the selective skin homing receptor, CLA (101). The CLA epitope is characterized by specific binding to the monoclonal antibody HECA-452 (101). CLA binds to its vascular counter receptor, E-selectin (CD62E), which is expressed on inflamed superficial dermal postcapillary venules and endothelial cells (102). CLA$^+$ CD45RO$^+$ T cells migrate across activated endothelium using CLA/E-selectin, VLA-4/VCAM-1, and LFA-1/ICAM-1 interactions (103). Selective inhibition of these interactions affects skin-selective T-cell homing. Lymphocyte function–associated antigen (LFA) is composed of integrins CD11a and CD18 (104). Treatment with the monoclonal antibody for CD11a (efalizumab) has reduced CLA$^+$ T cell numbers in lesional AD (105) and accumulated them in the circulation (106). In addition, CLA is expressed by the malignant T cells of chronic-phase cutaneous T-cell lymphoma (mycosis fungoides and Sezary syndrome) but not by nonskin-associated T-cell lymphomas (101). In both AD and contact dermatitis, T cells specific to skin-related allergens are confined to the CLA$^+$ T-cell population (11). The CLA$^+$ memory/effector cells demonstrate typical features of in vivo activation in AD (10). Freshly isolated, unstimulated CLA$^+$ T cells show significantly higher levels of CD25 (IL-2 receptor-α chain), CD40-ligand, and HLA-DR expression. Additional evidence for in vivo activation of CLA$^+$ T cells appears from the spontaneous proliferation immediately after purification without further activation. CLA$^+$ T cells contain and spontaneously release high amounts of preformed IL-5 and IL-13, but only very little IL-4 and IFN-γ in their cytoplasm as demonstrated by intracellular cytokine staining immediately after purification (2,10). Moreover, CLA$^+$ memory/effector T cells induce IgE production by B cells and enhance eosinophil survival by inhibiting eosinophil apoptosis in AD (2,10). In contrast, the CLA$^-$ population represents a resting memory T-cell fraction, induces rather IgG in B cells, and does not show any effect on eosinophil survival and apoptosis (2,10).

The CLA epitope consists of a sialyl-Lewis x carbohydrate and corresponds to a posttranslational modification of the P-selectin glycoprotein ligand 1 (PSGL-1) (107). The generation of CLA on T cells undergoing naive to memory transition in skin-draining lymph nodes requires α-(1,3)-fucosyltransferase (FucT-VII) activity (107,108). Thus, CLA expression predominantly reflects the regulated activity of the glycosyltransferase, FucT-VII (107,108). Studies in mice suggest that adaptively transferred Th1 cells are preferentially recruited to cutaneous DTH reactions compared with Th2 cells (109). In addition, in vitro differentiated Th1 but not Th2 cells have been shown to bind E-selectin, and expression of functional selectin ligands are upregulated by IL-12 and inhibited by IL-4 by opposite effects on FucT-VII gene expression in mice (40,110,111). Skin-selective homing ligand expression is regulated by the same mechanisms in both CD4$^+$ and CD8$^+$ T cells (14,40,110,111). The CLA molecule was expressed on Th1 cells during the differentiation process (14,40,110,111). More importantly, CLA can be induced on Th2 cells by T-cell stimulation with bacterial superantigen and/or IL-12 challenge (14). These Th2 cells demonstrate the same cytokine profile as the T cells found in skin biopsies and in peripheral blood of AD patients. They show high IFN-γ, IL-5, and IL-13 production with very little or no IL-4 production (7,54,112,113). By IL-12 stimulation, CLA could be expressed on the surface of allergen-specific Th1, Th2, Th0, and T regulatory 1 clones, representing a nonskin-related antigen-specific T cells (14). In addition, CLA could be reinduced on T cells that have lost CLA expression upon resting (14). Apparently, skin-selective homing is not restricted to functional and phenotypic T-cell subsets. IL-12 and/or superantigen responsiveness such as certain T-cell receptor variable β-chain expression or IL-12Rβ expression act as factors that control CLA expression on T cells.

CHEMOKINE NETWORK IN THE AD SKIN

Mechanisms that control infiltration of inflammatory cells into AD skin are intensely investigated. Multiple molecules, including families of adhesion molecules and chemokines, provide signals for the dynamic trafficking of T cells into inflammatory tissues. Transendothelial migration and influx into skin represent the first phase leading to dermal perivascular infiltration by T cells, and a second step of chemotaxis takes place in the migration of T cells closer to and into the epidermis where they augment T-cell–mediated effector functions in AD. Increased expression of C-C chemokines (monocyte chemoattractant protein 4, eotaxin, and RANTES) contributes to infiltration of macrophages, eosinophils, and T cells into acute and chronic AD skin lesions (114).

Cutaneous T-cell–attracting chemokine CTACK/CCL27 and its receptor CRP-2/CCR10 are demonstrated to play a role in preferential attraction of CLA$^+$ T cells to the skin (115,116). CTACK is predominantly expressed in the skin and selectively attracts a tissue-specific subpopulation of memory lymphocytes. It is also reported as ALP in mouse. The terms "Eskine" and "ILC" were also used for the same chemokine (116). It is designated as CCL27 in the new systematic chemokine nomenclature. CTACK is constitutively expressed in mouse skin suggesting that other mechanisms of chemoattraction during flares of AD must exist. CCL27 binds to the chemokine receptor CCR10, which is expressed almost exclusively on CLA$^+$ lymphocytes (115). Blocking CCL27 with antibodies abrogates the migration of lymphocytes to the skin in a CCR4$^{-/-}$ murine model (117). Expression of CCL27 is under the control of NF-κB pathway, which plays a vital role in controlling inflammation through its regulation of transcription of chemokines and proinflammatory cytokines (118).

In a mouse model of AD, the Th2-selective chemokine, the Thymus and activation-regulated chemokine (TARC), is selectively induced by mechanical injury. NC/Nga mice spontaneously develop AD-like lesions and TARC is highly expressed in the basal epidermis with lesions, whereas it is not expressed in the skin without lesions (119). On the other hand, TARC augments TNF-α–induced CTACK production in keratinocytes (120). Similarly, the expression of macrophage-derived chemokine (MDC/CCL22) was increased several fold in the mouse skin with AD-like lesions (119). CCL22 level reflects the disease activity of AD, and it

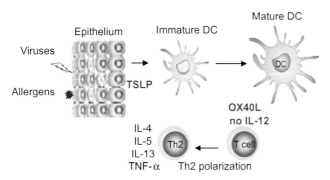

FIGURE 3 Thymic stromal lymphopoietin in T-cell differentiation. Thymic stromal lymphopoietin (TSLP) is an IL-7–like cytokine produced by epithelial cells, especially by keratinocytes. TSLP activate dendritic cell maturation to particularly dendritic cells that promote an inflammatory Th2 profile with TNF-α in naïve T cells. Expression of OX40L by TSLP-induced DCs trigger naïve CD4$^+$ T cells to produce IL-4, IL-5, IL-13, and TNF-α but not IL-10.

also plays an important role regarding the production of CCL22 in the pathogenesis of AD (121). Thymic stromal lymphopoietin (TSLP) is an IL-7–like cytokine highly expressed by keratinocytes in the lesions of acute and chronic AD. TSLP-treated CD11c$^+$ blood dendritic cells produce thymus and activation-regulated chemokine (TARC)/CCL17 and MDC (122). CD4$^+$ helper T cells as well as CD8$^+$ T cells (123) that are stimulated by TSLP-induced dendritic cells in an antigen-specific manner secrete a proallergic pattern of cytokines, that is, increased amounts of IL-4, IL-5, IL-13, and TNF-α, and reduced levels of IFN-γ and IL-10 (122). The high expression of TSLP is also associated with Langerhans cell migration and activation in situ as well. TSLP-induced dendritic cells mature and migrate into the draining lymph nodes to initiate the adaptive phase of allergic immune response. TSLP-induced dendritic cells express OX40L (124), which triggers the differentiation of allergen-specific naive CD4$^+$ T cells to inflammatory Th2 cells They can trigger this polarization even in the absence of IL-12. Afterwards, TARC and MDC recruit these Th2 cells to the site of inflammation (125). Thus, TSLP behaves as a master switch of allergic inflammation at the epithelial cell–dendritic cell interface (Fig. 3).

Eotaxin is a C-C chemokine and a potent activator of human eosinophils, basophils, and Th2 cells via the chemokine receptor CCR3. Immunohistologic staining and mRNA of eotaxin and its receptor CCR3 have been found to be significantly increased in lesional skin from AD but not in nonatopic controls. No significant difference in the expression of MCP-3, MIP-1α, and IL-8 has been observed between skin samples from AD patients and nonatopic controls (126). Also the role of TCIs in reducing the number of eosinophils in skin and suppressing the expression of eotaxin, CCR3, and RANTES has been reported (127).

IL-16 is a cytokine with selective chemotactic activity for CD4$^+$ T cells. An in situ hybridization study for IL-16 mRNA has demonstrated positive signals for IL-16 both in the basal layer of epidermis and in the dermis of AD skin samples (128). In addition, the numbers of epidermal and dermal IL-16 mRNA$^+$ cells were found significantly increased in acute in comparison to chronic AD skin lesions (128). Furthermore, the same study demonstrated that upregulation of IL-16 mRNA expression in acute AD was associated with increased numbers of CD4[+] cells. These results suggest that IL-16 may play a role in initiation of skin inflammation (128).

In the chronic stage of AD, the IFN-γ–induced chemokines particularly come to the scene. By IFN-γ stimulation, chemokines such as IFN-γ inducible protein-10 (IP-10), monokine induced by gamma-IFN (Mig), and IFN-γ inducible α-chemoattractant (iTac) are strongly upregulated in keratinocytes. These chemokines are highly upregulated in AD lesions and are assumed to attract T cells bearing the specific receptor CXCR3, which is highly expressed on T cells isolated from skin biopsies of AD patients towards the epidermis (129).

Transendothelial migration of skin-homing T cells was studied in a bilayer vascular construct consisting of a fibroblast matrix underneath an activated endothelial cell monolayer (103,130). Transmigration studies through IL-1β–activated and TNF-α–activated endothelium demonstrated that IL-8 and IL-8 receptor B, LFA1, and ICAM-1 were selectively involved in the enhanced transendothelial migration of CLA[+] T cells (130). Together these studies on chemokine network for skin homing of T cells demonstrate a complex system of different chemokines and chemokine receptors during different disease stages and for different T-cell subsets. The involvement of epidermal keratinocytes on the skin-homing process by releasing chemotactic substances requires further investigation. Similarly, the role of dendritic cells or Langerhans cells in generation of a chemokine network in the skin is not yet clearly elucidated.

EFFECTOR MECHANISMS IN AD

The Role of IL-5 and IL-13, IL-25, IL-31 and IL-33 in AD

Although most patients with AD show high concentrations of total and allergen-specific IgE in blood and skin, some of them express normal IgE levels and show no allergen-specific IgE antibodies. The diagnostic criteria of AD by Hanifin and Rajka (131) can also be fulfilled in the absence of elevated total IgE and specific IgE to food or environmental allergens. Even the atopy patch test can show that aeroallergens applied under occluded skin can induce a positive reaction in the absence of allergen specific-IgE (132). This suggests that elevated IgE levels and IgE sensitization are not prerequisites in the pathogenesis of the disease. The subgroup of AD patients with normal IgE levels and without specific IgE sensitization has been termed the nonatopic form of AD (NAD), nonatopic eczema, nonAD, or intrinsic-type AD (7,133). It has been suggested that T cells are likely involved in the pathogenesis of AD and NAD. CD4[+] and CD8[+] subsets of skin infiltrating T cells as well as skin homing CLA[+] T cells from peripheral blood, equally responded to superantigen, SEB, and produce IL-2, IL-5, IL-13, and IFN-γ in both forms of the disease (2,7). Interestingly, skin T cells from AD patients express higher IL-5 and IL-13 levels compared to NAD patients. Thus, T cells isolated from skin biopsies of AD, but not from the NAD, induced high IgE production in cocultures with normal B cells that is mediated by IL-13. In addition, B-cell activation with high CD23 expression is observed in the peripheral blood of AD, but not NAD patients (7). These findings suggest a lack of IL-13–induced B-cell activation and consequent IgE production in nonatopic eczema, although high numbers of T cells are present in lesional skin of both types (7). More importantly, IL-4 and IL-13 neutralization in B-cell cocultures with peripheral blood CLA[+] skin-homing T cells or skin-infiltrating T cells demonstrated that IL-13 represents the major cytokine for induction of hyper-IgE production in AD (2,7,10).

Cytokine determinations from peripheral blood CLA^+ T cells and skin biopsies of AD patients show increased IL-5 expression (2,7,54). Accordingly, supernatants from CLA^+ T cells of both $CD4^+$ and $CD8^+$ subsets extend the lifespan of freshly purified eosinophils in vitro, whereas supernatants of CLA^- T cells do not influence eosinophil survival. Neutralization of cytokines demonstrated the predominant role of CLA^+–T cell–IL-5 in prolonged eosinophil survival in AD (2).

IL-25, IL-31, and IL-33 represent novel targets to fight with Th2-mediated diseases. IL-25 (IL-17E) is a distinct member of the IL-17 cytokine family with important roles in triggering Th2 cell–mediated inflammation that features the infiltrations of eosinophils and Th2 memory cells (134). IL-25 promotes the initiation of Th2-type immune response against allergens and helminthes, which is mainly exerted by macrophages, eosinophils, and basophils (134,135). IL-31 is a novel T-cell cytokine that plays an important role in allergic skin inflammation and AD. IL-31 is associated with CLA^+ skin homing of T cells and also plays role in pruritus (136,137). Recently described cytokine IL-33 is a member of the IL-1 cytokine family, IL-1F11/IL-33. The four other members of the IL-1 cytokine family are IL-1a, IL-1b, IL-1 receptor antagonist, and IL-18. IL-33 is expressed on fibroblasts, smooth muscle cells, and epithelial cells of bronchus and small airways (138). IL-33 binds to IL-1 family receptor ST2, which is expressed by mast cells, Th2 cells, and eosinophils that may play important roles in eosinophil-mediated inflammation. Both IL-33 and its receptor may provide new therapeutic targets for controlling mucosal eosinophilic inflammation (139).

THE ROLE OF REGULATORY T CELLS IN AD

During the last decade, the concept of Treg cell–mediated immune suppression has been extensively explored. Two subsets of Treg cells with distinct phenotypes and mechanisms of action have been described (Fig. 4). Naturally occurring Treg cells are characterized by their $CD4^+CD25^+$ phenotype and have been suggested to develop under the control of the transcription factor FoxP3 (140). The second subset, the inducible Treg or T-regulatory type 1 (Tr1) cells are characterized by their secretion of high levels of IL-10 with or without TGF-β (141,142). They develop in the periphery under the influence of presumably immature dendritic cells (143) and/or in the presence of IL-10 and TGF-β, but also immunosuppressive drugs like glucocorticoids and vitamin D3 (144), and operate in a cytokine-mediated manner. In addition to these above-mentioned subsets, some of $CD8^+$ T cells, gammadelta T cells, dendritic cells, IL-10–producing B cells, natural killer (NK) cells, and resident tissue cells, which may promote the generation of Treg cells, can contribute to suppressive and regulatory events in inflammation (145).

To date a significant amount of data have accumulated on the role of Treg cells in the development of allergic diseases (146,147). However, there are still few studies evaluating the role of Treg cells in the pathogenesis of AD. Most research on the inhibitory capacities of Treg cells has focused on their ability to suppress proliferation of effector T cells. It can be speculated that regulatory T cells of either Tr1 or $CD4^+CD25^+$ Treg phenotype can suppress antigen-specific activation of T cells both in initial and reactivation stages of AD. The efficacy of both $CD4^+CD25^+$ Treg cells and Tr1 cells in the suppression of inflammation has engendered scientists to speculate that increasing Treg cell numbers may suppress an ongoing inflammation. It

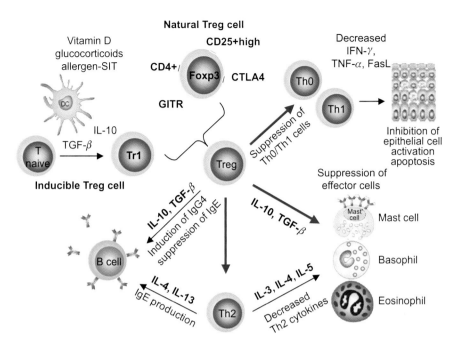

FIGURE 4 T regulatoy cells and allergy. Treg cells have immunosuppressive functions and cytokine profiles distinct from that of either Th1 or Th2 cells. Regulatory T cells are classified as naturally occurring and inducible Treg cells. Naturally occurring Treg cells express CD4, CD25high, GITR (glucocorticoid-induced TNFR-related protein), and CTLA-4 (intracytoplastimc T lymphocyte–associated antigen-4) in the outside membrane, and Foxp3 in the nucleus. The second subset, the inducible Treg or T-regulatory type 1 (Tr1) cells, is characterized by their secretion of high levels of IL-10. Tr1 cells develop in the periphery under the influence of presumably immature dendritic cells. Treg cell response is characterized by an abolished allergen-specific T-cell proliferation and the suppressed secretion of Th1- and Th2-type cytokines. Treg cells are able to inhibit the development of allergen-specific Th2 and Th1 cell responses and therefore play an important role in healthy immune response to allergens. Treg cells potently suppress IgE production and directly or indirectly suppress the activity of effector cells of allergic inflammation, such as eosinophils, basophils, and mast cells. In patients with atopic dermatitis, there is an increased pool of circulating regulatory T cells. Skin biopsies in AD patients also revealed overexpression of IL-10 and TGF-β but not CD4+CD25+. The efficacy of both CD4+CD25+ Treg cells and Tr1 cells in the suppression of inflammation has engendered the idea that migration of increased numbers of Treg cells to the inflammation area, or the induction of their local proliferation, may be beneficial in the treatment AD.

has been tempting to speculate that migration of increased numbers of Treg cells to the inflammation area, or the induction of their local proliferation, may be beneficial in the treatment of several inflammatory diseases, including AD.

   The idea supporting a possible role of Treg cells in AD has arisen as the dysfunction in CD4+CD25+ T-regulatory cell-specific transcription factor FoxP3, which acts as a master switch gene for Treg cell development and function (148), leads to immune dysregulation, polyendocrinopathy, enteropathy X-linked (IPEX) syndrome, often associates with AD (149). This suggests that there may be an essential role for CD4+CD25+FoxP3+ Treg cells in controlling inflammation of the skin, a system apparently malfunctioning in AD. There is an increased pool of circulating regulatory T cells in AD. It has previously been reported that the AD patients have more CD4$^+$CD25$^+$ Treg cells in peripheral blood samples than healthy control subjects (42). In association with Treg cells, overexpression of IL-10 was previously described in AD (150), and all isoforms of TGF-β have been described to be expressed in nonaffected skin, with an upregulation during wound repair (151). Recently, the presence and function of Treg cells in AD lesional skin was investigated. It was reported that the expression of IL-10, in addition to TGF-β receptor, is high in AD. Immunohistochemical analyses of lesional skin biopsies of AD patients revealed the presence of IL-10–secreting Tr1 cells, but not FoxP3$^+$CD4$^+$CD25$^+$ T cells (152). Devoid of functional Treg cells in skin lesions suggest an imbalance in T-cell regulation (152).

The role of IL-10–secreting Tr1 and CD4$^+$CD25$^+$ Treg cells in the control of keratinocyte apoptosis in AD is another important question to be clarified to understand the pathogenesis of the disease. This issue has been analyzed in both cell-to-cell contact and cytokine-mediated levels. Despite the presence of a considerable amount of IL-10–secreting Tr1 cells in lesional AD skin, isolated T cells from AD lesions induced apoptosis of keratinocytes. Studies on isolated Tr1 cells from peripheral blood of healthy donors have rendered that these cells and their cytokines IL-10 and TGF-β and CD4+CD25+ Treg cells do not have any suppressive role in already activated T-cell–induced keratinocyte apoptosis (152).

T HELPER 17 CELLS IN AD

T helper 17 cells (Th17) are subsets of Th cells that are distinct from Th1 and Th2 cells, with IL-17 producing capacity and mediate a variety of autoimmune diseases (153). IL-17 family cytokines (IL-17A to F) induce various signaling molecules and have crucial functions in immune regulation. Most notably, IL-17 coordinates local tissue inflammation through upregulation of proinflammatory cytokines and chemokines. IL-6 and TGF-β are necessary for induction of Th17 cells (154,155). These cells also participate in the pathogenesis of skin disorders. IL-17 plays a role in enhancing GM-CSF, TNF-α, IL-8, and vascular endothelial growth factor (VEGF) production by keratinocytes (156). IL-22, which belongs to IL-10 family, is expressed by Th17 cells. Its receptor is also expressed on various epithelial tissues (157). Koga et al. have recently evaluated the role of Th17 cells in AD and reported an increased percentage of IL-17$^+$CD4$^+$ T cells in PBMCs from severe AD patients. In immunohistochemical analyses, IL-17$^+$ cells infiltrating the papillary dermis are more marked in the acute than chronic lesions (156). Further studies will shed light on our current knowledge on Th17 cell–AD interaction.

DYSREGULATED APOPTOSIS IS A KEY PATHOGENETIC FACTOR IN AD

Increased Th1 Cell Apoptosis As a Mechanism of Th2 Predominance in Atopy

Although the death of certain cells can lead to functional deficiencies, prolonged survival of some effector cells can cause tissue injury and play a role on the pathogenesis of disease (158). Cell death by apoptosis is tightly regulated process that enables removal of unnecessary, aged, or damaged cells. During apoptosis a complex death program is initiated that ultimately leads to phagocytosis of the apoptotic cell. An interaction of specific receptors, termed *death receptors*, with their ligands is required for this process in which Fas (CD95) and Fas-ligand (CD178) interactions are essential for activation-induced cell death (AICD) of $CD4^+$ T cells (159–161). Interaction of Fas-ligand with Fas leads to the activation of cysteine proteases of the caspase family. This oligomerization triggers the activation of caspase-8 and caspase-3 (161). It has been demonstrated that caspase-3 expression levels are selectively upregulated in effector T cells, a population susceptible to AICD, which is dependent on early signaling events mediated by the TCR (162).

To assure self-tolerance and downregulation of an immune response, the elimination of T cells takes place in the periphery and involves induction of apoptosis (163). During the development of the immune response, T cells are stimulated by antigens presented by antigen-presenting cells that lead to T-cell activation and clonal expansion. Some of the activated T cells die by activation-induced T cell death under certain conditions (164). As stated before, circulating CLA^+ $CD45RO^+$ T cells with skin-specific homing property represent an activated memory/effector T-cell subset in AD (4). These cells express high levels of Fas and Fas ligand and undergo AICD, which is thought to play an important role in maintaining homeostasis of the immune response and prevention of excessive immune reactivity. Activated T cells can kill themselves (suicide) and other cells in the environment in a fratricidal way (159,165,166). Freshly purified CLA^+ $CD45RO^+$ T cells of atopic individuals displayed distinct features of in vivo triggered apoptosis such as procaspase degradation and active caspase-8 formation (4). The apoptosis of circulating CLA^+ memory/effector T cells was confined to atopic individuals, whereas nonatopic patients such as those with psoriasis, intrinsic-type asthma, contact dermatitis, intrinsic-type AD, and bee venom allergy, and healthy controls did not show any evidence for increased T-cell apoptosis. Hence, apoptosis is a powerful mechanism for deleting highly activated T cells; it raises the interesting possibility that unequal apoptosis of Th1 and Th2 effector cells may lead to preferential deletion of one subset over the other. Recently, it was demonstrated that Th1 cell apoptosis, particularly apoptosis of high IFN-γ–producing fraction of T cells, is much more prominent in atopic patients compared with healthy controls as a mechanism of Th2 predominance (167).

Differences in control of lifespan was observed between peripheral blood CLA^+ T cells and T cells infiltrating the eczema lesions. In peripheral blood of AD patients both $CD4^+$ and $CD8^+$ subsets of CLA^+ $CD45RO^+$ T cells expressed upregulated Fas and Fas ligand and undergo spontaneous AICD. CLA^- $CD45RO^+$ T cells are in a resting state, do not express Fas and Fas ligand, and are resistant to anti-Fas mAb-induced apoptosis (4). In contrast, T cells infiltrating the skin of AD patients expressed both Fas and Fas ligand; however, they do not show any signs of apoptosis in vivo suggesting prolonged survival in dermis. Apoptosis of CLA^+ $CD45RO^+$ T cells is inhibited by IL-2, IL-4, IL-15 as cytokines; fibronectin, tenascin, laminin, and collagen IV as extracellular matrix proteins (ECM), and transferrin demonstrating a multifactorial survival of skin infiltrating T cells in the tissue (4). Together, these results demonstrate the control of in vivo activated skin-homing T cell numbers in peripheral blood with increased apoptosis; in contrast, T-cell apoptosis is prevented by cytokines and extracellular matrix components in the eczematous skin.

Inflammatory cells reside in a protein network in the tissues, the ECM, which exerts a profound control over them. The effects of ECM are primarily mediated by integrins, a family of cell surface receptors that attach cells to the matrix and mediate mechanical and chemical signals from it. Many ECM signals converge on cell cycle regulation, directing cells to live or die, to proliferate, or to differentiate. Integrins can recognize several ECM proteins; conversely, individual ECM proteins can bind to several integrins (168). Most of the previous studies have concentrated on signaling pathways activated by integrins in adherent cells. Adherent cells must be anchored to an appropriate ECM to survive (169). During inflammation, leukocytes migrate into the affected tissue interacting with extracellular matrix proteins. Cell adhesion to the extracellular matrix has been implicated in protection from apoptosis in anchorage-dependent cell types. Apparently, integrin signaling by ECM represents an important survival signal in T cells, although they do not require anchorage in the tissues. Integrins activate various protein tyrosine kinases, including focal adhesion kinase (FAK), Src family kinases, Abl, a serine threonine kinase, and integrin-linked kinase (170,171). In AD skin, T cells express both Fas and Fas ligand but they are resistant to apoptosis. FAK appears to play a major role in conveying survival signals from the ECM (76,172). This is because FAK binds to phosphatidylinositol 3 (PI3)-kinase and the protective effect against apoptosis may be the result of PI3-kinase–mediated activation of protein kinase B (173).

In addition to ECM proteins, IL-2, IL-4, and IL-15 also prevent T-cell apoptosis (4). The common γc-chain is an essential signaling component shared by IL-2, IL-4, and IL-15 receptors as well as all other known T-cell growth factor receptors. IL-15 shares many biologic activities with IL-2 and signals through the IL-2 receptor β- and γ-chains (174). However, IL-15 and IL-2 differ in their controls of expression and secretion, their range of target cells, and their functional activities. IL-2 induces or inhibits T-cell apoptosis in vitro depending on T-cell activation, whereas IL-15 inhibits cytokine deprivation-induced apoptosis in activated T cells (161). Furthermore, blocking the γc-chain in mice inhibits T-cell proliferation and induces T-cell apoptosis that induces stable allograft survival (175).

Keratinocyte Apoptosis As a Mechanism of Spongiosis and Eczema in AD

The histologic hallmark of eczematous disorders is characterized by marked keratinocyte pathology. Spongiosis in the epidermis is identified by impairment or loss of cohesion between KC and the influx of fluid from dermis, sometimes progressing to vesicle formation. A study by Trautmann et al. delineated activated skin-infiltrating T-cell–induced epidermal keratinocyte apoptosis as a key pathogenic event in eczematous disorders (5). IFN-γ released from activated T cells upregulate Fas (CD95) on keratinocytes, which renders them susceptible to apoptosis. When the Fas number on keratinocytes reaches a threshold of approximately 40,000 Fas molecules per keratinocyte, the cells become susceptible to apoptosis. Keratinocytes exhibit a relatively low threshold for IFN-γ–induced Fas expression (0.1–1 ng/mL). This requirement is substantially achieved by low IFN-γ secreting T cells that also produce high amounts of IL-5 and IL-13 and thereby contribute to eosinophilia and IgE production (5). The lethal hit is delivered to keratinocytes by Fas ligand expressed on the surface of T cells that invade the epidermis and soluble Fas ligand released from T cells. In these studies, the involvement of cytokines other than IFN-γ was eliminated by experiments with different cytokines and anticytokine neutralizing antibodies. In addition, apoptosis pathways other than the Fas-pathway were ruled out by blocking T-cell–induced keratinocyte apoptosis with caspase inhibitors and soluble Fas-Fc protein. Keratinocyte apoptosis was demonstrated in situ in lesional eczematous skin and patch test lesions of both AD and allergic contact dermatitis. Exposure of normal human skin and cultured skin equivalents to activated

T cells demonstrated that keratinocyte apoptosis caused by skin infiltrating T cells represents a key event in the pathogenesis of eczematous dermatitis (5). Although allergic contact dermatitis and drug-induced skin rashes are not related to AD, the mechanism of epidermal injury shows histopathologic similarities. An exaggerated T-cell response to small-molecular-weight haptens plays a role in allergic contact dermatitis. It was demonstrated that keratinocytes could be the target of multiple hapten-specific cytotoxic T-cell responses, which play a role in epidermal injury during allergic contact dermatitis (176). Both nickel-reactive CD4$^+$ and CD8$^+$ T cells were exclusively cytotoxic against resting keratinocytes and IFN-γ treatment rendered keratinocytes susceptible to Th1 cytotoxicity. In addition, both Fas and perforin pathways play a role in keratinocyte killing (176). T-cell–mediated cytotoxicity against keratinocytes has also been studied in sulfamethoxazol-induced skin reactions (177). In addition, sulfamethoxazol-specific both CD4$^+$ and CD8$^+$ T cells expressed high perforin, and IFN-γ–pretreated keratinocytes were predominantly killed by CD4$^+$ T cells (177).

These studies demonstrate that both CD4$^+$ and CD8$^+$ T cells may play a role in keratinocyte injury according to their activation status. A direct contact of T cell to keratinocyte is not always required, and soluble Fas ligand released from activated T cells can also induce keratinocyte apoptosis if keratinocytes are susceptible to apoptosis. IFN-γ appears to be a decisive cytokine to render keratinocytes susceptible to apoptosis (5,176,177). Mice studies also provide evidence for the role of IFN-γ in eczema formation. IFN-γ knockout mice show significantly decreased allergic eczema formation (44,83) and transgenic mice expressing IFN-γ in the epidermis spontaneously developed eczema (178).

CONCLUSION

Activation and skin-selective homing of peripheral-blood T cells and effector functions in the skin represent sequential immunologic events in the pathogenesis of AD (Fig. 1). The CLA molecule represents a homing receptor involved in selective migration of memory/effector T cells to the skin. CLA is expressed on Th1 cells during the differentiation process and can be induced on Th2 cells by TcR stimulation. Both CD4$^+$ and CD8$^+$ T cells bearing CLA represent activated memory/effector T cell subsets in peripheral blood of AD patients. They induce IgE mainly by IL-13 and prolong eosinophil life span mainly by IL-5. On the other hand, the presence of IL-10–secreting Tr1 cells, but not FoxP3$^+$CD4$^+$CD25$^+$ T cells refers to devoid of functional regulatory T cells in infiltrate skin lesions, which demonstrates an imbalance in T-cell regulation. A chemokine network involving T cells, dendritic cells, and keratinocytes control the infiltration of inflammatory cells into AD skin. Dysregulated apoptosis in skin-infiltrating T cells and epidermal keratinocytes contributes to the elicitation and progress of AD. Activation-induced T-cell apoptosis plays a role in the control of circulating skin-homing memory/effector T cell numbers in peripheral blood. In contrast, T-cell apoptosis is prevented by cytokines and extracellular matrix components in the eczematous skin to form dermal T cell infiltrates and mediate effector functions. These activated T cells induce keratinocyte apoptosis via the Fas-dependent pathway representing a key pathogenetic factor in the formation of eczematous lesions. In this context, future studies for treatment of AD should be directed to T cells by inhibition of various modes of activation, inhibition of skin-homing, and inhibition of certain cytokines/chemokines that play a role in the pathogenesis. The immunoregulatory role of histamine and other mediators and novel cytokines such as IL-17, IL-22, IL-25, IL-26, IL-31, and IL-33 should be taken into consideration. The knowledge of the molecular basis of dysregulated apoptosis is pivotal in understanding the pathology in AD and may lead to more focused therapeutic applications in the future.

ACKNOWLEDGMENTS

The authors' laboratories are funded by the Swiss National Science Foundation (grants No. SNF-32–112306/1, 32–118226) and Global Allergy and Asthma European Network (GA²LEN).

REFERENCES

1. Akdis CA. Mechanisms of allergic disease. Curr Opin Immunol 2006; 18:718–726.
2. Akdis M, Simon HU, Weigl L, et al. Skin homing (cutaneous lymphocyte-associated antigen-positive) CD8 + T cells respond to superantigen and contribute to eosinophilia and igE production in atopic dermatitis. J Immunol 1999; 163:466–475.
3. Wollenberg A, Klein E. Current aspects of innate and adaptive immunity in atopic dermatitis. Clin Rev Allergy Immunol 2007; 33:35–44.
4. Akdis M, Trautmann A, Klunker S, et al. T helper (Th) 2 predominance in atopic diseases is due to preferential apoptosis of circulating memory/effector Th1 cells. FASEB J 2003; 17:1026–1035.
5. Trautmann A, Akdis M, Kleemann D, et al. T cell-mediated Fas-induced keratinocyte apoptosis plays a key pathogenetic role in eczematous dermatitis. J Clin Invest 2000; 106:25–35.
6. Schmid-Grendelmeier P, Simon D, Simon HU, et al. Epidemiology, clinical features, and immunology of the "intrinsic" (non-igE-mediated) type of atopic dermatitis (constitutional dermatitis). Allergy 2001; 56:841–849.
7. Akdis CA, Akdis M, Simon D, et al. T cells and T cell-derived cytokines as pathogenic factors in the nonallergic form of atopic dermatitis. J Invest Dermatol 1999; 113:628–634.
8. Weidinger S, O'Sullivan M, Illig T, et al. Filaggrin mutations, atopic eczema, hay fever, and asthma in children. J Allergy Clin Immunol 2008; 121:1203–1209 , E 1201.
9. Akdis CA, Akdis M, Trautmann A, et al. Immune regulation in atopic dermatitis. Curr Opin Immunol 2000; 12:641–646.
10. Akdis M, Akdis CA, Weigl L, et al. CLA+ memory T cells are activated in atopic dermatitis and regulate igE by an IL-13-dominated cytokine pattern: IgG4 counter-regulation by CLA− memory T cells. J Immunol 1997; 159:4611–4619.
11. Santamaria Babi LF, Picker LJ, Perez Soler MT, et al. Circulating allergen-reactive T cells from patients with atopic dermatitis and allergic contact dermatitis express the skin-selective homing receptor, the cutaneous lymphocyte-associated antigen. J Exp Med 1995; 181:1935–1940.
12. Shimada Y, Sato S, Hasegawa M, et al. Elevated serum L-selectin levels and abnormal regulation of L-selectin expression on leukocytes in atopic dermatitis: Soluble L-selectin levels indicate disease severity. J Allergy Clin Immunol 1999; 104:163–168.
13. Picker LJ, Terstappen LW, Rott LS, et al. Differential expression of homing-associated adhesion molecules by T cell subsets in man. J Immunol 1990; 145:3247–3255.
14. Akdis M, Klunker S, Schliz M, et al. Expression of cutaneous lymphocyte-associated antigen on human CD4(+) and CD8(+) Th2 cells. Eur J Immunol 2000; 30:3533–3541.
15. Leung DY, Gately M, Trumble A, et al. Bacterial superantigens induce T cell expression of the skin-selective homing receptor, the cutaneous lymphocyte-associated antigen, via stimulation of interleukin 12 production. J Exp Med 1995; 181:747–753.
16. Hoetzenecker W, Ecker R, Kopp T, et al. Pimecrolimus leads to an apoptosis-induced depletion of T cells but not langerhans cells in patients with atopic dermatitis. J Allergy Clin Immunol 2005; 115:1276–1283.

17. Van Reijsen FC, Bruijnzeel-Koomen CA, Kalthoff FS, et al. Skin-derived aeroallergen-specific T-cell clones of Th2 phenotype in patients with atopic dermatitis. J Allergy Clin Immunol 1992; 90:184–193.
18. Varney VA, Hamid QA, Gaga M, et al. Influence of grass pollen immunotherapy on cellular infiltration and cytokine mRNA expression during allergen-induced late-phase cutaneous responses. J Clin Invest 1993; 92:644–651.
19. Werfel T, Morita A, Grewe M, et al. Allergen specificity of skin-infiltrating T cells is not restricted to a type-2 cytokine pattern in chronic skin lesions of atopic dermatitis. J Invest Dermatol 1996; 107:871–876.
20. Frew AJ, Kay AB. The relationship between infiltrating CD4+ lymphocytes, activated eosinophils, and the magnitude of the allergen-induced late phase cutaneous reaction in man. J Immunol 1988; 141:4158–4164.
21. Abernathy-Carver KJ, Sampson HA, Picker LJ, et al. Milk-induced eczema is associated with the expansion of T cells expressing cutaneous lymphocyte antigen. J Clin Invest 1995; 95:913–918.
22. Kerschenlohr K, Decard S, Darsow U, et al. Clinical and immunologic reactivity to aeroallergens in "intrinsic" atopic dermatitis patients. J Allergy Clin Immunol 2003; 111:195–197.
23. Denkers EY, Caspar P, Sher A. Toxoplasma gondii possesses a superantigen activity that selectively expands murine T cell receptor V beta 5-bearing CD8 + lymphocytes. J Exp Med 1994; 180:985–994.
24. Chou MC, Lee SC, Lin YS, et al. V beta 8 + CD4−CD8− subpopulation induced by staphylococcal enterotoxin B. Immunol Lett 1997; 55:85–91.
25. Mothes N, Niggemann B, Jenneck C, et al. The cradle of igE autoreactivity in atopic eczema lies in early infancy. J Allergy Clin Immunol 2005; 116:706–709.
26. Natter S, Seiberler S, Hufnagl P, et al. Isolation of cDNA clones coding for igE autoantigens with serum igE from atopic dermatitis patients. FASEB J 1998; 12:1559–1569.
27. Valenta R, Seiberler S, Natter S, et al. Autoallergy: A pathogenetic factor in atopic dermatitis? J Allergy Clin Immunol 2000; 105:432–437.
28. Schmitt DA, Bieber T, Cazenave JP, et al. Fc receptors of human Langerhans cells. J Invest Dermatol 1990; 94:15S–21S.
29. Frohm M, Agerberth B, Ahangari G, et al. The expression of the gene coding for the antibacterial peptide LL-37 is induced in human keratinocytes during inflammatory disorders. J Biol Chem 1997; 272:15258–15263.
30. Harder J, Bartels J, Christophers E, et al. A peptide antibiotic from human skin. Nature 1997; 387:861.
31. Nizet V, Ohtake T, Lauth X, et al. Innate antimicrobial peptide protects the skin from invasive bacterial infection. Nature 2001; 414:454–457.
32. Ong PY, Ohtake T, Brandt C, et al. Endogenous antimicrobial peptides and skin infections in atopic dermatitis. N Engl J Med 2002; 347:1151–1160.
33. Morishita Y, Tada J, Sato A, et al. Possible influences of *Staphylococcus aureus* on atopic dermatitis—The colonizing features and the effects of staphylococcal enterotoxins. Clin Exp Allergy 1999; 29:1110–1117.
34. Leyden JJ, Marples RR, Kligman AM. *Staphylococcus aureus* in the lesions of atopic dermatitis. Br J Dermatol 1974; 90:525–530.
35. Strange P, Skov L, Lisby S, et al. Staphylococcal enterotoxin B applied on intact normal and intact atopic skin induces dermatitis. Arch Dermatol 1996; 132:27–33.
36. Herz U, Schnoy N, Borelli S, et al. A human-SCID mouse model for allergic immune response bacterial superantigen enhances skin inflammation and suppresses igE production. J Invest Dermatol 1998; 110:224–231.
37. Leung DY, Harbeck R, Bina P, et al. Presence of igE antibodies to staphylococcal exotoxins on the skin of patients with atopic dermatitis. Evidence for a New Group of Allergens. J Clin Invest 1993; 92:1374–1380.
38. Mandron M, Aries MF, Brehm RD, et al. Human dendritic cells conditioned with *Staphylococcus aureus* enterotoxin B promote Th2 cell polarization. J Allergy Clin Immunol 2006; 117:1141–1147.

39. Kang K, Kubin M, Cooper KD, et al. IL-12 synthesis by human Langerhans cells. J Immunol 1996; 156:1402–1407.
40. Lim YC, Henault L, Wagers AJ, et al. Expression of functional selectin ligands on Th cells is differentially regulated by IL-12 and IL-4. J Immunol 1999; 162:3193–3201.
41. Leung DY, Pober JS, Cotran RS. Expression of endothelial-leukocyte adhesion molecule-1 in elicited late phase allergic reactions. J Clin Invest 1991; 87:1805–1809.
42. Ou LS, Goleva E, Hall C, et al. T regulatory cells in atopic dermatitis and subversion of their activity by superantigens. J Allergy Clin Immunol 2004; 113:756–763.
43. Cardona ID, Goleva E, Ou LS, et al. Staphylococcal enterotoxin B inhibits regulatory T cells by inducing glucocorticoid-induced TNF receptor-related protein ligand on monocytes. J Allergy Clin Immunol 2006; 117:688–695.
44. Hauk PJ, Leung DY. Tacrolimus (FK506): New treatment approach in superantigen-associated diseases like atopic dermatitis? J Allergy Clin Immunol 2001; 107:391–392.
45. Schlievert PM, Case LC, Strandberg KL, et al. Superantigen profile of *Staphylococcus aureus* isolates from patients with steroid-resistant atopic dermatitis. Clin Infect Dis 2008; 46:1562–1567.
46. Schmid-Grendelmeier P, Fluckiger S, Disch R, et al. IgE-mediated and T cell-mediated autoimmunity against manganese superoxide dismutase in atopic dermatitis. J Allergy Clin Immunol 2005; 115:1068–1075.
47. Appenzeller U, Meyer C, Menz G, et al. IgE-mediated reactions to autoantigens in allergic diseases. Int Arch Allergy Immunol 1999; 118:193–196.
48. Valenta R, Duchene M, Pettenburger K, et al. Identification of profilin as a novel pollen allergen; igE autoreactivity in sensitized individuals. Science 1991; 253:557–560.
49. Mittermann I, Aichberger KJ, Bunder R, et al. Autoimmunity and atopic dermatitis. Curr Opin Allergy Clin Immunol 2004; 4:367–371.
50. Aichberger KJ, Mittermann I, Reininger R, et al. Hom S 4, an IgE-reactive autoantigen belonging to a new subfamily of calcium-binding proteins, can induce Th cell type 1-mediated autoreactivity. J Immunol 2005; 175:1286–1294.
51. Mittermann I, Reininger R, Zimmermann M, et al. The ige-reactive autoantigen Hom s 2 induces damage of respiratory epithelial cells and keratinocytes via induction of IFN-gamma. J Invest Dermatol 2008; 128:1451–1459.
52. Konur A, Schulz U, Eissner G, et al. Interferon (IFN)-gamma is a main mediator of keratinocyte (HaCaT) apoptosis and contributes to autocrine IFN-gamma and tumour necrosis factor-alpha production. Br J Dermatol 2005; 152:1134–1142.
53. Leung DY. Atopic Dermatitis: New insights and opportunities for therapeutic intervention. J Allergy Clin Immunol 2000; 105:860–876.
54. Hamid Q, Boguniewicz M, Leung DY. Differential in situ cytokine gene expression in acute versus chronic atopic dermatitis. J Clin Invest 1994; 94:870–876.
55. Kurahashi R, Hatano Y, Katagiri K. IL-4 suppresses the recovery of cutaneous permeability barrier functions in vivo. J Invest Dermatol 2008; 128:1329–1331.
56. Grewe M, Bruijnzeel-Koomen CA, Schopf E, et al. A role for Th1 and Th2 cells in the immunopathogenesis of atopic dermatitis. Immunol Today 1998; 19:359–361.
57. Thepen T, Langeveld-Wildschut EG, Bihari IC, et al. Biphasic response against aeroallergen in atopic dermatitis showing a switch from an initial Th2 response to a Th1 response in situ: An Immunocytochemical Study. J Allergy Clin Immunol 1996; 97:828–837.
58. Grewe M, Czech W, Morita A, et al. Human eosinophils produce biologically active IL-12: Implications for control of T cell responses. J Immunol 1998; 161:415–420.
59. Muller G, Saloga J, Germann T, et al. Identification and induction of human keratinocyte-derived IL-12. J Clin Invest 1994; 94:1799–1805.
60. Stoll S, Jonuleit H, Schmitt E, et al. Production of functional IL-18 by different subtypes of murine and human dendritic cells (DC): DC-derived IL-18 enhances IL-12-dependent Th1 development. Eur J Immunol 1998; 28:3231–3239.
61. Yawalkar N, Hunger RE, Pichler WJ, et al. Human afferent lymph from normal skin contains an increased number of mainly memory/effector CD4(+) T cells expressing activation, adhesion and co-stimulatory molecules. Eur J Immunol 2000; 30: 491–497.

62. Wollenberg A, Kraft S, Hanau D, et al. Immunomorphological and ultrastructural characterization of Langerhans cells and a novel, inflammatory dendritic epidermal cell (IDEC) population in lesional skin of atopic eczema. J Invest Dermatol 1996; 106:446–453.

63. Novak N, Bieber T. The role of dendritic cell subtypes in the pathophysiology of atopic dermatitis. J Am Acad Dermatol 2005; 53:S171–S176.

64. Bieber T, Braun-Falco O. IgE-bearing langerhans cells are not specific to atopic eczema but are found in inflammatory skin diseases. J Am Acad Dermatol 1991; 24:658–659.

65. Schuller E, Teichmann B, Haberstok J, et al. In situ expression of the costimulatory molecules CD80 and CD86 on langerhans cells and inflammatory dendritic epidermal cells (IDEC) in atopic dermatitis. Arch Dermatol Res 2001; 293:448–454.

66. Wollenberg A, Wen S, Bieber T. Phenotyping of epidermal dendritic cells: Clinical applications of a flow cytometric micromethod. Cytometry 1999; 37:147–155.

67. Kehry MR, Yamashita LC. Low-affinity IgE receptor (CD23) function on mouse B cells: Role in IgE-dependent antigen focusing. Proc Natl Acad Sci U S A 1989; 86:7556–7560.

68. Kinet JP. Atopic allergy and other hypersensitivities. Curr Opin Immunol 1999; 11:603–605.

69. Stingl G, Maurer D. IgE-mediated allergen presentation via Fc epsilon RI on antigen-presenting cells. Int Arch Allergy Immunol 1997; 113:24–29.

70. Maurer D, Stingl G. Immunoglobulin E-binding structures on antigen-presenting cells present in skin and blood. J Invest Dermatol 1995; 104:707–710.

71. Maurer D, Ebner C, Reininger B, et al. The high affinity IgE receptor (Fc Epsilon RI) mediates IgE-dependent allergen presentation. J Immunol 1995; 154:6285–6290.

72. Pirron U, Schlunck T, Prinz JC, et al. IgE-dependent antigen focusing by human B lymphocytes is mediated by the low-affinity receptor for IgE. Eur J Immunol 1990; 20:1547–1551.

73. Santamaria LF, Bheekha R, Van Reijsen FC et al. Antigen focusing by specific monomeric immunoglobulin E bound to CD23 on Epstein-Barr virus-transformed B cells. Hum Immunol 1993; 37:23–30.

74. Van Der Heijden FL, Joost Van Neerven RJ, Van Katwijk M, et al. Serum-IgE-facilitated allergen presentation in atopic disease. J Immunol 1993; 150:3643–3650.

75. Van Neerven RJ, Wikborg T, Lund G, et al. Blocking antibodies induced by specific allergy vaccination prevent the activation of CD4+ T cells by inhibiting serum-IgE-facilitated allergen presentation. J Immunol 1999; 163:2944–2952.

76. Bieber T. The pro- and anti-inflammatory properties of human antigen-presenting cells expressing the high affinity receptor for IgE (Fc Epsilon RI). Immunobiology 2007; 212:499–503.

77. Novak N, Bieber T, Katoh N. Engagement of Fc epsilon RI on human monocytes induces the production of IL-10 and prevents their differentiation in dendritic cells. J Immunol 2001; 167:797–804.

78. Achatz G, Nitschke L, Lamers MC. Effect of transmembrane and cytoplasmic domains of IgE on the IgE response. Science 1997; 276:409–411.

79. Fahy JV, Fleming HE, Wong HH, et al. The effect of an anti-IgE monoclonal antibody on the early- and late-phase responses to allergen inhalation in asthmatic subjects. Am J Respir Crit Care Med 1997; 155:1828–1834.

80. Coyle AJ, Wagner K, Bertrand C, et al. Central role of immunoglobulin (Ig) E in the induction of lung eosinophil infiltration and T helper 2 cell cytokine production: Inhibition by a non-anaphylactogenic anti-IgE antibody. J Exp Med 1996; 183:1303–1310.

81. Heusser C, Jardieu P. Therapeutic potential of anti-IgE antibodies. Curr Opin Immunol 1997; 9:805–813.

82. Belloni B, Ziai M, Lim A, et al. Low-dose anti-IgE therapy in patients with atopic eczema with high serum IgE levels. J Allergy Clin Immunol 2007; 120:1223–1225.

83. Spergel JM, Mizoguchi E, Oettgen H, et al. Roles of Th1 and Th2 cytokines in a murine model of allergic dermatitis. J Clin Invest 1999; 103:1103–1111.

84. Akdis CA, Simons FE. Histamine receptors are hot in immunopharmacology. Eur J Pharmacol 2006; 533:69–76.

85. Jutel M, Watanabe T, Klunker S, et al. Histamine regulates T-cell and antibody responses by differential expression of H1 and H2 receptors. Nature 2001; 413:420–425.
86. Oda T, Morikawa N, Saito Y, et al. Molecular cloning and characterization of a novel type of histamine receptor preferentially expressed in leukocytes. J Biol Chem 2000; 275:36781–36786.
87. Thurmond RL, Gelfand EW, Dunford PJ. The role of histamine H1 and H4 receptors in allergic inflammation: The search for new antihistamines. Nat Rev Drug Discov 2008; 7:41–53.
88. Bayram H, Devalia JL, Khair OA, et al. Effect of loratadine on nitrogen dioxide-induced changes in electrical resistance and release of inflammatory mediators from cultured human bronchial epithelial cells. J Allergy Clin Immunol 1999; 104:93–99.
89. Jeannin P, Delneste Y, Gosset P, et al. Histamine induces interleukin-8 secretion by endothelial cells. Blood 1994; 84:2229–2233.
90. Meretey K, Falus A, Taga T, et al. Histamine influences the expression of the interleukin-6 receptor on human lymphoid, monocytoid and hepatoma cell lines. Agents Actions 1991; 33:189–191.
91. Vannier E, Dinarello CA. Histamine enhances interleukin (IL)-1-induced IL-1 gene expression and protein synthesis via H2 receptors in peripheral blood mononuclear cells. Comparison with IL-1 receptor antagonist. J Clin Invest 1993; 92:281–287.
92. Fujikura T, Shimosawa T, Yakuo I. Regulatory effect of histamine H1 receptor antagonist on the expression of messenger RNA encoding CC chemokines in the human nasal mucosa. J Allergy Clin Immunol 2001; 107:123–128.
93. Berclaz PY, Shibata Y, Whitsett JA, et al. Regulates alveolar macrophage Fcgamma R-mediated phagocytosis and the IL-18/IFN-gamma-mediated molecular connection between innate and adaptive immunity in the lung. Blood 2002; 100:4193–4200.
94. Kanda N, Watanabe S. Histamine enhances the production of granulocyte-macrophage colony-stimulating factor via protein kinase calpha and extracellular signal-regulated kinase in human keratinocytes. J Invest Dermatol 2004; 122:863–872.
95. Kanda N, Watanabe S. Histamine enhances the production of human beta-defensin-2 in human keratinocytes. Am J Physiol Cell Physiol 2007; 293:C1916–C1923.
96. Caron G, Delneste Y, Roelandts E, et al. Histamine polarizes human dendritic cells into Th2 cell-promoting effector dendritic cells. J Immunol 2001; 167:3682–3686.
97. Gutzmer R, Langer K, Lisewski M, et al. Expression and function of histamine receptors 1 and 2 on human monocyte-derived dendritic cells. J Allergy Clin Immunol 2002; 109:524–531.
98. Idzko M, La Sala A, Ferrari D, et al. Expression and function of histamine receptors in human monocyte-derived dendritic cells. J Allergy Clin Immunol 2002; 109:839–846.
99. Ohtani T, Aiba S, Mizuashi M, et al .H1 and H2 histamine receptors are absent on Langerhans cells and present on dermal dendritic cells. J Invest Dermatol 2003; 121:1073–1079.
100. Dijkstra D, Stark H, Chazot PL, et al. Human inflammatory dendritic epidermal cells express a functional histamine H4 receptor. J Invest Dermatol 2008; 128:1696–1703.
101. Picker LJ, Michie SA, Rott LS, et al. A unique phenotype of skin-associated lymphocytes in humans. Preferential expression of the heca-452 epitope by benign and malignant T cells at cutaneous sites. Am J Pathol 1990; 136:1053–1068.
102. Picker LJ, Kishimoto TK, Smith CW, et al. ELAM-1 is an adhesion molecule for skin-homing T cells. Nature 1991; 349:796–799.
103. Santamaria Babi LF, Moser R, Perez Soler MT, et al. Migration of skin-homing T cells across cytokine-activated human endothelial cell layers involves interaction of the cutaneous lymphocyte-associated antigen (CLA), the very late antigen-4 (VLA-4), and the lymphocyte function-associated antigen-1 (LFA-1). J Immunol 1995; 154:1543–1550.
104. Kupper TS, Fuhlbrigge RC. Immune surveillance in the skin: Mechanisms and clinical consequences. Nat Rev Immunol 2004; 4:211–222.
105. Hassan AS, Kaelin U, Braathen LR, et al. Clinical and immunopathologic findings during treatment of recalcitrant atopic eczema with efalizumab. J Am Acad Dermatol 2007; 56:217–221.

106. Harper EG, Simpson EL, Takiguchi RH, et al. Efalizumab therapy for atopic dermatitis causes marked increases in circulating effector memory CD4+ T cells that express cutaneous lymphocyte antigen. J Invest Dermatol 2008; 128:1173–1181.
107. Fuhlbrigge RC, Kieffer JD, Armerding D, et al. Cutaneous lymphocyte antigen is a specialized form of PSGL-1 expressed on skin-homing T cells. Nature 1997; 389:978–981.
108. Knibbs RN, Craig RA, Natsuka S, et al. The fucosyltransferase FucT-VII regulates E-selectin ligand synthesis in human T cells. J Cell Biol 1996; 133:911–920.
109. Austrup F, Vestweber D, Borges E, et al. P- and E-selectin mediate recruitment of T-helper-1 but not T-helper-2 cells into inflammed tissues. Nature 1997; 385:81–83.
110. Blander JM, Visintin I, Janeway CA Jr, et al. Alpha(1,3)-fucosyltransferase VII and alpha(2,3)-sialyltransferase IV are up-regulated in activated CD4 T cells and maintained after their differentiation into Th1 and migration into inflammatory sites. J Immunol 1999; 163:3746–3752.
111. Wagers AJ, Waters CM, Stoolman LM, et al. Interleukin 12 and interleukin 4 control T cell adhesion to endothelial selectins through opposite effects on alpha1, 3-fucosyltransferase VII gene expression. J Exp Med 1998; 188:2225–2231.
112. Grewe M, Gyufko K, Schopf E, et al. Lesional expression of interferon-gamma in atopic eczema. Lancet 1994; 343:25–26.
113. Hamid Q, Naseer T, Minshall EM, et al. In vivo expression of IL-12 and IL-13 in atopic dermatitis. J Allergy Clin Immunol 1996; 98:225–231.
114. Taha RA, Minshall EM, Leung DY, et al. Evidence for increased expression of eotaxin and monocyte chemotactic protein-4 in atopic dermatitis. J Allergy Clin Immunol 2000; 105:1002–1007.
115. Homey B, Wang W, Soto H, et al. Cutting edge: The orphan chemokine receptor G protein-coupled receptor-2 (GPR-2, CCR10) binds the skin-associated chemokine CCL27 (CTACK/ALP/ILC). J Immunol 2000; 164:3465–3470.
116. Morales J, Homey B, Vicari AP, et al. A skin-associated chemokine that preferentially attracts skin-homing memory T cells. Proc Natl Acad Sci U S A 1999; 96:14470–14475.
117. Reiss Y, Proudfoot AE, Power CA, et al. CC chemokine receptor (CCR)4 and the CCR10 ligand cutaneous T cell-attracting chemokine (CTACK) in lymphocyte trafficking to inflamed skin. J Exp Med 2001; 194:1541–1547.
118. Vestergaard C, Johansen C, Otkjaer K, et al. Tumor necrosis factor-alpha-induced CTACK/CCL27 (cutaneous T-cell-attracting chemokine) production in keratinocytes is controlled by nuclear factor kappaB. Cytokine 2005; 29:49–55.
119. Vestergaard C, Yoneyama H, Murai M, et al. Overproduction of Th2-specific chemokines in NC/Nga mice exhibiting atopic dermatitis-like lesions. J Clin Invest 1999; 104:1097–1105.
120. Vestergaard C, Johansen C, Christensen U, et al. TARC augments TNF-alpha-induced CTACK production in keratinocytes. Exp Dermatol 2004; 13:551–557.
121. Hashimoto S, Nakamura K, Oyama N, et al. Macrophage-derived chemokine (MDC)/CCL22 produced by monocyte derived dendritic cells reflects the disease activity in patients with atopic dermatitis. J Dermatol Sci 2006; 44:93–99.
122. Soumelis V, Reche PA, Kanzler H, et al. Human epithelial cells trigger dendritic cell mediated allergic inflammation by producing TSLP. Nat Immunol 2002; 3:673–680.
123. Ebner S, Nguyen VA, Forstner M, et al. Thymic stromal lymphopoietin converts human epidermal Langerhans cells into antigen-presenting cells that induce proallergic T cells. J Allergy Clin Immunol 2007; 119:982–990.
124. Ito T, Wang YH, Duramad O, et al. TSLP-activated dendritic cells induce an inflammatory T helper type 2 cell response through OX40 ligand. J Exp Med 2005; 202:1213–1223.
125. Liu YJ. Thymic stromal lymphopoietin and OX40 ligand pathway in the initiation of dendritic cell-mediated allergic inflammation. J Allergy Clin Immunol 2007; 120:238–244 [Quiz 245–236].
126. Yawalkar N, Uguccioni M, Scharer J, et al. Enhanced expression of eotaxin and CCR3 in atopic dermatitis. J Invest Dermatol 1999; 113:43–48.
127. Park CW, Lee BH, Han HJ, et al. Tacrolimus decreases the expression of eotaxin, CCR3, rantes and interleukin-5 in atopic dermatitis. Br J Dermatol 2005; 152:1173–1181.

128. Laberge S, Ghaffar O, Boguniewicz M, et al. Association of increased CD4+ T-cell infiltration with increased IL-16 gene expression in atopic dermatitis. J Allergy Clin Immunol 1998; 102:645–650.
129. Klunker S, Trautmann A, Akdis M, et al. A second step of chemotaxis after transendothelial migration: Keratinocytes undergoing apoptosis release IFN-gamma-inducible protein 10, monokine induced by IFN-gamma, and IFN-gamma-inducible alpha-chemoattractant for T cell chemotaxis toward epidermis in atopic dermatitis. J Immunol 2003; 171:1078–1084.
130. Santamaria Babi LF, Moser B, Perez Soler MT, et al. The interleukin-8 receptor B and CXC chemokines can mediate transendothelial migration of human skin homing T cells. Eur J Immunol 1996; 26:2056–2061.
131. Hanifin JM, Rajka G. Diagnostic criteria for atopic dermatitis: Consider the context. Arch Dermatol 1999; 135:1551.
132. Ingordo V, D'Andria G, D'Andria C, et al. Results of atopy patch tests with house dust mites in adults with 'intrinsic' and 'extrinsic' atopic dermatitis. J Eur Acad Dermatol Venereol 2002; 16:450–454.
133. Wuthrich B. Serum IgE in atopic dermatitis: Relationship to severity of cutaneous involvement and course of disease as well as coexistence of atopic respiratory diseases. Clin Allergy 1978; 8:241–248.
134. Wang YH, Angkasekwinai P, Lu N, et al. IL-25 augments type 2 immune responses by enhancing the expansion and functions of TSLP-DC-activated Th2 memory cells. J Exp Med 2007; 204:1837–1847.
135. Kang CM, Jang AS, Ahn MH, et al. Interleukin-25 and interleukin-13 production by alveolar macrophages in response to particles. Am J Respir Cell Mol Biol 2005; 33:290–296.
136. Bilsborough J, Leung DY, Maurer M, et al. IL-31 is associated with cutaneous lymphocyte antigen-positive skin homing T cells in patients with atopic dermatitis. J Allergy Clin Immunol 2006; 117:418–425.
137. Dillon SR, Sprecher C, Hammond A, et al. Interleukin 31, a cytokine produced by activated T cells, induces dermatitis in mice. Nat Immunol 2004; 5:752–760.
138. Schmitz J, Owyang A, Oldham E, et al. IL-33, an interleukin-1-like cytokine that signals via the IL-1 receptor-related protein ST2 and induces T helper type 2-associated cytokines. Immunity 2005; 23:479–490.
139. Cherry WB, Yoon J, Bartemes KR, et al. A novel IL-1 family cytokine, IL-33, potently activates human eosinophils. J Allergy Clin Immunol 2008; 121:1484–1490.
140. Hori S, Nomura T, Sakaguchi S. Control of regulatory T cell development by the transcription factor Foxp3. Science 2003; 299:1057–1061.
141. Akdis CA, Blesken T, Akdis M, et al. Role of interleukin 10 in specific immunotherapy. J Clin Invest 1998; 102:98–106.
142. Groux H, O'Garra A, Bigler M, et al. A CD4+ T-cell subset inhibits antigen-specific T-cell responses and prevents colitis. Nature 1997; 389:737–742.
143. Roncarolo MG, Levings MK, Traversari C. Differentiation of T regulatory cells by immature dendritic cells. J Exp Med 2001; 193:F5–F9.
144. Barrat FJ, Cua DJ, Boonstra A, et al. In vitro generation of interleukin 10-producing regulatory CD4(+) T cells is induced by immunosuppressive drugs and inhibited by T helper type 1 (Th1)- and Th2-inducing cytokines. J Exp Med 2002; 195:603–616.
145. Bellinghausen I, Konig B, Bottcher I, et al. Inhibition of human allergic T-helper type 2 immune responses by induced regulatory T cells requires the combination of interleukin-10-treated dendritic cells and transforming growth factor-beta for their induction. Clin Exp Allergy 2006; 36:1546–1555.
146. Akdis M, Verhagen J, Taylor A, et al. Immune responses in healthy and allergic individuals are characterized by a fine balance between allergen-specific T regulatory 1 and T helper 2 cells. J Exp Med 2004; 199:1567–1575.
147. Taylor A, Verhagen J, Akdis CA, et al. Regulatory cells in allergy and health: A question of allergen specificity and balance. Int Arch Allergy Immunol 2004; 135:73–82.

148. Sakaguchi S, Sakaguchi N, Asano M, et al. Immunologic self-tolerance maintained by activated T cells expressing IL-2 receptor alpha-chains (CD25). Breakdown of a single mechanism of self-tolerance causes various autoimmune diseases. J Immunol 1995; 155:1151–1164.
149. Chatila TA. Role of regulatory T cells in human diseases. J Allergy Clin Immunol 2005; 116:949–959 [Quiz 960].
150. Ohmen JD, Hanifin JM, Nickoloff BJ, et al. Overexpression of Il-10 in atopic dermatitis. contrasting cytokine patterns with delayed-type hypersensitivity reactions. J Immunol 1995; 154:1956–1963.
151. Frank S, Madlener M, Werner S. Transforming growth factors beta1, beta2, and beta3 and their receptors are differentially regulated during normal and impaired wound healing. J Biol Chem 1996; 271:10188–10193.
152. Verhagen J, Akdis M, Traidl-Hoffmann C, et al. Absence of T-regulatory cell expression and function in atopic dermatitis skin. J Allergy Clin Immunol 2006; 117:176–183.
153. Harrington LE, Hatton RD, Mangan PR, et al. Interleukin 17-producing CD4+ effector T cells develop via a lineage distinct from the T helper type 1 and 2 lineages. Nat Immunol 2005; 6:1123–1132.
154. Bettelli E, Carrier Y, Gao W, et al. Developmental pathways for the generation of pathogenic effector Th17 and regulatory T cells. Nature 2006; 441:235–238.
155. Mangan PR, Harrington LE, O'Quinn DB, et al. Transforming growth factor-beta induces development of the T(H)17 lineage. Nature 2006; 441:231–234.
156. Koga C, Kabashima K, Shiraishi N, et al. Possible pathogenic role of Th17 cells for atopic dermatitis. J Invest Dermatol 2008; 128:2625–2630.
157. Wolk K, Kunz S, Witte E, et al. IL-22 increases the innate immunity of tissues. Immunity 2004; 21:241–254.
158. Simon HU, Blaser K. Inhibition of programmed eosinophil death: A key pathogenic event for eosinophilia? Immunol Today 1995; 16:53–55.
159. Ju ST, Panka DJ, Cui H, et al. Fas(CD95)/FasL interactions required for programmed cell death after T-cell activation. Nature 1995; 373:444–448.
160. Russell JH. Activation-induced death of mature T cells in the regulation of immune responses. Curr Opin Immunol 1995; 7:382–388.
161. Scaffidi C, Kirchhoff S, Krammer PH, et al. Apoptosis signaling in lymphocytes. Curr Opin Immunol 1999; 11:277–285.
162. Sabbagh L, Bourbonniere M, Sekaly RP, et al. Selective up-regulation of caspase-3 gene expression following TCR engagement. Mol Immunol 2005; 42:1345–1354.
163. Thompson CB. Apoptosis in the pathogenesis and treatment of disease. Science 1995; 267:1456–1462.
164. Green DR, Scott DW. Activation-induced apoptosis in lymphocytes. Curr Opin Immunol 1994; 6:476–487.
165. Brunner T, Mogil RJ, Laface D, et al. Cell-autonomous Fas (CD95)/Fas–ligand interaction mediates activation-induced apoptosis in T-cell hybridomas. Nature 1995; 373:441–444.
166. Dhein J, Walczak H, Baumler C, et al. Autocrine T-cell suicide mediated by APO-1/(Fas/CD95). Nature 1995; 373:438–441.
167. Akkoc T, De Koning PJ, Ruckert B, et al. Increased activation-induced cell death of high IFN-gamma-producing T(H)1 cells as a mechanism of T(H)2 predominance in atopic diseases. J Allergy Clin Immunol 2008; 121:652–658 E651.
168. Ruoslahti E, Pierschbacher Md. New perspectives in cell adhesion: RGD and integrins. Science 1987; 238:491–497.
169. Clark EA, Brugge JS. Integrins and signal transduction pathways: The road taken. Science 1995; 268:233–239.
170. Hannigan GE, Leung-Hagesteijn C, Fitz-Gibbon L, et al. Regulation of cell adhesion and anchorage-dependent growth by A new beta 1-integrin-linked protein kinase. Nature 1996; 379:91–96.
171. Wary KK, Mainiero F, Isakoff SJ, et al. The adaptor protein shc couples A class of integrins to the control of cell cycle progression. Cell 1996; 87:733–743.

172. Frisch SM, Vuori K, Ruoslahti E, et al. Control of adhesion-dependent cell survival by focal adhesion kinase. J Cell Biol 1996; 134:793–799.
173. Khwaja A, Rodriguez-Viciana P, Wennstrom S, et al. Matrix adhesion and ras transformation both activate a phosphoinositide 3-OH kinase and protein kinase B/Akt cellular survival pathway. EMBO J 1997; 16:2783–2793.
174. Giri JG, Kumaki S, Ahdieh M, et al. Identification and cloning of a novel IL-15 binding protein that is structurally related to the alpha chain of the IL-2 receptor. EMBO J 1995; 14:3654–3663.
175. Li XC, Ima A, Li Y, et al. Blocking the common gamma-chain of cytokine receptors induces T cell apoptosis and long-term islet allograft survival. J Immunol 2000; 164:1193–1199.
176. Traidl C, Sebastiani S, Albanesi C, et al. Disparate cytotoxic activity of nickel-specific CD8+ and CD4+ T cell subsets against keratinocytes. J Immunol 2000; 165:3058–3064.
177. Schnyder B, Frutig K, Mauri-Hellweg D, et al. T-cell-mediated cytotoxicity against keratinocytes in sulfamethoxazol-induced skin reaction. Clin Exp Allergy 1998; 28:1412–1417.
178. Carroll JM, Crompton T, Seery JP, et al. Transgenic mice expressing IFN-gamma in the epidermis have eczema, hair hypopigmentation, and hair loss. J Invest Dermatol 1997; 108:412–422.

8 Antigen-Presenting Cells

Natalija Novak and Thomas Bieber

Department of Dermatology and Allergy, University of Bonn, Bonn, Germany

INTRODUCTION AND BACKGROUND

Dendritic cells (DC) as antigen-presenting cells are outposts of our immune system, which are located at the interface to the environment. In particular, in diseases with an impaired epidermal skin barrier such as atopic dermatitis (AD), the properties of DC in terms of antigen-uptake and presentation as well as T-cell priming are of strong importance (1). Basically, antigens can be taken up by DC in three different ways: macropinocytosis for large particles, phagocytosis, and receptor-mediated endocytosis (2). The latter is important for antigen capture by immature DC. Antigens recognized by receptors are internalized and clustered in clathrin-coated pits. After digestion, peptides are uploaded onto a major histocompatibility class (MHC) II. Upon maturation, DC migrate from the peripheral organs to the lymph nodes, where they present the antigens to T cells and prime T cells to initiate primary immune responses (3,4).

Allergens as well as microbial antigens represent important trigger factors of AD (5). In regard to the clinical picture, allergen exposure is directly linked to severe flare-ups of eczematous skin lesions. The concept of allergen sensitization and challenge via the skin has been further supported by observations from atopy patch tests in which aeroallergens or food allergens applied to the skin induced an eczematous skin reaction within 24 to 48 hours in sensitized individuals (6,7). However, these observations raised the question, how allergen uptake is managed in the skin and which cells are mainly responsible for this phenomenon.

Some answers to these questions resulted from the discovery of IgE-bearing DC in the epidermal skin lesions of AD over two decades ago (8). A few years later, the high-affinity receptor for IgE (FcεRI) has been identified as the main IgE-binding structure on these cells (9,10). In this context, it is more than likely that IgE-receptor–mediated uptake of antigens plays an outstanding role in the pathophysiolocial network of AD.

In support of this concept, several FcεRI-bearing subtypes have been identified in human skin of AD patients so far. Concerning myeloid DC, both, CD207$^+$/CD1a$^+$, that is, Langerhans cells (LC) as well as CD207$^-$/CD1a$^+$/FcεRI$^+$ DC are located in the epidermis (11). Although low numbers of CD207$^+$/FcεRI$^+$/CD1a$^+$ DC occur in the dermis, CD1c$^+$/FcεRI$^+$ DC represent the major DC subpopulation of the dermal compartment (Table 1) (12).

STRUCTURAL AND FUNCTIONAL CHARACTERISTICS OF FcεRI ON DC

Structurally, FcεRI expressed by human antigen–presenting cells differs from FcεRI on the surface of effector cells of allergic reactions. FcεRI on DC has a trimeric structure and consists of the IgE-binding α-chain and the γ-chain dimer, which is

TABLE 1   Distribution of FcεRI-Bearing Dendritic Cells in the
Epidermis and Dermis in AD

	Epidermis	Dermis
FcεRI⁺/CD207⁺/CD1a⁺	+++	+
FcεRI⁺/CD207⁻/CD1a⁺	+++	+
FcεRI⁺/CD1c⁺/CD1a⁺	+	++
FcεRI+/CD123⁺/BDCA2⁺	−	++

Source: Adapted from Ref. 17.

responsible for downstream-signaling, while the β-chain, which stabilizes FcεRI on the cell surface is absent (13,14). Interestingly, FcεRI surface expression is regulated distinctly in APC of atopic and nonatopic donors in vitro. In APC of nonatopic individuals, most of the IgE-binding α-chain remains in the intracellular space, while only few γ-chain dimers are present (15). This variant of the α-chain is incompletely processed in terms of glycosylation and segregated in the endoplasmic reticulum. In contrast, in APC of atopic individuals, a second variant of the α-chain can be detected, which associates with the γ-chains present in high levels in these cells. The complete trimeric FcεRI complex is transported to the cell surface, which accounts most likely for the high IgE-binding capacity of APC in the skin of atopic individuals (15,16). Aggregation of FcεRI on DC induces NF-κb activation via p50 and p65 and the release of tumor necrosis factor (TNF)-α (17). Interestingly, upregulated protein-tyrosine kinase expression and phosphorylation of phospholipase C-gamma 1 occurs only after FcεRI cross linking of epidermal LC of atopic donors with high FcεRI expression (18). This implies that effective downstream signaling and calcium mobilization is restricted to DC in the context of atopic diseases. Further on, IgE-receptor expression in lesional skin of AD has been shown to correlate with serum IgE levels (11). A higher expression of FcεRI on epidermal DC in patients with the so-called extrinsic variant of AD, which goes along with high total serum IgE levels and a high number of sensitizations as opposed to lower FcεRI expression in patients with the intrinsic variant of AD, allows to distinguish epidermal DC of these two subgroups of AD by their phenotypic characteristics (19). Most interestingly, FcεRI overexpression on DC in the skin has been observed in both, involved as well as skin of patients with allergic rhinitis and asthma without AD (20).

THE ROLE OF MYELOID DC SUBTYPES

The most prominent members of myeloid DC in the epidermis are the classical LC, which are bone marrow derived, CD1a-, and MHCII-positive and characterized by the Birbeck granules. Birbeck granules are visible electron-microscopically as tennis-racket–shaped organelles originating from the accumulation of the C-type lectin Langerin (21). LC reside in both healthy and inflamed skin and are constantly renewed under steady-state conditions (22). The frequency of LC in healthy, noninflamed skin ranges between 0.5% and 2% of all epidermal cells, depending on the localization and age of the individual (23).

As a characteristic feature of AD, LC are equipped with FcεRI on their cell surface and it is supposed that this surface structure enables them to take up allergens penetrating the skin (24). In vitro studies of LC provide evidence that LC are in the foreground in the initial phase of AD (24). In view of the current disease concept, LC take up invading allergens and present these allergens to T cells. T cells of the Th2 type are primed by LC in vitro, which are characterized by the production of interleukin (IL)-4, IL-5, and IL-13, a cytokine profile which is typical for the initial phase of AD (25–26). Further on, allergen challenge and concomitant IgE-receptor cross linking on LC or activation by microbial products such as staphylococcal enterotoxins lead to the release of different chemotactic mediators, which might recruit other inflammatory cells including inflammatory dendritic epidermal cells (IDEC) from their precursors into the skin (27–29).

IDEC are only present at inflammatory epidermal sites and bear significantly high numbers of FcεRI in combination with CD11b molecules and the mannose receptor (CD206) (30) on their cell surface, but are Langerin (CD207) negative (12,31). In time kinetics acquired with the help of atopy patch tests, invasion of IDEC into the epidermis within 24 to 48 hours after allergen application and concomitant upregulation of FcεRI expression on both epidermal DC subtypes, LC, and IDEC has been observed (32), supporting the view of a two-step model directed by DC subtypes in AD. Chemokine receptors, such as CCR8 expressed by DC responding to CCL1 (33) or Thymic stromal lymphopoietin receptor (TSLPR), which responds to TSLP produced by keratinocytes (34) and IgE-receptor–challenged mast cells might represent other components of this recruitment process. Due to their high ability to release distinct proinflammatory mediators after IgE-receptor–mediated allergen challenge, it is assumed that IDEC are the main dendritic amplifiers of the epidermal allergic–inflammatory reaction in AD (35). Allergen challenge of IDEC in vitro leads, beside the release of proinflammatory cytokines and chemokines such as CCL17 and CLL18 (34), to the production of IL-12 and IL-18, which might alter the initial Th2 prone immune response into a micromilieu, which is more dominated by Th1 cytokines and leads to the chronification of the skin lesions (Fig. 1) (24,25).

THE IMPACT OF PLASMACYTOID DENDRITIC CELLS

Plasmacytoid DC (PDC) have a plasma-cell–like morphology, are MHCII+CD1a-, CD11c-negative, but positive for the α-chain of the IL-3 receptor (CD123) and the blood-dendritic cell antigen (BDCA)-2 (36). They are producers of type I interferons and are equipped with specific pattern recognition receptors of the innate immune system that enable them to sense microbial pathogens and thereby defend our organism against bacterial and viral infections, which represents besides linking innate and adaptive immunity, one of their major tasks (37). An increased number of PDC is detectable in the peripheral blood of AD patients (38) as compared to subjects with psoriasis. During acute viral infection of the skin, such as disseminated Herpes simplex virus infection, called Eczema herpeticatum, the number of PDC in the peripheral blood profoundly increases (39).

PDC in the peripheral blood of AD patients have been shown to bear the FcεRI receptor on their surface, which is occupied with IgE molecules (40–42). IgE-receptor expression of PDC correlates with the IgE serum levels, indicating that IgE in the micromilieu might be necessary to stabilize this structure on the cell surface of PDC. Further on, activation of FcεRI on PDC counterregulates the toll-like receptor (TLR)9 pathway (43). This counterregulation is mediated by tumor necrosis factor (TNF)-α released by PDC after IgE-receptor challenge, which downregulates in an endogenous way TLR9 expression (44). Aggregation of FcεRI on PDC induces the release of IL-10 (41,43) and IL-10–mediated apoptosis of PDC in vitro.

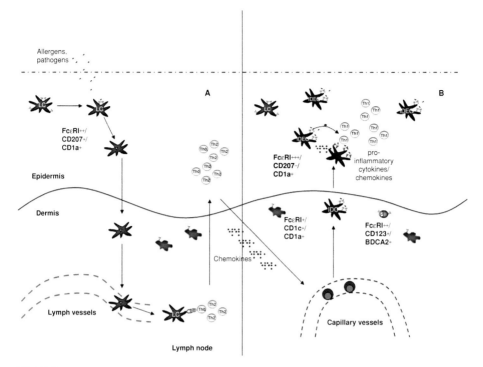

FIGURE 1   Network of LC and IDEC in the epidermis of AD patients. (**A**) LC residing in the epidermis capture pathogens, secrete cytokines/chemokines, process antigens, migrate to the lymph nodes, and present them to T cells. In the lymph node, LC prime large amounts of Th2 cells, which are characteristic for the initial phase of AD. (**B**) Allergen challenge and concomitant IgE-receptor cross linking on LC or activation by microbial products leads to the release of different chemotactic mediators by diverse skin cells, which together with soluble factors contribute to the recruitment of inflammatory dendritic epidermal cells (IDEC) into the skin. Allergen challenge of IDEC in vitro leads to the release of proinflammatory cytokines and chemokines, which might contribute to the amplification of the allergic–inflammatory reaction and alteration of the initial Th2 immune micromilieu to the predominance of Th1 T cells in the skin, which seem to be a crucial step for the chronification of the skin lesions. Distribution of IgE-receptor bearing DC subtypes in the epidermis and dermis is depicted.

Further on, the preactivation of PDC via allergen challenge significantly reduces the capacity of PDC to produce IFN-α and IFN-β in response to subsequent stimulation with viral DNA motifs (41). The decrease in the capacity to produce type I interferons correlates directly with the FcεRI expression of PDC (45). The reduced capacity of PDC to produce type I interferon after allergen challenge might be one of the reasons for the high susceptibility of AD patients to viral infections. There is also evidence for a reduced amount of PDC in the epidermis of AD patients in comparison to other chronic inflammatory skin diseases such as psoriasis, allergic contact dermatitis, or lupus erythematodes which might be based on a lower recruitment of these cells into the skin due to reduced expression of skin-homing molecules on PDC of atopic donors (41) or a higher rate of apoptosis of PDC in the Th2 prone micromilieu of AD skin (46). However, substantial numbers of PDC are present in the dermal compartment (12). Together, modifications on the level of PDC have been identified as important risk factors for the manifestation of bacterial and viral infections of the skin, which significantly aggravate the course of AD (47).

DC AS THERAPEUTIC TARGETS

Concerning DC as target cells for therapeutic measures for AD, two main mechanisms seem to be of major relevance for the efficacy of the treatment: first, down-regulation of the expression of FcεRI on epidermal DC, which might discontinue the vicious circle of allergen uptake, presentation, and inflammation in the skin and second, reduction of the number of proinflammatory DC subtypes in favor of a higher number and overbalance of LC. Reduction of FcεRI expression is observable after topical treatment with tacrolimus and glucocorticoids (48) as well as after systemic application of anti-IgE antibodies (49). Treatment with topical glucocorticoids induces the depletion of all DC subtypes, namely, of epidermal LC (50), IDEC (48), and dermal PDC (51).

In contrast, profound modulation of the LC/IDEC balance in a more selective way and without induction of DC apoptosis is observable during topical treatment with immunomodulators (48). Topical treatment with both tacrolimus or pimecrolimus leads to clinical improvement of histologic characteristics such as spongiosis, acanthosis, and density of the cellular infiltrate (52,53). Besides changes in the amount of IL-5, IL-13, and IL-10 in the skin, the number of CD1a$^+$ epidermal DC increases (52,53). Further on, the number of IDEC in the epidermis decreases below the detectable level and this phenomenon is not based on the apoptosis of these cells (48,54,55). One explanation for this could be that tacrolimus and TGF-β1 act synergistically on the generation of LC-like DC in vitro, lowering the stimulatory capacity of LC-like DC towards T cells and inhibiting LC maturation (56). This is partially achieved by the stabilization of the TGF-βRII expression on differentiating DC, which might increase their sensitivity to TGF-β produced by different cell types in the skin and might promote the generation of LC (56). The hypothesis of tacrolimus as a promoter of LC generation is in line with the observation that the number of CD1a$^+$ LC increases in the epidermis of AD patients after treatment with tacrolimus (52–54,56). Therefore, shifting the balance of differentiating DC to LC with more suppressive, tolerogenic properties might be of major importance for the therapeutic effect of tacrolimus and represents an attractive strategy for the treatment of AD (56).

Additional therapeutic approaches arise from recent observations, which show that IDEC in lesional skin of AD express high amounts of the histamine receptor 4 (HR4) (57). Specific stimulation of HR4 with HR4 agonists on IDEC in vitro reduced the amount of Th2-related chemokines and IL-12 released by these cells. Based on these observations, treatment with HR4 agonists might target IDEC and reduce the release of proallergic and proinflammatory mediators of this DC subtype (57).

FUTURE PERSPECTIVES

Without any doubt, we learned much about the phenotypic and functional characteristics of antigen-presenting cells in AD. However, several questions about the mechanisms by which DC in the skin and blood of AD patients prevent or initiate allergic inflammation remain to be answered. Detailed knowledge about the properties of these distinct DC subtypes would enable us to optimally target these multifaceted cells with the help of effective topical and systemic therapeutic strategies in the future.

REFERENCES

1. Cork MJ, Robinson DA, Vasilopoulos Y, et al. New perspectives on epidermal barrier dysfunction in atopic dermatitis: Gene–environment interactions. J Allergy Clin Immunol 2006; 118(1):3–21.
2. Sabatte J, Maggini J, Nahmod K, et al. Interplay of pathogens, cytokines and other stress signals in the regulation of dendritic cell function. Cytokine Growth Factor Rev 2007; 18(1–2):5–17.
3. Banchereau J, Briere F, Caux C, et al. Immunobiology of dendritic cells. Annu Rev Immunol 2000; 18:767–811.
4. Shortman K, Naik SH. Steady-state and inflammatory dendritic-cell development. Nat Rev Immunol 2007; 7(1):19–30.
5. Bieber T. Atopic dermatitis. N Engl J Med 2008; 358(14):1483–1494.
6. Turjanmaa K, Darsow U, Niggemann B, et al. EAACI/GA2LEN position paper: Present status of the atopy patch test. Allergy 2006; 61(12):1377–1384.
7. Darsow U, Laifaoui J, Kerschenlohr K, et al. The prevalence of positive reactions in the atopy patch test with aeroallergens and food allergens in subjects with atopic eczema: A European Multicenter Study. Allergy 2004; 59(12):1318–1325.
8. Bruijnzeel-Koomen C, van Wichen DF, Toonstra J, et al. The presence of IgE molecules on epidermal Langerhans cells in patients with atopic dermatitis. Arch Dermatol Res 1986; 278:199–205.
9. Bieber T, de la Salle H, Wollenberg A, et al. Human epidermal Langerhans cells express the high affinity receptor for immunoglobulin E (Fc epsilon RI). J Exp Med 1992; 175(5):1285–1290.
10. Wang B, Rieger A, Kilgus O, et al. Epidermal Langerhans cells from normal human skin bind monomeric IgE via Fc epsilon RI. J Exp Med 1992; 175(5):1353–1365.
11. Wollenberg A, Kraft S, Hanau D, et al. Immunomorphological and ultrastructural characterization of Langerhans cells and a novel, inflammatory dendritic epidermal cell (IDEC) population in lesional skin of atopic eczema. J Invest Dermatol 1996; 106(3):446–453.
12. Stary G, Bangert C, Stingl G, et al. Dendritic cells in atopic dermatitis: Expression of FcepsilonRI on two distinct inflammation-associated subsets. Int Arch Allergy Immunol 2005; 138(4):278–290.
13. Kraft S, Novak N. Fc receptors as determinants of allergic reactions. Trends Immunol 2005; 27(2):88–95.
14. Kraft S, Kinet JP. New developments in FcepsilonRI regulation, function and inhibition. Nat Rev Immunol 2007; 7(5):365–378.
15. Novak N, Kraft S, Bieber T. Unraveling the mission of FcepsilonRI on antigen-presenting cells. J Allergy Clin Immunol 2003; 111(1):38–44.
16. Novak N, Tepel C, Koch S, et al. Evidence for a differential expression of the FcepsilonRIgamma chain in dendritic cells of atopic and nonatopic donors. J Clin Invest 2003; 111(7):1047–1056.
17. Kraft S, Novak N, Katoh N, et al. Aggregation of the high-affinity IgE receptor Fc(epsilon)RI on human monocytes and dendritic cells induces NF-kappaB activation. J Invest Dermatol 2002; 118(5):830–837.
18. Kraft S, Wessendorf JH, Haberstok J, et al. Enhanced expression and activity of protein-tyrosine kinases establishes a functional signaling pathway only in FcepsilonRI high Langerhans cells from atopic individuals. J Invest Dermatol 2002; 119(4):804–811.
19. Oppel T, Schuller E, Gunther S, et al. Phenotyping of epidermal dendritic cells allows the differentiation between extrinsic and intrinsic forms of atopic dermatitis. Br J Dermatol 2000; 143(6):1193–1198.

20. Semper AE, Hartley JA, Tunon-De-Lara JM, et al. Expression of the high affinity receptor for Immunoglobulin E (IgE) by dendritic cells in normals and asthmatics. Adv Exp Med Biol 1995; 378:135–138.
21. Villadangos JA, Heath WR. Life cycle, migration and antigen presenting functions of spleen and lymph node dendritic cells: Limitations of the Langerhans cells paradigm. Semin Immunol 2005; 17(4):262–272.
22. Ginhoux F, Tacke F, Angeli V, et al. Langerhans cells arise from monocytes in vivo. Nat Immunol 2006; 7(3):265–273.
23. Berman B, Chen VL, France DS, et al. Anatomical mapping of epidermal Langerhans cell densities in adults. Br J Dermatol 1983; 109(5):553–558.
24. Novak N, Valenta R, Bohle B, et al. FcepsilonRI engagement of Langerhans cell-like dendritic cells and inflammatory dendritic epidermal cell-like dendritic cells induces chemotactic signals and different T-cell phenotypes in vitro. J Allergy Clin Immunol 2004; 113(5):949–957.
25. Grewe M, Walther S, Gyufko K, et al. Analysis of the cytokine pattern expressed in situ in inhalant allergen patch test reactions of atopic dermatitis patients. J Invest Dermatol 1995; 105(3):407–410.
26. Eyerich K, Huss-Marp J, Darsow U, et al. Pollen grains induce a rapid and biphasic eczematous immune response in atopic eczema patients. Int Arch Allergy Immunol 2008; 145(3):213–223.
27. Gunther C, Bello-Fernandez C, Kopp T, et al. CCL18 is expressed in atopic dermatitis and mediates skin homing of human memory T cells. J Immunol 2005; 174(3):1723–1728.
28. Pivarcsi A, Gombert M, Dieu-Nosjean MC, et al. CC chemokine ligand 18, an atopic dermatitis-associated and dendritic cell-derived chemokine, is regulated by staphylococcal products and allergen exposure. J Immunol 2004; 173(9):5810–5817.
29. Homey B, Steinhoff M, Ruzicka T, et al. Cytokines and chemokines orchestrate atopic skin inflammation. J Allergy Clin Immunol 2006; 118(1):178–189.
30. Wollenberg A, Mommaas M, Oppel T, et al. Expression and function of the mannose receptor CD206 on epidermal dendritic cells in inflammatory skin diseases. J Invest Dermatol 2002; 118(2):327–334.
31. Wollenberg A, Wen S, Bieber T. Langerhans cell phenotyping: A new tool for differential diagnosis of inflammatory skin diseases. Lancet 1995; 346(8990):1626–1627.
32. Kerschenlohr K, Decard S, Przybilla B, et al. Atopy patch test reactions show a rapid influx of inflammatory dendritic epidermal cells in patients with extrinsic atopic dermatitis and patients with intrinsic atopic dermatitis. J Allergy Clin Immunol 2003; 111(4):869–874.
33. Gombert M, eu-Nosjean MC, Winterberg F, et al. CCL1–CCR8 interactions: An axis mediating the recruitment of T cells and Langerhans-type dendritic cells to sites of atopic skin inflammation. J Immunol 2005; 174(8):5082–5091.
34. Guttman-Yassky E, Lowes MA, Fuentes-Duculan J, et al. Major differences in inflammatory dendritic cells and their products distinguish atopic dermatitis from psoriasis. J Allergy Clin Immunol 2007; 119(5):1210–1217.
35. Novak N, Peng W, Yu C. Network of myeloid and plasmacytoid dendritic cells in atopic dermatitis. Adv Exp Med Biol 2007; 601:97–104.
36. Cella M, Jarrossay D, Facchetti F, et al. Plasmacytoid monocytes migrate to inflamed lymph nodes and produce large amounts of type I interferon. Nat Med 1999; 5(8):919–923.
37. Soumelis V, Liu YJ. From plasmacytoid to dendritic cell: Morphological and functional switches during plasmacytoid pre-dendritic cell differentiation. Eur J Immunol 2006; 36(9):2286–2292.
38. Hashizume H, Horibe T, Yagi H, et al. Compartmental imbalance and aberrant immune function of blood CD123 + (plasmacytoid) and CD11c + (myeloid) dendritic cells in atopic dermatitis. J Immunol 2005; 174(4):2396–2403.
39. Kabashima K, Sugita K, Tokura Y. Increment of circulating plasmacytoid dendritic cells in a patient with Kaposi's varicelliform eruption. J Eur Acad Dermatol Venereol 2008; 22(2):239–241.

40. Foster B, Metcalfe DD, Prussin C. Human dendritic cell 1 and dendritic cell 2 subsets express FcepsilonRI: Correlation with serum IgE and allergic asthma. J Allergy Clin Immunol 2003; 112(6):1132–1138.
41. Novak N, Allam JP, Hagemann T, et al. Characterization of FcepsilonRI-bearing CD123 blood dendritic cell antigen-2 plasmacytoid dendritic cells in atopic dermatitis. J Allergy Clin Immunol 2004; 114(2):364–370.
42. Beeren IM, De Bruin-Weller MS, Ra C, et al. Expression of Fc(epsilon)RI on dendritic cell subsets in peripheral blood of patients with atopic dermatitis and allergic asthma. J Allergy Clin Immunol 2005; 116(1):228–229.
43. Schroeder JT, Bieneman AP, Xiao H, et al. TLR9- and FcepsilonRI-mediated responses oppose one another in plasmacytoid dendritic cells by down-regulating receptor expression. J Immunol 2005; 175(9):5724–5731.
44. Schroeder JT, Chichester KL, Bieneman AP. Toll-like receptor 9 suppression in plasmacytoid dendritic cells after IgE-dependent activation is mediated by autocrine TNF-alpha. J Allergy Clin Immunol 2008; 121(2):486–491.
45. Tversky JR, Le TV, Bieneman AP, et al. Human blood dendritic cells from allergic subjects have impaired capacity to produce interferon-alpha via Toll-like receptor 9. Clin Exp Allergy 2008; 38(5):781–788.
46. Wollenberg A, Wagner M, Gunther S, et al. Plasmacytoid dendritic cells: A new cutaneous dendritic cell subset with distinct role in inflammatory skin diseases. J Invest Dermatol 2002; 119(5):1096–1102.
47. Novak N, Bieber T. The role of dendritic cell subtypes in the pathophysiology of atopic dermatitis. J Am Acad Dermatol 2005; 53(2 suppl. 2):S171–S176.
48. Schuller E, Oppel T, Bornhovd E, et al. Tacrolimus ointment causes inflammatory dendritic epidermal cell depletion but no Langerhans cell apoptosis in patients with atopic dermatitis. J Allergy Clin Immunol 2004; 114(1):137–143.
49. Prussin C, Griffith DT, Boesel KM, et al. Omalizumab treatment downregulates dendritic cell FcepsilonRI expression. J Allergy Clin Immunol 2003; 112(6):1147–1154.
50. Hoetzenecker W, Ecker R, Kopp T, et al. Pimecrolimus leads to an apoptosis-induced depletion of T cells but not Langerhans cells in patients with atopic dermatitis. J Allergy Clin Immunol 2005; 115(6):1276–1283.
51. Hoetzenecker W, Meindl S, Stuetz A, et al. Both pimecrolimus and corticosteroids deplete plasmacytoid dendritic cells in patients with atopic dermatitis. J Invest Dermatol 2006; 126(9):2141–2144.
52. Simon D, Vassina E, Yousefi S, et al. Reduced dermal infiltration of cytokine-expressing inflammatory cells in atopic dermatitis after short-term topical tacrolimus treatment. J Allergy Clin Immunol 2004; 114(4):887–895.
53. Simon D, Vassina E, Yousefi S, et al. Inflammatory cell numbers and cytokine expression in atopic dermatitis after topical pimecrolimus treatment. Allergy 2005; 60(7):944–951.
54. Wollenberg A, Sharma S, Von Bubnoff D, et al. Topical tacrolimus (FK506) leads to profound phenotypic and functional alterations of epidermal antigen-presenting dendritic cells in atopic dermatitis. J Allergy Clin Immunol 2001; 107:519–525.
55. Panhans-Groß A, Novak N, Kraft S, et al. Human epidermal Langerhans' cells are targets for the immunosuppressive macrolide tacrolimus (FK506). J Allergy Clin Immunol 2001; 107(2):345–352.
56. Kwiek B, Peng WM, Allam JP, et al. Tacrolimus and TGF-beta act synergistically on the generation of Langerhans cells. J Allergy Clin Immunol 2008; 122(1):126–132.
57. Dijkstra D, Stark H, Chazot PL, et al. Human inflammatory dendritic epidermal cells express a functional histamine H4 receptor. J Invest Dermatol 2008; 128(7):1696–1703.

9 Mast Cells and Basophils

Anne-Marie Irani and Lawrence B. Schwartz

Virginia Commonwealth University, Richmond, Virginia, U.S.A.

INTRODUCTION

Mast cells and basophils are generally recognized as the principal cell types to initiate IgE-dependent, type I immediate hypersensitivity reactions. More recently, mast cells have been implicated as participants in innate immunity, additional aspects of acquired immunity, and tissue remodeling (Fig. 1). Mast cells originate from bone marrow progenitors but complete their maturation in tissues where they then reside. Basophils also originate from bone marrow progenitors but complete their maturation before being released from the bone marrow into the circulation, where they reside until called into tissues at sites of inflammation, particularly during the late phase of IgE-mediated immediate hypersensitivity reactions and during the early phase of cell-mediated, delayed-type hypersensitivity reactions. Mast cells and basophils are the only two cell types that constitutively express substantial quantities of the high-affinity, tetrameric receptor for IgE (FcεRI) and store histamine in their secretory granules. These two cell types are distinguished from one another by their respective pathways for growth, differentiation, and survival; patterns of cell-surface adhesion, cytokine and chemokine receptors; responses to non–IgE-dependent agonists; secretory granule proteoglycans and proteases; and morphologies. For example, nuclei of peripheral blood basophils have deeply divided lobes, whereas those of mast cells in normal tissues are rounded.

Atopic dermatitis is a genetically influenced chronic inflammatory disorder of the skin characterized by persistent pruritus that leads to scratching and lichenification. Atopic dermatitis is commonly seen in association with allergic rhinitis and asthma in families or individuals, suggesting that it is a cutaneous form of allergic disease. Although the participation of mast cells and basophils in allergic disorders is well established, their significance in atopic dermatitis still remains unclear. An experimental allergen challenge of an IgE-sensitized host reveals two phases to the subsequent immediate hypersensitivity reaction. The early phase of the IgE-dependent reaction (beginning 5–30 minutes postchallenge), depending on the target tissue and distribution of allergen, involves local edema, smooth muscle contraction, vasodilation, and increased permeability of postcapillary venules. These events represent the characteristic features of acute urticaria, but not of atopic dermatitis. The late phase of an immediate hypersensitivity reaction (4–12 hours postchallenge) involves the recruitment and activation of basophils, eosinophils, and other cell types. These late reactions can persist for at least two days in the challenged site, but eventually appear to completely resolve. Topical applications of allergen repeated daily for six days can result in an increased number of mast cells (1). Thus, chronic allergic inflammation can result from prolonged allergen exposure and may contribute to the pathophysiology of atopic dermatitis.

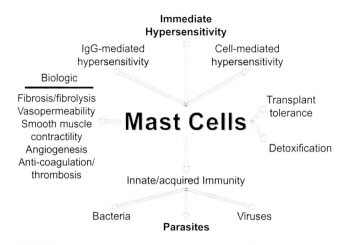

FIGURE 1 Immunologic effector roles of mast cells and basophils. Mast cells and basophils are the primary effector cells in immediate hypersensitivity reactions, but they also may participate in innate immune defense and in acquired immunity against certain microbes, as well as homeostatic processes in tissues.

Several studies suggest a relationship between atopic dermatitis and mast cells and basophils. First, in lichenified lesions of atopic dermatitis, the total number of mast cells may be increased [Fig. 2(A) and (B)], while in the acute phase of atopic dermatitis, mast cells are fragmented or degranulated but not notably increased in number (2–4). No significant correlation between clinical severity scores and mast cell numbers was found (5). Second, patients suffering from atopic dermatitis have markedly elevated levels of serum IgE. Mast cells and basophils are well-known target cells for this molecule, because they express abundant amounts of FcεRI on their surfaces. Third, certain genes associated with atopy are also expressed by mast cells. The β-subunit of FcεRI on chromosome 11q13 is linked to atopy, the state of enhanced IgE responsiveness (6,7). DNA sequences from atopic individuals show three base-pair substitutions converting Ile 181 to Leu 181. Although initially no such linkage was found in 95 English eczema families (8) linkage did emerge with later analyses (9). A significant association between the BstXI polymorphism in mast cell chymase on chromosome 14q11.2 and eczema has been reported (10–12).

This chapter will focus on the biology of human mast cells and basophils and the potential involvement of these cells in the pathogenesis of atopic dermatitis.

DIFFERENTIATION OF MAST CELLS AND BASOPHILS

Mast cells and basophils were initially thought to be developmentally related by virtue of their shared characteristic features, including metachromasia of their secretory granules, FcεRI on their surfaces, and histamine in their secretory granules. Both mast cells and basophils originate from hematopoietic stem cells, but they follow divergent pathways of differentiation. Basophils, like most myeloid cells, complete their differentiation in the bone marrow prior to entering the systemic circulation and develop largely under the influence of interleukin (IL)-3, a process that is augmented by transforming growth factor (TGF)-β. In contrast, mast cells

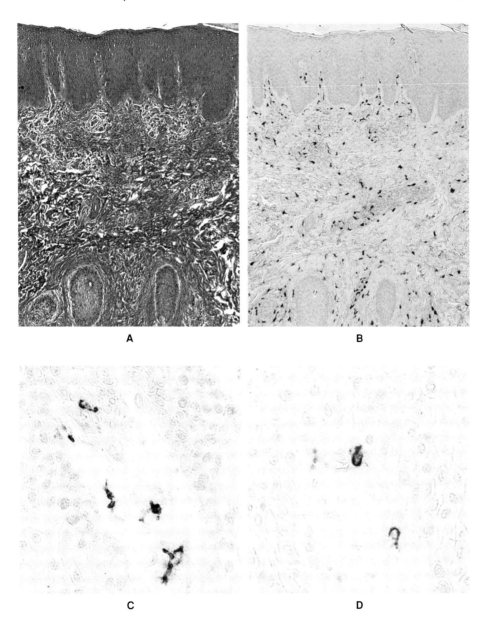

A B

C D

FIGURE 2 Mast cells in lesional skin of atopic dermatitis. Sequential sections of lichenified skin were stained with hematoxylin and eosin (**A**) and labeled with antitryptase mAb (**B**). Mast cells are difficult to identify in the hematoxylin and eosin-stained section, while immunohistochemistry for tryptase clearly reveals mast cell hyperplasia at this site. (**C**) Four MC$_{TC}$ cells are seen, one of which has penetrated into the epidermis. (**D**) Two MC$_T$ cells are observed in the dermis near the basement membrane.

destined to reside in peripheral tissues will leave the bone marrow as an immature mononuclear progenitor, probably with multipotential capabilities, enter the circulation still without characteristic secretory granules and surface FcεRI expression, but complete their differentiation into mature mast cells only after arriving in peripheral tissues such as lung, bowel, dermis, and nasal and conjunctival mucosa, largely under the influence of stem cell factor (SCF).

Murine Mast Cell Development

The evidence that tissue mast cells are derived from hematopoietic cells was first shown by using bg^J/bg^J mice (13). This beige mouse has a disorder similar to human Chediak-Higashi syndrome, characterized by marked enlargement of lysosomes and specific granules in various cell types. Transplantation of bg^J/bg^J mice bone marrow cells into irradiated $+/+$ mice resulted in the development of mast cells containing bg^J/bg^J-type giant granules. The origin of mast cells was also shown by in vitro suspension culture systems (14–18). When cells derived from hematopoietic tissues of mice were cultured with growth factors from stimulated T cells or with culture medium from a mouse myelomonocytic leukemia cell line WEHI-3, cells morphologically identified as mast cells appeared. Later, IL-3 was identified as the mast cell growth factor in the culture medium of WEHI-3 cells (19) and stimulated T cells (20). In suspension culture with IL-3, a large number of mast cells can be generated from murine hematopoietic progenitor cells. The importance of IL-3 for murine mast cell development in vivo has also been examined. Substantial IL-3–dependent hyperplasia of mast cells in the intestine after parasite infection has been observed for wild-type but not T cell–deficient (21) or IL-3–deficient mice (22). In the latter case, basophils were also deficient, but basal levels of mast cells were normal in both cases.

Genetically mast cell–deficient mice, named W/W^v (defective Kit) and Sl/Sl^d (defective SCF, also called Kit ligand), were identified by Kitamura and coworkers (23,24). These mice are anemic and also deficient in germ cells, melanocytes, and intestinal cells of Cajal. Despite the mast cell depletion in noninflamed tissues from W and Sl mutant mice, bone marrow–derived mast cells can be generated in vitro when bone marrow–derived progenitors are cultured with IL-3, and mast cells also can appear at tissue sites of inflammation. Fibroblasts derived from normal $+/+$ mouse embryos express SCF and thus can support the survival of bone marrow–derived mast cells derived from $+/+$ mice and those from Sl/Sl^d mice, but not those from W/W^v mice. W/W^v mice have been used to study the involvement of mast cells in various disease models, including anaphylaxis and allergic airway inflammation (25).

Human Mast Cell Development

Human mast cells differentiate under the influence of SCF (26–28). In contrast to rodent mast cells, IL-3 has little, if any, influence on the differentiation of human mast cells other than to expand the pool of hematopoietic progenitor cells (29). This is likely a consequence of mast cells from skin and lung being devoid of IL-3R (30), although it has been found on cord blood–derived (31,32) and intestinal (33) mast cells, where IL-3 partially protects against apoptosis due to SCF withdrawal and enhances degranulation and LTC$_4$ production (34).

Human mast cells originate from CD34+ bone marrow-derived progenitor cells (35). Using sorted cells isolated from cord blood or peripheral blood, mast cell progenitors were further characterized as multipotential cells positive for CD34 and CD38 (36) or for CD34, CD13, and Kit (37). However, less mature CD34+/CD38– precursor cells (38) did not give rise to mast cells when cultured with SCF, indicating a need for additional factors at this early stage of hematopoiesis. CD13, a membrane-bound zinc-dependent metalloprotease also known as aminopeptidase N, was originally recognized as a marker for subsets of normal and malignant myeloid cells (39) and later as a cell activation marker associated with proliferation. Thus, the early steps of hematopoietic commitment to a mast cell lineage still need further clarification.

When mast cells fail to develop in the bone marrow where SCF clearly affects the development of other cell types is an enigma. Either the bone marrow microenvironment lacks an accessory factor present in peripheral sites or the microenvironment contains additional factors that are not permissive for mast cell development to occur. The latter seems in part to be the case, because both granulocyte-macrophage colony-stimulating factor (GM-CSF) (40) and IL-4 (40,41) appear to diminish SCF-dependent development of mast cells from progenitors in vitro but have little effect on more mature mast cells.

Growth Factors That Affect Human Mast Cell Development

Unlike other myelocytes, which stop expressing Kit as they mature, mast cells express increasing amounts of Kit as they develop. SCF, the ligand for Kit, exerts various effects on mast cells throughout their development, including differentiation, survival, chemotaxis, activation, and priming. SCF is the only growth factor that by itself supports the growth and differentiation in vitro of human mast cells from hematopoietic precursors in bone marrow and peripheral blood (28), cord blood (27,42), and fetal liver (26,43). These in vitro–derived human-cultured mast cells now make possible further investigation about human mast cell characterization and their function, about the effect of cytokines on mast cell proliferation and development, and receptor expression during the maturation process. Removal of SCF from cultured mast cells (44) results in their apoptosis. Certain gain-of-function mutations in human Kit (45) are associated with systemic mastocytosis. However, less commonly, loss of function mutations in Kit (46) are also associated with this disease characterized by mast cell hyperplasia, perhaps indicating that there are factors other than Kit involved in mastocytosis. A different group of activating Kit mutations are associated with intestinal stromal cell tumors in which interstitial cells of Cajal are transformed (47).

IL-4 effects on human mast cells are pleiotropic. Human mast cell numbers are diminished by IL-4 after culturing progenitor cells obtained from peripheral blood, cord blood, and fetal liver with SCF (44,48,49). The ability of IL-4 to downregulate expression of Kit may help to explain the ability of this cytokine to attenuate mast cell development under some circumstances (44,48). On the other hand, IL-4 induces FcεRI expression on developing fetal liver–derived and cord blood–derived mast cells (49,50), enhances SCF-dependent proliferation of intestinal preparations of mast cells activated through FcεRI (51), and enhances the survival of cord blood–derived mast cells after withdrawal of SCF (32). For cord blood–derived mast cells obtained with the combination of SCF and IL-6, IL-4 did not affect total mast cell numbers in one study but did induce their homotypic aggregation and enhance the percentage of chymase-positive mast cells (52). Enhancement of the chymase-positive mast cells by IL-4 also was observed for those derived from fetal liver (49).

Using mast cells derived from fetal liver and cord blood progenitors cultured with SCF alone, IL-4 was shown to induce apoptosis only in the cord blood–derived mast cells, and this apoptotic effect on mast cells could be abolished if the cells were cultured with IL-6 in addition to SCF (41). IL-13, like IL-4 but with a weaker effect, downregulates Kit expression and upregulates adhesion molecule expression on HMC-1 cells, but has a negligible effect on SCF-dependent mast cell development from cord blood progenitors (53).

IL-6 has diverse effects on the development of human mast cells in vitro. IL-6 has been reported to both enhance (42) and attenuate (54) mast cell numbers obtained from cultures of cord blood progenitors and block IL-4–mediated apoptosis of cord blood–derived mast cells developed with SCF alone (35). IL-6 can enhance the percentage of mast cells expressing chymase (54).

IL-9 can enhance the SCF-dependent growth of mast cell progenitors from human cord blood (55), but does not protect them from apoptosis due to SCF withdrawal.

IL-10, in rodent systems, stimulates mast cell growth when added to other mast cell growth factors, including IL-3, SCF, and IL-4 (56). IL-10 also increases cellular levels of the β-chymases, mouse mast cell protease (mMCP)-1, and mMCP-2, principally by stabilizing the corresponding mRNA molecules (57–59). With human cells IL-10 alone did not promote the survival of cord blood–derived (32) or fetal liver–derived (60) mast cells. IL-33 accelerates the maturation of progenitors into tryptase$^+$ cells (61). Glucocorticosteroids inhibit mast cell development in vitro, but have minimal effects on mature mast cells.

Mast Cell Heterogeneity

Like lymphocytes and other hematopoietic cells, mast cell subtypes have also been described that display variations in their morphologic, biochemical, and functional properties. In mice, mast cells are often divided into connective tissue and mucosal mast cells. Connective tissue mast cells predominate in the skin, peritoneal cavity, and muscular propria of the stomach and express heparin proteoglycan; mucosal mast cells predominate in the mucosal layer of the gastrointestinal tract and express chondroitin sulfate proteoglycan. These different proteoglycan compositions probably account for differences in histochemical staining patterns. Both cell types can be stained by Alcian blue, but only those with heparin are stained with Safranin, a red dye, or Berberine sulfate, a fluorescent label.

In humans, two types of mast cells have been identified based on their protease composition (Fig. 3) (62). MC_{TC} cells contain tryptase, chymase, mast cell carboxypeptidase, and cathepsin G–like protease in their secretory granules. MC_T cells also contain tryptase in their granules but lack these other proteases. MC_{TC} cells are the predominant mast cell type in small bowel submucosa and in normal and urticaria pigmentosa skin as well as skin of atopic dermatitis, whereas MC_T cells are the predominant type found in the small bowel mucosa and normal airway, and appear to be selectively recruited near the surface of the airway during seasonal allergic disease. More recently, mature MC_{TC} cells obtained from human lung and skin preparations were shown to express surface CD88 (C5aR) and could be separated from MC_T cells by cell sorting (63). Of possible interest is the selective attenuation in numbers of MC_T cells in the small bowel of patients with end-stage immunodeficiency diseases (64). Mast cells from different tissues, irrespective of their protease phenotype, may exhibit functional differences in their response to

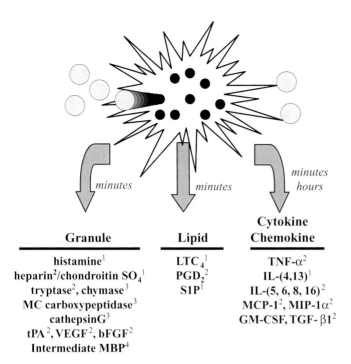

FIGURE 3 Mediators released by IgE-dependent activation of mast cells and basophils. Superscript numbers indicate the following cell types: 1, both mast cells and basophils; 2, MC_T and MC_{TC} cells; 3, MC_{TC} cells; and 4, basophils alone. *Abbreviation*: S1P, sphingosine 1 phosphate.

non–IgE-dependent activators and pharmacologic modulators of activation. The selected participation of basophils and different types of mast cells in various clinical conditions as well as the duration, intensity, and tissue distribution of a particular response will depend on various characteristics of the agonist, immunologic sensitivity of the host, the target tissue involved, and any underlying pathology.

Effect of Microenvironment on Mast Cell Phenotype

In murine systems, the microenvironment influences the phenotype of the mast cells. When immature bone marrow–derived mast cells from wild-type mice are transferred into the peritoneal cavity of mast cell–deficient W/W^v mice, the histamine content increased more than 20-fold and the proteoglycan class changed from chondroitin sulfate to heparin. The phenotypic change also occurred in the opposite direction (65). In contrast, after injection of a single connective tissue type of mast cell from the peritoneal cavity of a wild-type mouse into the stomach wall of a W/W^v mouse, mast cells with phenotypic features of mucosal mast cells appeared in the mucosa and of connective tissue mast cells in the muscularis propria (65,66). Similarly, immature bone marrow–derived mast cells cocultured with mouse 3T3 fibroblasts developed a connective tissue mast cell–like phenotype, becoming Safranin and carboxypeptidase A positive (67). SCF alone induces this phenotypic maturation of bone marrow–derived mast cells into connective tissue mast cell–like cells (68). However, because Kit-deficient mast cells that develop in inflammatory skin lesions of W/W^v mice have the connective tissue mast cell phenotype (69), factors other than SCF may influence mast cell development in mice. For example, nerve growth factor in association with IL-3 results in a connective tissue mast cell–like phenotype (70). However, the developmental pathway(s) of human mast cells may not parallel those of the mouse.

In humans, conditions that influence the selective development or recruitment of MC_{TC} and MC_T cells are not yet understood. SCF-dependent in vitro–derived mast cells generally are immature and express tryptase but little if any chymase. Cytokines such as IL-4 (71), IL-6 (54), and NGF (72) have been reported to induce modest levels of chymase expression. However, fetal liver–derived mast cells express chymase mRNA but not chymase protein, suggesting that the level of regulation of chymase expression in such cells may be beyond gene expression. On the other hand, chymase expression in vivo may be regulated at the level of gene expression, because MC_T cells isolated from lung appear to lack chymase mRNA as well as chymase protein. Furthermore, cultured MC_T cells from lung remained deficient in chymase protein and chymase mRNA (63).

In vivo observations suggest that MC_{TC} and MC_T cells develop along distinct pathways. Patients with inherited severe combined immunodeficiency disease and acquired immunodeficiency syndrome, both end-stage, exhibited marked and selective decreases in MC_T cell concentrations in the small bowel, whereas the concentration and distribution of MC_{TC} cells were unaffected (64). This suggests that the recruitment, development, or survival of MC_T cells is dependent on functional T lymphocytes and that MC_{TC} cell development proceeds independently. Also, an ultrastructural analysis of immature mast cells in various tissues indicated that at the time granules first form, they form either as MC_T or MC_{TC} cells (73).

Potential chemokine-dependent pathways for recruitment of mast cells or mast cell progenitors into tissues have been suggested. Chemokines are small proteins involved in the recruitment of various leukocytes by interacting with specific chemokine receptors. The presence of the CXCR2 chemokine receptor for IL-8 on HMC-1 cells (74) and on relatively mature cord blood–derived mast cells (75) and CCR3, CCR5, CXCR2, and CXCR4 on developing cord blood–derived mast cells (75) has been reported. Of potential interest is CCR3, which is expressed on eosinophils, basophils, and a subset of T cells with Th2-like features. CCR3 binds eotaxin, eotaxin-2, RANTES, and monocyte chemotactic proteins (MCP)-2 to -4. When tissue sections were subjected to immunohistochemical staining, high percentages of CCR3-expressing mast cells were found in the skin and in the intestinal submucosa; much lower percentages were found in the intestinal mucosa and in lung, suggesting preferential expression of CCR3 by MC_{TC} cells (76). Thus, selective chemokines may play an important role in the tissue distribution of different types of human mast cells.

MEDIATORS

Mast cells and basophils contain numerous potent and biologically active mediators that can exert many different effects in inflammation at sites of their activation. Mediators secreted by activated mast cells and basophils can be divided into those stored in secretory granules prior to cell activation and those that are newly generated after an activation signal. The former include histamine, proteoglycans, proteases, and certain cytokines; the latter include metabolites of arachidonic acid, cytokines, and chemokines, as summarized in Figure 3.

Histamine

Histamine, the sole biogenic amine in human mast cells and basophils, is the only preformed mediator of the cells with direct potent vasoactive and smooth muscle spasmogenic effects. Histamine, β-imidazolylethylamine, is formed from histidine by histidine decarboxylase and then stored in secretory granules. With degranulation, histamine is released, diffuses rapidly, and is metabolized within minutes after release, suggesting that it is destined to act quickly and locally. Human mast cells and basophils contain 1 to 3 pg of histamine per cell. Mast cells account for nearly all the histamine stored in normal tissues, with the exception of the glandular stomach and central nervous system. Histamine concentrations of about 0.1 M are estimated to exist inside secretory granules, whereas concentrations of about 2 nM exist in plasma. The amount of histamine present in circulating basophils, if released, could raise plasma histamine levels about 500-fold, so great care must be exercised to avoid disrupting basophils when collecting blood for a plasma histamine determination.

Histamine exerts its biologic and pathobiologic effects through its interaction with cell-specific receptors designated HI, H2, H3, and H4, which were initially denned with the recognition of specific agonists and antagonists. Both H1 (77) and H2 (78) receptors have seven regions predicted to span the plasma membrane and are G protein–coupled receptors. HI receptors are blocked by chlorpheniramine, H2 receptors are blocked by cimetidine, and H3 and H4 receptors are blocked by thioperamide. Examples of receptor-specific agonists include 2-methylhistamine at H1 receptors, dimaprit at H2 receptors, α-methylhistamine at H3 receptors, and clobenpropit at H4 receptors.

Effects of histamine mediated by H1 receptors include enhanced permeability of postcapillary venules, vasodilation, contraction of bronchial and gastrointestinal smooth muscle, and increased mucus secretion at mucosal sites. Increased vasopermeability will facilitate the tissue deposition of factors from plasma that may be important for tissue growth and repair and deposition of foreign material or immune complexes that result in tissue inflammation. Histamine by an H1 receptor–dependent mechanism in rodents also activates endothelial cells to transfer P-selectin from internal Weibel-Palade bodies to the cell surface, where neutrophil rolling is thereby enhanced (79,80). H1 receptor knock-out mice exhibit modest neurologic alterations but show no developmental abnormalities (81).

H2 receptor agonists stimulate gastric acid secretion by parietal cells. H2 agonists also inhibit secretion by cytotoxic lymphocytes and granulocytes, augment suppression by T lymphocytes, enhance epithelial permeability across human airways, stimulate chemokinesis of neutrophils and eosinophils and expression of eosinophil C3b receptors, and activate endothelial cells to release a potent inhibitor of platelet aggregation, PGI_2 (prostacyclin).

H1R are preferentially expressed on TH1 cells, and stimulate this type of helper T cell; H2R are preferentially expressed on TH2 cells, and inhibit this cell type. H1R$^{-/-}$ mice show a reduced Th1 response and enhanced TH2 response, while H2R$^{-/-}$ mice show increased TH1 and TH2 responses (82). Whether antihistamines used by humans affect their immune response in vivo in a similar manner remains to be determined. Stimulation of H3R affects neurotransmitter release and histamine formation in the central and peripheral nervous system. They are postulated to be involved in crosstalk between mast cells and peripheral nerves. Bronchial hyperreactivity in atopics with asthma to irritant stimuli may in part be mediated by histamine-mediated neurogenic hyperexcitability. H4R has been identified on hematopoietic cells and peripheral nerves (83,84). Mast cells express H1R, H2R, and H4R, but not H3R. H4R can directly mediate chemotaxis of mast cells (85) or enhance their migration to CXCL12 (86), indicating the possibility of paracrine recruitment. In animal studies, pharmacologic antagonists specific for the H4R have demonstrated their ability to modulate acute inflammation, hapten-mediated colitis, pruritus, and allergic airway inflammation (87,88).

The combined effects of H1 receptor– and H2 receptor–mediated activities of histamine are required for the full expression of vasoactivity. For example, the "triple response" caused by an intradermal injection of histamine, namely a central erythema within seconds (histamine arteriolar vasodilation), followed by circumferential erythema (axon reflex vasodilation mediated by neuropeptides) and a central wheal (histamine vasopermeability, edema) peaking at about 15 minutes, is mostly blocked by H1 receptor antagonists but is completely blocked only with a combination of H1 and H2 receptor antagonists (89). Analogous results have been observed for the tachycardia, widened pulse pressure, diastolic hypotension, flushing, and headaches resulting from intravenous infusion of histamine (90). Addition of a putative H4R antagonist may be useful for controlling the pruritus of urticaria.

Proteoglycans

The presence of highly sulfated proteoglycans in secretory granules of mast cells and basophils results in metachromasia when these cells are stained with basic dyes. The intracellular proteoglycans present in mast cells are heparin and chondroitin sulfate E. Chondroitin sulfate A is the predominant type in human basophils and eosinophils. Among bone marrow–derived cells, heparin is selectively expressed by mast cells and resides in the secretory granules of all mature human mast cells (91), but only in connective tissue mast cells in rodents. Glial cells are also capable of producing heparin (92). When mast cells are activated to degranulate, heparin proteoglycan is exocytosed along with other granule constituents in a complex with positively charged proteases, likely to include tryptase and chymase.

Proteoglycans are composed of glycosaminoglycan side chains, repeating unbranched disaccharide units of a uronic acid, and hexosamine moieties that are variably sulfated, which are covalently linked to a single-chain protein core via a specific trisaccharide–protein linkage region consisting of -Gal-Gal-Xyl-Ser. The average number of sulfate residues per respective disaccharide is 2.5, 1.5, and 1.0. The characteristic susceptibility of heparin to nitrous acid is due to attack at the N-sulfate residue; chondroitin sulfates lack this residue and are resistant to nitrous acid. On the other hand, the same peptide core is associated with heparin and chondroitin sulfate proteoglycans, and both proteoglycan types may reside in the same cell, even on the same peptide core. In humans the core protein is 17,600 Da in size and contains a glycosaminoglycan attachment region of 18 amino acids, where two to three glycosaminoglycans of about 20,000 Da are attached.

The biologic functions of endogenous mast cell proteoglycans include maturation and morphology of secretory granules (93–98), and maturation and stabilization of the active form of tryptase (99–101). These proteoglycans bind to histamine, neutral proteases, and acid hydrolases at the acidic pH inside mast cell secretory granules. The stabilizing effect of heparin and, to a lesser degree, chondroitin sulfate E on human tryptase activity may be crucial for the full expression of mast cell–mediated events. Heparin and, to a lesser extent, chondroitin sulfate E express anticoagulant, anticomplement, antikallikrein, and Hageman factor autoactivation activities. The anticoagulant activities of human and commercial porcine heparin are similar and depend on a specific pentasaccharide sequence. Heparin neutralizes the ability of eosinophil-derived major basic protein to kill schistosomula and enhances the binding of fibronectin to collagen. Heparin protects and facilitates basic fibroblast growth factor activity, which appears to reside in cutaneous mast cells (102), and modulates the cell adhesion properties of matrix proteins such as vitronectin, fibronectin, and laminin. Binding of heparin to L- and P-selectins inhibits inflammation (103), perhaps by blocking leukocyte rolling. However, when heparin is saturated with tryptase and other mast cell proteases, these activities may be attenuated. Disrupting the gene encoding glucosaminyl N-deacetylase/N-sulfotransferase-2 (NDST-2) (96,97) in mice yields mast cells exhibiting large vacuolated granules that were deficient in histamine and protease activities. In this NDST-2 knock-out mouse, only those mast cells that normally produce heparin, the so-called connective tissue mast cells, were affected, but coagulation-related problems were not noted.

Proteases

Proteases are enzymes that cleave peptide bonds, and certain ones are the dominant protein components of secretory granules in human and rodent mast cells. Basophils, compared to mast cells, are deficient in secretory granules protease activity. Some of these enzymes serve as selective markers that distinguish mast cells from other cell types, including basophils, and different mast cell subpopulations from one another.

Tryptase

Trypsin-like activity was first associated with human mast cells by histoenzymatic stains (104–106). Abundant and releasable trypsin-like activity was found in human lung mast cells in 1981 (107), followed by purification to homogeneity of the enzyme accounting for >90% of this activity, which was named tryptase (108). The enzyme was found to be a tetramer that spontaneously and irreversibly reverted to inactive monomers at neutral pH in a physiologic salt solution unless stabilized by heparin or dextran sulfate (109,110). In 1998, the crystal structure of lung-derived tryptase was solved (111), confirming the tetrameric structure and the length of the heparin-binding groove previously predicted (109). Two heparin grooves per tetramer were found, each spanning the two adjacent subunits bound to one another only through weak hydrophobic interactions. All of the active sites faced into the small, central pore of the planar tetramer, thereby restricting inhibitor and substrate access (112). Because tryptase is selectively concentrated in mast cell secretory granules, it has also been studied as a clinical marker of mast cell–mediated diseases.

Two genes encoding α and β-tryptases are clustered on the short arm of human chromosome 16; one gene, named TPSB, is monomorphic for β-tryptase, while the other gene, named TPSAB, is dimorphic and encodes either α- or β-tryptase (113–115). Each encodes a 30-amino-acid leader sequence and a 245-amino-acid catalytic portion. α-Tryptases show ~90% sequence identity to β-tryptases. Defining differences appear to include Arg^{-3} and Gly^{215} in β-tryptases and Gln^{-3} and Asp^{215} in α-tryptases. Each α- and β-tryptase has several subtypes, αI- and αII-tryptases and βI-, βII-, and βIII-tryptases show at least 98% identity within types.

Human Tryptases

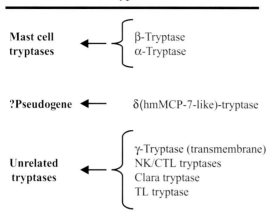

Mast cell   β-Tryptase
tryptases   α-Tryptase

?Pseudogene   ◀——   δ(hmMCP-7-like)-tryptase

Unrelated   γ-Tryptase (transmembrane)
tryptases   NK/CTL tryptases
                       Clara tryptase
                       TL tryptase

FIGURE 4 Proteases assigned the name tryptase are divided into those that are selectively expressed by mast cells, a possible pseudogene, and those that are biochemically and immunologically unrelated to α- and β-tryptases.

Each of these tryptase genes is organized into six exons and five introns. Tryptase genotypes exhibit 2:2 (βα/βα), 3:1 (ββ/βα), or 4:0 (ββ/ββ) molar ratios in approximately 25%, 50%, or 25% of individuals, respectively (116,117). A third closely related gene, δ-tryptase, encodes an mRNA for which translation terminates 40 amino acids earlier than α- and β-tryptases, also may be expressed by human mast cells (118), though precise quantitation has not yet been performed.

By comparison, mouse mast cell tryptases mMCP-6 and mMCP-7 (119,120), syntenic on mouse chromosome 17, have amino acid sequences 71% identical to one another, each of which shows ~75% sequence identity and a similar exon/intron organization to the human enzymes. Human α- and β-tryptases are more closely related to one another than to known nonhuman tryptases (121).

Confusion arose when the term tryptase was applied to other trypsin-like serine proteases (Fig. 4). These include trypsin-like enzymes in natural killer and cytotoxic T cells (NK tryptases) (122–124), a MOLT-4 T-helper-cell line (tryptase TL_2) (125), and lung Clara cells (tryptase Clara) (126). However, these enzymes do not show sufficient sequence homology or comparable biochemical properties to the mast cell tryptase family to be in the same family. A family of serine protease genes has been cloned near the tryptase locus on human chromosome 16 and mouse chromosome 17 and referred to as transmembrane tryptases because of a predicted transmembrane region near the C terminus and trypsin-like substrate specificity (127). Again, these enzyme appear to be biochemically and immunologically distinct from α- and β-tryptases. Herein the term tryptase will be used only for the α- and β-tryptases of human mast cells.

Purified recombinant αI-protryptase and βII-protryptase were used to study processing to the active enzyme(s) (101,128). βII-Protryptase was processed in two proteolytic steps. First, autocatalytic intermolecular cleavage at Arg^{-3} occurred optimally at acidic pH and in the presence of heparin or dextran sulfate. Second, the remaining prodipeptide was removed by dipeptidyl peptidase I, a cysteine peptidase found in most hematopoietic cells with an acidic pH optimum.

The mature peptide spontaneously formed enzymatically active tetramers, a process that seemed to require heparin or dextran sulfate. This processing mechanism might explain why tryptase and heparin are coexpressed in human mast cells and in mast cells of many other species. Two studies in mice assessed the impact of heparin on processing of mouse tryptases by disrupting the gene encoding glucosaminyl NDST-2 (96,97). In one study, those mast cells that normally produce heparin were markedly deficient in histamine and in chymase and tryptase enzymatic activities (96), suggesting that processing of certain mouse chymases and mouse tryptases was suboptimal in the absence of heparin.

On the other hand, a biologic processing mechanism for α-protryptase is still undefined. The presence of Gln^{-3} in αI-protryptase, instead of Arg^{-3} in β-tryptase, precludes optimal autocatalytic processing. Failure to process αI-protryptase to αI-protryptase might explain why human mast cells appear to spontaneously secrete enzymatically inactive α-protryptase, while βII-tryptase is stored in their secretory granules. Recombinant human αI-protryptase with an enterokinase peptide cleavage site inserted next to the mature portion was processed in vitro to a catalytically active enzyme (129), bypassing the need for a natural processing step. The resultant α-tryptase exhibited relatively little enzymatic activity against small synthetic substrates and no fibrinogen-cleaving activity.

The quantity of catalytically active tryptase per mast cell (10–35 pg) (130) is dramatically higher than the levels of proteases found in other cell types, such as neutrophils (~1–3 pg of elastase and of cathepsin G per cell). What regulates tryptase activity after its release into the extracellular milieu is uncertain, because the enzyme is resistant to classical biologic inhibitors of serine proteases (112).

A new possibility was raised after it was observed that lung and βII-tryptases degraded fibrinogen ~50-fold faster at pH 6 than at 7.4 (131). A similar acidic pH optimum was noted for processing of βII-protryptase (101) and for cleavage of low-molecular-weight kininogen (132) by lung-derived tryptase. Release of β-tryptase at sites of acidic pH, such as foci of inflammation and areas of poor vascularity, might be optimal for the enzyme, while diffusion away from such sites would result in reduced proteolytic activity. Such a mechanism would tend to limit the activity of β-tryptase to its local tissue site of release.

Catalytically active tetrameric tryptase loses enzymatic activity and converts to monomers at neutral pH and physiologic ionic strength in the absence of a stabilizing molecule like heparin. Placing inactive tryptase monomers (formed at neutral pH) into an acidic environment leads to the complete reassociation of these monomers into a catalytically active tetramer (100). Thus, at the acidic pH optimum for proteolysis, β-tryptase catalytic activity is stabilized, and inactive tryptase monomers theoretically could reassociate into catalytically active tetramers.

The biologic activities of enzymatically active tryptase are not obvious from the involvement of mast cells in diseases such as mastocytosis, anaphylaxis, urticaria, and asthma. The most relevant biologic substrate(s) of tryptase remains uncertain, though many potential ones have been evaluated, primarily in vitro. Predicted biologic outcomes might include anticoagulation, fibrosis and fibrolysis, kinin generation and destruction, cell surface protease–activated receptor (PAR)-2 activation, enhancement of vasopermeability, angiogenesis, inflammation, and airway smooth muscle hyperreactivity. Showing the importance of these potential activities in vivo remains a challenge. Studies on mice showed that the numbers of neutrophils increased >100-fold when enzymatically active β-tryptase was instilled into the lungs (133).

The emerging availability of pharmacologic inhibitors of tryptase, and preliminary studies suggesting they attenuate the bronchial response to an allergen challenge may facilitate identification of the most important biologic substrates.

Tryptase also has been used as a clinical biomarker, particularly for systemic anaphylaxis and systemic mastocytosis (134). Mature β-tryptase is stored in secretory granules, from where it is released by degranulation from activated mast cells. Mature tryptase can be measured by a specific ELISA. Accordingly, mature tryptase levels in serum or plasma are undetectable for healthy subjects (<1 ng/mL), but rise in those with insect sting–induced systemic anaphylaxis according to the clinical severity (hypotension). Levels of mature tryptase begin to rise within minutes of clinical symptoms, peak approximately one hour after onset and then decline with a half-time of about two hours. In the absence of hypotension, elevated mature tryptase levels are not usually observed. For comparison, histamine levels peak 5 to 10 minutes after onset, and then decline with a half-time of 1 to 2 minutes. Also of interest is the observation that anaphylaxis induced by ingestion of foods does not usually result in an elevated level of mature tryptase, suggesting that the pathogenesis of food-induced anaphylaxis may be different than other anaphylaxis induced by other stimuli.

Protryptases (α and β) are constitutively released by mast cells at rest. These tryptase precursors can be detected in serum or in plasma by an ELISA that measures all forms of tryptase (mature and pro), referred to as total tryptase. Total tryptase levels in serum from healthy subjects average ~5 ng/mL (1–15 ng/mL range) (Table 1). Individuals with systemic mastocytosis typically have a total tryptase level >20 ng/mL without an elevated level of mature tryptase when their disease is otherwise quiescent, which reflects the increased burden of mast cells. Other conditions associated with an elevated total tryptase level in the absence of an elevated mature include acute myelogenous leukemia, hypereosinophilic syndrome associated with the FIP1L1-PDGFRA mutation, end-stage renal failure, certain myelodysplastic conditions and refractory anemia, and iatrogenic administration of SCF. Cytoreductive therapy in conditions associated with elevated total tryptase levels can be monitored by following these levels. Interestingly, neither total nor mature tryptase levels are elevated in urticaria (135), unless urticaria is associated with systemic mastocytosis or systemic anaphylaxis. This is consistent with their being modest to no increases in mast cell numbers in cutaneous urticarial lesions (136,137).

Chymase

Chymase is one of the two principal enzymes accounting for the chymotrypsin-like activity present in human cutaneous mast cells. The enzyme was purified from human skin (138), and the corresponding gene cloned and localized to human chromosome 14 (139). Chymase was selectively localized to a subpopulation of mast cells by enzymatic (140) and immunohistochemical techniques (62). These MC_{TC} cells obtained from skin contain ~4.5 pg of chymase per cell.

Human chymase is a monomer of 30,000 Da whose crystal structure has been solved (141). Its chymotryptic substrate specificity prefers the motif nX-Pro-(Phe,Tyr,Trp)-Y-Y, where $n \geq 6$, X is any amino acid, and Y is any amino acid except Pro (142). Like tryptase, chymase is a serine esterase that is stored fully active in mast cell secretory granules, presumably bound to heparin and chondroitin sulfate E. Heparin facilitates processing of prochymase to active chymase by dipeptidyl peptidase I (143) and either attracts or repels potential chymase substrates based on ionic forces (144). Unlike tryptase, chymase stability is not substantially affected by heparin and its activity is inhibited by classical biologic inhibitors of serine proteinases, such as α_1-antichymotrypsin, α_1-proteinase inhibitor, and α_2-macroglobulin (145). Neither chymotrypsinlike enzymatic activity nor chymase mRNA were detected in lung MC_T cells (146).

Potential biologic activities of chymase, like those of tryptase, are based on in vitro observations. Chymase is a potent activator of angiotensin I, inactivates bradykinin and PAR-1 receptors (147), and attacks the lamina lucida of the basement membrane at the dermal–epidermal junction of human skin. The potential importance of angiotensin II generation by mast cell chymase in humans is of great interest. Chymase potently stimulates mucus production from glandular cells in vitro (148), suggesting a similar role in asthma and allergic rhinitis, where release of chymase in proximity to glandular tissue might be involved in the state of hypersecretion. Biologically active Kit can be released from the cell surface by chymase (149). Processing of type I procollagen by chymase to collagen-like fibrils has been demonstrated in vitro (150) and may relate to the finding of chymase-containing mast cells at sites of fibrosis in places such as rheumatoid synovium (151). Chymase degrades growth factors and cytokines such as Kit, pro–IL-18, IL-6, and IL-13 (149,152,153).

Cathepsin G

Human mast cell cathepsin G, like chymase, is a serine-class neutral protease with chymotryptic substrate specificity that is found in a subset of mast cells as well as in neutrophils and monocytes. The enzyme resides with chymase in MC_{TC} cells (154) and exhibits a molecular weight of 30,000 Da. Its crystal structure shows a similar polypeptide fold to that of rat mast cell proteinase II (155). Its proteolytic activity is controlled by serine proteinase inhibitors, $\alpha1$-antichymotrypsin in particular (156). Cathepsin G cleaves connective tissue and plasma proteins and exhibits modest microbicidal activities, and may act in concert with other proteases, such as neutrophil elastase and proteinase 3 (157). Like chymase, it stimulates mucous glandular secretion (148), of possible importance, in allergic asthma and rhinitis.

Mast Cell Carboxypeptidase

Human mast cell carboxypeptidase A3 resides with chymase and cathepsin G in secretory granules of MC_{TC} cells (158). Stored fully active, when released it cleaves the carboxy terminal His^9–Leu^{10} bond of angiotensin I and behaves like a zinc-dependent exopeptidase. Human mast cells dispersed from skin contain 5 to 16 pg of carboxypeptidase per cell. Human mast cell carboxypeptidase A3 is a monomer with a molecular weight of 34,500 Da (159) and substrate specificity for carboxy terminal Phe and Leu residues. Based on the analysis of the cDNA-derived amino-acid sequence and gene structure (160), the human enzyme is more homologous to human pancreatic carboxypeptidase B than that in A, but the catalytic site is more homologous to human pancreatic carboxypeptidase A, as are its substrate specificities for carboxy-terminal Phe and Leu residues.

Murine bone marrow–derived mast cells showed abnormality in maturation and morphology in the absence of carboxypeptidase A (161). Carboxypeptidase A3, in cooperation with chymase, is also involved in the formation and degradation of angiotensin II (162). Carboxypeptidase A3 also inactivates endogenous endothelin as well as exogenous snake and honey bee venoms (163,164).

Other Proteases and Enzymes
Tissue-type plasminogen activator has been identified in tissue-derived mast cells (165), potentially complementing mast cell antithrombotic and anticoagulant activities with the fibrinolytic properties of this protease. Mast cells also concentrate various acid hydrolases in their secretory granules, perhaps reflecting the lysosomal origin of this organelle, including β-galactosidase, aryl sulfatase, and β-hexosaminidase, the latter enzyme serving as a marker to evaluate degranulation of dispersed preparations of mast cells (107).

Matrix metalloproteinase-9 (MMP-9), a gelatinase B, has been identified in cord blood–derived mast cells, and by immunohistochemistry, human skin, lung, and synovial mast cells are strongly positive for MMP-9 (166). Because MMPs can promote the degradation of extracellular matrix, they are believed to play a role in the pathogenesis of certain disorders associated with tissue remodeling. Studies in dog mast cells suggest that SCF increases expression, whereas TGF-β downregulates expression of progelatinase B (167), while in mice SCF downregulates MMP-9 (168). Thus, external agents may influence the fibrolytic versus fibrotic capabilities of this cell type.

Mast cells from human lung tissue and HMC-1 cells reportedly express rennin, which generates angiotensin I from angiotensinogen (169,170). Mast cells also express small amounts of granzyme B in response to FcεRI-mediated cell activation (171,172).

Lipids
Metabolites of Arachidonic Acid
Human mast cells purified from lung incorporate exogenous arachidonic acid into neutral lipids and phospholipids and store these lipids in membranes and cytoplasmic lipid bodies. Liberation of the arachidonic acid destined for oxidative metabolism, as shown in mice, is dependent upon cytosolic phospholipase A_2 (173). In general, oxidation of arachidonic acid occurs through the cyclooxygenase (COX) pathway to prostaglandins (PGs) and thromboxanes (TXs), or the 5-, 12-, or 15-lipoxygenase (LO) pathways to monohydroxy fatty acids, leukotrienes (LTs) that include both LTB_4 and the sulfidopeptides LTC_4, LTD_4, and LTE_4, formerly known as slow-reacting substances of anaphylaxis (SRS-A), and lipoxins. Platelet-activating factor, made by acetylating the lysophospholipid remaining after arachidonic acid departs, has not been shown to be a major secretory product of human mast cells and basophils. The major eicosanoid products secreted by activated mast cells and basophils are summarized in Figure 3.

Activation of human mast cells obtained from lung, skin, and intestine results in PGD_2 production through the activity of PGD synthase and in LTC_4 production through the activity of LTC synthase in weight ratios of approximately 5:1, respectively. Smaller amounts of LTB_4 isomers are also produced. Ratios of these metabolites cannot be used to distinguish MC_T from MC_{TC} cell activation. In contrast, activation of peripheral blood basophils obtained from normal human subjects results in LTC_4, but not PGD_2 production. However, cells other than mast cells and basophils produce PGD_2 (e.g., platelets and certain antigen-presenting cells) and LTC$_4$ (e.g., eosinophils). Both leukotriene and prostaglandin production by activated mast cells can be blocked without altering release of granule mediators and cytokines.

The biologic importance of mast cell–derived and basophil-derived products of arachidonic acid metabolism has gained support with the advent of inhibitors of 5-LO and the cysLT1 receptor (174) for LTD$_4$, both of which are helpful in atopic and in aspirin-induced asthma, each condition also involving activation of mast cells as well as eosinophils, another major source of LTC$_4$. Of potential clinical interest was the finding that dexamethasone can upregulate 5-LO levels and LTC$_4$ production by HMC-1 cells in vitro (175). A metabolite of PGD$_2$ is elevated in the urine of patients with active systemic mastocytosis. The importance of PGD$_2$ production in the subgroup of these patients with recurrent hypotensive episodes was suggested when administration of aspirin inhibited generation of the PGD$_2$ metabolite and led to clinical improvement (176). PGD$_2$ is produced by mast cells during both the immediate and late phases of immediate hypersensitivity reactions, where COX-1 is responsible for PGD$_2$ production during the early phase and COX-2 during the late phase (177,178). The ability of PGD$_2$ to activate human eosinophils (179) and to play a role during induction of allergic airway disease in mice (180) suggests its potential importance in human allergic diseases at sites of mast cell–dependent inflammation. However, prostaglandin and leukotriene inhibitors exhibit minimal consistent benefit in urticaria and atopic dermatitis.

Metabolite of Sphingosine

Sphingosine-1-phosphate (S1P) is a newly appreciated lipid mediator that is both produced by mast cells and affects mast cell activation and recruitment. S1P is formed from sphingosine and ATP by the action of sphingosine kinases. S1P is produced and secreted by activated mast cells, and also acts on mast cells to enhance degranulation through binding to its S1P2 receptor and to enhance recruitment by binding to its S1P1 receptor, both of which are expressed on mast cells (181). In mice, S1P levels in the circulation affect the severity of IgE-mediated anaphylaxis (182).

Cytokines and Chemokines

There is no doubt that mast cells and basophils represent important sources of inflammatory mediators during acute, IgE-dependent reactions. Moreover, recent findings indicate that mast cells and basophils can also contribute to both the late-phase inflammation and the chronic tissue changes as potentially significant sources of several cytokines. Human mast cells and basophils, when activated, produce a diverse array of cytokines and chemokines (Fig. 3). These include tumor necrosis factor (TNF)-α, IL-3, -4, -5, -6, -8, -10, -13, and -16, lymphotactin, GM-CSF, MCP-1, TGF-β1, monocyte inflammatory peptide (MIP)-1α and nerve growth factor by mast cells, and at least IL-4 and IL-13 by basophils. In some cases cytokines may be stored in secretory granules and released with other preformed mediators. Mast cells have been noted to be the dominant IL-4–positive cell in allergic nasal mucosa (183), and in the skin lesion of atopic dermatitis (272), while basophils are the dominant IL-4–positive cell in the asthmatic airway 24 hours after allergen challenge (184) and in allergen-challenged peripheral blood cells (185). Cytokines also can be newly generated and released hours after mast cells or basophils are activated. These cytokines serve to recruit and activate other cell types, thereby amplifying the host response during immediate hypersensitivity events. For example, endothelial cells are activated by various mediators to recruit eosinophils and other cell types during the late phase response of immediate hypersensitivity reactions. Mast cells-derived TNF-α enhances T-cell activation and differentiation of naïve T cells into Th1 and Th2 subsets (186). Mast cells can thereby be involved in sustaining allergic inflammation hours after granule exocytosis is finished.

Interestingly, levels of FcεRI expression on mast cells and basophils can be regulated by IgE levels in vivo and in vitro in both mice (187,188) and humans (49,189,190). Because this process also can increase the ability of mast cells to produce IL-4, IL-13, and MIP-1α, all of which can promote IgE production from plasma cells, IgE-dependent upregulation of FcεRI expression may also be part of a positive feedback mechanism for further production of IgE (191) and thereby promote allergic reactions associated with high levels of IgE. In addition, mast cells have been reported to be able to express CD40 ligand on their surface (192), an important costimulatory factor for the B-cell switch to IgE production.

ACTIVATION AND REGULATED SECRETION

FcεRI-Mediated Activation

Mast cells and basophils are thought to play an important role in allergic disorders, primarily as a result of their expression of a high-affinity IgE receptor, FcεRI, that binds the Fc region of monomeric IgE with high specificity and affinity ($K_a = 10^9$ M^{-1}). At least under some circumstances, many other potential effector cells such as Langerhans cells, monocytes and macrophages, circulating dendritic cells, and eosinophils also may express small numbers of this receptor. In addition, another cell surface receptor, CD23, binds IgE, albeit with lower affinity ($K_a = 10^6$ M^{-1}). The expression of CD23 is widely distributed on B and T cells, monocytes, eosinophils, Langerhans cells, and platelets. However, the FcεRI expressed on mast cells and basophils is the principal molecule through which IgE exerts its characteristic biologic function: the release of various kinds of inflammatory mediators.

The complete FcεRI receptor is composed of four subunits, α, β, and two γ chains, which appear to float on the cell surface in lipid-based domains called rafts (193). The α-chain contains the extracellular IgE binding domain. Only the β-chain crosses the plasma membrane four times and has both N- and C-termini protruding into the cytoplasm. Each β and two disulfide-linked α-chains, located primarily in the membrane and cytoplasm, have one special intracytoplasmic activation motif composed of a twice-repeated Tyr-X-X-Leu sequence, designated as ITAM or immunoreceptor tyrosine activation motif. In humans, the presence of the β-chain, though not essential for surface receptor expression or signal transduction, markedly amplifies phosphorylation of the γ-chains and signal transduction, thereby increasing the magnitude of cell activation and host response (194,195). The γ-chains are shared with the CD16 and FcεRIII receptors of natural killer cells and may substitute for the T-cell receptor ζ chain.

Mast cells and basophils undergo regulated degranulation when FcεRI is dimerized by multivalent antigen or antireceptor antibody. The earliest biochemical events involved in signal transduction after FcεRI aggregation are tyrosine phosphorylation of ITAMs. The C-terminal of the β-subunit of FcεRI is constitutively associated with Src-family protein tyrosine kinases (PTKs) such as Lyn. ITAMs located in the β- and γ-subunits of FcεRI are phosphorylated by Lyn within seconds after receptor cross-linking. These ITAMs, when doubly phosphorylated, provide docking sites for the cytoplasmic PTK, Syk, which has SH-2 domains that recognize such motifs. Syk is then phosphorylated by Lyn and possibly by itself (196–198). The Syk dependence of IgE-mediated signal transduction in humans appears to be clinically relevant, because patients whose basophils have low levels of Syk expression are nonreleasers to FcεRI cross-linking. Incubation of basophils with IL-3 induces Syk expression and, when FcεRI is cross-linked, degranulation and IL-4 production and VCAM-1 binding (199,200). These early events are also regulated by signal inhibitory regulatory proteins (SIRPs) that contain ITIMs, immunotyrosine inhibition motifs. For example, SIRP-α is expressed in human mast cells and has been shown in mice to act in part by recruiting SH-2–bearing protein tyrosine phosphatases (SHP-1 and -2) that dephosphorylate ITAMs on β- and γ-chains of FcεRI, thereby downregulating signal transduction and mediator release (201). CD45, a protein tyrosine phosphatase, promotes mediator release; mast cells from mice that are deficient in this enzyme do not exhibit IgE-dependent activation (202).

Later events in the signal transduction pathway are mediated by phosphorylated Syk, which then recruits other signal transduction molecules, such as Btk in mice, though perhaps not in human mast cells (203). Defective Btk in mice attenuates degranulation and cytokine production by activated mast cells as well as the anaphylactic response of the animal (204,205). SLP-76 is an adapter protein known to be a substrate for both ZAP-70 and Syk. In SLP-76 knock-out mice, mast cells undergo phosphorylation of Syk with FcεRI cross-linking but do not release mediators (206). The activation signal is finally transmitted to pathways involving phospholipase C (PLC)γ, MAP kinase, protein kinase C, and phosphotidyl inositol (PI)-3 kinase.

Degranulation of mast cells and basophils is associated with activation of small G proteins that cause actin polymerization and actin relocalization (207,208). Metabolism of phospholipids, which mostly reside in secretory granules, occurs early during the secretory response, is necessary for the later secretion of lipid mediators and may be important for regulated secretion to ensue. Generation of inositol triphosphate (IP$_3$) and diacylglycerol after FcεRI receptor aggregation results in release of calcium from the endoplasmic reticulum. This in turn stimulates calcium-dependent isoforms of protein kinase C and may directly facilitate fusion of lipid bilayers as exocytosis proceeds. A cytoplasmic calcium sensor called synaptotagmin II also influences exocytosis by mast cells (209).

Activation by Other Immunologic Stimuli

Mast cells can also be activated through their pattern recognition receptors, which detect microbial-derived molecules. Among them are mammalian toll-like receptors (TLRs). A total of 11 TLRs have been reported. Bone marrow–derived murine mast cells degranulate and produce cytokines in response to bacterial peptidoglycan via TLR2 (210), while only cytokine production was noticed when they were activated by lipopolysaccharide via TLR4 (211). In addition, murine fetal skin-derived mast cells express functional TLR3, TLR7, and TLR9, which when engaged by ligands, lead to cytokine and chemokine production (212). Human in vitro–derived mast cells express TLRs 1–7, which when occupied by ligands, leads to the production of cytokines without degranulation (213).

Human mast cells at rest do not express FcγRI and RIII receptors (214). However, MC$_{TC}$ cells from skin express functional FcγRIIa, aggregation of which leads to degranulation and production of cytokines, PGD_2, and LTC_4 (215). These cells do not express inhibitory FcγRIIb. Treatment with IFN-γ induces the transient expression of FcγRI, which when aggregated also causes mast cells to release histamine, cytokines, PGD_2, and LTC_4 (216,217). These findings suggest that human mast cells can be involved in IgG-dependent immune responses and hypersensitivity.

Activation by Nonimmunologic Reagents

Regulated secretion by mast cells and basophils also may be induced by nonimmunologic agonists. Multivalent lectins, like bivalent concanavalin A, crosslink membrane FcεRI or IgE. Calcium ionophores activate by directly translocating calcium.

The secretory response to some nonimmunologic reagents varies between mast cells isolated from different tissues. Basic biomolecules such as compound 48/80, C3a, C5a, morphine, codeine, mellitin, eosinophil-derived major basic protein, and various neuropeptides such as substance P, vasoactive intestinal peptide (VIP), somatostatin, and calcitonin gene–related protein (CGRP) activate human mast cells isolated from skin, but are inactive against mast cells derived from most other tissues. Mast cells from heart respond to C5a, but not to substance P (218). In contrast, basophils respond to C5a and C3a, but not to the neuropeptides, compound 48/80, morphine, and codeine. The desArg derivatives of C3a and C5a are inactive on skin mast cells but still show limited agonist activity against basophils. Whether these basic peptides activate mast cells and basophils by stereospecific receptor interactions or by ionic perturbations of membrane components is not clear (219). Differences in the secretory response between mast cells isolated from different tissues may relate in part to microenvironmental influences. For example, the rat mucosal mast cell line RBL-2 H2 reversibly acquires responsiveness to substance P when cocultured with 3T3 fibroblasts without otherwise changing its phenotype.

Basophils also can be activated as well as primed to better respond to antigen by IL-3, an interleukin that does not affect human mast cell activation. The differences between basophils and mast cells with respect to their non–IgE-mediated pathways of activation, in theory, could lead to the activation of one cell type in the absence of the other. Basophils, like eosinophils but in contrast to mast cells, express surface Fc-αR and can be activated by an IgA-dependent pathway (220,221). The peptide f-Met-Leu-Phe activates human basophils, but not mast cells. HIV-1 gp120 activates IgE-armed basophils to secrete IL-4 and IL-13 (222), of possible interest to immediate hypersensitivity reactions commonly observed in HIV-infected individuals. Immunologic activation of mast cells can be enhanced by adenosine (223), possibly through the adenosine A2b receptor in humans (224). In contrast, mediator release from human basophils is inhibited by adenosine. ATP also can enhance mediator release from activated mast cells by binding to the P2Y surface purinoreceptor expressed on human lung mast cells (225).

Various histamine-releasing factors derived from monocytes, lymphocytes, platelets, and neutrophils also have been described that are of potential clinical significance. The protein termed p23, for example, has been shown to have IgE-dependent histamine, cytokine, and LTC_4-releasing activity on basophils, an effect on mast cells being uncertain (226,227). Chemokines, initially discovered because of their abilities to attract predominantly monocytes or neutrophils, include potent basophil histamine-releasing and histamine-attracting agents (228). Active chemokines include MCP-1 to -4, RANTES, MIP-1α and -1β, eotaxin and eotaxin-2, and ecalectin. Most of these chemokines affect eosinophils as well as basophils. The presence of the chemokine receptor CCR3 on basophils and eosinophils dovetails with the cellular specificity of these CC class chemokines (229). However, a further level of complexity was revealed for MCP-1, which when intact preferentially activates basophils over eosinophils but, after the N-terminal amino acid is removed, preferentially activates eosinophils over basophils. In contrast to the effects of these chemokines on basophils, mast cell mediator release appears to be unaffected (230,231), even though human mast cells express CCR3 (75,76). However, human mast cells appear to be capable of producing both MCP-1 and MIP-1α (191,232), suggesting a mechanism in which basophils may be recruited to and activated at tissue sites of mast cell activation.

CLINICAL MARKERS OF MAST CELLS AND BASOPHILS
Analysis of the cellular infiltration found in the skin of atopic dermatitis patients has provided important clues for understanding the pathogenesis of this disorder. The involvement of mast cells and basophils can be addressed in terms of both cell numbers and cell activation. Antibodies developed against cell-specific surface or granule components provide an immunohistologic means for detecting these cells in tissues with greater sensitivity and specificity than classic dye-based histologic stains.

Immunohistochemistry
The most selective surface marker phenotype for all human mast cells is the coexpression of high levels of Kit and FcεRI. This pattern is readily demonstrated on dispersed mast cells by flow cytometry. Tryptase serves as a granule marker for all human mast cells; the >100-fold smaller amounts present in basophils typically provide an adequate differential for distinguishing these two cell types from one another. Mast cells are difficult to identify in tissue specimens stained with hematoxylin and eosin [Fig. 2(A)], while tryptase provides a more sensitive and specific immunohistochemical marker for mast cells. Antitryptase immunohistochemistry reveals mast cell hyperplasia at sites of lichenification in atopic dermatitis [Fig. 2(B)]. Monoclonal antibodies (mAbs) against chymase and mast cell carboxypeptidase serve to identify the MC_{TC} type of mast cell, because no other normal cell type appears to express these products. No specific marker for the MC_T type of mast cell has been found; these cells being identified by the presence of tryptase in the absence of chymase as well as by the absence of CD88 on their surface (63).

By using metachromatic stains, the total number of mast cells has been shown to be increased in lichenified lesions of atopic dermatitis. In the acute phase of atopic dermatitis of four patients, MC_{TC} cells identified by immunohistochemistry, as in skin of normal subjects, were reported to be the predominant mast cell type. However, unlike skin of normal subjects, a substantial population (1–17%) of the mast cells displayed an MC_T phenotype [Fig. 2(D)] (3). These findings were confirmed by another study, which demonstrated that in the upper dermis of nonlesional and lesional atopic dermatitis skin, only 80% of tryptase-positive cells displayed chymase enzyme activity, whereas all the skin mast cells of normal control subjects contained chymase (4). Whether chymase inside mast cells is inhibited in vivo or simply as a result of processing tissue bathed in high levels of serum-derived protease inhibitors remains to be clarified. Within the epidermis of atopic dermatitis,

Tryptase immunoassays

	Mature tryptase (B12/G5 mAbs)	Total tryptase (B12/G4 mAbs)
Tryptase type recognized	β-Tryptase	α/β-Pro+mature tryptases
Normal serum (ng/mL)	<1	1–15
Systemic anaphylaxis (acute)	>1	(*Total*/β) *ratio* < *10* ↑
Systemic mastocytosis (nonacute)	±↑	≥ 20 (*Total*/β) *ratio* > *20*

FIGURE 5   Characteristics of the total tryptase and mature tryptase immunoassays performed on serum or plasma. β-Tryptase is preferentially measured when the G5 mAb is used for detection, while both immature and mature forms of α- and β-tryptases are measured when the G4 mAb is used for detection. The B12 mAb is used for capture in both immunoassays.

a few lesional samples were reported to contain chymase-positive cells [Fig. 2(C)] (3), a feature not seen in skin of healthy controls. In another report, mast cells were observed in the epidermis of 3 of 10 specimens of noninvolved skin from the upper arm of atopic dermatitis patients (233). However, the potential significance of epidermal mast cells is unclear.

Although an FcεRI⁺/Kit⁻ surface phenotype or FcεRI⁺/tryptase⁻ surface/granule phenotype has been considered to selectively represent basophils, the abilities of activated monocytes, eosinophils, and antigen-presenting cells such as Langerhans cells to express FcεRI make this consideration problematic, particularly at sites of inflammation (234). Two mAbs (235,236) that recognize components of basophil secretory granules but do not label other cell types, including mast cells and eosinophils, identify basophils in tissues by immunohistochemistry. The respective antigens are called 2D7 antigen and basogranin. The 2D7 antibody has been shown to recognize pro-MBP (237). Using such mAbs, basophil influx during the late phase of allergic reactions was shown to occur in the skin (238–240), lung (184,240,241), and nose (242). Basophil numbers were about fivefold lower than eosinophils, but appeared to account for a substantial portion of the IL-4–producing cells.

Serum Tryptase Levels

Immunoassays for cell-specific, releasable, and preformed granule mediators provide a more precise measure of either local or systemic activation of a particular cell type than is possible by either clinical criteria or documentation of antigen-specific IgE. Most mAbs against human tryptase recognize both α- and β-tryptase products, whereas one mAb called G5 (linear epitope) recognizes mature β-tryptase but not α-protryptase (Fig. 5). This is of clinical relevance because α-protryptase appears to be continuously secreted by human mast cells, and its levels in blood thereby serve as a measure of mast cell number. In contrast, β-tryptase is stored in secretory granules and is released only during granule exocytosis; its levels serve as a measure of mast cell activation. Therefore, elevated serum levels of α/β protryptases reflect mast cell hyperplasia such as occurs in systemic mastocytosis, whereas elevated serum levels of mature β-tryptase reflect mast cell activation such as occurs in systemic anaphylaxis (134). Because β-tryptase accounts for all of the tryptase enzymatic activity, it is the principal form measured by enzymatic assays whereas the currently commercially available tryptase immunoreactive assay (Pharmacia, Uppsala, Sweden) measures a combination of α and β tryptases.

Systemic mastocytosis is associated with mast cell hyperplasia in skin lesions (urticaria pigmentosa), liver, spleen, lymph nodes, and bone marrow (243). The disorder is subdivided into those with indolent mastocytosis, systemic mastocytosis associated with a hematologic disorder, and aggressive systemic mastocytosis (244). In a study of tryptase levels in subjects with biopsy-diagnosed mastocytosis, most of those with systemic mastocytosis indicated by a bone marrow biopsy (35 of 42) had levels of total tryptase >20 ng/mL and ratios of total tryptase to β-tryptase >20 (135). Normal subjects ($n = 55$) had total tryptase levels of <14 ng/mL (245). This suggested a specificity of >98% and a sensitivity of 83% for total tryptase levels when compared to a bone marrow biopsy. However, among the seven subjects with systemic mastocytosis and a serum total tryptase level below 20 ng/mL, all had total tryptase levels between 10 and 20 ng/mL, three had ambiguous bone marrow readings, and another had the bone marrow biopsy performed 5 years before the serum sample was collected. Most subjects with local cutaneous mast cell disease (10 of 13) had levels similar to normal controls (1–11 ng/mL; ratios ≤11). Among the three subjects with serum total tryptase levels above this range, one was an infant with diffuse cutaneous mastocytosis, and another had no bone marrow biopsy performed. The indolent group with urticaria pigmentosa and no evidence of systemic involvement had levels of total tryptase in the normal range. Thus, the level of total tryptase appears to distinguish those with local versus systemic disease. However, the absolute level of total tryptase did not predict clinical severity, suggesting that factors other than the mast cell burden alone are important in systemic mastocytosis.

β-Tryptase levels in serum or plasma are elevated in most subjects with systemic anaphylaxis of sufficient severity to result in hypotension (246). β-Tryptase is released from mast cells in parallel with histamine (107) but diffuses more slowly than histamine, presumably due to its association with the macromolecular protease–proteoglycan complex. During insect sting–induced anaphylaxis, β-tryptase levels in the circulation are maximal 15 to 120 minutes after the sting, while histamine levels peak at about 5 minutes and decline to baseline by 15 to 30 minutes (247,248). Peak β-tryptase levels decline with a half-time of 1.5 to 2.5 hours. In insect sting–induced systemic anaphylaxis, the ratios of total tryptase to β-tryptase were less than 6 in 16 of 17 subjects, being 23 in the one outlier (245). Thus, when β-tryptase is detectable in serum, a total to β-tryptase ratio ≤10 suggests systemic anaphylaxis. Mast cells also have been implicated in anaphylactic reactions to cyclooxygenase inhibitors by finding elevated levels of β-tryptase in blood (247). In cases of clinical anaphylaxis with a normal level of β-tryptase, pathogenetic mechanisms without mast cell activation should be considered. These might include basophil activation or complement anaphylatoxin generation.

An analysis of serum samples from patients with atopic dermatitis revealed no elevation of total or β-tryptase (273). However, this does not rule out local cutaneous increases in either mast cell number or mast cell activation. The dermal microdialysis technique may offer the ability to better assess local mediator production in lesional and nonlesional sites of atopic dermatitis (249).

MAST CELLS AND BASOPHILS AS THERAPEUTIC TARGETS IN ATOPIC DERMATITIS

The mediators for pruritus in atopic dermatitis are still unknown. Although histamine is the crucial mediator of pruritus in type I allergic reactions, particularly in urticaria where HI receptor blockade effectively abolishes itch and improves the skin condition, there is some controversy about the role of histamine in atopic dermatitis. Some authors report a significant reduction of pruritus by histamine H1-blockers (250–252), but others find no antipruritic effect or only a marginal effect probably due to sedative effects (253,254). Interestingly, the direct cutaneous application of histamine results in a lower itch rating (255) and smaller axon reflex flares in atopic dermatitis patients than control subjects (256), suggesting that histamine is not a crucial mediator for itch in atopic dermatitis (257). Pharmacologic responsiveness of mast cells varies depending on the tissue source and differs from that of basophils. Both disodium cromoglycate and nedocromil, used for the treatment of allergic asthma, rhinitis, and conjunctivitis, are weak inhibitors of lung mast cell activation but are ineffective against mast cells from skin and intestine.

Topical corticosteroids are the most established treatment for atopic dermatitis. Dexamethasone in vitro inhibits mediator secretion by human basophils, but not by human lung-derived mast cells. Dexamethasone also inhibits SCF-induced development of mast cells from fetal liver cells but shows no appreciable effect on developed mast cells (258). In vivo, local instillation of nasal glucocorticosteroids over a prolonged period of time diminished mediator release during the immediate response to nasal allergen challenge, perhaps due to the capacity for local steroids to diminish mast cell concentrations as demonstrated in the synovium (259), skin (260), and rectal mucosa (261), or to the prevention of the superficial migration of mast cells that apparently occurs in atopic subjects during the allergy season (262,263).

Macrolide immunosuppressants are potent immunosuppressive drugs that act primarily on T cells by inhibiting cytokine gene activation. Cyclosporin A and tacrolimus (FK-506) produce rapid and long-lasting inhibition of IgE-dependent histamine release from human basophils and skin- and lung-derived mast cells (264–266). Rapamycin interferes with the inhibitory activity of FK-506 by competing for the same FK-binding protein, but by itself does not inhibit mast cell or basophil activation. Oral treatment with cyclosporin A has proven to be effective in atopic dermatitis (267), perhaps due both to its inhibitory effects on T cells as well as mast cells and basophils. Topical treatment with tacrolimus also appears to provide effective treatment of atopic dermatitis (268).

SUMMARY

Mast cells and basophils, the two principal effector cells of immediate hypersensitivity, also appear to be involved in atopic dermatitis. Mast cells are increased in number at lesional sites. Occasionally, mast cells penetrate into epidermis in these lesions. Mast cells in lesions may also exhibit an MC_T phenotype. Basophils are difficult to observe with metachromatic stains in sites of inflammation, but appear to be present by immunohistochemistry that targets basophil-specific markers. By virtue of the high levels of antigen-specific IgE also present, mast cells and basophils are armed and capable of discharging their mediators upon encountering antigen. However, the pruritic component of atopic dermatitis is most of the time minimally dependent on histamine, unlike urticaria. Also, the inflammatory components clearly involve multiple cell types. On the other hand, using mast cell–deficient mice (W/W^v), mast cells were shown to regulate IFN-γ expression in the skin and circulating IgE levels in allergen-induced skin inflammation (269). More recently, a mouse lacking a negative regulator of FcεRI-dependent mast cell activation, Rab guanine nucleotide exchange factor I or RabGDF1 was found to display many of the characteristic features of human atopic dermatitis, such as elevated total IgE levels and chronic skin inflammation with mast cells in the dermis (270). Furthermore, omalizumab, a monoclonal anti-IgE antibody with the ability to markedly decrease free IgE levels, has shown benefit in the treatment of subjects with atopic dermatitis (271). Thus, the role and importance in atopic dermatitis of mast cells and basophils may vary at different stages of the disease. As we learn more about these cell types, develop better markers for them, and obtain therapeutic agents more precisely targeted at them, their contributions to atopic dermatitis will be understood with greater precision.

REFERENCES

1. Mitchell EB, Crow J, Williams G, et al. Increase in skin mast cells following chronic house dust mite exposure. Br J Dermatol 1986; 114:65–73.
2. Mihm M Jr, Soter N, Dvorak H, et al. The structure of normal skin and the morphology of atopic eczema. J Invest Dermatol 1976; 67:305–312.
3. Irani AA, Sampson HA, Schwartz LB. Mast cells in atopic dermatitis. Allergy 1989; 44(suppl. 9):31–34.
4. Järvikallio A, Naukkarinen A, Harvima IT, et al. Quantitative analysis of tryptase- and chymase-containing mast cells in atopic dermatitis and nummular eczema. Br J Dermatol 1997; 136:871–877.
5. Damsgaard TE, Olesen AB, Sorensen FB, et al. Mast cells and atopic dermatitis. Stereological quantification of mast cells in atopic dermatitis and normal human skin. Arch Dermatol Res 1997; 289:256–260.
6. Sandford AJ, Shirakawa T, Moffatt MF, et al. Localisation of atopy and beta subunit of high-affinity IgE receptor (Fc epsilon RI) on chromosome 11q [see comments]. Lancet 1993; 341:332–334.
7. Shirakawa T, Li A, Dubowitz M, et al. Association between atopy and variants of the beta subunit of the high-affinity immunoglobulin E receptor [see comments]. Nat Genet 1994; 7:125–129.
8. Coleman R, Trembath RC, Harper JI. Chromosome 11q13 and atopy underlying atopic eczema. Lancet 1993; 341:1121–1122.
9. Cox HE, Moffatt MF, Faux JA, et al. Association of atopic dermatitis to the beta subunit of the high affinity immunoglobulin E receptor [see comments]. Br J Dermatol 1998; 138:182–187.
10. Mao XQ, Shirakawa T, Yoshikawa T, et al. Association between genetic variants of mast-cell chymase and eczema [see comments] [published erratum appears in Lancet 1997 Jan 4 349(9044):64]. Lancet 1996; 348:581–583.
11. Mao XQ, Shirakawa T, Enomoto T, et al. Association between variants of mast cell chymase gene and serum IgE levels in eczema [published erratum appears in Hum Hered 1998 Mar–Apr; 48(2):91]. Hum Hered 1998; 48: 38–41.
12. Tanaka K, Sugiura H, Uehara M, et al. Association between mast cell chymase genotype and atopic eczema: Comparison between patients with atopic eczema alone and those with atopic eczema and atopic respiratory disease. Clin Exp Allergy 1999; 29:800–803.

13. Kitamura Y, Shimada M, Hatanaka K, et al. Development of mast cells from grafted bone marrow cells in irradiated mice. Nature 1977; 268:442–443.
14. Hasthorpe S. A hemopoietic cell line dependent upon a factor in pokeweed mitogen-stimulated spleen cell conditioning medium. J Cell Physiol 1980; 105:379–384.
15. Nabel GJ, Galli SJ, Dvorak AM, et al. Inducer T lymphocytes synthesize a factor that stimulates proliferation of cloned mast cells. Nature 1981; 291:332–334.
16. Nagao K, Yokoro K, Aaronson SA. Continuous lines of basophil mast cells derived from normal mouse bone marrow. Science 1981; 212:333–335.
17. Schrader JW, Lewis SJ, Clark-Lewis I, et al. The persisting (P) cell: Histamine content, regulation by a T cell-derived factor, origin from a bone marrow precursor, and relationship to mast cells. Proc Natl Acad Sci USA 1981; 78:323–327.
18. Yung YP, Eger R, Tertian G, et al. Long-term in vitro culture of murine mast cells. II. Purification of a mast cell growth factor and its dissociation from TCGF. J Immunol 1981; 127:794–799.
19. Ihle JN, Keller JR, Oroszlan S, et al. Biologic properties of homogeneous interleukin 3. I. Demonstration of WEHI-3 growth factor activity, mast cell growth factor activity, p cell-stimulating factor activity, colony-stimulating factor activity, and histamine-producing cell-stimulating factor activity. J Immunol 1983; 131:282–287.
20. Yokota T, Lee F, Rennick D, et al. Isolation and characterization of a mouse cDNA clone that expresses mast-cell growth-factor activity in monkey cells. Proc Natl Acad Sci U S A 1984; 81:1070–1074.
21. Ruitenberg EJ, Elgersma A. Absence of intestinal mast cell response in congenitally athymic mice during *Trichinella spiralis* infection. Nature 1976; 264:258–260.
22. Lantz CS, Boesiger J, Song CH, et al. Role for interleukin-3 in mast-cell and basophil development and in immunity to parasites. Nature 1998; 392:90–93.
23. Kitamura Y, Hatanaka K. Decrease of mast cells in W/W^v mice and their increase by bone marrow transplantation. Blood 1978; 52:447–452.
24. Kitamura Y, Go S. Decreased production of mast cells in Sl/Sl^d anemic mice. Blood 1979; 53:492–497.
25. Wedemeyer J, Tsai M, Galli SJ. Roles of mast cells and basophils in innate and acquired immunity. Curr Opin Immunol 2000; 12:624–631.
26. Irani AA, Nilsson G, Miettinen U, et al. Recombinant human stem cell factor stimulates differentiation of mast cells from dispersed human fetal liver cells. Blood 1992; 80:3009–3021.
27. Mitsui H, Furitsu T, Dvorak AM, et al. Development of human mast cells from umbilical cord blood cells by recombinant human and murine c-kit ligand. Proc Natl Acad Sci U S A 1993; 90:735–739.
28. Valent P, Spanblöchl E, Sperr WR, et al. Induction of differentiation of human mast cells from bone marrow and peripheral blood mononuclear cells by recombinant human stem cell factor/kit-ligand in long-term culture. Blood 1992; 80:2237–2245.
29. Shimizu Y, Matsumoto K, Okayama Y, et al. Interleukin-3 does not affect the differentiation of mast cells derived from human bone marrow progenitors. Immunol Invest 2008; 37:1–17.
30. Valent P, Besemer J, Sillaber C, et al. Failure to detect IL-3-binding sites on human mast cells. J Immunol 1990; 145:3432–3437.
31. Dahl C, Hoffmann HJ, Saito H, et al. Human mast cells express receptors for IL-3, IL-5 and GM-CSF; a partial map of receptors on human mast cells cultured in vitro. Allergy 2004; 59:1087–1096.
32. Yanagida M, Fukamachi H, Ohgami K, et al. Effects of T-helper 2-type cytokines, interleukin-3 (IL- 3), IL-4, IL-5, and IL-6 on the survival of cultured human mast cells. Blood 1995; 86:3705–3714.
33. Gebhardt T, Sellge G, Lorentz A, et al. Cultured human intestinal mast cells express functional IL-3 receptors and respond to IL-3 by enhancing growth and IgE receptor-dependent mediator release. Eur J Immunol 2002; 32:2308–2316.
34. Hsieh FH, Lam BK, Penrose JF, et al. T helper cell type 2 cytokines coordinately regulate immunoglobulin E-dependent cysteinyl leukotriene production by human cord

blood-derived mast cells: Profound induction of leukotriene C(4) synthase expression by interleukin 4. J Exp Med 2001; 193:123–133.
35. Rottem M, Okada T, Goff JP, et al. Mast cells cultured from the peripheral blood of normal donors and patients with mastocytosis originate from a CD34$^+$/FceRI$^-$ cell population. Blood 1994; 84:2489–2496.
36. Kempuraj D, Saito H, Kaneko A, et al. Characterization of mast cell-committed progenitors present in human umbilical cord blood. Blood 1999; 93:3338–3346.
37. Kirshenbaum AS, Goff JP, Semere T, et al. Demonstration that human mast cells arise from a progenitor cell population that is CD34(+), c-kit(+), and expresses aminopeptidase N (CD13). Blood 1999; 94:2333–2342.
38. Terstappen LW, Huang S, Safford M, et al. Sequential generations of hematopoietic colonies derived from single nonlineage-committed CD34+CD38− progenitor cells. Blood 1991; 77:1218–1227.
39. Civin CI. Human monomyeloid cell membrane antigens. Exp Hematol 1990; 18:461–467.
40. Du ZM, Li YL, Xia HZ, et al. Recombinant human granulocyte-macrophage colony-stimulating factor (CSF), but not recombinant human granulocyte CSF, down-regulates the recombinant human stem cell factor-dependent differentiation of human fetal liver-derived mast cells. J Immunol 1997; 159:838–845.
41. Oskeritzian CA, Wang Z, Kochan JP, et al. Recombinant human (rh)IL-4-mediated apoptosis and recombinant human IL-6-mediated protection of recombinant human stem cell factor-dependent human mast cells derived from cord blood mononuclear cell progenitors. J Immunol 1999; 163:5105–5115.
42. Saito H, Ebisawa M, Tachimoto H, et al. Selective growth of human mast cell induced by Steel factor, IL-6, and prostaglandin E$_2$ from cord blood mononuclear cells. J Immunol 1996; 157:343–350.
43. Kambe N, Kambe M, Chang HW, et al. An improved procedure for the development of human mast cells from dispersed fetal liver cells in serum-free culture medium. J Immunol Methods 2000; 240:101–110.
44. Nilsson G, Miettinen U, Ishizaka T, et al. Interleukin-4 inhibits the expression of Kit and tryptase during stem cell factor-dependent development of human mast cells from fetal liver cells. Blood 1994; 84:1519–1527.
45. Nagata H, Worobec AS, Oh CK, et al. Identification of a point mutation in the catalytic domain of the protooncogene c-kit in peripheral blood mononuclear cells of patients who have mastocytosis with an associated hematologic disorder. Proc Natl Acad Sci U S A 1995; 92:10560–10564.
46. Longley BJ Jr, Metcalfe DD, Tharp M, et al. Activating and dominant inactivating c-KIT catalytic domain mutations in distinct clinical forms of human mastocytosis. Proc Natl Acad Sci U S A 1999; 96:1609–1614.
47. Hirota S, Isozaki K, Moriyama Y, et al. Gain-of-function mutations of c-*kit* in human gastrointestinal stromal tumors. Science 1998; 279:577–580.
48. Sillaber C, Strobl H, Bevec D, et al. IL-4 regulates c-*kit* proto-oncogene product expression in human mast and myeloid progenitor cells. J Immunol 1991; 147:4224–4228.
49. Xia HZ, Du ZM, Craig S, et al. Effect of recombinant human IL-4 on tryptase, chymase, and Fce receptor type I expression in recombinant human stem cell factor-dependent fetal liver-derived human mast cells. J Immunol 1997; 159:2911–2921.
50. Toru H, Ra C, Nonoyama S, et al. Induction of the high-affinity IgE receptor (FceRI) on human mast cells by IL-4. Int Immunol 1996; 8:1367–1373.
51. Bischoff SC, Sellge G, Lorentz A, et al. IL-4 enhances proliferation and mediator release in mature human mast cells. Proc Natl Acad Sci U S A 1999; 96:8080–8085.
52. Toru H, Kinashi T, Ra C, et al. Interleukin-4 induces homotypic aggregation of human mast cells by promoting LFA-1/ICAM-1 adhesion molecules. Blood 1997; 89:3296–3302.
53. Nilsson G, Nilsson K. Effects of interleukin (IL)-13 on immediate-early response gene expression, phenotype and differentiation of human mast cells. Comparison with IL-4. Eur J Immunol 1995; 25:870–873.
54. Kinoshita T, Sawai N, Hidaka E, et al. Interleukin-6 directly modulates stem cell factor-dependent development of human mast cells derived from CD34(+) cord blood cells. Blood 1999; 94:496–508.

55. Matsuzawa S, Sakashita K, Kinoshita T, et al. IL-9 enhances the growth of human mast cell progenitors under stimulation with stem cell factor. J Immunol 2003; 170:3461–3467.
56. Thompson-Snipes L, Dhar V, Bond MW, et al. Interleukin 10: A novel stimulatory factor for mast cells and their progenitors. J Exp Med 1991; 173:507–510.
57. Ghildyal N, Friend DS, Nicodemus CF, et al. Reversible expression of mouse mast cell protease 2 mRNA and protein in cultured mast cells exposed to IL-10. J Immunol 1993; 151:3206–3214.
58. Ghildyal N, McNeil HP, Gurish MF, et al. Transcriptional regulation of the mucosal mast cell-specific protease gene, MMCP-2, by interleukin 10 and interleukin 3. J Biol Chem 1992; 267:8473–8477.
59. Ghildyal N, McNeil HP, Stechschulte S, et al. IL-10 induces transcription of the gene for mouse mast cell protease-1, a serine protease preferentially expressed in mucosal mast cells of *Trichinella spiralis*-infected mice. J Immunol 1992; 149:2123–2129.
60. Kambe M, Kambe N, Oskeritzian CA, et al. IL-6 attenuates apoptosis, while neither IL-6 nor IL-10 affect the numbers or protease phenotype of fetal liver-derived human mast cells. Clin Exp Allergy 2001; 31:1077–1085.
61. Allakhverdi Z, Smith DE, Comeau MR, et al. Cutting edge: The ST2 ligand IL-33 potently activates and drives maturation of human mast cells. J Immunol 2007; 179:2051–2054.
62. Irani AA, Schechter NM, Craig SS, et al. Two types of human mast cells that have distinct neutral protease compositions. Proc Natl Acad Sci U S A 1986; 83:4464–4468.
63. Oskeritzian CA, Zhao W, Min HK, et al. Surface CD88 functionally distinguishes the MCTC from the MCT type of human lung mast cell. J Allergy Clin Immunol 2005; 115:1162–1168.
64. Irani AM, Craig SS, DeBlois G, et al. Deficiency of the tryptase-positive, chymase-negative mast cell type in gastrointestinal mucosa of patients with defective T lymphocyte function. J Immunol 1987; 138:4381–4386.
65. Kanakura Y, Thompson H, Nakano T, et al. Multiple bidirectional alterations of phenotype and changes in proliferative potential during the in vitro and in vivo passage of clonal mast cell populations derived from mouse peritoneal mast cells. Blood 1988; 72:877–885.
66. Nakano T, Sonoda T, Hayashi C, et al. Fate of bone marrow-derived cultured mast cells after inracutaneous, intraperitoneal and intracenous transfer into genetically mast cell deficient W/W^V mice. Evidence that cultured mast cells can give rise to both connective tissue type and mucosal mast cells. J Exp Med 1985; 162:1025–1043.
67. Levi-Schaffer F, Austen KF, et al. Coculture of interleukin 3-dependent mouse mast cells with fibroblasts results in a phenotypic change of the mast cells [published erratum appears in Proc Natl Acad Sci U S A 1986 Oct; 83(20):7805]. Proc Natl Acad Sci U S A 1986; 83:6485–6488.
68. Tsai M, Shih LS, Newlands GF, et al. The rat c-kit ligand, stem cell factor, induces the development of connective tissue-type and mucosal mast cells in vivo. Analysis by anatomical distribution, histochemistry, and protease phenotype. J Exp Med 1991; 174:125–131.
69. Gordon JR, Galli SJ. Phorbol 12-myristate 13-acetate-induced development of functionally active mast cells in W/Wv but not Sl/Sld genetically mast cell-deficient mice. Blood 1990; 75:1637–1645.
70. Matsuda H, Kannan Y, Ushio H, et al. Nerve growth factor induces development of connective tissue- type mast cells in vitro from murine bone marrow cells. J Exp Med 1991; 174:7–14.
71. Toru H, Eguchi M, Matsumoto R, et al. Interleukin-4 promotes the development of tryptase and chymase double-positive human mast cells accompanied by cell maturation. Blood 1998; 91:187–195.
72. Tam SY, Tsai M, Yamaguchi M, et al. Expression of functional TrkA receptor tyrosine kinase in the HMC-1 human mast cell line and in human mast cells. Blood 1997; 90:1807–1820.
73. Craig SS, Schechter NM, Schwartz LB. Ultrastructural analysis of maturing human T and TC mast cells in situ. Lab Invest 1989; 60:147–157.

74. Nilsson G, Mikovits JA, Metcalfe DD, et al. Mast cell migratory response to interleukin-8 is mediated through interaction with chemokine receptor CXCR2/interleukin-8RB. Blood 1999; 93:2791–2797.

75. Ochi H, Hirani WM, Yuan Q, et al. T helper cell type 2 cytokine-mediated comitogenic responses and CCR3 expression during differentiation of human mast cells in vitro. J Exp Med 1999; 190:267–280.

76. Romagnani P, De Paulis A, Beltrame C, et al. Tryptase-chymase double-positive human mast cells express the eotaxin receptor CCR3 and are attracted by CCR3-binding chemokines. Am J Pathol 1999; 155:1195–1204.

77. Yamauchi K, Sato R, Tanno Y, et al. Nucleotide sequence of the cDNA encoding l-histidine decarboxylase derived from human basophilic leukemia cell line, KU-812-F. Nucleic Acids Res 1990; 18:5891.

78. Gantz I, Schaffer M, DelValle J, et al. Molecular cloning of a gene encoding the histamine H2 receptor [published erratum appears in Proc Natl Acad Sci U S A 1991 Jul; 88(13):5937]. Proc Natl Acad Sci U S A 1991; 88:429–433.

79. Asako H, Kurose I, Wolf R, et al. Role of H1 receptors and P-selectin in histamine-induced leukocyte rolling and adhesion in postcapillary venules. J Clin Invest 1994; 93:1508–1515.

80. Kubes P, Kanwar S. Histamine induces leukocyte rolling in post-capillary venules. A P-selectin-mediated event. J Immunol 1994; 152:3570–3577.

81. Inoue I, Yanai K, Kitamura D, et al. Impaired locomotor activity and exploratory behavior in mice lacking histamine H1 receptors. Proc Natl Acad Sci U S A 1996; 93:13316–13320.

82. Jutel M, Watanabe T, Klunker S, et al. Histamine regulates T-cell and antibody responses by differential expression of H1 and H2 receptors. Nature 2001; 413:420–425.

83. Zhu Y, Michalovich D, Wu H, et al. Cloning, expression, and pharmacological characterization of a novel human histamine receptor. Mol Pharmacol 2001; 59:434–441.

84. Nakaya M, Takeuchi N, Kondo K. Immunohistochemical localization of histamine receptor subtypes in human inferior turbinates. Ann Otol Rhinol Laryngol 2004; 113:552–557.

85. Hofstra CL, Desai PJ, Thurmond RL, et al. Histamine H4 receptor mediates chemotaxis and calcium mobilization of mast cells. J Pharmacol Exp Ther 2003; 305:1212–1221.

86. Godot V, Arock M, Garcia G, et al. H4 histamine receptor mediates optimal migration of mast cell precursors to CXCL12. J Allergy Clin Immunol 2007; 120:827–834.

87. Zhang M, Thurmond RL, Dunford PJ. The histamine H(4) receptor: A novel modulator of inflammatory and immune disorders. Pharmacol Ther 2007; 113:594–606.

88. Huang JF, Thurmond RL. The new biology of histamine receptors. Curr Allergy Asthma Rep 2008; 8:21–27.

89. Robertson I, Greaves MW. Responses of human skin blood vessels to synthetic histamine analogues. Br J Clin Pharmacol 1978; 5:319.

90. Kaliner M, Shelhamer JH, Ottesen EA. Effects of infused histamine: Correlation of plasma histamine levels and symptoms. J Allergy Clin Immunol 1982; 69:283–289.

91. Craig SS, Irani AM, Metcalfe DD, et al. Ultrastructural localization of heparin to human mast cells of the MC_{TC} and MC_T types by labeling with antithrombin III-gold. Lab Invest 1993; 69:552–561.

92. Stringer SE, Mayer-Proschel M, Kalyani A, et al. Heparin is a unique marker of progenitors in the glial cell lineage. J Biol Chem 1999; 274:25455–25460.

93. Braga T, Grujic M, Lukinius A, et al. Serglycin proteoglycan is required for secretory granule integrity in mucosal mast cells. Biochem J 2007; 403:49–57.

94. Abrink M, Grujic M, Pejler G. Serglycin is essential for maturation of mast cell secretory granule. J Biol Chem 2004; 279:40897–40905.

95. Ringvall M, Ronnberg E, Wernersson S, et al. Serotonin and histamine storage in mast cell secretory granules is dependent on serglycin proteoglycan. J Allergy Clin Immunol 2008; 121:1020–1026.

96. Forsberg E, Pejler G, Ringvall M, et al. Abnormal mast cells in mice deficient in a heparin-synthesizing enzyme. Nature 1999; 400:773–776.

97. Humphries DE, Wong GW, Friend DS, et al. Heparin is essential for the storage of specific granule proteases in mast cells. Nature 1999; 400:769–772.
98. Yamashita Y, Charles N, Furumoto Y, et al. Cutting edge: Genetic variation influences Fc epsilonRI-induced mast cell activation and allergic responses. J Immunol 2007; 179:740–743.
99. Fukuoka Y, Schwartz LB. Human beta-Tryptase: Detection and characterization of the active monomer and prevention of tetramer reconstitution by protease inhibitors. Biochemistry 2004; 43:10757–10764.
100. Ren S, Sakai K, Schwartz LB. Regulation of human mast cell beta-tryptase: Conversion of inactive monomer to active tetramer at acid pH. J Immunol 1998; 160:4561–4569.
101. Sakai K, Ren S, Schwartz LB. A novel heparin-dependent processing pathway for human tryptase. Autocatalysis followed by activation with dipeptidyl peptidase I. J Clin Invest 1996; 97:988–995.
102. Reed JA, Albino AP, McNutt NS. Human cutaneous mast cells express basic fibroblast growth factor. Lab Invest 1995; 72:215–222.
103. Nelson RM, Cecconi O, Roberts WG, et al. Heparin oligosaccharides bind L- and P-selectin and inhibit acute inflammation. Blood 1993; 82:3253–3258.
104. Lagunoff D, Chi EY. Effect of colchicine on rat mast cells. J Cell Biol 1976; 71:182–195.
105. Hopsu VK, Glenner GG. A histochemical enzyme kinetic system applied to the trypsin-like amidase and esterase activity in human mast cells. J Cell Biol 1963; 17:503–510.
106. Glenner GC, Cohen LA. Histochemical demonstration of species-specific trypsin-like enzyme in mast cells. Nature (London) 1960; 185:846–847.
107. Schwartz LB, Lewis RA, Seldin D, et al. Acid hydrolases and tryptase from secretory granules of dispersed human lung mast cells. J Immunol 1981; 126:1290–1294.
108. Schwartz LB, Lewis RA, Austen KF. Tryptase from human pulmonary mast cells. Purification and characterization. J Biol Chem 1981; 256:11939–11943.
109. Alter SC, Metcalfe DD, Bradford TR, et al. Regulation of human mast cell tryptase. Effects of enzyme concentration, ionic strength and the structure and negative charge density of polysaccharides. Biochem J 1987; 248:821–827.
110. Schwartz LB, Bradford TR. Regulation of tryptase from human lung mast cells by heparin. Stabilization of the active tetramer. J Biol Chem 1986; 261:7372–7379.
111. Pereira PJ, Bergner A, Macedo-Ribeiro S, et al. Human β-tryptase is a ring-like tetramer with active sites facing a central pore. Nature 1998; 392:306–311.
112. Alter SC, Kramps JA, Janoff A, et al. Interactions of human mast cell tryptase with biological protease inhibitors. Arch Biochem Biophys 1990; 276:26–31.
113. Miller JS, Westin EH, Schwartz LB. Cloning and characterization of complementary DNA for human tryptase. J Clin Invest 1989; 84:1188–1195.
114. Miller JS, Moxley G, Schwartz LB. Cloning and characterization of a second complementary DNA for human tryptase. J Clin Invest 1990; 86:864–870.
115. Pallaoro M, Fejzo MS, Shayesteh L, et al. Characterization of genes encoding known and novel human mast cell tryptases on chromosome 16p13.3. J Biol Chem 1999; 274:3355–3362.
116. Min HK, Moxley G, Neale MC, et al. Effect of sex and haplotype on plasma tryptase levels in healthy adults. J Allergy Clin Immunol 2004; 114:48–51.
117. Soto D, Malmsten C, Blount JL, et al. Genetic deficiency of human mast cell a-tryptase. Clin Exp Allergy 2002; 32:1000–1006.
118. Wang HW, McNeil HP, Husain A, et al. Delta tryptase is expressed in multiple human tissues, and a recombinant form has proteolytic activity. J Immunol 2002; 169:5145–5152.
119. McNeil HP, Reynolds DS, Schiller V, et al. Isolation, characterization, and transcription of the gene encoding mouse mast cell protease 7. Proc Natl Acad Sci U S A 1992; 89:11174–11178.
120. Reynolds DS, Gurley DS, Austen KF, et al. Cloning of the cDNA and gene of mouse mast cell protease-6. Transcription by progenitor mast cells and mast cells of the connective tissue subclass. J Biol Chem 1991; 266:3847–3853.

121. Caughey GH. Mast cell chymases and tryptases: Phylogeny, family relations, and biogenesis. In: Caughey GH, ed. Mast cell proteases in immunology and biology, vol 6. New York, NY: Marcel Dekker, Inc., 1995:305.
122. Baker E, Sayers TJ, Sutherland GR, et al. The genes encoding NK cell granule serine proteases, human tryptase-2 (TRYP2) and human granzyme A (HFSP), both map to chromosome 5q11–q12 and define a new locus for cytotoxic lymphocyte granule tryptases. Immunogenetics 1994; 40:235–237.
123. Hudig D, Allison NJ, Kam CM, et al. Selective isocoumarin serine protease inhibitors block RNK-16 lymphocyte granule-mediated cytolysis. Mol Immunol 1989; 26:793–798.
124. Sayers TJ, Lloyd AR, McVicar DW, et al. Cloning and expression of a second human natural killer cell granule tryptase, HNK-Tryp-2/granzyme 3. J Leukoc Biol 1996; 59:763–768.
125. Kido H, Fukutomi A, Katunuma N. A novel membrane-bound serine esterase in human T4+ lymphocytes immunologically reactive with antibody inhibiting syncytia induced by HIV-1. Purification and characterization. J Biol Chem 1990; 265:21979–21985.
126. Kido H, Yokogoshi Y, Sakai K, et al. Isolation and characterization of a novel trypsin-like protease found in rat bronchiolar epithelial Clara cells. A possible activator of the viral fusion glycoprotein. J Biol Chem 1992; 267:13573–13579.
127. Wong GW, Tang YZ, Stevens RL. Cloning of the human homolog of mouse transmembrane tryptase. Int Arch Allergy Immunol 1999; 118:419–421.
128. Sakai K, Long SD, Pettit DA, et al. Expression and purification of recombinant human tryptase in a baculovirus system. Protein Expr Purif 1996; 7:67–73.
129. Sherman MA, Secor VH, Lee SK, et al. STAT6-independent production of IL-4 by mast cells. Eur J Immunol 1999; 29:1235–1242.
130. Schwartz LB, Irani AAM, Roller K, et al. Quantitation of histamine, tryptase and chymase in dispersed human T and TC mast cells. J Immunol 1987; 138:2611–2615.
131. Ren S, Lawson AE, Carr M, et al. Human tryptase fibrinogenolysis is optimal at acidic pH and generates anticoagulant fragments in the presence of the anti-tryptase monoclonal antibody B12. J Immunol 1997; 159:3540–3548.
132. Proud D, Siekierski ES, Bailey GS. Identification of human lung mast cell kininogenase as tryptase and relevance of tryptase kininogenase activity. Biochem Pharmacol 1988; 37:1473–1480.
133. Huang C, De Sanctis GT, O'Brien PJ, et al. Evaluation of the substrate specificity of human mast cell tryptase beta I and demonstration of its importance in bacterial infections of the lung. J Biol Chem 2001; 276:26276–26284.
134. Schwartz LB. Diagnostic value of tryptase in anaphylaxis and mastocytosis. Immunol. Allergy Clin North Am 2006; 26:451–463.
135. Schwartz LB, Sakai K, Bradford TR, et al. The α form of human tryptase is the predominant type present in blood at baseline in normal subjects and is elevated in those with systemic mastocytosis. J Clin Invest 1995; 96:2702–2710.
136. Natbony SF, Phillips ME, Elias JM, et al. Histologic studies of chronic idiopathic urticaria. J Allergy Clin Immunol 1983; 71:177–183.
137. Smith CH, Kepley C, Schwartz LB, et al. Mast cell number and phenotype in chronic idiopathic urticaria. J Allergy Clin Immunol 1995; 96:360–364.
138. Schechter NM, Fraki JE, Geesin JC, et al. Human skin chymotryptic protease. Isolation and relation to cathepsin G and rat mast cell proteinase. J Biol Chem 1983; 258:2973–2978.
139. Caughey GH, Zerweck EH, Vanderslice P. Structure, chromosomal assignment, and deduced amino acid sequence of a human gene for mast cell chymase. J Biol Chem 1991; 266:12956–12963.
140. Osman IA, Garrett JR, Smith RE. Enzyme histochemical discrimination between tryptase and chymase in mast cells of human gut. J Histochem Cytochem 1989; 37:415–421.
141. Huber R, Bode W, Schechter NM, et al. The 2.2 Å crystal structure of human chymase in complex with succinyl-Ala-Ala-Pro-Phe-chloromethylketone: Structural explanation for its dipeptidyl carboxypeptidase specificity. J Mol Biol 1999; 286:163–173.

142. Kinoshita A, Urata H, Bumpus FM, et al. Multiple determinants for the high substrate specificity of an angiotensin II-forming chymase from the human heart. J Biol Chem 1991; 266:19192–19197.
143. Murakami M, Karnik SS, Husain A. Human prochymase activation. A novel role for heparin in zymogen processing. J Biol Chem 1995; 270:2218–2223.
144. Pejler G, Sadler JE. Mechanism by which heparin proteoglycan modulates mast cell chymase activity. Biochemistry 1999; 38:12187–12195.
145. Walter M, Sutton RM, Schechter NM. Highly efficient inhibition of human chymase by alpha (2)-macroglobulin. Arch Biochem Biophys 1999; 368:276–284.
146. Xia HZ, Kepley CL, Sakai K, et al. Quantitation of tryptase, chymase, FceRIα, and FceRIgamma mRNAs in human mast cells and basophils by competitive reverse transcription-polymerase chain reaction. J Immunol 1995; 154:5472–5480.
147. Schechter NM, Brass LF, Lavker RM, et al. Reaction of mast cell proteases tryptase and chymase with protease activated receptors (PARs) on keratinocytes and fibroblasts. J Cell Physiol 1998; 176:365–373.
148. Sommerhoff CP, Fang KC, Nadel JA, et al. Classical second messengers are not involved in proteinase-induced degranulation of airway gland cells. Am J Physiol 1996; 271:L796–L803.
149. Longley BJ, Tyrrell L, Ma Y, et al. Chymase cleavage of stem cell factor yields a bioactive, soluble product. Proc Natl Acad Sci U S A 1997; 94:9017–9021.
150. Kofford MW, Schwartz LB, Schechter NM, et al. Cleavage of type I procollagen by human mast cell chymase initiates collagen fibril formation and generates a unique carboxyl-terminal propeptide. J Biol Chem 1997; 272:7127–7131.
151. Gotis-Graham I, McNeil HP. Mast cell responses in rheumatoid synovium–Association of the MC_{TC} subset with matrix turnover and clinical progression. Arthritis Rheum 1997; 40:479–489.
152. Omoto Y, Tokime K, Yamanaka K, et al. Human mast cell chymase cleaves pro-IL-18 and generates a novel and biologically active IL-18 fragment. J Immunol 2006; 177:8315–8319.
153. Zhao W, Oskeritzian CA, Pozez AL, et al. Cytokine production by skin-derived mast cells: Endogenous proteases are responsible for degradation of cytokines. J Immunol 2005; 175:2635–2642.
154. Schechter NM, Irani AM, Sprows JL, et al. Identification of a cathepsin G-like proteinase in the MC_{TC} type of human mast cell. J Immunol 1990; 145:2652–2661.
155. Hof P, Mayr I, Huber R, et al. The 1.8 Å crystal structure of human cathepsin G in complex with Suc-Val-Pro-PheP-(OPh)2: A Janus-faced proteinase with two opposite specificities. EMBO J 1996; 15:5481–5491.
156. Travis J, Bowen J, Baugh R. Human alpha-1-antichymotrypsin: Interaction with chymotrypsin-like proteinases. Biochemistry 1978; 17:5651–5656.
157. Korkmaz B, Moreau T, Gauthier F. Neutrophil elastase, proteinase 3 and cathepsin G: Physicochemical properties, activity and physiopathological functions. Biochimie 2008; 90:227–242.
158. Irani AM, Goldstein SM, Wintroub BU, et al. Human mast cell carboxypeptidase: Selective localization to MC_{TC} cells. J Immunol 1991; 147:247–253.
159. Goldstein SM, Kaempfer CE, Kealey JT, et al. Human mast cell carboxypeptidase: Purification and characterization. J Clin Invest 1989; 83:1630–1636.
160. Reynolds DS, Gurley DS, Stevens RL, et al. Cloning of cDNAs that encode human mast cell carboxypeptidase A, and comparison of the protein with mouse mast cell carboxypeptidase A and rat pancreatic carboxypeptidases. Proc Natl Acad Sci U S A 1989; 86:9480–9484.
161. Feyerabend TB, Hausser H, Tietz A, et al. Loss of histochemical identity in mast cells lacking carboxypeptidase A. Mol Cell Biol 2005; 25:6199–6210.
162. Lundequist A, Tchougounova E, Abrink M, et al. Cooperation between mast cell carboxypeptidase A and the chymase mouse mast cell protease 4 in the formation and degradation of angiotensin II. J Biol Chem 2004; 279:32339–32344.

163. Metz M, Piliponsky AM, Chen CC, et al. Mast cells can enhance resistance to snake and honeybee venoms. Science 2006; 313:526–530.
164. Schneider LA, Schlenner SM, Feyerabend TB, et al. Molecular mechanism of mast cell mediated innate defense against endothelin and snake venom sarafotoxin. J Exp Med 2007; 204:2629–2639.
165. Sillalber C, Baghestanian M, Bevec DM, et al. The mast cell as site of tissue-type plasminogen activator expression and fibrinolysis. J Immunol 1999; 162:1032–1041.
166. Kanbe N, Tanaka A, Kanbe M, et al. Human mast cells produce matrix metalloproteinase 9. Eur J Immunol 1999; 29:2645–2649.
167. Fang KC, Wolters PJ, Steinhoff M, et al. Mast cell expression of gelatinases A and B is regulated by kit ligand and TGF-β. J Immunol 1999; 162:5528–5535.
168. Tanaka A, Arai K, Kitamura Y, et al. Matrix metalloproteinase-9 production, a newly identified function of mast cell progenitors, is downregulated by c-kit receptor activation. Blood 1999; 94:2390–2395.
169. Veerappan A, Reid AC, Estephan R, et al. Mast cell renin and a local renin–angiotensin system in the airway: Role in bronchoconstriction. Proc Natl Acad Sci U S A 2008; 105:1315–1320.
170. Silver RB, Reid AC, Mackins CJ, et al. Mast cells: A unique source of renin. Proc Natl Acad Sci U S A 2004; 101:13607–13612.
171. Strik MC, de Koning PJ, Kleijmeer MJ, et al. Human mast cells produce and release the cytotoxic lymphocyte associated protease granzyme B upon activation. Mol Immunol 2007; 44:3462–3472.
172. Pardo J, Wallich R, Ebnet K, et al. Granzyme B is expressed in mouse mast cells in vivo and in vitro and causes delayed cell death independent of perforin. Cell Death Differ 2007; 14:1768–1779.
173. Fujishima H, Sanchez Mejia RO, et al. Cytosolic phospholipase A2 is essential for both the immediate and the delayed phases of eicosanoid generation in mouse bone marrow-derived mast cells. Proc Natl Acad Sci U S A 1999; 96:4803–4807.
174. Lynch KR, O'Neill GP, Liu Q, et al. Characterization of the human cysteinyl leukotriene CysLT1 receptor. Nature 1999; 399:789–793.
175. Colamorea T, Di Paola R, Macchia F, et al. 5-Lipoxygenase upregulation by dexamethasone in human mast cells. Biochem Biophys Res Commun 1999; 265:617–624.
176. Roberts LJ II, Sweetman BJ, Lewis RA, et al. Increased production of prostaglandin D2 in patients with systemic mastocytosis. N Engl J Med 1980; 303:1400–1404.
177. Murakami M, Bingham CO III, Matsumoto R, et al. IgE-dependent activation of cytokine-primed mouse cultured mast cells induces a delayed phase of prostaglandin D_2 generation via prostaglandin endoperoxide synthase-2. J Immunol 1995; 155:4445–4453.
178. Underhill DM, Ozinsky A, Hajjar AM, et al. The Toll-like receptor 2 is recruited to macrophage phagosomes and discriminates between pathogens [In Process Citation]. Nature 1999; 401:811–815.
179. Raible DG, Schulman ES, DiMuzio J, et al. Mast cell mediators prostaglandin-D$_2$ and histamine activate human eosinophils. J Immunol 1992; 148:3536–3542.
180. Matsuoka T, Hirata M, Tanaka H, et al. Prostaglandin D-2 as a mediator of allergic asthma. Science 2000; 287:2013–2017.
181. Jolly PS, Bektas M, Olivera A, et al. Transactivation of sphingosine-1-phosphate receptors by FcepsilonRI triggering is required for normal mast cell degranulation and chemotaxis. J Exp Med 2004; 199:959–970.
182. Olivera A, Mizugishi K, Tikhonova A, et al. The sphingosine kinase-sphingosine-1-phosphate axis is a determinant of mast cell function and anaphylaxis. Immunity 2007; 26:287–297.
183. Wang M, Saxon A, Diaz-Sanchez D. Early IL-4 production driving Th2 differentiation in a human in vivo allergic model is mast cell derived. Clin Immunol Immunopathol 1999; 90:47–54.

184. Irani AM, Nouri-Aria KT, Jacobson MR, et al. Basophil, eosinophil and IL-4 mRNA-positive cell numbers increase in the bronchial mucosa of atopic asthmatics 24 h after segmental bronchial allergen challenge. J Allergy Clin Immunol 2001; 108:205–211.
185. Devouassoux G, Foster B, Scott LM, et al. Frequency and characterization of antigen-specific IL-4- and IL-13-producing basophils and T cells in peripheral blood of healthy and asthmatic subjects. J Allergy Clin Immunol 1999; 104:811–819.
186. Nakae S, Suto H, Iikura M, et al. Mast cells enhance T cell activation: Importance of mast cell costimulatory molecules and secreted TNF. J Immunol 2006; 176:2238–2248.
187. Lantz CS, Yamaguchi M, Oettgen HC, et al. IgE regulates mouse basophil FceRI expression in vivo. J Immunol 1997; 158:2517–2521.
188. Yamaguchi M, Lantz CS, Oettgen HC, et al. IgE enhances mouse mast cell FceRI expression in vitro and in vivo: Evidence for a novel amplification mechanism in IgE-dependent reactions. J Exp Med 1997; 185:663–672.
189. MacGlashan D, Schroeder JT. Functional consequences of Fc epsilon RI alpha up-regulation by IgE in human basophils. J Leukoc Biol 2000; 68:479–486.
190. Yamaguchi M, Sayama K, Yano K, et al. IgE enhances Fce receptor I expression and IgE-dependent release of histamine and lipid mediators from human umbilical cord blood-derived mast cells: Synergistic effect of IL-4 and IgE on human mast cell Fce receptor I expression and mediator release. J Immunol 1999; 162:5455–5465.
191. Yano K, Yamaguchi M, De Mora F, et al. Production of macrophage inflammatory protein-1 α by human mast cells: Increased anti-IgE-dependent secretion after IgE-dependent enhancement of mast cell IgE-binding ability. Lab Invest 1997; 77:185–193.
192. Gauchat JF, Henchoz S, Mazzei G, et al. Induction of human IgE synthesis in B cells by mast cells and basophils. Nature 1993; 365:340–343.
193. Baird B, Sheets ED, Holowka D. How does the plasma membrane participate in cellular signaling by receptors for immunoglobulin E? Biophys Chem 1999; 82:109–119.
194. Dombrowicz D, Lin SQ, Flamand V, et al. Allergy-associated FcRβ is a molecular amplifier of IgE- and lgG-mediated in vivo responses. Immunity 1998; 8:517–529.
195. Lin SQ, Cicala C, Scharenberg AM, et al. The FceRIβ subunit functions as an amplifier of FceRIgamma-mediated cell activation signals. Cell 1996; 85:985–995.
196. Bochner BS, Schleimer RP. The role of adhesion molecules in human eosinophil and basophil recruitment. J Allergy Clin Immunol 1994; 94:427–438.
197. Rivera VM, Brugge JS. Clustering of Syk is sufficient to induce tyrosine phosphorylation and release of allergic mediators from rat basophilic leukemia cells. Mol Cell Biol 1995; 15:1582–1590.
198. Vallé A, Kinet JP. N-acetyl-L-cysteine inhibits antigen-mediated Syk, but not Lyn tyrosine kinase activation in mast cells. FEBS Lett 1995; 357:41–44.
199. Kepley CL, Youssef L, Andrews RP, et al. Syk deficiency in nonreleaser basophils. J Allergy Clin Immunol 1999; 104:279–284.
200. Kepley CL, Youssef L, Andrews RP, et al. Multiple defects in Fc epsilon RI signaling in Syk-deficient nonreleaser basophils and IL-3-induced recovery of Syk expression and secretion. J Immunol 2000; 165:5913–5920.
201. Lienard H, Bruhns P, Malbec O, et al. Signal regulatory proteins negatively regulate immunoreceptor-dependent cell activation. J Biol Chem 1999; 274:32493–32499.
202. Berger SA, Mak TW, Paige CJ. Leukocyte common antigen (CD45) is required for immunoglobulin E-mediated degranulation of mast cells. J Exp Med 1994; 180:471–476.
203. Suzuki H, Takei M, Yanagida M, et al. Early and late events in FcεRI signal transduction in human cultured mast cells. J Immunol 1997; 159:5881–5888.
204. Hata D, Kawakami Y, Inagaki N, et al. Involvement of Bruton's tyrosine kinase in FcεRI-dependent mast cell degranulation and cytokine production. J Exp Med 1998; 187:1235–1247.
205. Setoguchi R, Kinashi T, Sagara H, et al. Defective degranulation and calcium mobilization of bone-marrow derived mast cells from Xid and Btk-deficient mice. Immunol Lett 1998; 64:109–118.
206. Pivniouk VI, Martin TR, Lu-Kuo JM, et al. SLP-76 deficiency impairs signaling via the high-affinity IgE receptor in mast cells. J Clin Invest 1999; 103:1737–1743.

207. Frigeri L, Apgar JR. The role of actin microfilaments in the down-regulation of the degranulation response in RBL-2 H3 mast cells. J Immunol 1999; 162:2243–2250.

208. Sullivan R, Price LS, Koffer A. Rho controls cortical F-actin disassembly in addition to, but independently of, secretion in mast cells. J Biol Chem 1999; 274:38140–38146.

209. Baram D, Adachi R, Medalia O, et al. Synaptotagmin II negatively regulates Ca^{2+}-triggered exocytosis of lysosomes in mast cells. J Exp Med 1999; 189:1649–1657.

210. Supajatura V, Ushio H, Nakao A, et al. Differential responses of mast cell Toll-like receptors 2 and 4 in allergy and innate immunity. J Clin Invest 2002; 109:1351–1359.

211. McCurdy JD, Lin TJ, Marshall JS. Toll-like receptor 4-mediated activation of murine mast cells. J Leukoc Biol 2001; 70:977–984.

212. Matsushima H, Yamada N, Matsue H, et al. TLR3-, TLR7-, and TLR9-mediated production of proinflammatory cytokines and chemokines from murine connective tissue type skin-derived mast cells but not from bone marrow-derived mast cells. J Immunol 2004; 173:531–541.

213. Kulka M, Alexopoulou L, Flavell RA, et al. Activation of mast cells by double-stranded RNA: Evidence for activation through Toll-like receptor 3. J Allergy Clin Immunol 2004; 114:174–182.

214. Okayama Y, Hagaman DD, Woolhiser M, et al. Further characterization of Fc gamma RII and Fc gamma RIII expression by cultured human mast cells. Int Arch Allergy Immunol 2001; 124:155–157.

215. Zhao W, Kepley CL, Morel PA, et al. Fc{gamma}RIIa, Not Fc{gamma}RIIb, is constitutively and functionally expressed on skin-derived human mast cells. J Immunol 2006; 177:694–701.

216. Okayama Y, Kirshenbaum AS, Metcalfe DD. Expression of a functional high-affinity IgG receptor, Fc gamma RI, on human mast cells: Up-regulation by IFN-gamma. J Immunol 2000; 164:4332–4339.

217. Okayama Y, Hagaman DD, Metcalfe DD. A comparison of mediators released or generated by IFN-gamma-treated human mast cells following aggregation of Fc gamma RI or Fc epsilon RI. J Immunol 2001; 166:4705–4712.

218. Sperr WR, Bankl HC, Mundigler G, et al. The human cardiac mast cell: Localization, isolation, phenotype, and functional characterization. Blood 1994; 84:3876–3884.

219. Mousli M, Hugli TE, Landry Y, et al. Peptidergic pathway in human skin and rat peritoneal mast cell activation. Immunopharmacology 1994; 27:1–11.

220. Iikura M, Yamaguchi M, Miyamasu M, et al. Secretory IgA-mediated basophil activation. Biochem Biophys Res Commun 1999; 264:575–579.

221. Iikura M, Yamaguchi M, Fujisawa T, et al. Secretory IgA induces degranulation of IL-3-primed basophils. J Immunol 1998; 161:1510–1515.

222. Patella V, Florio G, Petraroli A, et al. HIV-1 gp120 induces IL-4 and IL-13 release from human Fc epsilon RI+ cells through interaction with the V(H)3 region of IgE. J Immunol 2000; 164:589–595.

223. Peachell PT, Lichtenstein LM, Schleimer RP. Differential regulation of human basophil and lung mast cell function by adenosine. J Pharmacol Exp Ther 1991; 256:717–726.

224. Feoktistov I, Biaggioni I. Pharmacological characterization of adenosine A_{2B} receptors–Studies in human mast cells co-expressing A_{2A} and A_{2B} adenosine receptor subtypes. Biochem Pharmacol 1998; 55:627–633.

225. Schulman ES, Glaum MC, Post T, et al. ATP modulates anti-IgE-induced release of histamine from human lung mast cells. Am J Respir Cell Mol Biol 1999; 20:530–537.

226. MacDonald SM, Rafnar T, Langdon J, et al. Molecular identification of an IgE-dependend histamine-releasing factor. Science 1995; 269:688–690.

227. Schroeder JT, Lichtenstein LM, MacDonald SM. Recombinant histamine-releasing factor enhances IgE-dependent IL-4 and IL-13 secretion by human basophils. J Immunol 1997; 159:447–452.

228. Baggiolini M, Uguccioni M, Loetscher P. Chemokines and chemokine receptors in allergic inflammation. In: Marone G, Lichtenstein LM, Austen KF, Holgate ST, eds. Asthma and Allergic Diseases: Physiology, Immunopharmacology and Treatment. London, UK: Academic Press, 1998:157.

229. Uguccioni M, Mackay CR, Ochensberger B, et al. High expression of the chemokine receptor CCR3 in human blood basophils–Role in activation by eotaxin, MCP-4, and other chemokines. J Clin Invest 1997; 100:1137–1143.
230. Hartmann K, Beiglböck F, Czarnetzki BM, et al. Effect of CC chemokines on mediator release from human skin mast cells and basophils. Int Arch Allergy Immunol 1995; 108:224–230.
231. Silverstein MD, Reed CE, O'Connell EJ, et al. Long-term survival of a cohort of community residents with asthma. N Engl J Med 1994; 331:1537–1541.
232. Baghestanian M, Hofbauer R, Kiener HP, et al. The c-kit ligand stem cell factor and anti-IgE promote expression of monocyte chemoattractant protein-1 in human lung mast cells. Blood 1997; 90:4438–4449.
233. Imayama S, Shibata Y, Hori Y. Epidermal mast cells in atopic dermatitis. Lancet 1995; 346:1559.
234. Rajakulasingam K, Durham SR, O'Brien F, et al. Enhanced expression of high-affinity IgE receptor (FceRI) a chain in human allergen-induced rhinitis with co-localization to mast cells, macrophages, eosinophils, and dendritic cells. J Allergy Clin Immunol 1997; 100:78–86.
235. Kepley CL, Craig SS, Schwartz LB. Identification and partial characterization of a unique marker for human basophils. J Immunol 1995; 154:6548–6555.
236. McEuen AR, Buckley MG, Compton SJ, et al. Development and characterization of a monoclonal antibody specific for human basophils and the identification of a unique secretory product of basophil activation. Lab Invest 1999; 79:27–38.
237. Plager DA, Weiss EA, Kephart GM, et al. Identification of basophils by a mAb directed against pro-major basic protein 1. J Allergy Clin Immunol 2006; 117:626–634.
238. Irani AM, Huang C, Xia HZ, et al. Immunohistochemical detection of human basophils in late-phase skin reactions. J Allergy Clin Immunol 1998; 101:354–362.
239. Ying S, Robinson DS, Meng Q, et al. C-C chemokines in allergen-induced late-phase cutaneous responses in atopic subjects: Association of eotaxin with early 6-hour eosinophils, and of eotaxin-2 and monocyte chemoattractant protein-4 with the later 24-hour tissue eosinophilia, and relationship to basophils and other C-C chemokines (monocyte chemoattractant protein-3 and RANTES). J Immunol 1999; 163:3976–3984.
240. Macfarlane AJ, Kon OM, Smith SJ, et al. Basophils, eosinophils, and mast cells in atopic and nonatopic asthma and in late-phase allergic reactions in the lung and skin. J Allergy Clin Immunol 2000; 105:99–107.
241. KleinJan A, McEuen AR, Dijkstra MD, et al. Basophil and eosinophil accumulation and mast cell degranulation in the nasal mucosa of patients with hay fever after local allergen provocation. J Allergy Clin Immunol 2000; 106:677–686.
242. Wilson DR, Irani AM, Walker SM, et al. Grass pollen immunotherapy inhibits seasonal increases in basophils and eosinophils in the nasal epithelium. Clin Exp Allergy 2001; 31:1705–1713.
243. Travis WD, Li CY, Bergstralh EJ, et al. Systemic mast cell disease. Analysis of 58 cases and literature review. Medicine (Baltimore) 1988; 67:345–368.
244. Metcalfe DD. Classification and diagnosis of mastocytosis: Current status. J Invest Dermatol 1991; 96:2S–4S.
245. Schwartz LB, Bradford TR, Rouse C, et al. Development of a new, more sensitive immunoassay for human tryptase: Use in systemic anaphylaxis. J Clin Immunol 1994; 14:190–204.
246. Schwartz LB, Metcalfe DD, Miller JS, et al. Tryptase levels as an indicator of mast-cell activation in systemic anaphylaxis and mastocytosis. N Engl J Med 1987; 316:1622–1626.
247. Schwartz LB, Yunginger JW, Miller JS, et al. The time course of appearance and disappearance of human mast cell tryptase in the circulation after anaphylaxis. J Clin Invest 1989; 83:1551–1555.
248. Van der Linden PWG, Hack CE, Poortman J, et al. Insect-sting challenge in 138 patients: Relation between clinical severity of anaphylaxis and mast cell activation. J Allergy Clin Immunol 1992; 90:110–118.
249. Church MK, Skinner SP, Burrows LJ, et al. Microdialysis in human skin. Clin Exp Allergy 1995; 25:1027–1029.

250. Behrendt H, Ring J. Histamine, antihistamines and atopic eczema. Clin Exp Allergy 1990; 20(suppl. 4):25–30.
251. Hannuksela M, Kalimo K, Lammintausta K, et al. Dose ranging study: Cetirizine in the treatment of atopic dermatitis in adults. Ann Allergy 1993; 70:127–133.
252. Langeland T, Fagertun HE, Larsen S. Therapeutic effect of loratadine on pruritus in patients with atopic dermatitis. A multi-crossover-designed study. Allergy 1994; 49:22–26.
253. Hanifin JM. The role of antihistamines in atopic dermatitis. J Allergy Clin Immunol 1990; 86:666–669.
254. Wahlgren CF. Itch and atopic dermatitis: Clinical and experimental studies. Acta Derm Venereol Suppl (Stockh) 1991; 165:1–53.
255. Heyer G, Hornstein OP, Handwerker HO. Skin reactions and itch sensation induced by epicutaneous histamine application in atopic dermatitis and controls. J Invest Dermatol 1989; 93:492–496.
256. Giannetti A, Girolomoni G. Skin reactivity to neuropeptides in atopic dermatitis. Br J Dermatol 1989; 121:681–688.
257. Rukwied R, Lischetzki G, McGlone F, et al. Mast cell mediators other than histamine induce pruritus in atopic dermatitis patients: A dermal microdialysis study. Br J Dermatol 2000; 142:1114–1120.
258. Irani AM, Nilsson G, Ashman LK, et al. Dexamethasone inhibits the development of mast cells from dispersed human fetal liver cells cultured in the presence of recombinant human stem cell factor. Immunology 1995; 84:72–78.
259. Malone DG, Wilder RL, Saavedra-Delgado AM, et al. Mast cell numbers in rheumatoid synovial tissues. Correlations with quantitative measures of lymphotic infiltration and modulation by anti-inflammatory therapy. Arthritis Rheum 1987; 30:130–137.
260. Lavker RM, Schechter NM. Cutaneous mast cell depletion results from topical corticosteroid usage. J Immunol 1985; 135:2368–2373.
261. Goldsmith P, McGarity B, Walls AF, et al. Corticosteroid treatment reduces mast cell numbers in inflammatory bowel disease. Dig Dis Sci 1990; 35:1409–1413.
262. Bentley AM, Jacobson MR, Cumberworth V, et al. Immunohistology of the nasal mucosa in seasonal allergic rhinitis: Increases in activated eosinophils and epithelial mast cells. J Allergy Clin Immunol 1992; 89:877–883.
263. Enerbäck L, Pipkorn U, Granerus G. Intraepithelial migration of nasal mucosal mast cells in hay fever. Int Arch Allergy Appl Immunol 1986; 80:44–51.
264. Stellato C, De Paulis A, Ciccarelli A, et al. Anti-inflammatory effect of cyclosporin A on human skin mast cells. J Invest Dermatol 1992; 98:800–804.
265. Marone G, Triggiani M, Cirillo R, et al. Cyclosporin A inhibits the release of histamine and peptide leukotriene C4 from human lung mast cells. Ric Clin Lab 1988; 18:53–59.
266. Cirillo R, Triggiani M, Siri L, et al. Cyclosporin A rapidly inhibits mediator release from human basophils presumably by interacting with cyclophilin. J Immunol 1990; 144:3891–3897.
267. Naeyaert JM, Lachapelle JM, Degreef H, et al. Cyclosporin in atopic dermatitis: Review of the literature and outline of a Belgian consensus. Dermatology 1999; 198:145–152.
268. Ruzicka T, Bieber T, Schopf E, et al. A short-term trial of tacrolimus ointment for atopic dermatitis. European Tacrolimus Multicenter Atopic Dermatitis Study Group. N Engl J Med 1997; 337:816–821.
269. Alenius H, Laouini D, Woodward A, et al. Mast cells regulate IFN-gamma expression in the skin and circulating IgE levels in allergen-induced skin inflammation. J Allergy Clin Immunol 2002; 109:106–113.
270. Tam SY, Tsai M, Snouwaert JN, et al. RabGEF1 is a negative regulator of mast cell activation and skin inflammation. Nat Immunol 2004; 5:844–852.
271. Vigo PG, Girgis KR, Pfuetze BL, et al. Efficacy of anti-IgE therapy in patients with atopic dermatitis. J Am Acad Dermatol 2006; 55:168–170.
272. Obara W, Kawa Y, Ra C, Nishioka K, Sowa Y, Mizoguchi M. T cells and mast cells as a major source of Interleukin-13 in atopic dermatitis. Br J Dermatol 2002; 205:11–17.
273. Gerdesb S, Kurral W, Mrowietz U. Br J Dermatol 2008, Dec. 12, Epub ahead of print.

Kristin M. Leiferman

Departments of Dermatology and Medicine, University of Utah, Salt Lake City, Utah, U.S.A.

Margot S. Peters

Rochester, Minnesota, U.S.A.

Douglas A. Plager

Department of Dermatology, Mayo Clinic and Mayo Foundation, Rochester, Minnesota, U.S.A.

Gerald J. Gleich

Departments of Dermatology and Medicine, University of Utah, Salt Lake City, Utah, U.S.A.

INTRODUCTION

Atopic dermatitis has been linked with allergies since it was established as a disease entity (1). Eosinophils are prominently associated with allergic reactions, and evidence for a pathogenic role for eosinophils in atopic dermatitis has accumulated. Dating back to early descriptions of the disease, atopic dermatitis patients had peripheral blood eosinophilia. Although only a paucity of eosinophils are found in affected skin, eosinophil granule proteins are widely deposited in lesions of atopic dermatitis, providing evidence that eosinophil degranulation occurs in this disease (2,3). Eosinophils elaborate injurious toxins and inflammatory mediators. The potent effects that eosinophil mediators have on cells and tissues point to a pathogenic role in diseases that exhibit cutaneous eosinophil infiltration and prominent granule protein deposition. Observations demonstrating eosinophil involvement in atopic dermatitis are reviewed herein, summarized in Table 1, and schematically represented in Figure 1.

PHLOGISTIC PROPERTIES OF EOSINOPHILS

Studies over the past few decades have shown that eosinophils have the potential for multiple inflammatory activities. The eosinophil contains several cationic granule proteins including major basic protein (MBP)-1 and -2, eosinophil peroxidase (EPO), eosinophil cationic protein (ECP), and eosinophil-derived neurotoxin (EDN). MBP, EPO, and ECP are toxic to various targets including helminths, protozoa, bacteria, and normal mammalian cells (4). These proteins are cytostimulants for basophil and mast cell mediator release (4,5), for neutrophil (6) and platelet (7) activation, and for activation of eosinophils themselves (8). MBP-1, EPO, ECP, and EDN increase microvascular permeability (9) and induce wheal-and-flare reactions in human skin (10). EDN and ECP are ribonucleases that also have antiviral activity (11). Based on its ability to serve as a chemoattractant and activator of dendritic cells, as well as the capacity to enhance antigen-specific immune responses, EDN has properties of an endogenous alarmin that alerts the adaptive immune system for preferential enhancement of antigen-specific Th2 immune responses (12).

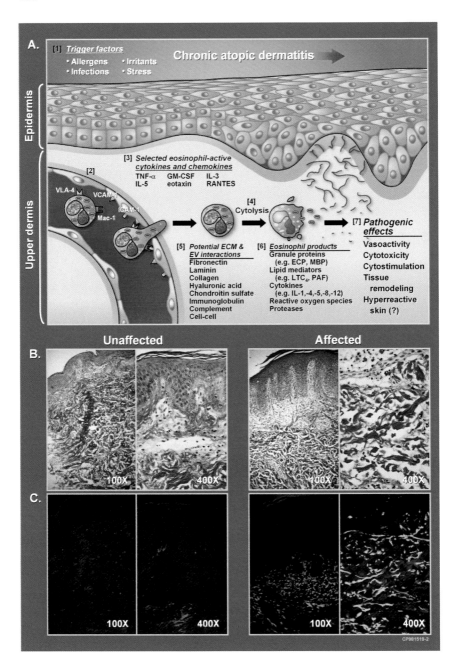

TABLE 1 Evidence for Eosinophil Involvement in Atopic Dermatitis

Eosinophils and eosinophil granule proteins possess phlogistic activities and cytotoxic effects that are associated with allergic inflammation
Eosinophil granule proteins are extensively deposited in lesional skin with evidence of cytolytic eosinophil degeneration
Eosinophil granule proteins are increased in peripheral blood and correlate with disease activity
Peripheral blood eosinophils are increased in severe disease, decrease with therapeutic improvement: "activated" hypodense eosinophils with prolonged survival (delayed programmed cell death) correlate best with disease activity
Th2 immunologic reactivity is present and associated with IL-5 expression; IL-5 has specific activities on eosinophils inducing eosinophilopoiesis, activation, and chemotaxis
Adhesion molecule expression specific for eosinophil transendothelial migration is present
Eosinophil chemotaxins are expressed
Eosinophil infiltration and extracellular eosinophil granule protein deposition occur in patch test allergen models

Activated eosinophils not only release granule proteins but also generate lipid mediators such as leukotriene (LT) C_4 and platelet-activating factor (PAF), generate reactive oxygen species, and participate in antibody-dependent cytotoxicity reactions. The oxidative products of eosinophils, including superoxide anions, hydroxyl radicals, and singlet oxygen (13,14), like the granule proteins, are damaging to cells. Low-molecular-weight mediators produced by eosinophils, PAF, and LTC_4 (15,16), increase vascular permeability. Other properties of PAF include leukocyte activation and recruitment to areas of inflammation. LTC_4 stimulates smooth muscle contraction. Eosinophils are also capable of synthesizing and secreting important inflammatory and regulatory cytokines (17–19); these include interleukin (IL)-1α, transforming growth factor (TGF)-α and -β_1, granulocyte-macrophage colony-stimulating factor (GM-CSF), IL-3, IL-4, IL-5, IL-6, IL-8, IL-12, tumor necrosis factor

---

FIGURE 1 Eosinophil involvement in atopic dermatitis. (**A**) As cutaneous inflammation develops, a variety of factors (1) lead to infiltration of eosinophils (2) and other immune cells (e. g., CD4$^+$ T cells and macrophages, not shown). The mechanisms of eosinophil activation and infiltration into tissues are not fully understood but are dependent on the interaction of eosinophil CD49 d/CD29 (i.e., VLA-4 or α4β1 integrin) with endothelial cell VCAM-1 and eosinophil CD1 lb/CDl8 (i.e., Mac-l, αMβ2 integrin) with endothelial cell ICAM-1. Cytokines and chemokines (3) derived from various cellular sources also contribute to eosinophil chemotaxis and activation. The timing and mechanism of eosinophil degranulation (4) following vascular transmigration remain largely unknown. Deposition of eosinophil granule proteins in the upper dermis likely occurs by cytolysis. Interactions with extracellular matrix (ECM) or extravascular (EV) immune molecules may mediate eosinophil activation (5). Activation followed by degranulation results in mediator release and deposition of eosinophil granule proteins (6). Release of eosinophil-derived IL-12 could contribute to the Th2 to Th1 cytokine profile shift observed in chronic atopic dermatitis lesions. Eosinophils also may function as antigen-presenting cells (APC). Cutaneous eosinophil activation and degranulation may contribute to disease pathology via several mechanisms (7). (**B**) H & E-stained sections of clinically unaffected (two left panels) and affected (two right panels) skin (left l00× and right 400× original magnification, respectively). Affected skin shows perivascular inflammation and upper-dermal edema with a dense band of hyalinization at the epidermal–dermal junction, and the epidermis is thickened with elongated rete ridges. Clinically unaffected skin shows slight perivascular inflammatory cell infiltration. (**C**) Indirect immunofluorescence staining for MBP in serial sections of affected and normal-appearing skin as in B. MBP is deposited extracellularly in an extensive fibrillar pattern in the upper dermis of affected skin with minimal MBP deposition in the upper-dermis of unaffected tissue. Skin from a healthy individual shows no MBP staining. Control sections from all three specimens stained with protein A purified rabbit IgG were negative (not shown).

(TNF)-α, and macrophage inhibitory protein (MIP)-1α. The stimuli that trigger eosinophils to produce cytokines are being elucidated, but chemotactic factors C5a and N-formyl-methionyl-leucyl-phenylalanine (FMLP) induce production of IL-8 and GM-CSF by eosinophils (20). Through expression of MHC class II molecules and IL-lα production, eosinophils may act as specialized antigen-presenting cells (18,21) and may be important in innate viral immunity, promoting clearance of respiratory syncytial virus (22). Eosinophils may be involved in tissue repair by promoting collagen synthesis through release of TGF-α and -β₁ (23); they also may promote fibrosis by stimulating fibroblast DNA synthesis and extracellular matrix protein production (24). Therefore, the functional diversity of the eosinophil has manifold implications for its role in disease. Moreover, eosinophil-derived cytokines may interact with other eosinophil mediators or other cell types to enhance inflammatory consequences (19,25).

Eosinophil activation with deposition of toxic cationic proteins occurs in many diseases (3,26,27). Peripheral blood levels of eosinophil granule proteins are increased in patients with asthma (28), diseases such as episodic angioedema with eosinophilia (10) and the eosinophilia-myalgia syndrome (29), and in the blood of patients receiving IL-2 in cancer protocols (30). In episodic angioedema with eosinophilia and IL-2–treated patients, increased IL-5 concentrations temporally precede increases in blood eosinophil counts (30,31).

Eosinophil granule proteins are detected in tissues by immunohistologic staining (32–39). Immunofluorescence methods are useful in determining eosinophil involvement because granule protein deposition is generally not detectable by histologic evaluation of hematoxylin and eosin (H & E) or Giemsa-stained sections. Using indirect immunofluorescence with polyclonal antibodies to purified eosinophil granule proteins injected in surgical waste skin, the detectable concentrations in tissue are as follows: EPO, 0.05 μM; MBP, 0.1 μM; ECP, 0.25 μM; and EDN, 1.0 μM (40). These concentrations result in minimal staining, and it is likely that much greater concentrations are deposited in diseased tissues that exhibit extensive staining. However, even minimal concentrations are capable of inducing biologic effects. The granule proteins appear to be deposited in some lesions, not through classical exocytotic degranulation but by cytolytic degranulation. As detected by electron microscopy, disrupted eosinophils with free membrane-bound granules are present in lesional tissues (10,36,41). Peripheral blood eosinophils from patients with allergies appear to have the same granule morphology as those from healthy subjects; however, eosinophils in diseased tissues show cytolysis as well as loss of granule matrix and core structures (41), suggesting that circulating blood eosinophils retain their granule contents until they reach their target organs (42).

EOSINOPHIL-RELATED CLINICAL, HISTOLOGIC AND IMMUNOPATHOLOGIC FEATURES OF ATOPIC DERMATITIS

Several schemes of diagnostic criteria for atopic dermatitis have been used for clinical definition and investigations of the disorder (43–45). The principal, basic features of the disease are pruritus and scratching, characteristic morphology and distribution of skin lesions, chronic or chronically relapsing course, and personal or family history of atopy. Other diagnostic features include facial pallor and erythema, itch with sweating, white dermographism, and delayed blanch to acetylcholine injection. No specific clinical feature or laboratory test is diagnostic for atopic dermatitis. Inclusion of the various additional features for diagnosis of atopic dermatitis emphasizes the importance of cutaneous inflammation in association with aberrant pharmacophysiologic responses in the disease.

IgE-mediated inflammation is associated with eosinophils, and several observations suggest that IgE and allergens contribute to the pathogenesis of atopic dermatitis. Serum IgE levels are elevated in approximately 80% of patients with atopic dermatitis and correlate with the extent of skin involvement (46). In a study of 102 atopic dermatitis patients and 107 age-matched controls, absolute eosinophil counts and IgE levels were significantly higher in the atopics and varied with disease activity (47). Allergen-specific IgE antibodies are common in atopic dermatitis patients and may contribute to disease exacerbations. When prick or intradermal skin tests are performed, patients with atopic dermatitis often show wheal-and-flare responses to multiple allergens and frequently have serum IgE antibodies to multiple allergens.

Controlled studies have shown that ingestion of foods by children with atopic dermatitis sensitive to these foods provokes cutaneous pruritus and erythema, leading to scratching and, subsequently, eczematous lesions (48). Furthermore, cutaneous exacerbations after food challenges are associated with significant increases in plasma histamine concentrations, indicative of mast cell degranulation. These and other findings (chap. 13) support the concept that repeated ingestion of provocative foods that result from such exposure contribute to the development of chronic atopic dermatitis.

The role of inhaled allergens in atopic dermatitis has been observed in numerous studies. Exacerbations of atopic dermatitis have been reported after inhalational exposure to a variety of allergens including horse dander, ragweed pollen, and mold [(49–51); chap. 12]. Recent studies have focused on the role of direct skin contact by aeroallergens in the development of atopic dermatitis lesions; eczematoid lesions were provoked by application of allergens to superficially abraded skin (52) and, subsequently, eczematous reactions were demonstrated in nonabraded skin to a variety of aeroallergens (53). Development of these reactions requires the presence of epidermal cells that coexpress IgE receptors and CD1a (54). Avoidance of aeroallergens that elicit eczematous reactions at patch test sites or cause immediate hypersensitivity reactions has been reported to improve atopic dermatitis (53,55,56).

Approximately 50% of patients with chronic atopic dermatitis have circulating IgE directed against staphylococcal enterotoxins; these toxins have been identified on skin of atopic dermatitis patients colonized with *Staphylococcus aureus* (57,58). Also, atopic dermatitis patients' own basophils release histamine on exposure to relevant staphylococcal enterotoxins. These findings indicate that local production of enterotoxin by *S. aureus* on the skin surface could induce IgE-mediated histamine release and trigger an inflammatory reaction that exacerbates atopic dermatitis (58). In addition, staphylococcal enterotoxin superantigens augment allergen-specific IgE synthesis and eosinophil infiltration through Th2 activity (59,60). IgE antibodies to skin proteins also have been reported in atopic dermatitis (61). Thus, autoreative IgE antibodies represent another mechanism that may contribute to cutaneous inflammation in atopic dermatitis.

The histopathologic changes in atopic dermatitis which can be observed by examination of H & E stained tissue sections are nonspecific (1). With Giemsa staining of epon-embedded lesional tissues, additional histopathologic features have been observed (62). Acute lesions show epidermal spongiosis and dermal perivascular inflammatory cell infiltration. Chronic lesions exhibit thickening of the epidermis with elongation of and fibrosis around the rete ridges. Langerhans cells and mast cells are increased in chronic lesions, and endothelial cells are enlarged (62). Eosinophils may be found at any stage. Immunohistologic staining shows that most infiltrating inflammatory cells in the dermis are T-lymphocytes that express the CD4 phenotype (63,64) as well as activation and memory markers (57). Mast cells [(62); chap. 9] and other cells present in atopic dermatitis lesions, such as Langerhans cells and macrophages, bear high-affinity (FcεRI) and low-affinity (FcεRII) IgE receptors (65,66); IgE antibody binds to these receptors (66–68). Surface FcεRI receptor expression correlates with serum IgE levels (69). Some reports have claimed that eosinophils, like mast cells and basophils, express high-affinity IgE receptors (70), while others have failed to confirm this (71–73). Eosinophils, however, do possess low-affinity IgE receptors (73,74). These receptors may be important in the role of eosinophils in parasite immunity, but their role in IgE-mediated allergic inflammation is unclear.

Circulating IgE antibodies in atopic dermatitis patients bind to and activate IgE receptor-bearing cells (63,75). Allergen presentation in the disease appears to be mediated by epidermal Langerhans cells bearing IgE (76) and other cutaneous dendritic cells (77), and allergens are capable of stimulating IgE-bearing macrophages to synthesize and secrete leukotrienes, PAF, IL-1, and TNF-α (78,79). Antigen-presenting cells (chap. 8) and mast cells likely regulate the local accumulation of inflammatory cells and/or preferentially influence infiltration of T-cells that express Th2 activity (chap. 7), which includes IL-5 production. The contribution of eosinophils to atopic dermatitis pathophysiology has been appreciated only recently, as the factors associated with Th2 activity that attract and activate eosinophils have been recognized in association with prominent eosinophil granule protein deposition.

CYTOKINE EXPRESSION AND EOSINOPHILS IN ATOPIC DERMATITIS

Several lines of investigation indicate that eosinophils are recruited to and activated in tissue sites by Th2 cytokines derived primarily from lymphocytes and mast cells (80,81). Deposition of granule proteins then occurs as a function of eosinophil activation and/or cytolytic degranulation (82). IL-3, IL-5, and GM-CSF stimulate eosinophil growth, maturation, and differentiation. These cytokines, along with TNF-α and interferon (IFN)-γ, activate and prime eosinophils for various functions. IL-5, for example, affects eosinophils by increasing their viability, decreasing their density, decreasing their granule content, and inducing release of their cytoplasmic granule proteins into the extracellular environment (83,84). In addition, IL-5 stimulates eosinophilopoiesis and eosinophil release from bone marrow (85); it also is chemotactic for eosinophils (86), albeit relatively weakly compared to other eosinophil chemokines such as eotaxin (87). IL-5 likely accounts for the frequent presence of eosinophils in allergic inflammation.

The existence of a functional IL-4 receptor has been identified on eosinophils, through which IL-4 primes eosinophils to certain chemotactic stimuli (88,89). Peripheral blood eosinophil counts and have been analyzed prospectively in children, at ages three months, eighteen months and six years; over 40% of subjects had demonstrable allergic disease by age six years (90). Most of the patients with allergic disease at age six years had peripheral blood eosinophilia at age three months. In addition, children with detectable serum IL-4 at 18 months were more often allergic at six years. At age six years, only nine children had detectable IL-4 and five of the nine had allergic disease. The findings suggest that eosinophilia during infancy and increased serum IL-4 at age 18 months are associated with development of allergic disease during the first six years of life.

Other eosinophil-influencing cytokines produced by Th2 lymphocytes following antigen exposure include IL-1, IL-9, IL-10, and IL-13. IL-1 is a proinflammatory cytokine functioning as a lymphocyte activator (91); IL-1 stimulates enhancement of IL-2 production and IL-2 receptor expression. IL-2 induces eosinophilia and capillary leak syndrome (30). IL-9 potentiates certain IL-4 and IL-5 activities, functioning to stimulate IgE production by B-cells and eosinophil development, as well as to increase IL-5 receptor expression (92,93). In situ hybridization analysis of IL-9 mRNA demonstrated a progressive increase in IL-9, with a peak at 48 hours after antigen exposure, in atopic dermatitis lesional skin (94). The increase in IL-9 mRNA production correlated with increasing numbers of eosinophils in these specimens. IL-10, typically an inhibitory cytokine, may be involved in allergic inflammation, based on observations that IL-10 deficient (IL-10−/−) mice have decreased eosinophil infiltration, IL-4, IL-5, and eotaxin secretion (95). IL-13 is located within the gene cluster on chromosome 5, which contains IL-4, IL-5, and granulocyte-macrophage colony stimulating factor (GM-CSF) (96–98). IL-13 is functionally similar to IL-4 in its ability to induce B-cell proliferation and IgE production and is a cofactor with IL-4 in the induction of vascular cell adhesion molecule-1 (VCAM-1) expression.

IL-17A and IL-17F are members of the IL-17 cytokine family (99) that may play crucial roles in allergic inflammation (100). IL-17A and IL-17F are produced from the distinct lymphocyte subset Th17, which is specifically induced by IL-23 from dendritic cells and macrophages in response to microbial stimuli. It is now clear that Th17 cells are involved in the pathogenesis of various chronic inflammatory diseases that were formerly categorized as Th1-mediated disorders (101). Human eosinophils constitutively express receptors for IL-17A, IL-17F, and IL-23; these three interleukins induce release of chemokines, GRO-α/CXCL1, IL-8/CXCL8, MIP-1β/CCL4, from eosinophils, while IL-17F and IL-23 also increase the production of proinflammatory cytokines, IL-1 and IL-6. Synergistic effects on the release of proinflammatory cytokines were found during combined treatment with IL-17F and IL-23; effects were enhanced in a dose-dependent manner by IL-23, but not IL-17F. Furthermore, IL-17A, IL-17F, and IL-23 differentially activated the ERK, p38 MAPK, and NF-kappaB signal transduction pathways; selective inhibition of these pathways significantly abolished IL-17A, IL-17F, and IL-23 cytokine release and the synergistic increases in IL-1 and IL-6 production by combined treatment with IL-17F and IL-23 (100). These studies, therefore, demonstrate Th17 lymphocyte-mediated eosinophil activation by differential intracellular signaling cascades in allergic inflammation. In addition, the number of Th17 cells is increased in the peripheral blood and acute skin lesions of atopic dermatitis (102). Taken together, these findings provide evidence for IL-23/IL-17 effects on eosinophils and further suggest a link between infections and allergic diseases through these mediators.

While several cytokines enhance eosinophil differentiation, survival, and activation, TGF-β_1 (a multifunctional cell growth-regulating cytokine) counteracts the survival-enhancing activities of IL-5, IL-3, GM-CSF, and IFN-γ on eosinophils (71). TGF-β_1 inhibits eosinophil survival in a dose-dependent manner and appears to act by inducing apoptosis of eosinophils (103). As noted, eosinophils elaborate TGF-β_1, as well as IL-3 and GM-CSF (104), revealing that activated eosinophils produce factors that both enhance and inhibit their own longevity in inflammatory conditions.

Another cytokine that affects eosinophils, brain-derived neurotrophic factor (BDNF), is increased in serum, plasma, eosinophils, and supernatants of stimulated eosinophils from patients with atopic dermatitis compared with controls; p75 neurotrophin receptor as well as tyrosine kinase B expression are higher on eosinophils from atopic dermatitis patients (105). Eosinophil apoptosis may be inhibited by BDNF, and the chemotactic index is high in BDNF-stimulated eosinophils from patients with atopic dermatitis but not controls. Screening differentially expressed genes in peripheral blood eosinophils from atopic dermatitis patients and healthy volunteers showed increased expression of *h*uman *s*uppressor of *c*ytokine *s*ignaling *p*rotein (HSOCP)-1 in cultured peripheral blood eosinophils after IL-4 stimulation as well as increased HSOCP-1-induced cell death in the eosinophil-like tumor cell line, AML15.3D10. These findings suggest that HSOCP-1 also plays a role in cell cycle control and apoptosis (106).

Various patterns of cytokine production in atopic dermatitis have been reported. Comparison of typical or "atopic" atopic dermatitis (with evidence for IgE involvement) to "nonatopic" atopic dermatitis (without an identifiable IgE relationship) demonstrated increased spontaneously released IL-4 and IL-5 (Th2-type cytokine expression) from peripheral blood lymphocytes in patients with "atopic" atopic dermatitis, whereas "nonatopic" atopic dermatitis patients displayed increased IL-5 but low IL-4 levels (107). Supernatants from lesional skin biopsy specimens showed similar findings; increased IL-4 levels were present only in "atopic" atopic dermatitis biopsies, whereas IL-5 was increased in both "atopic" atopic dermatitis and "nonatopic" atopic dermatitis specimens. A subsequent study showed that expression of IL-5 and IL-13 as well as the capacity of cutaneous T-cells to produce these cytokines is reduced in "nonatopic" atopic dermatitis patients compared with "atopic" atopic dermatitis (107,108). Cytokine mRNA expression in acute and chronic atopic dermatitis lesions (109) also has been studied; both acute and chronic lesions had significantly greater numbers of cells positive for IL-4 and IL-5 mRNA than did uninvolved skin, but chronic atopic dermatitis lesions had significantly fewer IL-4 mRNA-expressing cells and significantly more IL-5 mRNA-expressing cells than did acute lesions; the chronic lesions also showed greater eosinophil infiltration (109). In the peripheral blood and lesional skin of atopic dermatitis patients, CD4-positive and CD8-positive T-cells that express cutaneous lymphocyte-associated antigen (CLA) proliferate in response to superantigen stimulation and produce IL-5 and IL-13 (108). IL-5 and IL-5 receptor genetic polymorphisms are present in atopic dermatitis patients with high IL-5, peripheral blood eosinophilia and "atopic" or extrinsic atopic dermatitis (110,111). Considering the ability of IL-5 to promote differentiation, adhesion, and enhanced survival of eosinophils, these studies emphasize that inductive factors affect eosinophil involvement in atopic dermatitis.

EOSINOPHIL INFILTRATION INTO ATOPIC DERMATITIS SKIN

At least three interrelated signals are responsible for eosinophil infiltration into tissues: chemoattractants, adhesion molecules, and activating cytokines such as GM-CSF, IL-3, and IL-5. A combination of these signals likely determines the presence and degree of eosinophil infiltration, activation, and degranulation. Several members of the C-C chemokine gene superfamily are chemotactic for eosinophils (112–115), including eotaxins (116–119) and regulated upon activation, *n*ormal T-cell *e*xpressed and *s*ecreted (RANTES) (112,120). Eotaxins are specifically chemotactic for eosinophils; the effect of eotaxin on eosinophil infiltration appears to be dependent on IL-5 (87). Eotaxin-1, -2, and -3 bind to the CCR3 receptor, which is expressed on eosinophil, basophil, and mast cell surfaces. Other chemokines such as RANTES, macrophage chemotactic protein (MCP)-3, and MCP-4 bind to the CCR3 receptor, leading to eosinophil and basophil chemotaxis, and also bind the CCR1 receptor located on neutrophils, eosinophils, monocytes, T-cells, and basophils.

Following introduction of antigen into skin of sensitized subjects, expression of eotaxin mRNA and protein product occurred at six hours, suggesting that eotaxin regulates eosinophil infiltration at this time point (121). At 24 hours, expression of eotaxin-2 and MCP-4 mRNA correlated with eosinophil infiltration (121). Expression of eotaxin mRNA was paralleled by the occurrence of the eotaxin receptor, CCR3, on 83% of eosinophils. Peak expression of MCP-3 occurred at six hours after antigen injection; MCP-4 and RANTES peaked later, at 24 hours. No significant correlations were observed between basophil infiltrates, detected by BB1 (a basophil-specific antibody) staining, which peaked at 24 hours, and expression of eotaxin, eotaxin-2, RANTES, MCP-3, or MCP-4 (122). These findings suggest that eotaxin has a role in early recruitment of eosinophils after antigen exposure, whereas eotaxin-2 and MCP-4 are involved in later infiltration (24 hours) of eosinophils. In another study, investigation of a different chemokine that acts on the CCR1 receptor, MIP-1α (which also stimulates histamine release from mast cells and basophils and induces cellular motility), revealed peak expression of MIP-1α at six hours after antigen challenge with continued elevation through 24 hours (123). At six hours, there was colocalization of MIP-1α mRNA to neutrophils and basophils and, at 24 hours, colocalization with macrophages. Expression of the CCR1 receptor also correlated with MIP-1α expression.

The effects of intradermal allergen challenge and histamine injection on eotaxin mRNA and protein generation in atopics have been examined more closely with respect to endothelial production of eotaxin (124); 60 minutes after allergen challenge, there was a prompt increase in degranulating cutaneous mast cells with a simultaneous increase in eosinophils. The number of eotaxin-positive cells in tissues increased and peaked three hours postchallenge. In vitro, endothelial cells produced dose- and time-dependent eotaxin mRNA and protein after incubation with histamine. Preincubation of endothelial cells with histamine induced a significant increase in eosinophil adherence, which was inhibited by eotaxin-blocking monoclonal antibody (124). Thus, antigen-induced eotaxin expression by endothelial cells, and adherence and migration of eosinophils from microvasculature to tissues occur rapidly and are influenced by histamine from mast cells.

The dermis contains a high proportion of CD4-positive T-cells in atopic dermatitis, with a similar ratio of CD4/CD8 in extrinsic (atopic) and intrinsic (nonatopic)[1] lesions (125). Although other T-cell and epidermal Langerhans cell markers also were comparable in both groups, dermal eosinophil infiltration and eosinophil granule protein deposition were more prominent in extrinsic than intrinsic atopic dermatitis, as was expression of eotaxin immunoreactivity (125). Thus, differences in cytokine production may contribute to differences in tissue eosinophilia in the two types of atopic dermatitis.

---

[1] Here atopic and extrinsic refer to inflammation stimulated by antigen whereas nonatopic and intrinsic refer to inflammation in which antigen stimulation is not evident.

In children with atopic dermatitis, investigation of single-nucleotide polymorphisms (SNP) of the eotaxin gene revealed a significant difference in the genotype frequency of the -426 C–> T SNP between children with extrinsic atopic dermatitis and those with intrinsic atopic dermatitis, and between children with extrinsic atopic dermatitis and controls. In the children with extrinsic atopic dermatitis, there was no difference in the genotype frequency of -426 C–> T SNP between the groups with mild, moderate, and severe extrinsic atopic dermatitis (126). In addition, there appeared to be no significant association between -384 A–> G and 67G–> A SNP in the groups of children with extrinsic and intrinsic atopic dermatitis compared with controls. Evaluation of 32 trios (mother, father, offspring) from 68 extrinsic atopic dermatitis families pointed toward preferential transmission of the -426 T allele from parents to affected offspring, suggesting that the eotaxin gene may be important in the development of extrinsic atopic dermatitis (126).

RANTES is potently chemotactic for eosinophils and also is chemotactic for monocytes, T-lymphocytes, natural killer (NK) cells, and basophils, but not neutrophils (127). In addition to their chemotactic properties, eotaxin and RANTES stimulate production of reactive oxygen species by eosinophils, indicating that they have chemotactic and functional activation effects on eosinophils (128). Eotaxin is similar in potency to RANTES as an eosinophil chemoattractant, but more strongly stimulates production of reactive oxygen species by eosinophils (129). Both eotaxin and RANTES are produced by dermal fibroblasts (115,130), and RANTES also is inducibly produced by keratinocytes (131,132). Endothelial cells are a major source of eotaxin (124). Enhanced production of RANTES has been found in both keratinocytes (132) and fibroblasts from atopic dermatitis patients (115). Enhanced production of CC chemokines, including RANTES, eotaxin, MCP-1 and MIP-1, and CCR3 receptors occurs in patients with atopic dermatitis (133,134). IL-4 induces eotaxin expression (135,136). Eosinophils themselves express mRNA for RANTES (137), and RANTES upregulates expression of the CCR3 receptor on keratinocytes (138). Taken together, these findings show an intricate network of chemokine activities for eosinophil involvement in allergic inflammation.

Intradermal injection of RANTES into both nonallergic and allergic subjects is attended with a concentration- and time-dependent recruitment of eosinophils (139). However, a difference in the kinetics of eosinophil recruitment and degranulation (detected by MBP staining) has been observed between nonallergic and allergic subjects; nonallergic subjects showed virtually no eosinophil infiltration at 30 minutes and 6 hours, whereas significant eosinophil recruitment and degranulation were observed in allergic subjects by 30 minutes, reaching near maximum levels by 6 hours. However, by 24 hours, eosinophil infiltration and degranulation peaked in both groups and were similar. RANTES injections resulted in E-selectin expression in both subject groups; however, RANTES had no effect on adhesion molecule expression by endothelial cells in vitro, suggesting that the in vivo effects may be indirect (139). In another study, 24 hours after challenge with mite patch test, an increased number of RANTES-positive, CCR3-positive, and CCR5-positive cells as well as activated EG2 (anti-EDN)-positive eosinophils and CD3-positive T-cells were present in challenged lesional skin compared to unchallenged lesional skin of atopic dermatitis, which also was increased over normal skin of healthy volunteers (140). Eosinophils (EG2-positive cells) in nonchallenged lesional skin correlated with disease severity. In a murine model, *S. aureus* peptidoglycan applied percutaneously induced eosinophil infiltration through RANTES production by Langerhans cells (141). These results indicate that RANTES and its receptors, CCR3 and CCR5, may contribute to eosinophil involvement in chronic atopic dermatitis and also may be linked to staphylococcal colonization.

In order for eosinophils to migrate from peripheral blood into tissues, they must transmigrate blood vessels (142). The migratory response and activation of eosinophils require reorganization of the cytoskeleton. Stimulation of eosinophils with chemotaxins C5a, RANTES/CCL5, and platelet activating factor induces reversible polymerization of actin. Normodense eosinophils from patients with atopic dermatitis exhibit a lesser chemotaxin-induced actin response than do normodense eosinophils from healthy controls and hypodense eosinophils from atopic dermatitis patients. Stimulation of eosinophils with Th2-cytokines IL-3, IL-5, and GM-CSF does not appear to have a significant effect on actin polymerization, but pretreatment with IL-3, IL-5, or GM-CSF potentiates chemotaxin-induced actin polymerization (143).

Three gene superfamilies that regulate expression of eosinophil-surface proteins (144,145) contribute to the signaling needed for transmigration. First, selectins are involved in the early, high-sheer force stage of leukocyte adhesion to endothelium. Second, integrins, another gene superfamily of adhesion molecules, recognize counter-receptor members of the third gene superfamily, namely, the immunoglobulin gene superfamily. Together, members of these families interact to promote flattening and migration of cells onto and through the endothelium. In a murine antigen sensitization model, treatment with antibodies to ICAM-1, VCAM-1, and VLA-4 reduced eosinophil infiltration by 66.2%, 61.0%, and 54.0%, respectively, emphasizing the importance of these molecules for eosinophil infiltration (146). Following migration through vessels, eosinophils are present in the extracellular matrix where their cell surface integrins recognize substances such as the fibrous proteins, fibronectin, and laminin as well as collagen and the glycosaminoglycans, hyaluronic acid and chondroitin sulfate, and interact to further modulate eosinophil activity (147).

The importance of E-selectin expression by endothelial cells for tissue infiltration of lymphocytes is supported by the observation that T-cells in atopic dermatitis express the skin-specific homing receptor, cutaneous lymphocyte antigen (CLA). CLA is a ligand for E-selectin, and E-selectin expression also is associated with neutrophil adherence. In addition, endothelial cell expression of vascular cell adhesion molecule-1 (VCAM-1) is important in atopic dermatitis; VCAM-1, but not E-selectin, is found after IL-4 stimulation of endothelial cells (148) with adherence of eosinophils expressing very late antigen (VLA)-4 (a counterligand for VCAM-1). The number of eosinophils and degree of MBP, EPO, and ECP deposition are significantly and strongly correlated with the staining intensity of VCAM-1 (149). These findings implicate VCAM-1 expression in eosinophil recruitment in atopic dermatitis.

Evidence supports an important role for adhesion molecules in both leukocyte transmigration and function. Simultaneous monitoring of eosinophil adhesion and degranulation has shown that degranulation is always preceded by cellular adhesion (150). Human eosinophils express β_2-integrin CD1lb/CD18 (Mac-1). Cell–cell interactions between eosinophils and endothelial cells induce upregulation of CD11b and CD35 on eosinophils and an increased capacity of eosinophils to generate an oxidative burst (151). Monoclonal antibodies to CD18 markedly inhibit eosinophil adhesion, degranulation, and superoxide production induced by PAF or GM-CSF; monoclonal antibodies to CD1lb also inhibit eosinophil adhesion and degranulation (150). These findings indicate that CD1lb/CD18-dependent cellular adhesion plays a crucial role in eosinophil degranulation and superoxide production, which is of importance when eosinophils contact tissues after transmigrating vessels.

Migratory responses of eosinophils to C5a and TNF-α are the same in normal individuals and in patients with atopic dermatitis. Following IL-5 exposure, eosinophils from normal donors show potentiation of migratory responses to PAF and platelet factor 4 (152,153). However, in patients with atopic dermatitis given intracutaneous injection of PAF or allergen, there is much greater cutaneous eosinophilia at allergen-injected sites than at PAF-injected sites, indicating that PAF alone does not account for eosinophil mobilization in this disease. Taken together, these findings suggest in vivo priming of eosinophils in atopic dermatitis; however, this priming for migratory responses is apparently not maximal because it can be further potentiated by IL-5 (153).

EOSINOPHIL DEGRANULATION IN ATOPIC DERMATITIS

The common presence of peripheral blood eosinophilia in atopic dermatitis, the histologic finding of few infiltrating tissue eosinophils, and the prominent increases in a granule protein from eosinophils in peripheral blood prompted numerous studies, especially focused on determining whether eosinophils degranulate in this disease. Peripheral blood eosinophilia is found in many diseases and, specifically, has been associated with atopic dermatitis (1). Measurement of serum MBP levels and peripheral blood eosinophil counts in normal controls and individuals with various diseases, including 16 patients with atopic dermatitis, showed normal eosinophil numbers and low MBP levels in controls; but over half of the patients with atopic dermatitis had increased MBP levels in the peripheral blood, some with normal eosinophil counts and some with increased eosinophil numbers (154). These results suggest that the toxic eosinophil granule MBP "escapes" from eosinophils through degranulation, secretion, or another process.

Immunohistologic staining for eosinophil MBP, as a marker of eosinophil degranulation (34), revealed extracellular MBP deposition in 20 biopsy specimens from 18 patients with atopic dermatitis (43). Nineteen of the specimens were from chronic atopic dermatitis lesions (34); one specimen was from unaffected skin and had been obtained at the same time as a specimen of affected skin from that patient—two lesional specimens had been obtained from the same patient two years apart. Using affinity chromatography purified polyclonal antibody to MBP in an indirect immunofluorescence staining procedure, the dominant staining pattern in the 19 affected skin specimens was extracellular fibrillar fluorescence in the upper dermis, often with scattered extracellular granules involving the upper and mid-dermis. Both affected skin specimens from the same patient two years apart showed marked upper dermal fibrillar MBP fluorescence (34). Comparison of affected and unaffected skin from one patient showed marked upper dermal fibrillar MBP fluorescence in affected lesional skin and minimal fluorescence with fine, fibrillar extracellular MBP staining in the upper dermis in normal-appearing skin (Fig. 1). These studies demonstrated eosinophil activity in atopic dermatitis through deposition of granule products. A striking observation in the atopic dermatitis lesional specimens was extensive extracellular MBP staining but a paucity of intact eosinophils. Identifiable eosinophils were located predominantly within perivascular foci of mononuclear cell infiltration. Yet, in many of the specimens, extracellular MBP deposition was prominent throughout the upper dermis. With increased

MBP levels (154) and low-density eosinophils in the peripheral blood (155), dermal MBP deposition in lesions of atopic dermatitis could have resulted from tissue deposition of granule proteins from activated circulating eosinophils. However, the focal patchy localization of MBP principally in the upper dermis and the minimal staining of uninvolved skin argue against this and suggest that eosinophils deposit granule proteins directly in the skin in atopic dermatitis. Degranulated cells may not be recognizable morphologically, yet their granule proteins may be exerting biologic effects.

Following initial demonstration of marked extracellular MBP deposition in affected skin (34), additional atopic dermatitis patients were studied (38). Lesional skin biopsy specimens were obtained from 22 patients; blood and urine samples were collected the same day from 19 and 14 of the patients, respectively. Fifteen of the 22 patients showed prominent extracellular deposition of at least one eosinophil granule protein in lesional skin, which was markedly out of proportion to the few infiltrating intact cells. Only 4 of 19 patients had peripheral blood eosinophilia greater than 760 cells/μL; however, serum MBP, EDN, and ECP levels were increased in more than half of the sera (15 of 19, 14 of 19, and 10 of 19 specimens, respectively), and mean MBP, EDN, and ECP levels were increased compared to levels in 50 nonatopic normal subjects. Urine levels of MBP, EDN, and ECP were increased in 3 of 14, 7 of 14, and 0 of 14 specimens, respectively (38). Statistical comparisons showed significant positive correlations between serum levels of MBP and EDN and serum levels of EDN and ECP. In addition, tissue deposits of MBP correlated with those of EDN, as did MBP with ECP and EDN with ECP tissue deposits. Urine MBP levels correlated with serum EDN levels. Peripheral blood eosinophils counts correlated with the degree of MBP deposition in tissues. A relationship between the magnitude of body surface involvement and peripheral blood MBP levels was also found (38). In a separate study of atopic dermatitis, urine EDN concentrations correlated with disease severity and with pruritus but not with peripheral blood eosinophil counts, suggesting that urine EDN concentration may be a useful clinical marker of atopic dermatitis activity (156). Taken together, these studies demonstrate eosinophil products in skin lesions, peripheral blood and urine, and correlation with extent of atopic dermatitis. In a related condition, atopic keratoconjunctivitis, the presence of eosinophils and/or neutrophils in the cornea also correlated with the disease (157).

Monoclonal antibodies to ECP and MBP are commercially available and have been used in studies to delineate eosinophil involvement in atopic dermatitis. However, EG2 (Pharmacia & Upjohn, Uppsala, Sweden), a monoclonal antibody to ECP, stains ECP in and/or from eosinophils and/or neutrophils (158). The sensitivity in detecting extracellular MBP deposition with monoclonal MBP antibody BMK13 (Biodesign International, Kennebunk, ME) appears to be less than with polyclonal antibodies. Figure 2 illustrates the prominent extracellular eosinophil granule MBP staining observed in chronic atopic dermatitis lesions by both indirect immunofluorescence and immunoperoxidase staining methods. Figure 2 also demonstrates relative staining with monoclonal and polyclonal antibodies to MBP. Considerably less MBP is detected in tissues stained with monoclonal than with polyclonal antibodies using either method. Therefore, eosinophil involvement may be underestimated in tissue assays that use monoclonal MBP antibodies. Moreover, the detectable eosinophil granule protein staining with polyclonal antibodies likely indicates levels of granule proteins with pathogenic effects in tissues (40).

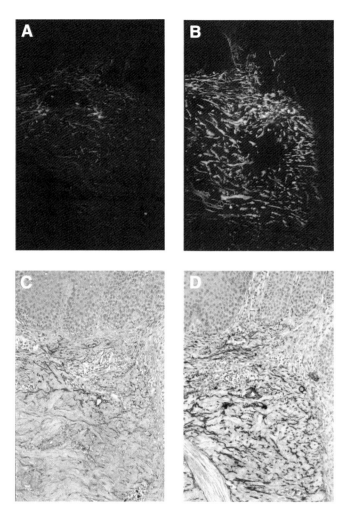

FIGURE 2 Eosinophil granule MBP deposition in an atopic dermatitis lesion as detected by different antibodies and indirect staining techniques. Lesional skin stained by: (**A**) indirect immunofluorescence with monoclonal MBP antibody (BMK13, Biodesign International, Kennebunk, ME); (**B**) indirect immunofluorescence with affinity-chromatography purified polyclonal MBP antibody; (**C**) immunoperoxidase with BMK13 monoclonal MBP antibody; and (**D**) immunoperoxidase with affinity-chromatography purified polyclonal MBP antibody. Polyclonal MBP antibodies (panels **B** and **D**) revealed greater MBP staining than did monoclonal antibodies (panels **A** and **C**) with both immunofluorescence and immunoperoxidase methods. Comparable fields from serial sections show extensive extracellular MBP deposition in the dermis with few intact infiltrating cells. In addition, the features of chronic dermatitis are evident with epidermal thickening, hyalinization at the epidermal-dermal junction and perivascular mononuclear cell infiltration in dermis (160× original magnification). Negative controls using protein A purified rabbit IgG and irrelevant monoclonal antibodies showed no staining (not shown).

Additional studies demonstrating relationships between eosinophils and atopic dermatitis disease activity are reviewed elsewhere (159,160). Results of these include the findings that peripheral blood eosinophil counts are increased in severe disease and decrease with therapeutic improvement (47,56,161–167). Such studies show that blood eosinophil counts roughly correlate with disease severity. Patients with severe disease may have normal counts, but these usually are individuals with atopic dermatitis alone, while those who have severe atopic dermatitis and concomitant respiratory or other allergies, with IgE specific antibodies, commonly have increased numbers of eosinophils in their peripheral blood (164,168). Eosinophils lose density with activation, and atopic dermatitis patients have significantly increased numbers of hypodense eosinophils (169). Neonates who develop infantile eczema appear to have significantly higher number eosinophils in cord blood compared to babies with seborrheic dermatitis, intertrigo, and diaper dermatitis (170). Eosinophilia during infancy is associated with allergic disease during the first six years of life (90).

CD69, also known as activation inducer molecule (AIM), is involved in early activation of lymphocytes, monocytes, and platelets; it also is expressed early by activated eosinophils in atopic dermatitis (171). Atopic dermatitis patients with CD69-positive eosinophils had significantly greater numbers of eosinophils and platelets, total IgE, and eosinophil nuclear lobes (172); they also exhibited growth failure, developmental delay, low serum albumin, and electrolyte abnormalities. EDN and IL-18 levels were significantly increased in this group, but not levels of IL-4, IL-5, and IL-12 (172). These observations suggest that CD69 surface expression on eosinophils may be a marker for severe abnormalities in atopic dermatitis.

In addition to established relationships between eosinophil counts and atopic dermatitis severity, serum levels of eosinophil granule proteins are increased in atopic dermatitis and correlate with disease activity (159,161,163,169,173–183) in adults (175,180,181) and children (174,179,184), although children typically have lower ECP levels (160). Correlations between ECP levels and peripheral blood eosinophil counts have yielded variable results (174,179), and ECP may be correlated best with hypodense eosinophils representative of activation (169). Eosinophil counts, ECP levels, and dermal infiltration of eosinophils and granule proteins (125) appear to be reduced in intrinsic compared with extrinsic atopic dermatitis; clinical severity seems to correlate with eosinophil counts and serum ECP levels in both types of atopic dermatitis (184). The relationship between peripheral blood ECP levels and clinical activity of atopic dermatitis provides additional strong support for the eosinophil's role in the disease. However, caution must be exercised in attributing detection of ECP solely to eosinophil activity, because, as noted, ECP may be derived from neutrophils (158). Like ECP, EDN is present in both neutrophils and eosinophils (158), but peripheral blood EDN may correlate better with disease severity than does ECP (185).

The presence of ECP in human breast milk has been associated with development of cow's milk allergy and atopic dermatitis in breast-fed infants (186). Breast-feeding mothers (58 atopic, 36 nonatopic) and their infants were studied prospectively from birth; colostrum and milk samples obtained at three months of lactation and the mothers' peripheral blood were examined. Evaluation at two-year follow-up showed that 51 mothers had children with cow's milk allergy, 24 had children with atopic dermatitis, and 19 had healthy children. ECP was undetectable in milk from all mothers with healthy infants, while ECP was found in 27% of mothers who had children with cow's milk allergy and 42% whose babies had atopic dermatitis. ECP was detected in breast milk in 26% of atopic and 25% of nonatopic mothers. The findings suggest that ECP in human breast milk is associated with development of cow's milk allergy and atopic dermatitis in breast-fed infants, but not with maternal atopy (186).

FATE OF EOSINOPHILS IN ATOPIC DERMATITIS

The striking extracellular deposition of eosinophil granule proteins in lesions of atopic dermatitis and increases in peripheral blood granule protein levels that correlate with disease activity suggest that these granule-associated proteins are released from eosinophils during the disease process. In the IgE-mediated late-phase reaction (LPR), extracellular eosinophil granule protein deposition corresponds with electron microscopic (EM) evidence of eosinophil disruption and free granules (36). EM studies of specimens from 10 patients with atopic dermatitis revealed disrupted eosinophils and/or free eosinophil granules in lesions from seven patients, but revealed no normal-appearing eosinophils. The dermis contained eosinophils exhibiting various degrees of degeneration, including intact cells with abnormal granules, intact cells with prominent pseudopod-like extensions with abnormal granules, eosinophils with degenerating cell and/or nuclear membranes, and free eosinophil granules in proximity to or in the absence of nearby degenerating eosinophils. Free granules and granules within degenerating eosinophils showed lucency and loss of core density (41). Although this EM study showed a spectrum of disrupted eosinophils in atopic dermatitis, there was no evidence of classical granule exocytosis (piecemeal degranulation) or vesicular transport. Thus, deposition of eosinophil granules and granule proteins in atopic dermatitis may be mainly the result of a cytolytic process. However, examination of eosinophils with sensitive techniques to identify granule proteins in vesicles might show evidence of piecemeal degranulation or the presence of sombrero vesicles (187,188).

Programmed cell death of peripheral blood eosinophils is delayed in atopic dermatitis to an even greater extent than in inhalant allergy (189), but is the same in "atopic" and "nonatopic" atopic dermatitis subjects, indicating that it is not specifically related to sensitization. On the other hand, apoptosis in eosinophils from atopic dermatitis patients can be induced in a dose-dependent manner with glucocorticoids (190).

Nur77 and NOR1, two genes that are members of NR4A orphan steroid nuclear receptor family, show greater expression in atopic dermatitis patients than in healthy individuals (191). Expression of Nurr1, another gene in the NR4A receptor family, also is greater in atopic dermatitis. In fractionated peripheral blood leukocytes from controls, NOR1 expression is the highest in eosinophils, but expression of Nur77 and Nurr1 genes is not eosinophil-specific. Increased apoptosis could be induced in both eosinophils and the eosinophil-like tumor cell line, AML14.3D10, by treatment with antibody against CD30 and Fas, which, with anti-CD30, was associated with rapid expression of NR4A receptor family genes (191). Thus, expression of the NR4A receptor family genes through CD30 signaling may regulate eosinophil apoptosis in atopic dermatitis.

In a proteomic approach to analyze eosinophilia in atopic dermatitis, 51 proteins were identified: 19 related to signaling, 8 involved in regulation of metabolism, 4 related to apoptosis, 3 involved in inflammation, and the others associated with transcription, RNA processing, translation, the cytoskeleton, and unknown functions. Eosinophils from atopic dermatitis patients had increased expression of cyclinA2, voltage-dependent anion channel protein 2, and 38 kDa FK506 binding protein 8 (192). In contrast, low viability eosinophils from healthy donors or cultured eosinophil-like tumor cells (AML14.3D10 cells) treated with dexamethasone showed increased phosphorylation of Grb7 and its upstream signaling protein, focal adhesion kinase (FAK) (192). These observations suggest that expressions of cyclinA2, voltage-dependent anion channel protein 2, and 38 kDa FK506 binding protein 8 as well as phosphorylation of Grb7 may be associated with antiapoptosis of eosinophils.

It is difficult to reconcile the delayed eosinophil apoptosis, or programmed cell death, observed in atopic dermatitis (189) with the prominence of cytolytic eosinophil degeneration observed in this disease (41). However, delayed programmed cell death may be an indicator of eosinophil activation that, once eosinophils transmigrate cutaneous vessels and infiltrate tissues (42), is associated with granule release and cytolytic cell death.

IgE-MEDIATED LATE-PHASE REACTIONS, EOSINOPHILS, AND ATOPIC DERMATITIS

Eosinophil degranulation occurs in several in vivo models of hypersensitivity including the IgE-mediated late-phase reaction (LPR) (36). Intradermal allergen injection in allergic patients causes the LPR and release of eosinophil granule proteins into tissues (and into blister fluids bathing these lesions) (193,194) with marked disruption of eosinophils and extracellular deposition of eosinophil granule proteins (36). Eosinophil survival-enhancing cytokines are also present in LPR blister fluids (195), and increased mRNA expression of the cytokine gene cluster IL-3, IL-4, IL-5, and GM-CSF is found in the cutaneous LPR (196). Similarly, after nasal challenge with antigen, the LPR is accompanied by a dramatic increase in eosinophils and eosinophil degranulation, as indicated by increases in MBP and EDN in nasal lavage fluids (197). Furthermore, eosinophil-active cytokines are present in nasal secretions (198). In studies of cytokine expression during allergen-induced late nasal responses, expression of IL-4 and IL-5 mRNA was found predominantly in eosinophils early (at six hours) (199). Analyses of eosinophil granule proteins in the pulmonary LPR induced by segmental challenge with ragweed extract have shown that MBP, EDN, EPO, and ECP are elevated in bronchoalveolar lavage (BAL) fluids (200), and IL-5 is the predominant eosinophil-active cytokine (201). Thus, allergen challenge of sensitized persons causes eosinophil infiltration and degranulation into the skin, nose, and lungs.

The late phase of the IgE-mediated reaction has been proposed as a model for chronic allergic inflammation, including that seen in atopic dermatitis (202,203). Immediate hypersensitivity reactions in the skin are characterized by development of a wheal and flare, which peaks in 10 to 20 minutes; the LPR is an inflammatory reaction developing hours later at the same site, but over a much larger area, and is associated with painful, pruritic edema. Pathologic examination of the cutaneous LPR has shown infiltration with mononuclear cells, neutrophils, basophils, and eosinophils along with edema and mast cell degranulation (204–206). Eosinophil infiltration occurs quickly after antigen challenge, with eosinophils marginating in blood vessels within 15 minutes after antigen challenge; eosinophil infiltration into tissues is maximal approximately six to eight hours postchallenge (36). Extracellular deposition of eosinophil and neutrophil granule proteins in the LPR begins within one hour after antigen challenge and persists up to 56 hours. Extracellular eosinophil and neutrophil granule protein deposition are prominent at the peak of the clinical reaction, six- to eight hours after antigen challenge (36).

The IgE-mediated cutaneous LPR and atopic dermatitis lesions both are associated with the induction of leukocyte adhesion molecules including E-selectin, VCAM-1, and intercellular adhesion molecule-1 (ICAM-1). In children with atopic dermatitis, increased circulating soluble ICAM-1 levels are found (207), and soluble E-selectin correlates with disease activity (208). Induction of these leukocyte adhesion molecules can be blocked by neutralizing antibodies to IL-1 and TNF-α (148) suggesting that these cytokines participate in the expression of leukocyte adhesion molecules. Therefore, release of such cytokines likely is involved in regulating the local accumulation of inflammatory cells at sites of allergic reactions.

As previously reviewed, eotaxin is an important chemokine for attracting eosinophils to inflammatory sites, particularly, in the LPR. Before allergen exposure, eotaxin is not present as mRNA or protein, but injection of allergen (into the skin of an allergic subject) stimulates eotaxin production (122). Eotaxin has a role in early recruitment of eosinophils after antigen exposure, whereas eotaxin-2 and MCP-4 are involved in later (24 hours) infiltration of eosinophils (122). Eotaxin production appears to be stimulated by IL-4, TNF-α, and IL-13 production, and both mast cells and T-lymphocytes are able to produce these molecules. IL-4 induces eotaxin mRNA in human dermal fibroblasts (135,136). IL-4 and TNF-α stimulate eotaxin-1 and eotaxin-3 production in human dermal fibroblasts and keratinocytes (209,210). Remarkably, IL-4 transgenic mice spontaneously develop a pruritic inflammatory disease similar to atopic dermatitis, associated with eosinophilia and expression of IgE and IgG1 (211). In contrast, IL-4 deficient (IL-4−/−) mice show a reduction in eosinophils in an experimental murine model of atopic dermatitis (212). Notably, levels of eotaxin-3 are high in patients with atopic dermatitis (213).

Immunohistologic studies have shown differences between atopic dermatitis and the cutaneous LPR. In the LPR, extracellular deposition of both eosinophil and neutrophil granule proteins is found (36). In contrast, in atopic dermatitis lesions, there is prominent extracellular eosinophil granule protein deposition but not neutrophil granule protein deposition (38). By immunoassay, serum levels of eosinophil granule proteins, but not neutrophil elastase, are increased in atopic dermatitis compared to normal controls (35,38). Overall, the results indicate that eosinophils are involved in established lesions of atopic dermatitis, but, unlike the IgE-mediated LPR, neutrophils do not appear to play a role.

The differences that are observed in the inflammatory cell activity of atopic dermatitis and LPR may have several explanations (Table 2). The mode of antigen exposure may be linked to the pathophysiologic outcome. For example, in atopic dermatitis, antigens are likely ingested, inhaled, or contacted rather than intradermally injected as in the LPR. The inflammatory response may be modified depending on antigen presentation and processing in different anatomical areas. Moreover, atopic dermatitis skin may differ from essentially normal skin of patients who have respiratory allergies (in whom LPRs are elicited); patients with atopic dermatitis show altered pharmacophysiologic responsiveness and aberrant skin barrier composition and function. Finally, repeated or continuous antigen exposure may induce a different inflammatory response pattern than does single exposure.

TABLE 2 Atopic Dermatitis and the IgE-Mediated Late-Phase Reaction: Possible Explanations for Differences in Inflammatory Markers

Different mode of antigen exposure
  Ingested, inhaled, or contacted vs. intradermal
Possible modification of disease expression depending on antigen processing and
  presentation
Atopic dermatitis skin may be constitutionally different than skin of patients with
  respiratory allergies
Repeated or continuous antigen exposure shows a progressive inflammatory
  response compared to single exposure

Allergen challenge models other than the LPR have been helpful in delineating the pathogenesis of atopic dermatitis and further establishing links between eosinophils and the pathophysiology of this disease. A different mode of antigen exposure, namely, the epicutaneous route, compares favorably to the intradermal route. Biopsies of aeroallergen patch test sites of atopic dermatitis patients show that lymphocytes and eosinophils infiltrate the dermis two to six hours after allergen application (214). By 24 to 48 hours after patch test application, eosinophils have infiltrated the epidermis and released ECP (214). Activated eosinophils also are present in the epidermis and dermis, in contact with antigen-presenting (OKT6-positive) cells (215). Furthermore, extracellular eosinophil granules are detected and ECP is found in macrophage-like dermal cells (215). In other studies of house dust mite patch test sites, biopsy specimens reveal that eosinophils localize in dermal postcapillary venules at two hours and infiltrate tissues at six hours; the process peaks at 24 to 48 hours with epidermal spongiosis at 48 hours. Endothelial cell expression of E-selectin and ICAM-1 is upregulated as infiltrating eosinophils increase (216). Increased expression of IL-4, IL-5, IL-6, IL-7, and TNF-α also has been observed (217,218). Taken together, these studies demonstrate a relationship between eosinophil activity and eczematous dermatitis and indicate that cutaneous eosinophil infiltration and degranulation may be induced by epicutaneous allergen contact.

Evidence also indicates that repeated or constant allergen exposure may be associated with a changing inflammatory pattern. In monkeys, for example, repeated allergen challenge by inhalation is attended with early accumulation of neutrophils, followed by a prolonged inflammatory reaction and a marked increase in airway eosinophils associated with greater airway hyperresponsiveness (219). Similarly, repeated or continual antigen challenge of skin probably results in further development of the IgE-mediated reaction (220) including eosinophil involvement (221). Moreover, chronic lesions of atopic dermatitis that may result from chronic allergen exposure show significantly fewer IL-4 and more IL-5 mRNA-expressing cells, and contain more eosinophils, than acute lesions (109). IL-12 mRNA-expressing cells also are more numerous in chronic lesions. Because eosinophils have been found to express IL-12 (222,223), they may be the IL-12–producing cells. A corresponding increase in IL-12 may promote a switch from Th0 to Th1, resulting in the IFN-γ production found in chronic atopic dermatitis lesions (57). Although the role of eosinophils in delayed-type hypersensitivity has not been well characterized, IFN-γ is a prominent cytokine in delayed-type hypersensitivity reactions, and IL-4 mRNA is expressed in contact dermatitis (224). Because eosinophils possess both functional IFN-γ and IL-4 receptors, they may be involved in Type IV, delayed hypersensitivity, and allergic contact dermatitis, as well as in Type I, IgE-mediated, and immediate hypersensitivity. Results from recent studies indicate that Th2 cells require signals in addition to antigen for maximal inflammatory cell recruitment and that Th1 and Th2 cells together promote a robust eosinophil-predominant inflammatory response (225).

POTENTIAL EOSINOPHIL-DIRECTED THERAPEUTIC INTERVENTIONS

Pathogenic pathways involved in atopic dermatitis continue to be investigated. IgE-bearing antigen-presenting cells, IgE-bearing mast cells and basophils, Th2 lymphocytes, and monocytes are implicated in the pathogenic process. Eosinophils also appear to be intricately involved, although they may not be central for initiating but rather for perpetrating or affecting the immunologic response. As such, therapeutic interference in eosinophil activity may ameliorate the end results of the inflammatory process but will likely not have as potentially grave consequences as would alteration of more centrally acting immunoresponsive cells. Glucocorticoids are the mainstay of treatment for eosinophil-related diseases and, especially in topical form, are widely used to treat atopic dermatitis. Lidocaine mimics certain activities of glucocorticoids in blocking IL-5 activity on eosinophils in vitro. Beneficial effects of nebulized lidocaine have been demonstrated in patients with asthma (226–228), but this agent has not been studied in atopic dermatitis.

Topical calcineurin inhibitors are effective in atopic dermatitis and are associated with changes in eosinophil-associated parameters. Short-term 0.1% tacrolimus ointment therapy induced significant improvement in atopic dermatitis, both clinically and histopathologically, and was associated with reduced infiltration of T-cells, B-cells, and eosinophils and reduced expression of IL-5, IL-10, and IL13 by CD4-positive T-cells, but with an increase in number of epidermal CD1a-positive dendritic cells (229). In another study, patients with atopic dermatitis treated with 0.03% tacrolimus ointment twice daily for eight weeks exhibited decreased numbers of eosinophils in affected skin, as well as suppression of eotaxin, CCR3, RANTES, and IL-5 (230). Three weeks after the treatment of acute atopic dermatitis with topical pimecrolimus, clinical improvement was associated with a decrease in the density of the inflammatory infiltrate containing lymphocytes and eosinophils, decrease in peripheral blood lymphocyte and eosinophil counts, reduced expression of IL-5, IL-10, and IL-13 in both CD4-positive and CD8-positive T-cells in tissues, reduced interferon-γ (a Th1 cytokine), and increased epidermal CD1-positive dendritic cells (231).

IFN-α effectively reduces total leukocyte and eosinophil counts in patients with the hypereosinophilic syndrome (HES) (232), and studies in atopic dermatitis have shown that improvement with IFN-γ treatment correlates with decreased eosinophil counts (166,233). IL-4 is important in Th2 development and eosinophil infiltration, therefore, soluble IL-4 receptor has been considered as treatment for eosinophil-associated diseases (234,235).

Omalizumab, a humanized IgE monoclonal antibody, inhibits early and late phase cutaneous reactions including tissue eosinophilia (236,237). The priming effect of repeated allergen challenge on eosinophil infiltration was abrogated in patients receiving omalizumab. In allergic asthma, omalizumab treatment reduced sputum eosinophil counts significantly (238). Treatment of atopic dermatitis with omalizumab has been tested only in small case series with variable results

(239,240) and without assessment of effects on eosinophil involvement, particularly eosinophil granule protein deposition.

The IL-5 monoclonal antibody, mepolizumab, reduces eosinophils and tenascin deposition (a marker of repair and remodeling) in allergen-challenged atopic skin (241). In a randomized double-blind, placebo-controlled design, skin biopsies were obtained from 24 atopics at allergen- and diluent-injected sites before six hours after and 48 hours following three intravenous doses of mepolizumab; this agent significantly inhibited eosinophil infiltration at 6 and 48 hours. Despite this, mepolizumab had no significant influence on the size of the 6 hours or 48 hours LPR. The results suggest that eosinophils probably do not play a role in inducing the redness, swelling, and induration characteristic of the peak (six hours) LPR, although the effect of mepolizumab on deposition of eosinophil granule proteins was not determined. At 48 hours, decreases in tenascin-positive cells correlated with reduction in eosinophil infiltration, providing evidence that eosinophils participate in the tissue remodeling process that characterizes allergic inflammation.

In a double-blind placebo-controlled study using the atopic patch test and designed to evaluate the ability of inhalant allergens to induce eczema in patients with atopic dermatitis, mepolizumab induced a significant decrease in peripheral blood eosinophil counts but did not inhibit the development of eczema (242). Although cutaneous eosinophils were decreased in the mepolizumab-treated group at day 16 compared with placebo, the difference was not significant; deposition of eosinophil granule proteins was not evaluated.

The efficacy of two 750 mg doses of mepolizumab, given one week apart, was evaluated in a randomized, placebo-controlled study of moderate-to-severe atopic dermatitis (243). Success was defined as marked improvement after two weeks of treatment, based on disease severity scoring with the Physician's Global Assessment of Improvement (PGA); pruritus and peripheral eosinophil counts were among the secondary endpoints. Eighteen patients received mepolizumab and 22 were given placebo. Peripheral blood eosinophil counts were significantly reduced in the treatment group compared with controls. Although no mepolizumab-treated patient achieved the marked improvement PGA endpoint set in this two-dose, two-week treatment protocol, modest ($<50\%$) improvement was scored significantly more often in the mepolizumab-treated patients (243). No assessment of tissue eosinophils or eosinophil granule proteins was conducted. Considering how long eosinophil granule proteins persist in tissues [e.g., six weeks for MBP (40)], the study was likely of insufficient duration.

Clinical trials of mepolizumab in patients with HES who were negative for the *FIP1L1–PDGFRA* fusion gene have been conducted (244). The primary end point, reduction of the prednisone dose to 10 mg or less per day for eight or more consecutive weeks, was achieved in 84% of patients given mepolizumab as compared with 43% administered placebo. Peripheral blood eosinophil counts decreased in 95% of patients (45% of placebo), and treatment with mepolizumab was associated with reduction in glucocorticoid therapy. Almost half of the patients were able to discontinue glucocorticoids during treatment with mepolizumab (244). Also, of note, anti-IL5 therapy has been helpful in treating the pruritic dermatitis that may accompany HES (245).

Clinical trials have been established to evaluate the efficacy of mepolizumab in asthma, nasal polyposis, and eosinophilic esophagitis (246). Thus far in asthma trials, mepolizumab has been shown to induce significant reductions in peripheral blood and sputum eosinophil counts, but has not improved allergen-induced airway inflammation (247). However, tissue eosinophilia and/or eosinophil granule protein deposition may not be sufficiently diminished to reduce their biologic effects (248); therefore, studies are ongoing, particularly in patients with increased eosinophils in sputum.

Agents that block eosinophil chemotaxins, including eotaxin, and chemotaxin receptor blockers (234,249,250) are under development as are agents that prevent eosinophil adhesion and, hence, activation. A CCR3 receptor antagonist has been shown to inhibit both early and late phase allergic inflammation in the conjunctiva in a mouse model (251), and a combined CCR3 receptor and H1 (histamine 1) receptor antagonist is in development (252). The leukotriene receptor antagonist, zafirlukast, appears to be beneficial in treating atopic dermatitis (253,254) as does montelukast in children (255), with associated reduction in peripheral blood eosinophil counts. Finally, polyanions, such as heparin and polyglutamic acid, can neutralize the toxicity of the intensely cationic eosinophil granule proteins and have been shown to block bronchial hyperreactivity caused by MBP (256). Thus, analyses of the therapeutic effects of neutralizing acidic substances are warranted.

CONCLUSION

Strong evidence supports a role for eosinophils in the pathogenesis of atopic dermatitis. The cutaneous inflammatory reaction in atopic dermatitis involves recruitment, activation, and degranulation of eosinophils with release of cytotoxic granule proteins and other mediators, which contribute to disease expression. The IgE-mediated reaction, as currently understood, is an incomplete or inadequate model for atopic dermatitis; however, repeated or continuous allergen challenge may be a multiphasic response beyond the classical dual-phase IgE response, with persistent inflammation and eosinophil involvement (Fig. 1). Understanding the role of eosinophils, including whether blocking the effects of eosinophil activity will modify the manifestations of atopic dermatitis, is important for continuing investigations into the pathophysiology of this challenging disease.

REFERENCES

1. Rajka G. Natural history and clinical manifestations of atopic dermatitis. Clin Rev Allergy 1986; 4:3–26.
2. Leiferman KM, Gleich, GJ. The role of eosinophils in atopic dermatitis. In: Leung DYM, ed. Atopic Dermatitis: From Pathogenesis to Treatment. Austin, TX: Landes Company, 1996:145–183.
3. Leiferman KM. Eosinophil granule proteins in cutaneous disease. In: Gleich GJ, Kay AB, ed. Eosinophils in Allergy and Inflammation. New York, NY: Marcel Dekker, Inc., 1994:455–469.
4. Gleich GJ, Adolphson CR, Leiferman KM. Eosinophils. In: Gallin JI, Goldstein IM, Snyderman R, ed. Inflammation, Basic Principles and Clinical Correlates. New York, NY: Raven Press, 1992:663–700.
5. Zheutlin LM, Ackerman SJ, Gleich GJ, et al. Stimulation of basophil and rat mast cell histamine release by eosinophil granule-derived cationic proteins. J Immunol 1984; 133:2180–2185.

6. Moy JN, Gleich GJ, Thomas LL. Noncytotoxic activation of neutrophils by eosinophil granule major basic protein. Effect on superoxide anion generation and lysosomal enzyme release. J Immunol 1990; 145:2626–2632.
7. Rohrbach MS, Wheatley CL, Slifman NR, et al. Activation of platelets by eosinophil granule proteins. J Exp Med 1990; 172:1271–1274.
8. Kita H, Abu-Ghazaleh RI, Sur S, et al. Eosinophil major basic protein induces degranulation and IL-8 production by human eosinophils. J Immunol 1995; 154:4749–4758.
9. Minnicozzi M, Duran WN, Gleich GJ, et al. Eosinophil granule proteins increase microvascular macromolecular transport in the hamster cheek pouch. J Immunol 1994; 153:2664–2670.
10. Gleich GJ, Schroeter AL, Marcoux JP, et al. Episodic angioedema associated with eosinophilia. N Engl J Med 1984; 310:1621–1626.
11. Rosenberg HF, Domachowske JB. Eosinophils, eosinophil ribonucleases, and their role in host defense against respiratory virus pathogens. J Leukoc Biol 2001; 70:691–698.
12. Yang D, Chen Q, Su SB, et al. Eosinophil-derived neurotoxin acts as an alarmin to activate the TLR2-MyD88 signal pathway in dendritic cells and enhances Th2 immune responses. J Exp Med 2008; 205:79–90.
13. Kanofsky JR, Hoogland H, Wever R, et al. Singlet oxygen production by human eosinophils. J Biol Chem 1988; 263:9692–9696.
14. Petreccia DC, Nauseef WM, Clark RA. Respiratory burst of normal human eosinophils. J Leukoc Biol 1987; 41:283–288.
15. Lee T, Lenihan DJ, Malone B, et al. Increased biosynthesis of platelet-activating factor in activated human eosinophils. J Biol Chem 1984; 259:5526–5530.
16. Shaw RJ, Walsh GM, Cromwell O, et al. Activated human eosinophils generate SRS-A leukotrienes following IgG-dependent stimulation. Nature 1985; 316:150–152.
17. Hansel TT, Braun RK, De Vries IJ, et al. Eosinophils and cytokines. Agents Actions Suppl 1993; 43:197–208.
18. Moqbel R. Eosinophils, cytokines, and allergic inflammation. Ann N Y Acad Sci 1994; 725:223–233.
19. Moqbel R, Levi-Schaffer F, Kay AB. Cytokine generation by eosinophils. J Allergy Clin Immunol 1994; 94:1183–1188.
20. Miyamasu M, Hirai K, Takahashi Y, et al. Chemotactic agonists induce cytokine generation in eosinophils. J Immunol 1995; 154:1339–1349.
21. Shi HZ, Humbles A, Gerard C, et al. Lymph node trafficking and antigen presentation by endobronchial eosinophils. J Clin Invest 2000; 105:945–953.
22. Phipps S, Lam CE, Mahalingam S, et al. Eosinophils contribute to innate antiviral immunity and promote clearance of respiratory syncytial virus. Blood 2007; 110:1578–1586.
23. Elovic A, Wong DT, Weller PF, et al. Expression of transforming growth factors-alpha and beta 1 messenger RNA and product by eosinophils in nasal polyps. J Allergy Clin Immunol 1994; 93:864–869.
24. Birkland TP, Cheavens MD, Pincus SH. Human eosinophils stimulate DNA synthesis and matrix production in dermal fibroblasts. Arch Dermatol Res 1994; 286:312–318.
25. Ochi H, De Jesus NH, Hsieh FH, et al. IL-4 and -5 prime human mast cells for different profiles of IgE-dependent cytokine production. Proc Natl Acad Sci U S A 2000; 97:10509–10513.
26. Butterfield JH, Leiferman KM. Eosinophil-associated diseases. In: Page CP, ed. The Handbook of Immunopharmacology, Immunopharmacology of Eosinophils. New York, NY: Academic Press, 1993:151–192.
27. Leiferman KM. A current perspective on the role of eosinophils in dermatologic diseases. J Am Acad Dermatol 1991; 24:1101–1112.
28. Gleich GJ. The eosinophil and bronchial asthma: Current understanding. J Allergy Clin Immunol 1990; 85:422–436.
29. Hertzman PA, Blevins WL, Mayer J, et al. Association of the eosinophilia-myalgia syndrome with the ingestion of tryptophan. N Engl J Med 1990; 322:869–873.

30. van Haelst Pisani C, Kovach JS, Kita H, et al. Administration of interleukin-2 (IL-2) results in increased plasma concentrations of IL-5 and eosinophilia in patients with cancer. Blood 1991; 78:1538–1544.

31. Butterfield JH, Leiferman KM, Abrams J, et al. Elevated serum levels of interleukin-5 in patients with the syndrome of episodic angioedema and eosinophilia. Blood 1992; 79:688–692.

32. Filley WV, Ackerman SJ, Gleich GJ. An immunofluorescent method for specific staining of eosinophil granule major basic protein. J Immunol Methods 1981; 47:227–238.

33. Filley WV, Holley KE, Kephart GM, et al. Identification by immunofluorescence of eosinophil granule major basic protein in lung tissues of patients with bronchial asthma. Lancet 1982; 2:11–16.

34. Leiferman KM, Ackerman SJ, Sampson HA, et al. Dermal deposition of eosinophil-granule major basic protein in atopic dermatitis. Comparison with onchocerciasis. N Engl J Med 1985; 313:282–285.

35. Leiferman KM, Peters MS, Gleich GJ. The eosinophil and cutaneous edema. J Am Acad Dermatol 1986; 15:513–517.

36. Leiferman KM, Fujisawa T, Gray BH, et al. Extracellular deposition of eosinophil and neutrophil granule proteins in the IgE-mediated cutaneous late phase reaction. Lab Invest 1990; 62:579–589.

37. Peters MS, Schroeter AL, Kephart GM, et al. Localization of eosinophil granule major basic protein in chronic urticaria. J Invest Dermatol 1983; 81:39–43.

38. Ott NL, Gleich GJ, Peterson EA, et al. Assessment of eosinophil and neutrophil participation in atopic dermatitis: Comparison with the IgE-mediated late-phase reaction. J Allergy Clin Immunol 1994; 94:120–128.

39. Perez GL, Peters MS, Reda AM, et al. Mast cells, neutrophils, and eosinophils in prurigo nodularis. Arch Dermatol 1993; 129:861–865.

40. Davis MD, Plager DA, George TJ, et al. Interactions of eosinophil granule proteins with skin: Limits of detection, persistence, and vasopermeabilization. J Allergy Clin Immunol 2003; 112:988–994.

41. Cheng JF, Ott NL, Peterson EA, et al. Dermal eosinophils in atopic dermatitis undergo cytolytic degeneration. J Allergy Clin Immunol 1997; 99:683–692.

42. Malm-Erjefalt M, Greiff L, Ankerst J, et al. Circulating eosinophils in asthma, allergic rhinitis, and atopic dermatitis lack morphological signs of degranulation. Clin Exp Allergy 2005; 35:1334–1340.

43. Hanifin JM, Rajka G. Diagnostic features of atopic dermatitis. Acta Derm Venereol (Stockh) 1980; 92 (suppl.):44–47.

44. Williams HC. What is atopic dermatitis and how should it be defined in epidemiological studies? In: Williams HC, ed. Atopic Dermatitis: The Epidemiology, Causes and Prevention of Atopic Eczema. Cambridge, UK: Cambridge University Press, 2000:3–24.

45. Archer CB. The pathophysiology and clinical features of atopic dermatitis. In: Williams HC, ed. Atopic Dermatitis: The Epidemiology, Causes and Prevention of Atopic Eczema. Cambridge, UK: Cambridge University Press, 2000:25–40.

46. Stone SP, Muller SA, Gleich GJ. IgE levels in atopic dermatitis. Arch Dermatol 1973; 108:806–811.

47. Dhar S, Malakar R, Chattopadhyay S, et al. Correlation of the severity of atopic dermatitis with absolute eosinophil counts in peripheral blood and serum IgE levels. Indian J Dermatol Venereol Leprol 2005; 71:246–249.

48. Sampson HA. The immunopathogenic role of food hypersensitivity in atopic dermatitis. Acta Derm Venereol Suppl (Stockh) 1992; 176:34–37.

49. Tuft L, Heck VM. Studies in atopic dermatitis. IV. Importance of seasonal inhalant allergens, especially ragweed. J Allergy 1952; 23:528–540.

50. Tuft L, Tuft HS, Heck VM. Atopic dermatitis: An experimental clinical study of the role of inhalant allergens. J Allergy 1950; 21:181–186.

51. Walker IC. Causation of eczema, urticaria, and angioneurotic edema by proteins other than those derived from foods. J Am Med Assoc 1918; 70:897–900.

52. Mitchell EB, Crow J, Chapman MD, et al. Basophils in allergen-induced patch test sites in atopic dermatitis. Lancet 1982; 1:127–130.

53. Clark RA, Adinoff AD. The relationship between positive aeroallergen patch test reactions and aeroallergen exacerbations of atopic dermatitis. Clin Immunol Immunopathol 1989; 53:S132–S140.
54. Langeveld-Wildschut EG, Bruijnzeel PL, Mudde GC, et al. Clinical and immunologic variables in skin of patients with atopic eczema and either positive or negative atopy patch test reactions. J Allergy Clin Immunol 2000; 105:1008–1016.
55. Platts-Mills TAE, Chapman MD, Mitchell B, et al. Role of inhalant allergens in atopic eczema. In: Ruzicka T, Ring J, Przybilla B, ed. Handbook of Allergens in Atopic Eczema. Heidelberg, Germany, Switzerland: Springer-Verlag, 1991:192–203.
56. Sanda T, Yasue T, Oohashi M, et al. Effectiveness of house dust-mite allergen avoidance through clean room therapy in patients with atopic dermatitis. J Allergy Clin Immunol 1992; 89:653–657.
57. Leung DY. Pathogenesis of atopic dermatitis. J Allergy Clin Immunol 1999; 104:S99–S108.
58. Leung DY, Harbeck R, Bina P, et al. Presence of IgE antibodies to staphylococcal exotoxins on the skin of patients with atopic dermatitis. Evidence for a new group of allergens. J Clin Invest 1993; 92:1374–1380.
59. Laouini D, Kawamoto S, Yalcindag A, et al. Epicutaneous sensitization with superantigen induces allergic skin inflammation. J Allergy Clin Immunol 2003; 112:981–987.
60. Hofer MF, Harbeck RJ, Schlievert PM, et al. Staphylococcal toxins augment specific IgE responses by atopic patients exposed to allergen. J Invest Dermatol 1999; 112:171–176.
61. Altrichter S, Kriehuber E, Moser J, et al. Serum IgE autoantibodies target keratinocytes in patients with atopic dermatitis. J Invest Dermatol 2008; 128:2232–2239.
62. Mihm MC Jr, Soter NA, Dvorak HF, et al. The structure of normal skin and the morphology of atopic eczema. J Invest Dermatol 1976; 67:305–312.
63. Leung DYM. Immunopathology of atopic dermatitis. Springer Semin Immunopathol 1992; 13:427–440.
64. Lever R, Turbitt M, Sanderson A, et al. Immunophenotyping of the cutaneous infiltrate and of the mononuclear cells in the peripheral blood in patients with atopic dermatitis. J Invest Dermatol 1987; 89:4–7.
65. Vercelli D, Jabara HH, Lee BW, et al. Human recombinant interleukin 4 induces Fc epsilon R2/CD23 on normal human monocytes. J Exp Med 1988; 167:1406–1416.
66. Wang B, Rieger A, Kilgus O, et al. Epidermal Langerhans cells from normal human skin bind monomeric IgE via Fc epsilon RI. J Exp Med 1992; 175:1353–1365.
67. Bruijnzeel-Koomen CA, Mudde GC, Bruijnzeel PL. The presence of IgE molecules on epidermal Langerhans cells in atopic dermatitis and their significance for its pathogenesis. Allerg Immunol (Paris) 1989; 21:219–223.
68. Barker JN, Alegre VA, MacDonald DM. Surface-bound immunoglobulin E on antigen-presenting cells in cutaneous tissue of atopic dermatitis. J Invest Dermatol 1988; 90:117–121.
69. Saini SS, Klion AD, Holland SM, et al. The relationship between serum IgE and surface levels of FcepsilonR on human leukocytes in various diseases: Correlation of expression with FcepsilonRI on basophils but not on monocytes or eosinophils. J Allergy Clin Immunol 2000; 106:514–520.
70. Gounni AS, Lamkhioued B, Delaporte E, et al. The high-affinity IgE receptor on eosinophils: From allergy to parasites or from parasites to allergy? J Allergy Clin Immunol 1994; 94:1214–1216.
71. Kita H, Kaneko M, Bartemes KR, et al. Does IgE bind to and activate eosinophils from patients with allergy? J Immunol 1999; 162:6901–6911.
72. Seminario MC, Saini SS, MacGlashan DW Jr, et al. Intracellular expression and release of Fc epsilon RI alpha by human eosinophils. J Immunol 1999; 162:6893–6900.
73. Kita H, Gleich GJ. Eosinophils and IgE receptors: A continuing controversy. Blood 1997; 89:3497–3501.
74. Sur S, Adolphson CR, Gleich GJ. Eosinophils: Biochemical and cellular aspects. In: Middleton EJ, Reed CE, Ellis EF, Adkinson NF, Yunginger JW, Busse WW, eds. Allergy: Principles and Practice, 4th ed. St. Louis, MO: Mosby, 1993.

75. Quinti I, Brozek C, Wood N, et al. Circulating IgG autoantibodies to IgE in atopic syndromes. J Allergy Clin Immunol 1986; 77:586–594.
76. Mudde GC, Van Reijsen FC, Boland GJ, et al. Allergen presentation by epidermal Langerhans' cells from patients with atopic dermatitis is mediated by IgE. Immunology 1990; 69:335–341.
77. Bieber T. The pro- and anti-inflammatory properties of human antigen-presenting cells expressing the high affinity receptor for IgE (Fc epsilon RI). Immunobiology 2007; 212:499–503.
78. Fuller RW, Morris PK, Richmond R, et al. Immunoglobulin E-dependent stimulation of human alveolar macrophages: Significance in type 1 hypersensitivity. Clin Exp Immunol 1986; 65:416–426.
79. Rouzer CA, Scott WA, Hamill AL, et al. Secretion of leukotriene C and other arachidonic acid metabolites by macrophages challenged with immunoglobulin E immune complexes. J Exp Med 1982; 156:1077–1086.
80. Bradding P, Roberts JA, Britten KM, et al. Interleukin-4, -5, and -6 and tumor necrosis factor-alpha in normal and asthmatic airways: Evidence for the human mast cell as a source of these cytokines. Am J Respir Cell Mol Biol 1994; 10:471–480.
81. Bradding P, Walls AF, Holgate ST. The role of the mast cell in the pathophysiology of asthma. J Allergy Clin Immunol 2006; 117:1277–1284.
82. Abu-Ghazaleh RI, Gleich GJ, Prendergast FG. Interaction of eosinophil granule major basic protein with synthetic lipid bilayers: A mechanism for toxicity. J Membr Biol 1992; 128:153–164.
83. Kita H, Weiler DA, Abu-Ghazaleh R, et al. Release of granule proteins from eosinophils cultured with IL-5. J Immunol 1992; 149:629–635.
84. Rothenberg ME, Petersen J, Stevens RL, et al. IL-5-dependent conversion of normodense human eosinophils to the hypodense phenotype uses 3T3 fibroblasts for enhanced viability, accelerated hypodensity, and sustained antibody-dependent cytotoxicity. J Immunol 1989; 143:2311–2316.
85. Silberstein DS, Austen KF, Owen WF Jr. Hemopoietins for eosinophils. Glycoprotein hormones that regulate the development of inflammation in eosinophilia-associated disease. Hematol Oncol Clin North Am 1989; 3:511–533.
86. Yamaguchi Y, Hayashi Y, Sugama Y, et al. Highly purified murine interleukin 5 (IL-5) stimulates eosinophil function and prolongs in vitro survival. IL-5 as an eosinophil chemotactic factor. J Exp Med 1988; 167:1737–1742.
87. Collins PD, Marleau S, Griffiths-Johnson DA, et al. Cooperation between interleukin-5 and the chemokine eotaxin to induce eosinophil accumulation in vivo. J Exp Med 1995; 182:1169–1174.
88. Dubois GR, Bruijnzeel-Koomen CA, Bruijnzeel PL. IL-4 induces chemotaxis of blood eosinophils from atopic dermatitis patients, but not from normal individuals. J Invest Dermatol 1994; 102:843–846.
89. Dubois GR, Schweizer RC, Versluis C, et al. Human eosinophils constitutively express a functional interleukin-4 receptor: Interleukin-4-induced priming of chemotactic responses and induction of PI-3 kinase activity. Am J Respir Cell Mol Biol 1998; 19:691–699.
90. Borres MP, Bjorksten B. Peripheral blood eosinophils and IL-4 in infancy in relation to the appearance of allergic disease during the first 6 years of life. Pediatr Allergy Immunol 2004; 15:216–220.
91. Borish L RL. Cytokines in Allergic Inflammation. In: Middleton E Jr, Reed CE, Ellis EF, Adkinson NF, Yunginger JW, Busse WW, eds. Allergy: Principles and Practice, 5th ed. vol 1. St Louis, MO: Mosby, 1998:108–119.
92. Fawaz LM, Sharif-Askari E, Hajoui O, et al. Expression of IL-9 receptor alpha chain on human germinal center B cells modulates IgE secretion. J Allergy Clin Immunol 2007; 120:1208–1215.
93. Gounni AS, Gregory B, Nutku E, et al. Interleukin-9 enhances interleukin-5 receptor expression, differentiation, and survival of human eosinophils. Blood 2000; 96:2163–2171.

94. Ying S, Meng Q, Kay AB, et al. Elevated expression of interleukin-9 mRNA in the bronchial mucosa of atopic asthmatics and allergen-induced cutaneous late-phase reaction: Relationships to eosinophils, mast cells and T lymphocytes. Clin Exp Allergy 2002; 32:866–871.
95. Laouini D, Alenius H, Bryce P, et al. IL-10 is critical for Th2 responses in a murine model of allergic dermatitis. J Clin Invest 2003; 112:1058–1066.
96. McKenzie AN, Culpepper JA, de Waal Malefyt R, et al. Interleukin 13, a T-cell-derived cytokine that regulates human monocyte and B-cell function. Proc Natl Acad Sci U S A 1993; 90:3735–3739.
97. Minty A, Chalon P, Derocq JM, et al. Interleukin-13 is a new human lymphokine regulating inflammatory and immune responses. Nature 1993; 362:248–250.
98. Bochner BS, Klunk DA, Sterbinsky SA, et al. IL-13 selectively induces vascular cell adhesion molecule-1 expression in human endothelial cells. J Immunol 1995; 154:799–803.
99. Moseley TA, Haudenschild DR, Rose L, et al. Interleukin-17 family and IL-17 receptors. Cytokine Growth Factor Rev 2003; 14:155–174.
100. Cheung PF, Wong CK, Lam CW. Molecular mechanisms of cytokine and chemokine release from eosinophils activated by IL-17 A, IL-17 F, and IL-23: Implication for Th17 lymphocytes-mediated allergic inflammation. J Immunol 2008; 180:5625–5635.
101. van Beelen AJ, Teunissen MB, Kapsenberg ML, et al. Interleukin-17 in inflammatory skin disorders. Curr Opin Allergy Clin Immunol 2007; 7:374–381.
102. Koga C, Kabashima K, Shiraishi N, et al. Possible Pathogenic Role of Th17 Cells for Atopic Dermatitis. J Invest Dermatol 2008; 128:2625–2630.
103. Atsuta J, Fujisawa T, Iguchi K, et al. Inhibitory effect of transforming growth factor beta 1 on cytokine-enhanced eosinophil survival and degranulation. Int Arch Allergy Immunol 1995; 108(suppl. 1):31–35.
104. Kita H, Ohnishi T, Okubo Y, et al. Granulocyte/macrophage colony-stimulating factor and interleukin 3 release from human peripheral blood eosinophils and neutrophils. J Exp Med 1991; 174:745–748.
105. Raap U, Goltz C, Deneka N, et al. Brain-derived neurotrophic factor is increased in atopic dermatitis and modulates eosinophil functions compared with that seen in nonatopic subjects. J Allergy Clin Immunol 2005; 115:1268–1275.
106. Ogawa K, Itoh M, Miyagawa M, et al. Expression of a human SOCS protein, HSOCP-1, in peripheral blood eosinophils from patients with atopic dermatitis. Int Arch Allergy Immunol 2004; 134(suppl. 1):2–6.
107. Kagi MK, Wuthrich B, Montano E, et al. Differential cytokine profiles in peripheral blood lymphocyte supernatants and skin biopsies from patients with different forms of atopic dermatitis, psoriasis and normal individuals. Int Arch Allergy Immunol 1994; 103:332–340.
108. Akdis CA, Akdis M, Simon D, et al. T cells and T cell-derived cytokines as pathogenic factors in the nonallergic form of atopic dermatitis. J Invest Dermatol 1999; 113:628–634.
109. Hamid Q, Boguniewicz M, Leung DY. Differential in situ cytokine gene expression in acute versus chronic atopic dermatitis. J Clin Invest 1994; 94:870–876.
110. Namkung JH, Lee JE, Kim E, et al. IL-5 and IL-5 receptor alpha polymorphisms are associated with atopic dermatitis in Koreans. Allergy 2007; 62:934–942.
111. Yamamoto N, Sugiura H, Tanaka K, et al. Heterogeneity of interleukin 5 genetic background in atopic dermatitis patients: Significant difference between those with blood eosinophilia and normal eosinophil levels. J Dermatol Sci 2003; 33:121–126.
112. Kaplan AP, Kuna P, Reddigari SR. Chemokines and the allergic response. Exp Dermatol 1995; 4:260–265.
113. Baggiolini M, Dahinden CA. CC chemokines in allergic inflammation. Immunol Today 1994; 15:127–133.
114. Schroder JM. Cytokine networks in the skin. J Invest Dermatol 1995; 105:20S–24S.
115. Schroder JM, Noso N, Sticherling M, et al. Role of eosinophil-chemotactic C-C chemokines in cutaneous inflammation. J Leukoc Biol 1996; 59:1–5.

116. Jose PJ, Griffiths-Johnson DA, Collins PD, et al. Eotaxin: A potent eosinophil chemoattractant cytokine detected in a guinea pig model of allergic airways inflammation. J Exp Med 1994; 179:881–887.
117. Ganzalo JA, Jia GQ, Aguirre V, et al. Mouse eotaxin expression parallels eosinophil accumulation during lung allergic inflammation but it is not restricted to a Th2-type response. Immunity 1996; 4:1–14.
118. Ponath PD, Qin S, Ringler DJ, et al. Cloning of the human eosinophil chemoattractant, eotaxin. Expression, receptor binding, and functional properties suggest a mechanism for the selective recruitment of eosinophils. J Clin Invest 1996; 97:604–612.
119. Hein H, Schluter C, Kulke R, et al. Genomic organization, sequence, and transcriptional regulation of the human eotaxin gene. Biochem Biophys Res Commun 1997; 237:537–542.
120. Kameyoshi Y, Dorschner A, Mallet AI, et al. Cytokine RANTES released by thrombin-stimulated platelets is a potent attractant for human eosinophils. J Exp Med 1992; 176:587–592.
121. Ying S, Meng Q, Zeibecoglou K, et al. Eosinophil chemotactic chemokines (eotaxin, eotaxin-2, RANTES, monocyte chemoattractant protein-3 (MCP-3), and MCP-4), and C-C chemokine receptor 3 expression in bronchial biopsies from atopic and nonatopic (intrinsic) asthmatics. J Immunol 1999; 163:6321–6329.
122. Ying S, Robinson DS, Meng Q, et al. C-C chemokines in allergen-induced late-phase cutaneous responses in atopic subjects: Association of eotaxin with early 6-hour eosinophils, and of eotaxin-2 and monocyte chemoattractant protein-4 with the later 24-hour tissue eosinophilia, and relationship to basophils and other C-C chemokines (monocyte chemoattractant protein-3 and RANTES). J Immunol 1999; 163:3976–3984.
123. Ying S, Meng Q, Barata LT, et al. Macrophage inflammatory protein-1alpha and C-C chemokine receptor-1 in allergen-induced skin late-phase reactions: relationship to macrophages, neutrophils, basophils, eosinophils and T lymphocytes. Clin Exp Allergy 2001; 31:1724–1731.
124. Menzies-Gow A, Ying S, Phipps S, et al. Interactions between eotaxin, histamine and mast cells in early microvascular events associated with eosinophil recruitment to the site of allergic skin reactions in humans. Clin Exp Allergy 2004; 34:1276–1282.
125. Rho NK, Kim WS, Lee DY, et al. Immunophenotyping of inflammatory cells in lesional skin of the extrinsic and intrinsic types of atopic dermatitis. Br J Dermatol 2004; 151:119–125.
126. Rigoli L, Caminiti L, Di Bella C, et al. Investigation of the eotaxin gene -426 C−> T, -384 A−> G and 67G−> a single-nucleotide polymorphisms and atopic dermatitis in Italian children using family-based association methods. Clin Exp Dermatol 2008; 33:316–321.
127. Ebisawa M, Bochner BS, Georas SN, et al. Eosinophil transendothelial migration induced by cytokines. I. Role of endothelial and eosinophil adhesion molecules in IL-1 beta-induced transendothelial migration. J Immunol 1992; 149:4021–4028.
128. Kapp A, Zeck-Kapp G, Czech W, et al. The chemokine RANTES is more than a chemoattractant: Characterization of its effect on human eosinophil oxidative metabolism and morphology in comparison with IL-5 and GM-CSF. J Invest Dermatol 1994; 102:906–914.
129. Elsner J, Hochstetter R, Kimmig D, et al. Human eotaxin represents a potent activator of the respiratory burst of human eosinophils. Eur J Immunol 1996; 26:1919–1925.
130. Bartels J, Schluter C, Richter E, et al. Human dermal fibroblasts express eotaxin: Molecular cloning, mRNA expression, and identification of eotaxin sequence variants. Biochem Biophys Res Commun 1996; 225:1045–1051.
131. Li J, Ireland GW, Farthing PM, et al. Epidermal and oral keratinocytes are induced to produce RANTES and IL-8 by cytokine stimulation. J Invest Dermatol 1996; 106:661–666.
132. Yamada H, Matsukura M, Yudate T, et al. Enhanced production of RANTES, an eosinophil chemoattractant factor, by cytokine-stimulated epidermal keratinocytes. Int Arch Allergy Immunol 1997; 114(suppl. 1):28–32.

133. Kaburagi Y, Shimada Y, Nagaoka T, et al. Enhanced production of CC-chemokines (RANTES, MCP-1, MIP-1alpha, MIP-1beta, and eotaxin) in patients with atopic dermatitis. Arch Dermatol Res 2001; 293:350–355.
134. Yawalkar N, Uguccioni M, Scharer J, et al. Enhanced expression of eotaxin and CCR3 in atopic dermatitis. J Invest Dermatol 1999; 113:43–48.
135. Mochizuki M, Bartels J, Mallet AI, et al. IL-4 induces eotaxin: A possible mechanism of selective eosinophil recruitment in helminth infection and atopy. J Immunol 1998; 160:60–68.
136. Mochizuki M, Schroder J, Christophers E, et al. IL-4 induces eotaxin in human dermal fibroblasts. Int Arch Allergy Immunol 1999; 120(suppl. 1):19–23.
137. Chihara J, Oyamada H, Yamada H, et al. Expression of mRNA for RANTES in human eosinophils. Int Arch Allergy Immunol 1997; 114(suppl. 1):33–35.
138. Wakugawa M, Nakamura K, Akatsuka M, et al. Expression of CC chemokine receptor 3 on human keratinocytes in vivo and in vitro—Upregulation by RANTES. J Dermatol Sci 2001; 25:229–235.
139. Beck LA, Dalke S, Leiferman KM, et al. Cutaneous injection of RANTES causes eosinophil recruitment: Comparison of nonallergic and allergic human subjects. J Immunol 1997; 159:2962–2972.
140. Kato Y, Pawankar R, Kimura Y, et al. Increased expression of RANTES, CCR3 and CCR5 in the lesional skin of patients with atopic eczema. Int Arch Allergy Immunol 2006; 139:245–257.
141. Matsui K, Wirotesangthong M, Nishikawa A. Percutaneous application of peptidoglycan from *Staphylococcus aureus* induces eosinophil infiltration in mouse skin. Clin Exp Allergy 2007; 37:615–622.
142. Gleich GJ. Mechanisms of eosinophil-associated inflammation. J Allergy Clin Immunol 2000; 105:651–663.
143. Kaatz M, Berod L, Czech W, et al. Interleukin-5, interleukin-3 and granulocyte-macrophage colony-stimulating factor prime actin-polymerization in human eosinophils: A study with hypodense and normodense eosinophils from patients with atopic dermatitis. Int J Mol Med 2004; 14:1055–1060.
144. Springer TA. Adhesion receptors of the immune system. Nature 1990; 346:425–434.
145. Bochner BS, Schleimer RP. The role of adhesion molecules in human eosinophil and basophil recruitment. J Allergy Clin Immunol 1994; 94:427–38 [quiz 39].
146. Hakugawa J, Bae SJ, Tanaka Y, et al. The inhibitory effect of anti-adhesion molecule antibodies on eosinophil infiltration in cutaneous late phase response in Balb/c mice sensitized with ovalbumin (OVA). J Dermatol 1997; 24:73–79.
147. Teti A. Regulation of cellular functions by extracellular matrix. J Am Soc Nephrol 1992; 2:S83–S87.
148. Schleimer RP, Ebisawa M, Georas SN, et al. The role of adhesion molecules and cytokines in eosinophil recruitment. In: Gleich GJ, Kay AB, eds. Eosinophils in Allergy and Inflammation. New York, NY: Marcel Dekker, Inc., 1994:99–112.
149. Wakita H, Sakamoto T, Tokura Y, et al. E-selectin and vascular cell adhesion molecule-1 as critical adhesion molecules for infiltration of T lymphocytes and eosinophils in atopic dermatitis. J Cutan Pathol 1994; 21:33–39.
150. Horie S, Kita H. CD11b/CD18 (Mac-1) is required for degranulation of human eosinophils induced by human recombinant granulocyte-macrophage colony-stimulating factor and platelet-activating factor. J Immunol 1994; 152:5457–5467.
151. Walker C, Rihs S, Braun RK, et al. Increased expression of CD11b and functional changes in eosinophils after migration across endothelial cell monolayers. J Immunol 1993; 150:4061–4071.
152. Morita E, Schroder JM, Christophers E. Chemotactic responsiveness of eosinophils isolated from patients with inflammatory skin diseases. J Dermatol 1989; 16:348–351.
153. Bruijnzeel PL, Kuijper PH, Rihs S, et al. Eosinophil migration in atopic dermatitis. I: Increased migratory responses to *N*-formyl-methionyl-leucyl-phenylalanine, neutrophil-activating factor, platelet-activating factor, and platelet factor 4. J Invest Dermatol 1993; 100:137–142.

154. Wassom DL, Loegering DA, Solley GO, et al. Elevated serum levels of the eosinophil granule major basic protein in patients with eosinophilia. J Clin Invest 1981; 67:651–661.

155. Miyasato M, Iryo K, Kasada M, et al. Varied density of eosinophils in patients with atopic dermatitis reflecting treatment with anti-allergic drug (abstr). J Invest Dermatol 1988; 90:589.

156. Goto T, Morioka J, Inamura H, et al. Urinary eosinophil-derived neurotoxin concentrations in patients with atopic dermatitis: A useful clinical marker for disease activity. Allergol Int 2007; 56:433–438.

157. Takano Y, Fukagawa K, Dogru M, et al. Inflammatory cells in brush cytology samples correlate with the severity of corneal lesions in atopic keratoconjunctivitis. Br J Ophthalmol 2004; 88:1504–1505.

158. Sur S, Glitz DG, Kita H, et al. Localization of eosinophil-derived neurotoxin and eosinophil cationic protein in neutrophilic leukocytes. J Leukoc Biol 1998; 63:715–722.

159. Simon D, Braathen LR, Simon HU. Eosinophils and atopic dermatitis. Allergy 2004; 59:561–570.

160. Kapp A. The role of eosinophils in the pathogenesis of atopic dermatitis—eosinophil granule proteins as markers of disease activity. Allergy 1993; 48:1–5.

161. Kagi MK, Joller-Jemelka H, Wuthrich B. Correlation of eosinophils, eosinophil cationic protein and soluble interleukin-2 receptor with the clinical activity of atopic dermatitis. Dermatology 1992; 185:88–92.

162. Mukai H, Noguchi T, Kamimura K, et al. Significance of elevated serum LDH (lactate dehydrogenase) activity in atopic dermatitis. J Dermatol 1990; 17:477–481.

163. Suagai T, Shoji A, Nagareda T. Changes of ECP values, number of eosinophils and EG2 eosinophils in the peripheral blood following oral ketotifen in patients with atopic dermatitis. Skin Res 1992; 34:368–386.

164. Uehara M, Izukura R, Sawai T. Blood eosinophilia in atopic dermatitis. Clin Exp Dermatol 1990; 15:264–266.

165. Businco L, Meglio P, Ferrara M. The role of food allergy and eosinophils in atopic dermatitis. Pediatr Allergy Immunol 1993; 4:33–37.

166. Stevens SR, Hanifin JM, Hamilton T, et al. Long-term effectiveness and safety of recombinant human interferon gamma therapy for atopic dermatitis despite unchanged serum IgE levels. Arch Dermatol 1998; 134:799–804.

167. Schneider LC, Baz Z, Zarcone C, et al. Long-term therapy with recombinant interferon-gamma (rIFN-gamma) for atopic dermatitis. Ann Allergy Asthma Immunol 1998; 80:263–268.

168. Jenerowicz D, Czarnecka-Operacz M, Silny W. Peripheral blood eosinophilia in atopic dermatitis. Acta Dermatovenerol Alp Panonica Adriat 2007; 16:47–52.

169. Miyasato M, Tsuda S, Nakama T, et al. Serum levels of eosinophil cationic protein reflect the state of in vitro degranulation of blood hypodense eosinophils in atopic dermatitis. J Dermatol 1996; 23:382–388.

170. Matsumoto K, Shimanouchi Y, Kawakubo K, et al. Infantile eczema at one month of age is associated with cord blood eosinophilia and subsequent development of atopic dermatitis and wheezing illness until two years of age. Int Arch Allergy Immunol 2005; 137(suppl. 1):69–76.

171. Thurau AM, Schylz U, Wolf V, et al. Identification of eosinophils by flow cytometry. Cytometry 1996; 23:150–158.

172. Toma T, Mizuno K, Okamoto H, et al. Expansion of activated eosinophils in infants with severe atopic dermatitis. Pediatr Int 2005; 47:32–38.

173. Jenerowicz D, Czarnecka-Operacz M, Silny W. Selected eosinophil proteins as markers of inflammation in atopic dermatitis patients. Acta Dermatovenerol Croat 2006; 14:73–80.

174. Paganelli R, Fanales-Belasio E, Carmini D, et al. Serum eosinophil cationic protein in patients with atopic dermatitis. Int Arch Allergy Appl Immunol 1991; 96:175–178.

175. Kapp A, Czech W, Krutmann J, et al. Eosinophil cationic protein in sera of patients with atopic dermatitis. J Am Acad Dermatol 1991; 24:555–558.

176. Czech W, Krutmann J, Schopf E, et al. Serum eosinophil cationic protein (ECP) is a sensitive measure for disease activity in atopic dermatitis. Br J Dermatol 1992; 126:351–355.
177. Juhlin L, Venge P. Eosinophilic cationic protein (ECP) in skin disorders. Acta Derm Venereol 1991; 71:495–501.
178. Krutmann J, Diepgen TL, Luger TA, et al. High-dose UVA1 therapy for atopic dermatitis: Results of a multicenter trial. J Am Acad Dermatol 1998; 38:589–593.
179. Sugai T, Sakiyama Y, Matumoto S. Eosinophil cationic protein in peripheral blood of pediatric patients with allergic diseases. Clin Exp Allergy 1992; 22:275–281.
180. Tsuda S, Kato K, Miyasato M, et al. Eosinophil involvement in atopic dermatitis as reflected by elevated serum levels of eosinophil cationic protein. J Dermatol 1992; 19:208–213.
181. Jakob T, Hermann K, Ring J. Eosinophil cationic protein in atopic eczema. Arch Dermatol Res 1991; 283:5–6.
182. Caproni M, D'Agata A, Cappelli G, et al. Modulation of serum eosinophil cationic protein levels by cyclosporin in severe atopic dermatitis. Br J Dermatol 1996; 135:336–337.
183. Halmerbauer G, Frischer T, Koller DY. Monitoring of disease activity by measurement of inflammatory markers in atopic dermatitis in childhood. Allergy 1997; 52:765–769.
184. Park JH, Choi YL, Namkung JH, et al. Characteristics of extrinsic vs. intrinsic atopic dermatitis in infancy: Correlations with laboratory variables. Br J Dermatol 2006; 155:778–783.
185. Taniuchi S, Chihara J, Kojima T, et al. Serum eosinophil derived neurotoxin may reflect more strongly disease severity in childhood atopic dermatitis than eosinophil cationic protein. J Dermatol Sci 2001; 26:79–82.
186. Osterlund P, Smedberg T, Hakulinen A, et al. Eosinophil cationic protein in human milk is associated with development of cow's milk allergy and atopic eczema in breast-fed infants. Pediatr Res 2004; 55:296–301.
187. Melo RC, Spencer LA, Dvorak AM, et al. Mechanisms of eosinophil secretion: Large vesiculotubular carriers mediate transport and release of granule-derived cytokines and other proteins. J Leukoc Biol 2008; 83:229–236.
188. Melo RC, Spencer LA, Perez SA, et al. Human eosinophils secrete preformed, granule-stored interleukin-4 through distinct vesicular compartments. Traffic 2005; 6:1047–1057.
189. Wedi B, Raap U, Lewrick H, et al. Delayed eosinophil programmed cell death in vitro: A common feature of inhalant allergy and extrinsic and intrinsic atopic dermatitis. J Allergy Clin Immunol 1997; 100:536–543.
190. Matsukura M, Yamada H, Yudate T, et al. Corticosteroid-induced apoptosis of eosinophils in atopic dermatitis patients. J Clin Lab Immunol 1996; 48:109–122.
191. Kagaya S, Hashida R, Ohkura N, et al. NR4 A orphan nuclear receptor family in peripheral blood eosinophils from patients with atopic dermatitis and apoptotic eosinophils in vitro. Int Arch Allergy Immunol 2005; 137(suppl. 1):35–44.
192. Yoon SW, Kim TY, Sung MH, et al. Comparative proteomic analysis of peripheral blood eosinophils from healthy donors and atopic dermatitis patients with eosinophilia. Proteomics 2005; 5:1987–1995.
193. Zweiman B, Atkins PC, von Allmen C, et al. Release of eosinophil granule proteins during IgE-mediated allergic skin reactions. J Allergy Clin Immunol 1991; 87:984–992.
194. Nish WA, Charlesworth EN, Davis TL, et al. The effect of immunotherapy on the cutaneous late phase response to antigen. J Allergy Clin Immunol 1994; 93:484–493.
195. Charlesworth EN, Nish WA, Charlesworth MG, et al. Standard high dose immunotherapy decreases the production of IL-3, IL-5 and GM-CSF during the cutaneous late phase response (LPR) to antigen (abstr). J Allergy Clin Immunol 1993; 91:252.
196. Kay AB, Ying S, Varney V, et al. Messenger RNA expression of the cytokine gene cluster, interleukin 3 (IL-3), IL-4, IL-5, and granulocyte/macrophage colony-stimulating factor, in allergen-induced late-phase cutaneous reactions in atopic subjects. J Exp Med 1991; 173:775–778.
197. Bascom R, Pipkorn U, Proud D, et al. Major basic protein and eosinophil-derived neurotoxin concentrations in nasal-lavage fluid after antigen challenge: Effect of systemic corticosteroids and relationship to eosinophil influx. J Allergy Clin Immunol 1989; 84:338–346.

198. Sim TC, Grant JA, Hilsmeier KA, et al. Proinflammatory cytokines in nasal secretions of allergic subjects after antigen challenge. Am J Respir Crit Care Med 1994; 149:339–344.
199. Nouri-Aria KT, O'Brien F, Noble W, et al. Cytokine expression during allergen-induced late nasal responses: IL-4 and IL-5 mRNA is expressed early (at 6 h) predominantly by eosinophils. Clin Exp Allergy 2000; 30:1709–1716.
200. Sedgwick JB, Calhoun WJ, Gleich GJ, et al. Immediate and late airway response of allergic rhinitis patients to segmental antigen challenge. Characterization of eosinophil and mast cell mediators. Am Rev Respir Dis 1991; 144:1274–1281.
201. Ohnishi T, Kita H, Weiler D, et al. IL-5 is the predominant eosinophil-active cytokine in the antigen-induced pulmonary late-phase reaction. Am Rev Respir Dis 1993; 147:901–907.
202. Gleich GJ. The late phase of the immunoglobulin E-mediated reaction: A link between anaphylaxis and common allergic disease? J Allergy Clin Immunol 1982; 70:160–169.
203. Sampson HA. Late-phase response to food in atopic dermatitis. Hosp Pract (Off Ed) 1987; 22:111–118, 21–22, 27–28.
204. Charlesworth EN, Hood AF, Soter NA, et al. Cutaneous late-phase response to allergen. Mediator release and inflammatory cell infiltration. J Clin Invest 1989; 83:1519–1526.
205. Dolovich J, Hargreave FE, Chalmers R, et al. Late cutaneous allergic responses in isolated IgE-dependent reactions. J Allergy Clin Immunol 1973; 52:38–46.
206. Solley GO, Gleich GJ, Jordon RE, et al. The late phase of the immediate wheal and flare skin reaction. Its dependence upon IgE antibodies. J Clin Invest 1976; 58:408–420.
207. Kojima T, Ono A, Aoki T, et al. Circulating ICAM-1 levels in children with atopic dermatitis. Ann Allergy 1994; 73:351–355.
208. Wolkerstorfer A, Laan MP, Savelkoul HF, et al. Soluble E-selectin, other markers of inflammation and disease severity in children with atopic dermatitis. Br J Dermatol 1998; 138:431–435.
209. Dulkys Y, Schramm G, Kimmig D, et al. Detection of mRNA for eotaxin-2 and eotaxin-3 in human dermal fibroblasts and their distinct activation profile on human eosinophils. J Invest Dermatol 2001; 116:498–505.
210. Igawa K, Satoh T, Hirashima M, et al. Regulatory mechanisms of galectin-9 and eotaxin-3 synthesis in epidermal keratinocytes: Possible involvement of galectin-9 in dermal eosinophilia of Th1-polarized skin inflammation. Allergy 2006; 61:1385–1391.
211. Chan LS, Robinson N, Xu L. Expression of interleukin-4 in the epidermis of transgenic mice results in a pruritic inflammatory skin disease: An experimental animal model to study atopic dermatitis. J Invest Dermatol 2001; 117:977–983.
212. Spergel JM, Mizoguchi E, Oettgen H, et al. Roles of TH1 and TH2 cytokines in a murine model of allergic dermatitis. J Clin Invest 1999; 103:1103–1111.
213. Kagami S, Kakinuma T, Saeki H, et al. Significant elevation of serum levels of eotaxin-3/CCL26, but not of eotaxin-2/CCL24, in patients with atopic dermatitis: Serum eotaxin-3/CCL26 levels reflect the disease activity of atopic dermatitis. Clin Exp Immunol 2003; 134:309–313.
214. Bruijnzeel PL, Kuijper PH, Kapp A, et al. The involvement of eosinophils in the patch test reaction to aeroallergens in atopic dermatitis: Its relevance for the pathogenesis of atopic dermatitis. Clin Exp Allergy 1993; 23:97–109.
215. Maeda K, Yamamoto K, Tanaka Y, et al. The relationship between eosinophils, OKT6-positive cells and house dust mite (HDM) antigens in naturally occurring lesions of atopic dermatitis. J Dermatol Sci 1992; 3:151–156.
216. Wakugawa M, Nakagawa H, Yamada N, et al. Chronologic analysis of eosinophil granule protein deposition and cell adhesion molecule expression in mite allergen-induced dermatitis in atopic subjects. Int Arch Allergy Immunol 1996; 111(suppl. 1):5–11.
217. Yamada N, Wakugawa M, Kuwata S, et al. Changes in eosinophil and leukocyte infiltration and expression of IL-6 and IL-7 messenger RNA in mite allergen patch test reactions in atopic dermatitis. J Allergy Clin Immunol 1996; 98:S201–S206.
218. Yamada N, Wakugawa M, Kuwata S, et al. Chronologic analysis of in situ cytokine expression in mite allergen-induced dermatitis in atopic subjects. J Allergy Clin Immunol 1995; 96:1069–1075.

219. Gundel RH, Gerritsen ME, Gleich GJ, et al. Repeated antigen inhalation results in a prolonged airway eosinophilia and airway hyperresponsiveness in primates. J Appl Physiol 1990; 68:779–786.
220. de Bruin-Weller MS, Weller FR, De Monchy JG. Repeated allergen challenge as a new research model for studying allergic reactions. Clin Exp Allergy 1999; 29:159–165.
221. Wang G, Savinko T, Wolff H, et al. Repeated epicutaneous exposures to ovalbumin progressively induce atopic dermatitis-like skin lesions in mice. Clin Exp Allergy 2007; 37:151–161.
222. Grewe M, Czech W, Morita A, et al. Human eosinophils produce biologically active IL-12: Implications for control of T cell responses. J Immunol 1998; 161:415–420.
223. Nutku E, Gounni AS, Olivenstein R, et al. Evidence for expression of eosinophil-associated IL-12 messenger RNA and immunoreactivity in bronchial asthma. J Allergy Clin Immunol 2000; 106:288–292.
224. Ohmen JD, Hanifin JM, Nickoloff BJ, et al. Overexpression of IL-10 in atopic dermatitis. Contrasting cytokine patterns with delayed-type hypersensitivity reactions. J Immunol 1995; 154:1956–1963.
225. Randolph DA, Stephens R, Carruthers CJ, et al. Cooperation between Th1 and Th2 cells in a murine model of eosinophilic airway inflammation. J Clin Invest 1999; 104:1021–1029.
226. Decco ML, Neeno TA, Hunt LW, et al. Nebulized lidocaine in the treatment of severe asthma in children: A pilot study. Ann Allergy Asthma Immunol 1999; 82:29–32.
227. Hunt LW, Frigas E, Butterfield JH, et al. Treatment of asthma with nebulized lidocaine: A randomized, placebo-controlled study. J Allergy Clin Immunol 2004; 113:853–859.
228. Hunt LW, Swedlund HA, Gleich GJ. Effect of nebulized lidocaine on severe glucocorticoid-dependent asthma. Mayo Clin Proc 1996; 71:361–368.
229. Simon D, Vassina E, Yousefi S, et al. Reduced dermal infiltration of cytokine-expressing inflammatory cells in atopic dermatitis after short-term topical tacrolimus treatment. J Allergy Clin Immunol 2004; 114:887–895.
230. Park CW, Lee BH, Han HJ, et al. Tacrolimus decreases the expression of eotaxin, CCR3, RANTES and interleukin-5 in atopic dermatitis. Br J Dermatol 2005; 152:1173–1181.
231. Simon D, Vassina E, Yousefi S, et al. Inflammatory cell numbers and cytokine expression in atopic dermatitis after topical pimecrolimus treatment. Allergy 2005; 60:944–951.
232. Butterfield JH, Gleich GJ. Interferon-alpha treatment of six patients with the idiopathic hypereosinophilic syndrome. Ann Intern Med 1994; 121:648–653.
233. Chang TT, Stevens SR. Atopic dermatitis: The role of recombinant interferon-gamma therapy. Am J Clin Dermatol 2002; 3:175–183.
234. Chantry D, Burgess LE. Chemokines in allergy. Curr Drug Targets Inflamm Allergy 2002; 1:109–116.
235. Nasert S, Millner M, Herz U, et al. Therapeutic interference with interferon-gamma (IFN-gamma) and soluble IL-4 receptor (sIL-4R) in allergic diseases. Behring Inst Mitt 1995:118–130.
236. Ong YE, Menzies-Gow A, Barkans J, et al. Anti-IgE (omalizumab) inhibits late-phase reactions and inflammatory cells after repeat skin allergen challenge. J Allergy Clin Immunol 2005; 116:558–564.
237. D'Amato G. Role of anti-IgE monoclonal antibody (omalizumab) in the treatment of bronchial asthma and allergic respiratory diseases. Eur J Pharmacol 2006; 533:302–307.
238. Djukanovic R, Wilson SJ, Kraft M, et al. Effects of treatment with anti-immunoglobulin E antibody omalizumab on airway inflammation in allergic asthma. Am J Respir Crit Care Med 2004; 170:583–593.
239. Krathen RA, Hsu S. Failure of omalizumab for treatment of severe adult atopic dermatitis. J Am Acad Dermatol 2005; 53:338–340.
240. Lane JE, Cheyney JM, Lane TN, et al. Treatment of recalcitrant atopic dermatitis with omalizumab. J Am Acad Dermatol 2006; 54:68–72.
241. Phipps S, Flood-Page P, Menzies-Gow A, et al. Intravenous anti-IL-5 monoclonal antibody reduces eosinophils and tenascin deposition in allergen-challenged human atopic skin. J Invest Dermatol 2004; 122:1406–1412.

242. Oldhoff JM, Darsow U, Werfel T, et al. No effect of anti-interleukin-5 therapy (mepolizumab) on the atopy patch test in atopic dermatitis patients. Int Arch Allergy Immunol 2006; 141:290–294.
243. Oldhoff JM, Darsow U, Werfel T, et al. Anti-IL-5 recombinant humanized monoclonal antibody (mepolizumab) for the treatment of atopic dermatitis. Allergy 2005; 60:693–696.
244. Rothenberg ME, Klion AD, Roufosse FE, et al. Treatment of patients with the hypereosinophilic syndrome with mepolizumab. N Engl J Med 2008; 358:1215–1228.
245. Plotz SG, Simon HU, Darsow U, et al. Use of an anti-interleukin-5 antibody in the hypereosinophilic syndrome with eosinophilic dermatitis. N Engl J Med 2003; 349:2334–2339.
246. Mepolizumab: 240563, Anti-IL-5 Monoclonal Antibody—GlaxoSmithKline, Anti-Interleukin-5 Monoclonal Antibody—GlaxoSmithKline, SB 240563. Drugs in R & D 2008; 9:125–130.
247. Leckie MJ, ten Brinke A, Khan J, et al. Effects of an interleukin-5 blocking monoclonal antibody on eosinophils, airway hyper-responsiveness, and the late asthmatic response. Lancet 2000; 356:2144–2148.
248. O'Byrne PM, Inman MD, Parameswaran K. The trials and tribulations of IL-5, eosinophils, and allergic asthma. J Allergy Clin Immunol 2001; 108:503–508.
249. De Lucca GV. Recent developments in CCR3 antagonists. Curr Opin Drug Discov Devel 2006; 9:516–524.
250. Elsner J, Escher SE, Forssmann U. Chemokine receptor antagonists: A novel therapeutic approach in allergic diseases. Allergy 2004; 59:1243–1258.
251. Nakamura T, Ohbayashi M, Toda M, et al. A specific CCR3 chemokine receptor antagonist inhibits both early and late phase allergic inflammation in the conjunctiva. Immunol Res 2005; 33:213–221.
252. Suzuki K, Morokata T, Morihira K, et al. A dual antagonist for chemokine CCR3 receptor and histamine H1 receptor. Eur J Pharmacol 2007; 563:224–232.
253. Carucci JA, Washenik K, Weinstein A, et al. The leukotriene antagonist zafirlukast as a therapeutic agent for atopic dermatitis. Arch Dermatol 1998; 134:785–786.
254. Chari S, Clark-Loeser L, Shupack J, et al. A role for leukotriene antagonists in atopic dermatitis? Am J Clin Dermatol 2001; 2:1–6.
255. Ehlayel MS, Bener A, Sabbah A. Montelukast treatment in children with moderately severe atopic dermatitis. Eur Ann Allergy Clin Immunol 2007; 39:232–236.
256. Barker RL, Gundel RH, Gleich GJ, et al. Acidic polyamino acids inhibit human eosinophil granule major basic protein toxicity. Evidence of a functional role for ProMBP. J Clin Invest 1991; 88:798–805.

Pathophysiology of Pruritus

Sonja Ständer and Thomas A. Luger

Department of Dermatology and Competence Center Pruritus, University of Münster, Münster, Germany

INTRODUCTION

Pruritus, regularly defined as an unpleasant sensation provoking the desire to scratch (1), is an essential feature of atopic dermatitis (AD) (2,3). Because of the high impact on life quality, most of the patients measure the severity of the eczema by the intensity of pruritus rather than of the appearance of skin lesions (4,5). Although pruritus is a cardinal symptom of atopic dermatitis, its neuromechanism is still not fully understood. As a cutaneous sensory perception, itch is excited on neuropeptide-containing free nerve endings of unmyelinated C-fibers. It is known that several mediators such as neuropeptides, interleukins, proteases, or cytokines provoke itch by directly binding to itch receptors or indirectly via histamine release. Interestingly, some variations of this complex pathophysiology could be demonstrated in patients with atopic dermatitis.

SENSORY CUTANEOUS NERVES

Sensory Nerves

The skin is equipped with an effective communication and control system designed to protect the organism in a constantly changing environment. For this purpose a dense network of highly specialized afferent sensory and efferent autonomic nerve branches occurs in all cutaneous layers, especially in the epidermis. The sensory system contains receptors for touch, temperature, pain, itch, and various other physical and chemical stimuli (236). The information is either processed in the central nervous system (CNS) or may directly elicit an inflammatory reaction by antidromic propagation of these impulses. The effector function of a nerve may be determined by secreted neuropeptides and the corresponding receptors of target structures [reviewed in Ref. (6)]. In addition, there is accumulating evidence that neuropeptides exert multiple effects on immunocompetent cells suggesting a strong interaction between the nervous and the immune systems (7–9).

Micrographic recordings have clearly shown that the sensation of itch is transmitted by a subpopulation of unmyelinated thin neurons (10,11). It is assumed that their terminals are free nerve endings located in the epidermis and around skin appendages. In humans, "free" nerve endings do not represent naked axons but remain covered by small cytoplasmic extensions of Schwann cells and a basement membrane that may show continuity with that of the epidermis (6). Multiple sensory modalities such as touch, temperature, pain, and itch may be attributed to the free nerve endings of "polymodal" C-fibers. However, some of the myelinated Aδ-fibers may account for particular subqualities of pain and itch. It can be hypothesized that pruritogenic agents specifically bind to itch receptors on the surface of chemosensitive nerve endings and thereby cause firing of axons. Since some weak mechanical and electrical stimuli often promote itch whereas more intense injury evokes pain, it was previously believed that itch is an altered form of pain. However, recent investigations clearly demonstrate that itch and pain should be considered as independent sensory modalities (10,11). During the past decade it was postulated that sensory C-fibers that may transmit pruritus, are a mechano-insensitive subset with slow conduction velocity (11). However, recent studies have shown that mechano-sensitive nerves also signal itch, for example, induced by cowhage (237).

Autonomic Nerves in the Skin

In contrast to sensory nerve fibers, the distribution of autonomic nerves is restricted to the dermis, innervating blood vessels, arteriovenous anastomoses, lymphatic vessels, glands, hair follicles, and stimulating immune cells to release neurotransmitters. Although autonomic nerves represent only a minority of cutaneous fibers, which predominantly generate neurotransmitters such as acetylcholine (Ach) and catecholamines, recent observations have revealed a potential role for neuropeptides released from sympathetic and parasympathetic neurons during cutaneous inflammation. Moreover, autonomic nerve fibers participate in the regulation of vascular effects in the skin by releasing Ach and vasoactive intestinal peptide (VIP) (12–16). In addition, muscarinic and nicotinergic Ach receptor expression has been described on keratinocytes, melanocytes, fibroblasts, and lymphocytes indicating a regulatory role of both the autonomic and sensory nervous system in the pathophysiology of AD [reviewed in Refs. (17–20)].

Nervous System in Atopic Dermatitis

Several investigators demonstrated that the number of cutaneous nerve fibers is altered in atopic skin lesions. An increase of sensory but decrease of adrenergic autonomic nerve fibers was observed (21), indicating a differential role of primary afferent and autonomic nerve fibers in pruritus pathophysiology. Therefore, immunohistochemical analysis of neuropeptide distribution in cutaneous nerve fibers was performed. Lesional atopic skin showed an increased number of neurofilament-, PGP 9.5-, calcitonin gene-related peptide (CGRP)-, and substance P (SP)-positive nerve fibers in the papillary dermis (22), at the dermoepidermal junction (23,24), in the epidermis (21), and around sweat glands (25). One group additionally described the presence of neuropeptide Y (NPY) in dendritic epidermal cells (24), while another group was unable to reproduce these findings (21). During chronic stress, the epidermal fraction of 5-hydroxytryamine 1A (5-HT1A) receptor and serotonin transporter protein (SERT) immunoreactivity in the involved skin was enhanded in atopic dermatitis patients (238). The authors concluded that a changed innervation and modulation of the serotonergic system are also indicated in chronic atopic eczema during chronic stress. In a semiquantitative analysis, Sugiura et al. (22) found different densities of PGP 9.5-positive peripheral nerves in early acute lesions of AD (2.5×10^3 $\mu m^2/\Delta s$), in subacute lesions (3.8×10^3 $\mu m^2/\Delta s$), in lichenified lesions (4.9×10^3 $\mu m^2/\Delta s$), and in prurigo lesions (7.1×10^3 $\mu m^2/\Delta s$) in comparison to noninvolved skin of patients with AD (2.0×10^3 $\mu m^2/\Delta s$). Hypertrophy of nerve fibers in atopic dermatitis is possibly stimulated by an increased release of nerve growth factor secreted by basal keratinocytes (26,27). Mihm et al. (28) described cutaneous myelinated nerves appearing demyelinated and sclerotic. However, other groups were not able to confirm these pathologic changes upon lightmicroscopical level (23,29). Electron microscopical investigation of lesional skin revealed an increased content of hyperplastic nerve fibers with enlarged axons (22,23). Terminal Schwann cells seem to migrate closer to the epidermis as in normal controls (23). In addition, axons lost their surrounding cytoplasm of Schwann cells in some areas and may thus communicate directly with dermal cells (22). These axons contained many mitochondria and neurofilaments with abundant neurovesicles (22) confirming immunohistologic findings. Finally, a higher immunoreactivity for most neuronal markers like CGRP and SP and altered nerve structures suggests that peripheral nerve fibers may play a role in the pathophysiology of itching in AD (24).

Central Transmission of Pruritus

Peripheral pruritogenic stimuli may be directly sensed as an inflammatory reaction by antidromic propagation of the impulses in the periphery or transmitted to the CNS (6). In atopic dermatitis, a decreased ability of sensory nerves to signal itching to the CNS was suggested (37). Several observations are in favor of an important role of the CNS in modulating itch responses. First, intraventricular injection of morphine induces heavy itch responses. One major possibility is opioid receptors to mediate these effects that are located on peripheral nerves and in the CNS (30,31). In support of this idea, it was shown that naloxone and naltrexone significantly inhibit itching in patients with different inflammatory dermatoses (32–34). The lower part of the medulla oblongata was proposed as an itch center, albeit a direct evidence for this location is still lacking (35). Recent investigations suggested the left primary sensory cortex to be involved in central itch perception as demonstrated by positron emission tomography and recent magnet resonance studies (36,239). Activation of motor-associated areas reflects probably the intention to pruritofensive movements (36). Interestingly, one study compared the central activation of an acute experimental histamine-induced itch stimulus in healthy volunteers and patients with history of atopic dermatitis. The study showed that more brain sites were activated in patients with AD. Activation in AD was significantly higher in the contralateral thalamus, ipsilateral caudate, and pallidum. The authors concluded that the observed changes in the motor system in subjects with chronic itch, along with activation of the basal ganglia, possibly correlate to the vicious itch–scratch circle in subjects with chronic itching skin diseases (239). In summary, the anatomy and physiology of the central perception and regulation of pruritus is still fragmentary and awaits further investigation.

NOCICEPTION IN ATOPIC SKIN

Itching reflects a distinct quality of cutaneous nociception elicited by chemical mediators and other stimuli to neuronal receptors. Several studies could demonstrate that itch in individuals with AD follow different pathways as compared to nonatopic individuals. For example, while normal volunteers experience intense pruritus after injection of histamine or SP, patients with AD only remark weak itch sensations. On the other hand, application of Ach results in pruritus rather than pain in AD patients (Table 1; Fig. 1).

TABLE 1   Mediators of Pruritus in Atopic Dermatitis

Substrate	Induction of itch	Mechanism
Amine		
Histamine	(+)	Direct binding to itch receptor, neurogenic inflammation
Neuropeptides		
Substance P	+	Histamine liberator
Calcitonin gene-related peptide	+	Histamine liberator, increase of IL-8
Vasoactive intestinal peptide	+	Histamine liberator
Somatostatin	+	m.n.n.
Neurotensin	+	Histamine liberator
Acetylcholine	+	m.n.n.
Proteases		
Tryptase	+	Activates protease-activated receptor-2
Chymase	+	m.n.n.
Papain	+	m.n.n.
Opioid peptides		
Endorphines	+	
Enkephalines	+	Central and peripheral modulation of itch perception, histamine-independent
Morphine	+	
Eicosanoids		
Prostaglandins	(+)	Potentiate histamin-, serotonin-, papain-induced pruritus, lowered itch threshold
Leukotriens	+	m.n.n.
Platelet activating factor	+	Histamine liberator
Cytokines		
Interleukin 2	+	Possibly release of various mediators
Interleukin 6	−	
Interleukin 8	−	
Interleukin 31	+	Activates IL3A-receptor
Interferon gamma	Relief pruritus	m.n.n.
Neurotrophin-4	+	m.n.n.
Eosinophils	+	Release mediators like PAF, leucotiens; Histamine liberation?
Basophils	−	

−, No induction of itch; (+), induction of weak itch; +, clear induction of itch; m.n.n., mechanism not known.

Histamine

Many mediators triggering itch have been investigated in AD. Among them, histamine has been a persistent candidate and is the most thoroughly studied pruritogen for decades. About 80 years ago, Lewis already reported that intradermal injections of histamine provoke redness, wheal, and flare (so-called triple response of neurogenic inflammation) accompanied with pruritus (38,39). Williams (40) suggested that histamine may play a role in the pathogenesis of AD since intramuscular histamine injections resulted in pruritus. Elevated histamine levels in both lesional and uninvolved skin in AD patients were also reported (41,42). However, recent investigations were not able to detect increased histamine levels in the skin (43). Uehara and Heyer (37,44–46) noticed reduced itch sensations in response to either intracutaneously injected or iontophoretically applied histamine when compared to nonatopic healthy subjects. Interestingly, histamine may not only

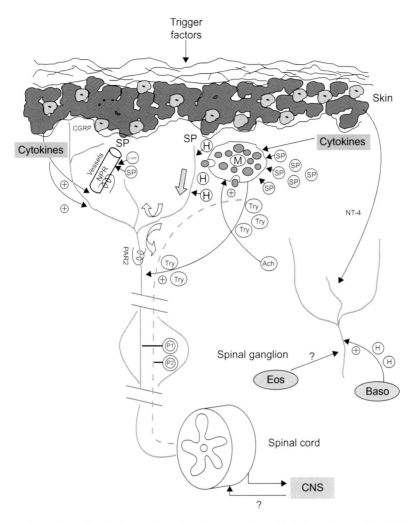

FIGURE 1 Pathophysiology of pruritus in atopic dermatitis. Trigger factors (Table 2) may directly activate neuropeptide release from sensory nerves or indirectly by stimulating mediators (Table 1) from mast cells or keratinocytes. Activation of primary afferent nerve fibers may either result in antidromic stimulation of neuropeptide release or will be processed to the central nervous system. Neuropeptides, proteases, or cytokines may provoke itch by direct binding to itch receptors or indirectly via histamine release from mast cells or basophils. *Abbreviations*: Ach, acetylcholine; Baso, basophils; CGRP, calcitonin gene-related peptide; CNS, central nervous system; Eos, eosinophils; H, histamine; M, mast cells; NPR, neuropeptide receptor; NT-4, neurotrophin-4; PAR2, proteinase-activated receptor-2; SP, substance P; Try, tryptase.

induce itch but also perifocal alloknesis (itch elicited by a slight mechanical, otherwise nonitching stimulus). Furthermore, intradermally injected SP releases histamine and provokes diminished itch perception in patients with AD in comparison to healthy subject, which underlines the minor capacity of histamine to induce pruritus in AD (47). These conflicting results of elevated levels of histamine and diminished itching after histamine application may indicate either an intrinsic downregulation of neuronal H1-receptor density or affinity, or increased histamine degradation in atopic skin (48). Consequently, antihistamines are often not efficient in AD, as demonstrated in experimental studies as well as double-blind, crossover trials. Recently, Rukwied et al. (49) demonstrated that pruritus induced by the mast cell degranulating substance compound C48/80 in AD patients could not be relieved by cetirizine H1 blockade. Wahlgren et al. (50) compared the antipruritic effect of H1 antagonist and placebo in AD patients and found no difference between these two agents. Recently, histamine 4 receptors were found in human skin (234). Interestingly, a mouse model suggests that a combination of H4 and H1 receptor antagonism might be a new strategy to treat pruritus related to allergic diseases like atopic dermatitis. In their experiments, the authors showed that H4 receptor antagonism fails to reduce the allergic inflammatory response but strongly inhibits allergen-induced itch (235). In sum, these results support the idea that not histamine and histamine 1 receptor but other mediators such as proteases and cytokines may mainly be involved in the pathophysiology of itch response during AD.

Neuropeptides

Several observations support the idea of an important role of neuropeptides for the pathophysiology of itching in various skin diseases (8,9,20,51). Neuropeptides such as SP, VIP, somatostatin, and neurotensin provoke itch along with the characteristics of neurogenic inflammation such as erythema, wheal, and flare (52–55). SP induces itch responses in human and mice, which are probably mediated via activation of the neurokinin 1 receptor (NK1R) (56,57), supporting a direct effect of SP in mediating pruritus in vivo. In contrast, CGRP does not mediate pruritogenic effects (58,59). Opioids have been also demonstrated to induce pruritus, which can be blocked using naloxone, a μ-opioid receptor antagonist (60,61).

In patients with atopic dermatitis, alterations in the nerve fiber containing neuropeptide profile could be demonstrated. Somatostatin-immunoreactive nerve fibers were decreased in AD patients (62). NPY-positive nerve fibers and Langerhans cells are increased as compared to healthy controls (21,24,62). Moreover, tissue concentrations of VIP were decreased, while SP concentrations were increased in lesional skin of AD patients (63–65). In contrast, staining pattern for CGRP was not altered in comparison to controls (62). These observations support the idea that an imbalance of the cutaneous nervous system including nerve fibers, neuropeptides, and their receptors as well as neuropeptide-degrading enzymes may play a crucial role in the pathophysiology of pruritus in AD (66).

Acetylcholine

Ach is very likely to play an important role in producing itch sensations in patients suffering from atopic dermatitis. Ach is a major neurotransmitter activating sweat glands, which may explain generalized itching during and after sweating in patients with AD. Ach is not only a neurotransmitter in glandular epithelium like eccrine sweat glands, it has also been shown to activate muscarinic receptors on cultured human keratinocytes and can be synthesized, released, and degraded by human keratinocytes in vitro (67,68). Interestingly, several authors found increased Ach levels in biopsies of patients with AD suggesting that increased production or release of Ach is involved in the pathophysiology of pruritus in AD (69,240). A recent study describes reduced expression of various subgroups of nicotinic Ach receptors (nAChRs) in lesional AD skin suggesting dysregulation of the cholinergic system in AD independently from inflammation (241). Intradermal application of Ach elicits pruritus instead of pain in patients with AD (16,46). While all healthy control subjects reported on burning pain after Ach administration, patients with AD complained of pure itching that developed shortly after Ach injection and lasted significantly longer than in controls (16). In addition, injection of Ach evoked pruritus in eczematous atopic lesions and intermingled burning as well as itching sensations in uninvolved areas (46), which underlines a different physiologic pruritus pathway in lesional as compared to nonlesional or healthy skin. Combined intracutaneous injections of VIP and Ach induce wheal, flare, and a dose-dependent pruritus in both lesional skin in AD and normal healthy controls (49,70). However, the subjective pruritus score did not differ between combined injections of VIP and Ach from Ach-injections alone in patients with AD (49). These results suggest a predominant role of Ach over VIP and a cholinerg, histamine-independent mechanism in the pathophysiology of pruritus in AD. Interestingly, it was speculated that the induction of intradermally injected Ach is not due to the substance itself but a spinal hypersensitivity for itch in patients with chronic pruritus, so-called central sensitization (242). To date, no studies abandon one theory.

Mast Cells, Proteinases, and Proteinase-Activated Receptors

A role of proteinases such as trypsin, chymotrypsin, and papain as pruritogenic agents has been proposed for over 40 years (71). Moreover, the pruritogenic effect and triple response of neurogenic inflammation induced by proteinases can be blocked by antihistamines (72), indicating an interaction of proteinases and mast cells in pruritus. Intradermal injection of mast cell tryptase into human and rabbit skin results in pruritus, vasodilatation, and erythema, followed by leukocyte infiltration and local induration (73), suggesting a role for tryptase in cutaneous inflammation and itching. Importantly, tryptase but not chymase is enhanced in lesional and nonlesional skin of patients with atopic dermatitis (74,243) and has been suggested to induce itch responses in human skin (49,75,243,). Other studies support a role of tryptase in itch responses of patients with AD (74,76–78). Thus, tryptase may be an important regulator of inflammatory and itch responses in the skin of patients with atopic dermatitis. Tryptase mediates some of its cellular effects via activating a proteinase-activated receptor-2 (PAR-2). Tryptase activates PAR-2 on keratinocytes (79), dermal endothelial cells (244), and sensory nerves (75) thereby contributing to inflammatory effects of mast cells. PAR-2 is markedly enhanced on primary afferent nerve fibers in skin biopsies of AD patients (243). Intracutaneous injection of PAR-2 agonists provoked enhanced and prolonged itch when applied intralesionally. Moreover, itch upon mast cell degranulation was abolished by local antihistamines in controls but prevailed in AD patients. Thus, PAR-2 signaling is one link between inflammatory and sensory phenomena in AD patients.

CYTOKINES AND INFLAMMATORY CELLS INVOLVED IN PATHOGENESIS OF PRURITUS IN ATOPIC DERMATITIS

Cytokines are released from various cutaneous and immune cells during inflammation. Certain cytokines have been demonstrated to induce pruritus and activate neuropeptide release from sensory nerves in the skin of patients with atopic dermatitis (Fig. 1).

Interleukin 2 (IL-2)

Although IL-1 does not seem to correlate with itching, IL-2 is claimed to be a potent inducer of pruritus. As observed upon therapeutical application, high doses of recombinant interleukin-2, as given in cancer patients, provoke frequently redness and cutaneous itching (80). Furthermore, AD patients treated with oral cyclosporin A, a drug that inhibits the production of various cytokines including IL-2, experience attenuation of itch (81,82). Additionally, a single intracutaneus injection of interleukin-2 induced a low-intensity intermittent local itch with maximal intensity between 6 and 48 hours as well as erythema in both atopic and healthy individuals (83,84). Interestingly, in patients with AD, this reaction tends to appear earlier than in healthy controls. Moreover, bradykinin appears to enhance the effect of IL-2–induced pruritus on sensory nerves (85). Upon prick testing, supernatants of mitogen-stimulated leucocytes were pruritic in AD patients but not in controls, probably due to increased concentration of IL-2 and IL-6 (86). The mechanism for the induction of itch by IL-2 remains to be established, but the latency preceding the itch response after injection in AD patients suggests an indirect pruritogenic effect of IL-2 via other mediators.

Interleukin 6 (IL-6)

IL-6 and IL-6 receptor are expressed in nerve and Schwann cells (87), and IL-6–like immunoreactivity was increased in nerve fibers of patients with positive epicutaneous patch tests and prurigo nodularis (88) suggesting a role for this cytokine in pruritus. Several studies suggest that IL-6 does not play a major role for pruritus in AD (86,89,90,91). In a clinical trial with AD patients, decreased sleep efficiency was associated with increasing disease severity, scratching, and IL-6 levels suggesting an important relationship between sleep and IL-6 (245).

Interleukin 8 (IL-8)

Recently, various studies revealed increased levels of the proinflammatory chemokine IL-8 in lesional skin (92), plasma (93), and blood mononuclear cells (89,94), especially eosinophils (95) of AD patients. However, the capacity of IL-8 to induce pruritus is questionable because prick testing with IL-8 does not induce whealing or pruritus (89). Further studies will have to clarify the influence of IL-8 in the pathophysiology of pruritus.

Interleukin 31 (IL-31)

Much attention is currently drawn to a new discovered interleukin, IL-31, which is very likely to play a major role in pathophysiology of AD pruritus. Discovered a couple of years ago, mice models suggested the role of pruritus induction (246,247). For example, IL-31 mRNA in the skin of NC/Nga mice with scratching behavior was found to be significantly higher than that in NC/Nga mice without scratching behavior (246). Moreover, IL-31 was significantly overexpressed in human AD skin compared with nonpruritic psoriatic skin inflammation (248). The authors could also demonstrate a link between bacterial colonization and induction of pruritus. Staphylococcal superantigen rapidly induced IL-31 expression in atopic individuals. In vitro, staphylococcal enterotoxin B but not viruses or T(H)1 and T(H)2 cytokines induced IL-31 in leukocytes. In patients with atopic dermatitis, activated leukocytes expressed significantly higher IL-31 levels compared with control subjects. IL-31 receptor A showed most abundant expression in dorsal root ganglia representing the site where the cell bodies of cutaneous sensory neurons reside. These results suggest a direct link among staphylococcal colonization, subsequent T-cell recruitment/activation, and pruritus induction in patients with atopic dermatitis (248).

Interferon Gamma (INF-γ)
Interferon gamma appears to have a beneficial effect on pruritus in AD (96). In a double-blind study, pruritus was reduced by 50% even one to two years after long-term treatment with recombinant human INF-γ (97). It is well known that INF-γ production is profoundly diminished in peripheral blood mononuclear cells of AD patients (98), which may contribute to the development of pruritus. Although an important role of INF-γ in the pathophysiology of pruritus in AD is likely, the underlying mechanism by which low INF-γ levels induce pruritus, however, has to be identified.

Neurotrophin-4 (NT-4)
Recent observations indicate that NT-4 may be involved in inflammatory and itch responses of patients with AD. NT-4 is a keratinocyte-derived agent which is highly expressed under inflammatory conditions and which exerts growth-promoting effects on nerve cells. Accordingly, NT-4 expression was found to be significantly increased in lesional skin of patients with atopic dermatitis and in prurigo lesions of atopic dermatitis skin (99,249). A recent study suggests that Prostaglandin E2 (PGE2) enhances neurotrophin-4 production via the EP3 receptor (249). It was suggested that PGE2 may promote innervation in skin lesions with atopic dermatitis via the induction of NT-4. NT-4 production can also be induced by INF-γ, which itself is known to have a beneficial effect on pruritus. These findings suggest a close relationship between immune and neurotrophic factors in the pathophysiology of pruritus in AD.

Nerve Growth Factor
Nerve growth factor (NGF) is released from keratinocytes, mast cells, and eosinophilic granulocytes and increased in atopic dermatitis skin (250–252). NGF is discussed to sensitize peripheral nerve endings resulting in facilitated induction of pruritus (236). Sprouting of epidermal nerve fibers as found in lesional AD skin is attributed to increased NGF expression in atopic dermatitis (23). In addition, remarkably increased serum levels of NGF and SP have been found to correlate with the severity of the disease in atopic dermatitis (252,253). In an animal model for AD (NC/Nga mice) increased epidermal NGF expression has been confirmed. Moreover, therapeutic anti-NGF approaches reduced pruritus successfully and represent a future therapy option of pruritus in AD (254,255).

Eosinophils
The role of eosinophils in the pathogenesis of AD has not been fully understood, however, it seems likely that they contribute to induction and maintenance of pruritus. Eosinophils may have direct contacts to nerve fibers (256) and release factors which may have a direct pruritogenic effect such as eosinophil-derived neurotoxin (EDN), NGF, brain-derived neurotrophic factor (BDNF), neurotrophin-3 (NT3), platelet-activating factor (PAF), leucotrienes, prostanoids, kinins, cytokines, and proteases (100–105,257). They may also exert an indirect itch response by

activating mast cells to release histamine or proteinases from eosinophils. In summary, it may be speculated that eosinophils and their mediators contribute to direct induction of pruritus and also to sensitization and nerve fiber sprouting in AD.

Basophils

In patients with AD, peripheral blood basophils are normal in number, but in vitro studies revealed abnormal function with increased or faster histamine releasability (106,107). However, Bull et al. could demonstrate that basophils and basophil release of histamine do not contribute to induction of itch and erythema in patients with AD (108).

EXPERIMENTALLY INDUCED PRURITUS IN ATOPIC DERMATITIS EXPLAINING NEW APPROACHES IN THE THERAPY

Platelet-activating factor (PAF) is a lipid mediator with a potent proinflammatory activity. PAF is released by several inflammatory cells such as mast cells, eosinophils, basophils, and neutrophils (74). PAF could be demonstrated to increase vascular permeability. Consequently, a wheal and flare reaction as well as pruritus resulted after intradermal injection suggesting release of histamine by PAF (109). Several PAF antagonists have been developed so far, and preliminary results of a double-blind study applying a synthetic PAF antagonist topically could demonstrate a statistically significant reduction of pruritus in patients with AD during the first two weeks of therapy (110). However, further studies will have to clarify the practicability of PAF antagonists upon daily use.

So far, the role of leukotriens in the pathogenesis of pruritus is speculative, although there is increasing evidence about their relevance in elicitation itch. Andoh and Kuraishi (111) demonstrated that intradermally injected leukotriene E4 is able to provoke scratching in mice. Additionally, a correlation of nocturnal itch and high urinary leukotriene E4 levels was demonstrated suggesting that increased production of leukotriens may contribute to nocturnal itch induction in AD (112). Preliminary studies showed reduce of pruritus in patients with AD during treatment with the leukotriene receptor antagonists, zafirlukast and zileuton (113–115).

Capsaicin, a naturally occurring alkaloid and the principal pungent of hot chilli peppers, has been advocated to be antipruritic in various dermatoses (116,117). Repeated topical application of capsaicin releases and prevents specifically the reaccumulation of neuropeptides in unmyelinated, C-type cutaneous nerves. Capsaicin exerts its functions via binding to a capsaicin-specific receptor, that is, the vanilloid receptor (TRPV1), which is located on free nerve endings (118). Receptor binding of capsaicin opens cation-specific ion channels, leads to depolarization of nerve fibers, and release of secretory granules containing neuropeptides, such as SP, CGRP, VIP, and neurokinin A. Because nociceptive sensations are mediated by unmyelinated C-fibers, depletion of neuropeptides upon continuous application of capsaicin impedes the perception of pain and itch sensations (119). Consequently, topical application of capsaicin appears to be helpful in AD (120, 121).

Morphine and opioids are known to play an intriguing part in itch elicited not only by receptor-independent histamine release from cutaneous mast cells (122), but also by a direct central and peripheral pruritogenic effect besides their predominant role in pain (30–32,60,123,124). Generalized pruritus after systemic application of morphine is a rare side effect, but epidural or in particular paraspinal application of

TABLE 2   Trigger Factors Inducing and Aggravating Pruritus in Atopic Dermatitis

Trigger factors	Examples
Endogenous trigger factors	Perspiration (most common trigger factor in AD)
	Xerosis
	Cutaneous microvasculature
	Emotional stress
Exogenous irritants	Scratching
	Wool fibers
	Lipid solvents (soap, detergents)
	Desinfectants
Contact and aero allergens	Dust mites
	Furry animals
	Pollens
	Molds
	Human dander
Microbial agents	Viral infections
	Staphylococcus aureus
	Pityrosporon yeast, Candida, Dermatophytes
Food	Hot, spicy food
	Hot drinks
	Alcoholics

Sources: Adapted from Refs. 166, 225.

opioid analgesics frequently induce itching. Consequently, opiate receptor antagonists have been demonstrated to have an inhibitory effect on pruritus (33,34,61,125–127). Recent experiments revealed that the oral opiate antagonist naltrexone is more effective to suppress histamine-induced itch and alloknesis than the antihistamine cetirizine (46,128) in patients with AD. However, although β-endorphin serum levels were demonstrated to be significantly elevated in children with pruritic AD (129), results of a therapy with opiate receptor antagonists were not reproducible. Although a few case reports demonstrated diminished pruritus using opiate antagonist naloxone and nalmefene (130), other groups could not reproduce these effects using nalmefene and nemexine in AD (34,131,132). Further controlled studies with μ-opioid antagonists and the new group of κ-opioid agonists have to clarify their relevance in the treatment of AD itch.

TRIGGER FACTORS MODULATING PRURITUS PERCEPTION IN ATOPIC DERMATITIS

The skin of AD patients reveals a higher tendency to itch upon minimal provocation due to reduced itch threshold and prolonged itch duration to pruritic stimuli as compared to healthy skin (133–135). A series of pruritus triggering factors are known (135) that release mast cell mediators or vasomotor and sweat reactions to cause itch, and all may be subjected to emotional influences (134) (Table 2).

Xerosis

Xerosis of the skin in patients with AD reflects a disturbed epidermal barrier and is a well-known activator of pruritus in AD patients of all ages. An increased transepidermal water loss and a decreased ability of the stratum corneum to bind water were measured (136), which may result from incomplete arrangement of intercellular lipid lamellae in the stratum corneum (137,138). A decrease of water content below 10% seems to be crucial for induction of itch and scratching (139). This generalized dryness of the skin triggers pruritus by unknown mechanisms (136,137). One possibility may be that an impaired barrier function in the skin supports the entrance of irritants and itchy agents (140,141). Additionally, pH changes within the skin may activate itch receptors (118).

Sweating

Generalized itching initiated by any stimulus to sweating (thermal, emotional stimuli) is a typical hallmark and represents the most common trigger factor of itch in patients with AD (134,142,143). Interestingly, increased sweating in lichenified skin was observed in AD patients suggesting a decreased threshold for sweat stimulation in chronic pruritic and altered skin (144). The underlying mechanism of sweat-induced pruritus remains to be explored, but there is raising evidence that Ach is involved. Ach induces eccrine sweating (6), is found to be increased in the skin of AD patients (69), and finally acts pruritogenic in AD patients (16).

Microcirculation

There is considerable evidence that the cutaneous microvasculature contributes to pruritus. Clinically, itching is mostly associated with erythema and hyperthermia. Most mediators for itching such as histamine, tryptase, Ach, SP, and prostaglandins are potent vasodilatators, rarely vasoconstrictors such as NPY or catecholamines. Interestingly, while neuropeptide-induced itching does not vary between atopic and nonatopic patients, vascular responses obviously showed a significant difference between these two groups. Moreover, patients with AD were more susceptible to stress and showed increased vasodilatation as compared to controls (145).

Exogenous Factors

Pruritus produced by direct contact with wool in patients with AD is a characteristic and reproducible phenomenon (91,146). It is likely that the irritation is caused by the spiky nature of wool fibers itself while wearing wool garments close to the skin. Mechanical vibration seems not to be responsible for induction of itch, because it inhibits experimental, histamine-induced itch (147). Thicker wool fibers were found to provoke more intense itching than thinner fibers and an additional redness after application of wool samples (148). Other irritants like lipid solvents, desinfectants (149) may additionally contribute to aggravate xerosis. Contact- and aeroallergens as dust mites or pollens [reviewed in Refs. (142)] may also provoke pruritus. Microbiologic agents like bacteria (*Staphylococcus aureus*) or yeast may exacerbate both dermatitis and pruritus (135,142).

Pruritus and erythema may also be triggered by substances increasing blood flow, conduct vasodilatation, or release histamine. Among those, heat, hot and spicy foods, hot drinks, and alcohol are most likely to generate itch in AD patients (135,142,150). In early childhood, food allergies exacerbate eczematous skin lesions, although food allergies mostly resolve during ageing in older children and adults (150).

Stress and Psychiatric Conditions

In general, itch can be induced or modified by cognitive stress perception like fatigue, anxiety, repressed emotions as well as psychiatric diseases like depression (151–158). Consequently, in atopic dermatitis, a correlation between the intensity of pruritus, scratching, and mental stress factors and psychiatric conditions could be demonstrated upon experimental studies (153,154,159–161). Furthermore, AD patients experienced a more intensive pruritus in comparison to healthy persons and patients with psoriasis under equal study conditions (159). Consistently, upon clinical examinations, up to 81% of AD patients acknowledge their pruritus to be aggravated by emotional stress (54). Relaxation therapies like autogenic training or hypnosis indirectly prove these findings by revealing a significant improvement of itching and eczema in AD patients (162,163). The mechanism of psychogen-triggered pruritus is unknown, but activation of the psychoneuroendocrine system is likely (8,9,153,154). Moreover, there is evidence from a recent study for a stress-induced pertubation of the epidermal barrier function resulting in inflammation and pruritus (164).

It is well established for several years that animals respond to external noxious stimuli resulting in alarm reaction followed by a resistance phase and potentially exhaustion of the biologic system. In a rat model, it was recently demonstrated that immobilization stress triggers mast cell degranulation, which was reduced by pretreatment with capsaicin (165). Thus, increased release of pruritogenic mediators by mast cells may result in scratching and skin lesions following stress tension (153). Pruritus intensity may also be increased by vasodilator responses and increased skin temperature to emotional stress as demonstrated by psychophysiologic studies (134,166). Thus, stress is connected with the production of mediators that influence several tissue organs including the skin (159). Neuropeptides such as SP, VIP, NPY, somatostatin, or CGRP released from sensory afferent nerves or neurotransmitters such as catecholamines and Ach generated by autonomic nerve fibers may be associated with emotional distress and cutaneous symptoms. For example, more pronounced release of neuropeptides like SP, CGRP, and neurotensin as well as vascular changes could be demonstrated during itching and scratching in AD patients as compared to normal controls (24,62,66). Furthermore, increased mast cell degranulation (165) and elevated count of blood granulocytes and leucocytes (167) were found in patients with AD upon stress stimuli. Finally, adrenaline may influence pruritus in a reverse mode. Patients with AD judge a preexisting pruritus to be less intensive in stress situations with high adrenaline levels (153,154,160).

CLINICAL ASPECTS

The diagnosis of active AD cannot be made if there is no history of itching (2). There are several aspects defining pruritus in patients with AD. Besides pruritus associated with erythema, alloknesis and atmoknesis are phenomena often observed in atopic dermatitis probably due to altered itch threshold. Many patients complain on nocturnal itch associated with sleep disturbance. All these types of pruritus may lead to a vigorous itch–scratch cycle.

Clinical Manifestation of Pruritus

It has long been debated whether itch precedes visible skin lesions or if otherwise erythema and accompanied inflammatory reaction appears first to evoke pruritus (140,142,143). However, both theories can be assumed to fit with clinical observations and furthermore to maintain the itch–scratch cycle. It is well known that various triggering factors like stress result first in appearance of erythema followed by itch (143,168,169). Furthermore, itch may be followed by vasodilatation and

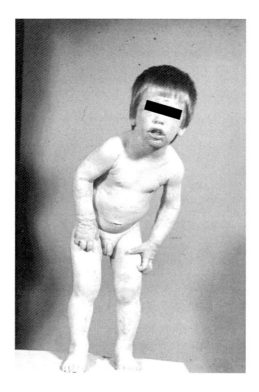

FIGURE 2 Child with atopic dermatitis and pruritus which pinches and kneads its skin instead of scratching.

inflammation due to scratching (140,142). However, pruritus in AD is regularly intense but intermittent with greater intensity in the evening and at night. Usually, itching is generalized, but localized forms are also known with preferential appearance in flexures, wrist, face, and neck (170). As a consequence, permanent itch leads to an intense scratch behavior and patients often resort to towels, combs, back-scratchers, brushes, and even scissors to combat pruritus (91,171). Interestingly, children with atopic dermatitis regularly pinch, knead, and roll their skin slowly instead of scratching or rubbing (G. Bonsmann, personal communication, 2001) (Fig. 2). Consistently scratching is at times so vigorous that it evokes pain and leads to an "antipruritic state" due to suppression of pruritus-conducting C-fibers by pain-conducting A-fibers. Intense and permanent pinching, rubbing, and scratching causes many of the skin lesions observed in patients with AD (140,172) such as acute skin traumatization like excoriations, erosions, bleeding, and crusts. Moreover, secondary skin changes like lichenifications, nodules, pigment shift, and scars may reflect chronic scratching (155,171). Now it is generally accepted that lichen simplex and prurigo nodularis as often seen in AD represent a cutaneous reaction pattern to repeated scratching (172). Interestingly, in areas not accessible for patients with AD like the upper back, unaffected skin without scratch lesions appears leading to the so-called "butterfly sign" (140).

Alloknesis, Atmoknesis
Alloknesis is a phenomenon occurring not only in AD but also in other dermatoses and defines pruritus that is evoked by usually nonpruritogenic, mechanical

stimuli (91). The clinical observation that once an itch has started in AD patients, it increases the liability of the surrounding skin resulting in itch is explainable by alloknesis. Another phenomenon is atmoknesis defining pruritus caused by exposure to air or undressing particularly notable in patients with AD. Both alloknesis and atmoknesis possibly result from an altered itch threshold in the periphery or central sensitization (171,242). Regarding pruritus and alloknesis, 52% of patients with AD complain about itch without a rash in comparison to 6% of nonatopic patients (143).

Nocturnal Itch

Several authors report on frequent sleep disturbances caused by nocturnal scratching (173–175). Upon scratch-monitor analysis and infrared video camera system, a higher nocturnal scratch frequency in patients with severe AD was demonstrated resulting in a serious sleep disturbance as compared to patients with moderate AD or healthy controls (173,174). Two types of scratching activity appeared, one during the time when patients were not asleep with various scratching movements like rubbing or pinching. The second scratching activity appeared during sleep, when scratch movements started abruptly, were monotonous and rhythmic, suggesting that scratch during sleep has the nature of a reflex. Most scratch movements appear during early and mid-night periods; rare movements were observed before daybreak possibly due to physiologic release of corticosteroids or melatonin (173,176,177). Finally, the scratching rate was reduced upon successful therapy (174,178).

Itch–Scratch Cycle

Severe pruritus in atopic dermatitis elicits reflectory scratching, resulting often in a vicious circle of itch and scratch. Increased amounts of neuropeptides, cytokines, and other inflammatory mediators are released by scratching and contribute to aggravation of both itch and erythema (54,140,169). Thus, the itch–scratch cycle is perpetuated. Various other pruritogenic triggers like wool fibers additionally maintain the itch–scratch circle (140,179). Furthermore, it could be demonstrated that patients with AD developed conditioned scratch responses earlier than control subjects (179), which is in favor of an additional factor perpetuating the itch–scratch cycle. Patients with AD tend to frequently act out anger and hostility or other emotional stress by scratching, rather than verbalizing their feelings (134,161,168,179,180). In addition, they are more likely to respond to minor signals and stimuli by scratching than that of nonatopic individuals, and many patients describe an emotionally disturbing event before occurrence of a flare reaction (54,181).

THERAPEUTICAL CONSIDERATIONS

Nonspecific Antipruritic Modalities

Some general principles are helpful during therapy of pruritus of any origin including atopic dermatitis (Table 3). First of all, elimination of identified provocative factors like wool fibers must be appreciated as the primary goal of the management (155,182,183). Furthermore, since scratching also represents a trigger factor and maintains the itch–scratch cycle, it must be interrupted by education of the patient to control scratch behavior (184). For example, the behavior method "habit

TABLE 3 Therapeutic Strategies Combating Pruritus in Atopic Dermatitis

Therapeutical modalities	Examples
General principles	Interruption of itch–scratch cycle
	Elimination of provocative factors
	Skin care to reduce sweating-induce itch
Unspecific topical preparations	Emollients
	Lotions containing cooling additives, menthol
	Bathing with oily additives
Unspecific physical modalities	Physical exercise[a]
	Acupuncture
	Cutaneous field stimulation
Japanese traditional medicine	Kampo herbals
Anti-inflammatory therapy	Corticosteroids, t and o[a]
	Cyclosporin A, o[a]
	Tacrolimus, t[a]
	Pimecrolimus, t[a]
	Palmitoylethanolamine (PEA), t
	Ultraviolet light
	Interferon gamma, i.c.[a]
	Macrolide antibiotics, o
Interfering with pathophysiology of pruritus in AD	Capsaicin, t
	Dinitrochlorobenzene, t
	Eicosapentaenoic acid, t
	Type 4 phosphodiesterase inhibitors
	Doxepin (but contact allergy upon long-term application), t
	PAF antagonists, t[a]
	Leukotriene antagonists, o (e.g., zafirlukast)
	Immunoglobulin therapy, i.v.
Contradictory results	Antihistamines, o
	Mycophenolat mofetil, o
	Opiate antagonists, o (e.g., naltrexone)
No antipruritic effect	Topical anesthetics
	Nitrazepam, o

[a]As proven by randomized, controlled studies.
Abbreviations: t, topically; o, orally; i.c., intracutaneously; i.v., intravenously.

reversal" can be employed (185). First, patients become aware of their scratching behavior by counting scratch movements. In a second step, they learn a new behavior by reacting to scratch impulses. Also controlled physical exercises like gymnastics or ball games were demonstrated in a controlled study to teach patients to cope better with itch attacks (186). Scratch induced skin damage caused by nocturnal scratch movements may be improved by using cotton gloves. To reduce sweating-induced itch, simple skin care such as clearing by warm shower and application of ointment has been recommended (46). Cooling the skin with lotions containing, for example, menthol results in relief of itch (187). To combat skin dryness, application of hydrophilic emollients and bathing with oily bath additives is helpful (182,183). Topical anaesthetics are reported to be useful in pruritus (188), albeit no effect was observed in AD patients (189). Unspecific physical modalities are described to be beneficial like acupuncture (190) and cutaneous field stimulation (191,192). A new ethnomedical approach is the oral application of the Japanese traditional kampo medicine formula "Byakkokaninjinto." Studies in NC mice, an animal model for atopic dermatitis, revealed a significant reduction of scratching activity possibly due to a cooling effect on skin temperature (193). However, only one abstract reports a successful treatment with this substance so far (194).

Specific Antipruritic Therapies

Although various symptomatic treatments were employed to relieve pruritus and scratching in patients with AD, no specific therapies are available as of yet (140). Because lesional AD skin shows a dense inflammatory cell infiltrate known to mediate or aggravate pruritus, anti-inflammatory therapies often result in cessation of pruritus. So far, most effective and consistent antipruritics remain systemic and topical immunomodulators such as glucocorticoids, cyclosporin A, tacrolimus, pimecrolimus, and ultraviolet light therapy (81,195–197). Moreover, there are no evident and efficient alternatives to topical application of *corticosteroids* for the control of acute episodes in atopic dermatitis (198–200). With reduction of skin lesions, a decreased itch intensity results probably due to reduction of inflammatory cells and protection of depolarization of nerve fibers mediated directly by the steroid (201). *Cyclosporin A* (CyA), a cyclic polypeptide with potent immunosuppressive effects, has been reported to have an itch-reliving effect in various diseases including atopic dermatitis. In a randomized study, CyA was demonstrated to significantly reduce itch intensity (81,202). After discontinuation of this therapy, pruritus recurred immediately suggesting that CyA represents a symptomatic and not causal therapy of pruritus. A case series reported on relief of itch and scratch lesions in prurigo forms of AD (258). Since oral cyclosporin A has demonstrated to be effective in atopic dermatitis, a topical CyA formulation has been developed to avoid systemic adverse effects. However, no significant improvement of atopic dermatitis was found upon clinical application (203).

The topical immunomodulators *tacrolimus* and *pimecrolimus* were frequently demonstrated to reduce erythema as well as pruritus and excoriations (197,204,205,210,211). Randomized studies confirmed topical administration of both to be antipruritic in adults and children (2–15 years) with AD (194,206–209). As both induce inhibitory effects on the production of proinflammatory cytokines from T cells and mast cells (210), the specific improvement of pruritus suggests interference of calcineurininhibitors with the neuroimmunologic network in the skin of patients with AD. In addition, it is speculated, that they bind to the capsaicin receptor TRPV1 to mediate initial burning (neurogenic inflammation) followed by rapid reduction of pruritus (259,260).

Endogenous and synthetic cannabinoids are known for their psychotic and analgetic potency upon systemic administration. Recently, both cannabinoid receptors CB1 and CB2 were found to be expressed on cutaneous sensory nerve fibers, mast cells, and keratinocytes (261). It was demonstrated that injections of the CB2 agonist *N-palmitoylethanolamine (PEA)* may inhibit experimental NGF-induced thermal hyperalgesia (262). First pilot trials with PEA–containing cream could relief pruritus in a large collection of pruritic AD patients (>2456 patients aged 2–70 years) (263). These preliminary data show that topically applied cannabinoid agonists may be an interesting future concept of antipruritic therapy.

Mycophenolat mofetil (MMF) is a novel immunosuppressive drug, which selectively inhibits lymphocyte proliferation. Uncontrolled studies with patients suffering from AD exhibit contradictory results. Some authors report on effective treatment of erythema and pruritus (212,213), while others found MMF to increase pruritus (214).

Treatment with INF-γ has been shown to be effective not only for the improvement of erythema, excoriations, and lichenifications, but also for pruritus (97,215,216). In addition, this effect is maintained up to two years after therapy (97).

Arachidonic acid metabolites are released from mast cells and are involved in the onset of AD. It has been demonstrated that eicosapentaenoic acid (EPA) may inhibit the activity of arachidonic acid metabolites. A recent study reported topical EPA administration to significantly reduce pruritus in AD (217).

Studies concerning the pathophysiology of pruritus clearly demonstrated that different nociceptive mechanisms are involved in AD. Thus, conventional therapeutic modalities like antihistamines often fail to ameliorate pruritus in AD (200). This is comprehensive with the idea that histamine is not the major mediator of pruritus in AD (49). Placebo-controlled studies concerning the antipruritic effect of oral *antihistamines* have shown conflicting results in AD. In some studies, no superior effect was observed as compared to placebo (50,218,219), while others showed a significant antipruritic effect (46,220–222). In recent experimental studies, the H1-antihistamine cetirizine could be demonstrated to focally reduce itch (46). However, an evidence-based review concerning the efficacy of antihistamines in relieving pruritus in atopic dermatitis concluded that little objective evidence exists for H1-antihistamines to demonstrate improvement of pruritus (223). Other modalities also failed to show an antipruritic effect in AD. Moreover, a placebo-controlled study with *nitrazepam* was initiated that claimed to reduce the nocturnal scratching behavior. However, the substance failed to influence the total duration of nocturnal scratching in patients with AD (224).

Topical application of the tricyclic antidepressant *doxepin* suggested having antipruritic effects because of its high affinity to H1 histamine receptors. In fact, 5% doxepin cream not only revealed improvement of histamine-induced and SP-mediated cutaneous responses but also evoked sedative effects in some patients (225,226). Unfortunately, doxepin was accompanied by contact allergies after long-term application (227).

Oral administration of *macrolide antibiotics* was reported to have an antipruritic effect in atopic dermatitis possibly due to their capacity to inhibit production of cytokines like IL-6 and IL-8 (228). Amelioration of pruritus has also been described under intravenous *immunoglobulin* therapy in few cases of AD (229,230). As of yet, however, no controlled studies were performed. Lately, contact sensitization to *dinitrochlorobenzene* (DNCB) claimed to significantly improve the clinical status of severe AD (231,232). There is also recent evidence that type 4 phosphodiesterase inhibitors have anti-inflammatory and antipruritic activities in patients with AD (233). Therapeutical modalities such as *capsaicin* (120,121), μ-*opiate antagonists/*κ-*opioid agonists* (34,127), *PAF antagonist* (110), and *leukotriene antagonists* (113–115) and possibly also PAR2- or IL31-antagonists appear to be promising new approaches in the therapy of atopic dermatitis (see section, experimentally induced pruritus in atopic dermatitis explaining new approaches in the therapy), but will have to prove their safety and practicability in future controlled studies. In conclusion, no completely effective and safe antipruritic agent has been successfully approved by controlled studies for the therapy of pruritus in atopic dermatitis so far. Further investigations are necessary to establish antipruritic substances influencing the centrally and peripherally altered itch perception in order to interfere with the complex pathophysiology of pruritus in atopic dermatitis.

REFERENCES

1. Rothman S. Physiology of itching. Physiol Rev 1941; 21:357–381.
2. Hanifin JM, Rajka G. Diagnostic features of atopic dermatitis. Acta Derm Venereol Suppl (Stockh) 1980; 92(suppl.):44–47.
3. Koblenzer CS. Itching and the atopic skin. J Allergy Clin Immunol 1999; 104:S109–S113.
4. Schnyder UW. Neurodermatitis vom klinisch dermatologischen Standpunkt. Acta Allergol 1961; 16:463–474.
5. Jemec GBE, Wulf HC. Patient-physician consensus on quality of life in dermatology. Clin Exp Dermatol 1996; 21:177–179.
6. Metze D, Luger T. Nervous system in the skin. In: Freinkel RK, Woodley D (Eds). The biology of the skin, Taylor and Francis 2001; 153–176.
7. Schmelz M, Michael K, Weidner C, et al. Which nerve fibres mediate the axon reflex flare in human skin? Neuroreport 2000; 11:645–648.
8. Scholzen T, Armstrong CA, Bunnett NW, et al. Neuropeptides in the skin: Interactions between the neuroendocrine and the skin immune system. Exp Dermatol 1998; 7:81–96.
9. Roosterman D, Goerge T, Schneider SW, Bunnett NW, Steinhoff M. Neuronal control of skin function: the skin as a neuroimmunoendocrine organ. *Physiol Rev.* 2006; 86(4):1309–1379.
10. Handwerker HO. Sixty years of C-fiber recordings from animal and human skin nerves: Historical notes. Prog Brain Res 1996; 113:39–51.
11. Schmelz M, Schmidt R, Bickel A, et al. Specific C-receptors for itch in human skin. J Neurosci 1997; 17:8003–8008.
12. Kaji A, Shigematsu H, Fujita K, et al. Parasympathetic innervation of cutaneous blood vessels by vasoactive intestinal polypeptide-immunoreactive and acetylcholinesterase-positive nerves: Histochemical and experimental study on rat lower lip. Neuroscience 1988; 25:353.
13. Advenier C, Devillier P. Neurokinins and the skin. Allerg Immunol (Paris) 1993; 25:280–282.
14. Brain SD, Williams TJ. Inflammatory oedema induced by synergism between calcitonin gene-related peptide (CGRP) and mediators of increased vascular permeability. Br J Pharmacol 1985; 86:855–860.
15. Wallengren J, Badendick K, Sundler F, et al. Innervation of the skin of the forearm in diabetic patients: Relation to nerve function. Acta Derm Venereol 1995; 75:37–42.
16. Heyer G, Vogelsang M, Hornstein OP. Acetylcholine is an inducer of itching in patients with atopic dermatitis. J Dermatol 1997; 24:621–625.
17. Schallreuter KU. Epidermal adrenergic signal transduction as part of the neuronal network in the human epidermis. J Investig Dermatol Symp Proc 1997; 2:37–40.
18. Röcken M, Schallreuter K, Renz H, et al. What exactly is "atopy"? Exp Dermatol 1998; 7:97–104.
19. Grando SA. Biological functions of keratinocyte cholinergic receptors. J Investig Dermatol Symp Proc 1997; 2:41–48.
20. Slominski A, Wortsman J. Neuroendocrinology of the skin. Endocr Rev 2000; 21:457–487.
21. Tobin D, Nabarro G, de la Faille HB, et al. Increased number of immunoreactive nerve fibers in atopic dermatitis. J Allergy Clin Immunol 1992; 90:613–622.

22. Sugiura H, Omoto M, Hirota Y, et al. Density and fine structure of peripheral nerves in various skin lesions at atopic dermatitis. Arch Derm Res 1997; 289:125–131.
23. Urashima R, Mihara M. Cutaneous nerves in atopic dermatitis. A histological, immuno-histochemical and electron microscopic study. Virchows Arch 1998; 432:363–370.
24. Pincelli C, Fantini F, Massimi P, et al. Neuropeptides in skin from patients with atopic dermatitis: An immunohistochemical study. Br J Dermatol 1990; 122:745–750.
25. Osterle LS, Cowen T, Rustin MH. Neuropeptides in the skin of patients with atopic dermatitis. Clin Exp Dermatol 1995; 20:462–467.
26. Albers KM, Wright DE, Davis BM. Overexpression of nerve growth factor in epidermis of transgenic mice causes hypertrophy of peripheral nerve system. J Neurosci 1994; 14:1422–1432.
27. Pincelli C, Sevignani C, Manfredini R, et al. Expression and function of nerve growth factor and nerve growth factor receptor on cultured keratinocytes. J Invest Dermatol 1994; 103:13–18.
28. Mihm MC, Soter NA, Dvorak HF, et al. The structure of normal skin and the morphology of atopic eczema. J Invest Dermatol 1976; 67:305–312.
29. Prose PH, Sedlis E. Morphologic and histochemical studies of atopic eczema in infants and children. J Invest Dermatol 1960; 34:149–165.
30. Fjellner B, Hägermark Ö. The influence of the opiate antagonist naloxone on experimental pruritus. Acta Derm Venereol 1984; 64:73–75.
31. Stein C. The control of pain in peripheral tissue by opiods. N Engl J Med 1995; 332:1685–1690.
32. Bernstein JE, Swift RM. Relief of intractable pruritus with naloxone. Arch Dermatol 1979; 115:1366–1367.
33. Summerfield JA. Naloxone modulates the perception of itch in man. Br J Clin Pharmacol 1980; 10:180–183.
34. Metze D, Reimann S, Beissert S, et al. Efficacy and safety of naltrexone, an oral opiate receptor antagonist, in the treatment of pruritus in internal and dermatological diseases. J Am Acad Dermatol 1999; 41:533–539.
35. Königstein H. Experimental study of itch stimuli in animals. Arch Dermatol Syph 1948; 57:829–849.
36. Darsow U, Drzezga A, Fritsch M, et al. Processing of histamine-induced itch in the human cerebral cortex: A correlation analysis with dermal reactions. J Invest Dermatol 2000; 115:1029–1033.
37. Heyer G, Hornstein OP, Handwerker HO. Skin reactions and itch sensation induced by epicutaneous histamine application in atopic dermatitis and controls. J Invest Dermatol 1989; 93:492–496.
38. Lewis T. The Blood Vessels of the Human Skin and Their Responses. London, UK: Shaw and Sons, 1927.
39. Lewis T, Grant RT, Marvin HM. Vascular reactions of the skin to injury. Heart 1929; 14:139–160.
40. Williams DH. Skin temperature reaction to histamine in atopic dermatitis (disseminated neurodermatitis). J Invest Dermatol 1938; 1:119–129.
41. Johnson HH, DeOreo GA, Lascheid WP, et al. Skin histamine levels in chronic atopic dermatitis. J Invest Dermatol 1960; 34:237–238.
42. Juhlin L. Localization and content of histamine in normal and diseased skin. Acta Derm Venereol Suppl (Stockh) 1967; 47:383–391.
43. Ruzicka T, Glück S. Cutaneous histamine levels in histamine releasability from the skin in atopic dermatitis and hyper-IgE-syndrome. Arch Dermatol Res 1983; 275:41–44.
44. Uehara M. Reduced histamine reaction in atopic dermatitis. Arch Dermatol (Chic) 1982; 118:244–245.
45. Heyer G, Koppert W, Martus P, et al. Histamine and cutaneous nociception: Histamine-induced responses in patients with atopic eczema, psoriasis and urticaria. Acta Derm Venereol Suppl (Stockh) 1998; 78:123–126.
46. Heyer GR, Hornstein OP. Recent studies of cutaneous nociception in atopic and non-atopic subject. J Dermatol 1999; 26:77–86.

47. Heyer G, Hornstein OP, Handwerker HO. Reactions to intradermally injected substance P and topically applied mustard oil in atopic dermatitis patients. Acta Derm Venerol Suppl (Stockh) 1991; 71:291–295.
48. Heyer G. Abnormal cutaneous neurosensitivity in atopic skin. Acta Derm Venereol Suppl (Stockh) 1992; 176(suppl.):93–94.
49. Rukwied R, Lischetzki G, McGlone F, et al. Mast cell mediators other than histamine induce pruritus in atopic dermatitis patients: A dermal microdialysis study. Br J Dermatol 2000; 142:1114–1120.
50. Wahlgren CF, Hägermark Ö, Bergström R. The antipruritic effect of a sedative and a non-sedative antihistamine in atopic dermatitis. Br J Dermatol 1990; 122:545–551.
51. Ansel JC, Kaynard AH, Armstrong CA, et al. Skin–nervous system interactions. J Invest Dermatol 1996; 106:198–204.
52. Rukwied R, Heyer G. Cutaneous reactions and sensations after intracutaneous injection of vasoactive intestinal polypeptide and acetylcholine in atopic eczema patients and healthy controls. Arch Dermatol Res 1998; 290:198–204.
53. Heyer G, Ulmer FJ, Schmitz J, et al. Histamine-induced itch and alloknesis (itchy skin) in atopic eczema patients and controls. Acta Derm Venereol 1995; 75:348–352.
54. Wahlgren CF. Pathophysiology of itching in urticaria and atopic dermatitis. Allergy 1992; 47:65–75.
55. Wahlgren CF. Measurement of itch. Semin Dermatol 1995; 14:284.
56. Andoh T, Nagasawa T, Satoh M, et al. Substance P induction of itch-associated response mediated by cutaneous NK1 tachykinin receptors in mice. J Pharmacol Exp Ther 1998; 286:1140–1145.
57. Scholzen TE, Steinhoff M, Bonaccorsi P, et al. Neutral endopeptidase terminates substance P-induced inflammation in allergic contact dermatitis. J Immunol 2001; 166:1285–1291.
58. Fjellner B, Hägermark Ö. Studies on pruritogenic and histamine-releasing effects of some putative peptide neurotransmitters. Acta Derm Venereol Suppl (Stockh) 1981; 61:245–250.
59. Fantini F, Pincelli C, Massimi P, et al. Neuropeptide-like immunoreactivity in skin lesions of atopic dermatitis and psoriasis. Br J Dermatol 1990; 122:838–839.
60. Fjellner B, Hägermark Ö. Potentiation of histamine-induced itch and flare responses in human skin by the encephalin analogue FK 33–824, β-endorphin and morphine. Arch Dermatol Res 1982; 274:29–37.
61. Bernstein JE, Grinzi RA. Butorphanol-induced pruritus antagonized by naloxone. J Am Acad Dermatol 1981; 5:227–228.
62. Pincelli C, Fantini F, Massimi P, et al. Neuropeptide Y-like immunoreactivity in Langerhans cells from patients with atopic dermatitis. Int J Neurosci 1990; 51:219–220.
63. Anand P, Springall DR, Blank MA, et al. Neuropeptides in skin disease: Increased VIP in eczema and psoriasis but not axillary hyperhidrosis. Br J Dermatol 1991; 124:547–549.
64. Pincelli C, Fantini F, Romualdi P, et al. Skin levels of vasoactive intestinal polypeptide in atopic dermatitis. Arch Dermatol Res 1991; 283:230–232.
65. Fantini F, Pincelli C, Romualdi P, et al. Substance P levels are decreased in lesional skin of atopic dermatitis. Exp Dermatol 1992; 1:127–128.
66. Giannetti A, Fantini F, Cimitan A, et al. Vasoactive intestinal polypeptide and substance P in the pathogenesis of atopic dermatitis. Acta Derm Venereol Suppl (Stockh) 1992; 176(suppl.):90–92.
67. Grando SA, Kist DA, Qui M, et al. Human keratinocytes synthesize, secrete and degrade acetylcholine. J Invest Dermatol 1993; 101:32–36.
68. Grando SA, Zelickson BD, Kist DA. Keratinocyte muscarinic acetylcholine reports: Immunolocalisation and partial characterization. J Invest Dermatol 1995; 104:95–100.
69. Scott A. Acetylcholine in normal and disease skin. Br J Dermatol 1962; 74:317–322.
70. Rukwied R, Heyer G. Administration of acetylcholine and vasoactive intestinal polypeptide to atopic eczema patients. Exp Dermatol 1999; 8:39–45.
71. Shelley W, Arthur R. The neurohistology and neurophysiology of the itch sensation in man. Arch Dermatol 1957; 76:296–323.

72. Hägermark Ö, Rajka G, Bergvist U. Experimental itch in human skin elicited by rat mast cell chymase. Acta Derm Venereol 1972; 52:125–128.
73. Bernstein JE. Capsaicin in dermatological disease. Semin Dermatol 1988; 7:304–309.
74. Jarvikallio A, Naukkarinen A, Harvima IT, et al. Quantitative analysis of tryptase- and chymase-containing mast cells in atopic dermatitis and nummular eczema. Br J Dermatol 1997; 136:871–877.
75. Steinhoff M, Vergnolle N, Young SH, et al. Agonists of proteinase-activated receptor 2 induce inflammation by a neurogenic mechanism. Nat Med 2000; 6:151–158.
76. Harvima IT, Naukkarinen A, Harvima RJ, et al. Enzyme- and immunohistochemical localization of mast cell tryptase in psoriatic skin. Arch Dermatol Res 1989; 281:387–391.
77. Naukkarinen A, Harvima IT, Aalto ML, et al. Mast cell tryptase and chymase are potential regulators of neurogenic inflammation in psoriatic skin. Int J Dermatol 1994; 33:366.
78. Damsgaard TE, Olesen AB, Sorensen FB, et al. Mast cells and atopic dermatitis. Stereological quantification of mast cells in atopic dermatitis and normal human skin. Arch Dermatol Res 1997; 289:256–260.
79. Steinhoff M, Corvera CU, Thoma MS, et al. Proteinase-activated receptor-2 in human skin: Tissue distribution and activation of keratinocytes by mast cell tryptase. Exp Dermatol 1999; 8:282–294.
80. Gaspari AA, Lotze MT, Rosenberg SA, et al. Dermatologic changes associated with interleukin 2 administration. JAMA 1987; 258:1624–1629.
81. Wahlgren CF, Scheynius A, Hägermark Ö. Antipruritic effect of oral cyclosporin A in atopic dermatitis. Acta Derm Venereol Suppl (Stockh) 1990; 70:323–329.
82. van Joost T, Stolz E, Heule F. Efficacy of low-dose cyclosporine in severe atopic skin disease. Arch Dermatol 1987; 123:166–167.
83. Wahlgren CF, Tengvall M Linder, Hägermark Ö, et al. Itch and inflammation induced by intradermally injected interleukin-2 in atopic dermatitis patients and healthy subjects. Arch Dermatol Res 1995; 287:572–580.
84. Darsow U, Scharein R, Bromm B, et al. Skin testing of the pruritogenic activity of histamine and cytokines (interleukin-2 and tumor nekrosis factor-alpha) at the dermal–epidermal junction. Br J Dermatol 1997; 137:415–417.
85. Martin HA. Bradykinin potentiates the chemoresponsiveness of rat cutaneous C-fibre polymodal nociceptors to interleukin-2. Arch Physiol Biochem 1996; 104:229–238.
86. Cremer B, Heimann A, Dippel E, et al. Pruritogenic effects of mitogen stimulated peripheral blood mononuclear cells in atopic eczema. Acta Derm Venerol Suppl (Stockh) 1995; 75:426–428.
87. Grothe C, Heese K, Meisinger C, et al. Expression of interleukin-6 and its receptor in the sciatic nerve and cultured Schwann cells: Relation to 18-kD fibroblast growth factor-2. Brain Res 2000; 885:172–181.
88. Nordlind K, Chin LB, Ahmed AA, et al. Immunohistochemical localization of interleukin-6-like immunoreactivity to peripheral nerve-like structures in normal and inflamed human skin. Arch Dermatol Res 1996; 288:431–435.
89. Lippert U, Hoer A, Möller A, et al. Role of antigen-induced cytokine released in atopic pruritus. Int Arch Allergy Immunol 1998; 116:36–39.
90. Kanai H, Nagashima A, Hirakata E, et al. The effect of azelastin hydrochloride on pruritus and leukotriene B4 in hemodialysis patients. Life Sci 1995; 57:207–213.
91. Wahlgren CF, Hägermark Ö, Bergstrom R. Patients' perception of itch induced by histamine, compound 48/80 and wool fibres in atopic dermatitis. Acta Derm Venereol 1991; 71:488–494.
92. Sticherling M, Bornscheuer E, Schröder JM, et al. Immunohistochemical studies on NAP-1/Il-8 in contact eczema and atopic dermatitis. Arch Dermatol Res 1992; 284:82–85.
93. Kimata H, Lindley I. Detection of plasma interleukin-8 in atopic dermatitis. Arch Dis Child 1994; 70:119–122.
94. Hatano Y, Katagiri K, Takayasu S. Increased levels in vivo of mRNAs for IL-8 and macrophage inflammatory protein-1 alpha (MIP-1 alpha), but not of RANTES mRNA

in peripheral blood mononuclear cells of patients with atopic dermatitis (AD). Clin Exp Immunol 1999; 117:237–243.

95. Yousefi S, Hemmann S, Weber M, et al. IL-8 is expressed by human peripheral blood eosinophils. Evidence for incresased secretion in asthma. J Immunol 1995; 154:5481–5490.

96. Reinhold U, Kukel S, Brzoska J, et al. Systemic interferon gamma treatment in severe atopic dermatitis. J Am Acad Dermatol 1993; 29:58–63.

97. Stevens SR, Hanifin JM, Hamilton T, et al. Long-term effectiveness and safety of recombinant human interferon gamma therapy for atopic dermatitis despite unchanged serum IgE levels. Arch Dermatol 1998; 134:799–804.

98. Reinhold U, Wehrmann W, Kukel S, et al. Evidence that defective interferon-gamma production in atopic dermatitis patients is due to intrinsic abnormalities. Clin Exp Immunol 1990; 79:374–379.

99. Grewe M, Vogelsang K, Ruzicka T, et al. Neurotrophin-4 production by human epidermal keratinocytes: Increased expression in atopic dermatitis. J Invest Dermatol 2000; 114:1108–1112.

100. Velaquez JR, Lacy P, Moqbel R. Replenishment of RANTES mRNA expression in activated eosinophils from atopic asthmatics. Immunology 2000; 99:591–599.

101. Akdis CA, Akdis M, Trautmann A, et al. Immune regulation in atopic dermatitis. Curr Opin Immunol 2000; 12:641–646.

102. Yamamoto J, Adachi Y, Onoue Y, et al. CD 30 expression on circulation memory CD4+ T cells as a Th2-dominated situation in patients with atopic dermatitis. Allergy 2000; 55:1011–1018.

103. Czarnetzki BM, Csato M. Comparative studies on human eosinophil migration towards platelet-activating factor and leukotriene B4. Int Arch Allergy Appl Immunol 1989; 88:191–193.

104. Sigal CE, Valone FH, Holtzmann MJ, et al. Preferential human eosinophil chemotactic activity of the platelet-activating factor (PAF) 1-0-hexadecyl-2-acetyl-sn-glyceryl-3-phosphocholine (AGEPC). J Clin Immunol 1987; 7:179–184.

105. Weller PF, Lee CW, Foster DW, et al. Generation and metabolism of 5-lipoxygenase pathway leukotriens by human eosinophils: Predominant production of leukotriene C4. Proc Natl Acad Sci U S A 1983; 80:7626–7630.

106. Lebel B, Venencie PY, Saurat JH, et al. Anti-IgE induced histamine release from basophils in children with atopic dermatitis. Acta Derm Venereol Suppl (Stockh) 1980; 92(suppl.):57–59.

107. von der Helm D, Ring J, Dorsch W. Comparison of histamine release and prostaglandin E2 production of human basophils in atopic and normal individuals. Arch Dermatol Res 1987; 279:536–542.

108. Bull HA, Courtney PF, Bunker CB, et al. Basophil mediator release in atopic dermatitis. J Invest Dermatol 1993; 100:305–309.

109. Fjellner B, Hägermark Ö. Experimental pruritus evoked by platelet activating factor (PAF-acether) in human skin. Acta Derm Venereol Suppl (Stockh) 1985; 65:409–412.

110. Abeck D, Andersson T, Grosshans E, et al. Topical application of a platelet-activating factor (PAF) antagonist in atopic dermatitis. Acta Derm Venereol Suppl (Stockh) 1997; 77:449–451.

111. Andoh T, Kuraishi Y. Intradermal leukotriene B4, but not prostaglandin E2, induces itch-associated responses in mice. Eur J Pharmacol 1998; 353:93–96.

112. Miyoshi M, Sakurai T, Kodama S. Clinical evaluation of urinary leukotriene E4 levels in children with atopic dermatitis. Arerugi 1999; 48:1148–1152.

113. Carruci JA, Washenik K, Weinstein A, et al. The leukotriene antagonist zafirlukast as a therapeutic agent for atopic dermatitis. Arch Dermatol 1998; 134:785–786.

114. Zabawski EJ, Kahn MA, Gregg LJ. Treatment of atopic dermatitis with zafirlukast. Dermatol Online J 1999; 5:10.

115. Woodmanse DP, Simon RA. A pilot study examining the role of zileuton in atopic dermatitis. Ann Allergy Asthma Immunol 1999; 83:548–552.

116. Bernstein JE, Parish LC, Rapaport M, et al. Effects of topically applied capsaicin on moderate and severe psoriasis vulgaris. J Am Acad Dermatol 1986; 15:504–507.

117. Ellis CN, Berberian B, Sulica VI, et al. A double-blind evaluation of topical capsaicin in pruritic psoriasis. J Am Acad Dermatol 1993; 29:438–442.
118. Caterina MJ, Schumacher MA, Tominaga M, et al. The capsaicin receptor: A heat-activated ion channel in the pain pathway. Nature 1997; 389:816–824.
119. Dray A. Neuropharmacological mechanisms of capsaicin and related substances. Biochem Pharmacol 1992; 44:611–615.
120. Reimann S, Luger T, Metze D. Topische Anwendung von Capsaicin in der Dermatologiezur Therapie von Juckreiz und Schmerz. Hautarzt 2000; 51:164–172.
121. Ständer S, Luger T, Metze D. Treatment of prurigo nodularis with topical capsaicin. J Am Acad Dermatol, 2001; 44:471–478.
122. Leung DV, Schneeberger EE, Gerha RS. The presence of IgE in macrophages and dendritic cells infiltrating into the skin lesions of atopic dermatitis. Clin Immunol Immunopathol 1987; 42:328.
123. Summerfield JA. Pain, itch and endorphins. Br J Dermatol 1981; 105:725–726.
124. Hägermark Ö. Peripheral and central mediators of itch. Skin Pharmacol 1992; 5:1–8.
125. Penning JP, Samson B, Baxter AD. Reversal of epidural morphine-induced respiratory depression and pruritus with nalbuphine. Can J Anaesth 1988; 35:559–604.
126. Bergasa NV, Alling DW, Talbot TL, et al. Effects of naloxone infusions in patients with the pruritus of cholestasis. A double-blind, randomized, controlled trial. Ann Intern Med 1995; 123:161–167.
127. Metze D, Reimann S, Luger TA. Effective treatment of pruritus with naltrexone, an orally active opiate antagonist. Ann N Y Acad Sci 1999; 885:430–432.
128. Heyer GR, Dotzer M, Diepgen TL, et al. Opiate and H1 antagonsits effects on histamine induced pruritus and alloknesis. Pain 1997; 73:239–243.
129. Georgala S, Schulpis KH, Papaconstantinou ED, et al. Raised β-endorphin serum levels in children with atopic dermatitis and pruritus. J Dermatol Sci 1994; 8:125–128.
130. Monroe EW. Efficacy and safety of nalmefene in patients with severe pruritus caused by chronic urticaria and atopic dermatitis. J Am Acad Dermatol 1989; 21:135–136.
131. Banerji D, Fox R, Seleznick M, et al. Controlled antipruritic trial of nalmefene in chronic urticaria and atopic dermatitis (abst.). J Allergy Clin Immunol 1988; 81:252.
132. Burch JR, Harrison PV. Opiates, sleep and itch. Clin Exp Dermatol 1988; 13:418–419.
133. Rajka G. Essential Aspects of Atopic Dermatitis. Berling: Springer-Verlag, 1989; 57–69.
134. Hanifin JM. Pharmacophysiology of atopic dermatitis. Clin Rev Allergy 1986; 4:43–65.
135. Morren MA, Przybilla B, Bamelis M, et al. Atopic dermatitis: Triggering factors. J Am Acad Dermatol 1994; 31:467–473.
136. Werner Y. The water content of the stratum corneum in patients with atopic dermatits. Measurement with the corneometer CM 420. Acta Derm Venereol Suppl (Stockh) 1986; 66:281–284.
137. Werner Y, Lindberg M, Forslind B. Membrane-coating granules in "dry" non-eczematous skin of patients with atopic dermatitis. A quantitative electron microscopic study. Acta Derm Venereol Suppl (Stockh) 1987; 67:385–390.
138. Fartasch M, Diepgen TL. The barrier function in atopic dry skin. Disturbance of membrane-coating granule exocytosis and formation of epidermal lipids? Acta Derm Venereol Suppl (Stockh) 1992; 176(suppl.):26–31.
139. Hägermark Ö. The pathophysiology of itch. In: Handbook of Atopic Eczema. Berlin, Germany: Springer Verlag, 1991; 278–286.
140. Wahlgren CF. Itch and atopic dermatitis. J Dermatol 1999; 26:770–779.
141. Yoshiike T, Aikawa Y, Sindhvananda J, et al. Skin barrier defect in atopic dermatitis: Increased permeability of the stratum corneum using dimethyl dulfoxide and theophylline. J Dermatol Sci 1993; 5:92–96.
142. Beltrani VS. The clinical spectrum of atopic dermatitis. J Allergy Clin Immunol 1999; 104:S87–S98.
143. Hanifin JM. Basic and clinical aspects of atopic dermatitis. Ann Allergy 1984; 52:386–393.
144. Rovensky J, Saxl O. Differences in the dynamics of sweat secretion in atopic children. J Invest Dermatol 1964; 43:171–176.

145. Graham DT, Wolf S. The relation of eczema to attitude and vascular reactions of the human skin. J Lab Clin Med 1953; 42:238.
146. Bendsoe N, Bjornberg A, Asnes H. Itching from wool fibres in atopic dermatitis. Contact Dermatitis 1987; 17:21–22.
147. Ekblom A, Fjellner B, Hansson P. The influence of mechanical vibratory stimulation and transcutaneous electrical nerve stimulation on experimental pruritus induced by histamine. Acta Physiol Scand 1984; 122:361–367.
148. Fisher AA. Nonallergic "itch" and "prickly" sensation to wool fibers in atopic and nonatopic persons. Cutis 1996; 58:323–324.
149. Hogan D, Danaker C, Maibach HI. Contact dermatitis risk factors and rehabilitation. Semin Dermatol 1994; 31:467–473.
150. Sicherer SH, Sampson HA. Food hypersensitivity and atopic dermatitis: Pathophysiology, epidemiology, diagnosis, and management. J Allergy Clin Immunol 1999; 104:114–122.
151. Griesemer RD. Emotionally triggered disease in a dermatological practice. Psychiatr Ann 1978; 8:49–56.
152. Niemeier V, Kupfer J, Gieler U. Observations during an itch-inducing lecture. Dermatol Psychosom 2000; 1:15–18.
153. Fjellner B, Arnetz BB, Eneroth P, et al. Pruritus during standardized mental stress. Relationship to psychoneuroendocrine and metabolic parameters. Acta Derm Venerol 1985; 65:199–205.
154. Fjellner B, Arnetz BB. Psychological predictors of pruritus during mental stress. Acta Derm Venereol Suppl (Stockh) 1985; 65:504–508.
155. Metze D, Reimann S, Luger T. Juckreiz-Symptom oder Krankheit. Berlin, Germany: Springer Verlag, 1997:77–86.
156. Koblenzer CS. Psychologic and Psychiatric Aspects of Itching. New York, NY: McGraw-Hill, 1994:347–365.
157. Gupta MA, Gupta AK, Schork NJ, et al. Depression modulates pruritus perception. A study of pruritus in psoriasis, atopic dermatitis and chronic idiopathic urticaria. Psychosom Med 1994; 56:36–40.
158. Cormia FE. Experimental histamine pruritus I. Influence of physical and psychological factors on threshold reactivity. J Invest Dermatol 1952; 19:21–34.
159. Arnetz BB, Fjellner B, Eneroth P, et al. Endokrine and dermatological concomitants of mental stress. Acta Derm Venereol Suppl (Stockh) 1991; 156:9–12.
160. Buhk H, Muthny FA. Psychophysiologische und psychoneuroimmunologische Ergebnisse zur Neurodermitis. Hautarzt 1997; 48:5–11.
161. Hermanns N, Scholz OB. Kognitive Einflüsse auf einen histamininduzierten Juckreiz und Quaddelbildung bei der atopischen Dermatitis. Verhaltensmod Verhaltensmed 1992; 13:171–194.
162. Ehlers A, Stangier U, Gieler U. Treatment of atopic dermatitis: A comparison of psychological and dermatological approaches to relapse prevention. J Consult Clin Psychol 1995; 63:624–635.
163. Shenefelt PD. Hypnosis in dermatology. Arch Dermatol 2000; 136:393–399.
164. Garg A, Chren MM, Sands LP, et al. Psychological stress pertubs epidermal permeability barrier homeostasis. Arch Dermatol 2001; 137:53–59.
165. Singh LK, Pang X, Alexacos N, et al. Acute immobilization stress triggers skin mast cell degranulation via corticotropin relasining hormone, neurotensin, and substance P: A link to neurogenic skin disorders. Brain Behav Immun 1999; 13:225–239.
166. Münzel K, Schandry R. Atopisches Ekzem: Psychophysiologische Reaktivität unter standarisierter Belastung. Hautarzt 1990; 41:606–611.
167. Schwarzer A, Scholz OB. Auswirkungen unterschiedlicher Aktivierungsbedingungen auf Patienten mit atopischer Dermatits. Verhaltensmod Verhaltensmed 1990; 11:45–58.
168. Graham DT, Wolf S. The relation of eczema to attitude and to vascular reactions of the human skin. J Lab Clin Med 1953; 42:238–254.
169. Leung DY. The immunologic basis of atopic dermatits. Clin Rev Allergy 1993; 11:447–469.

170. Heyer G, Magerl W. Pruritus Als Leit- Und Leidsymptom Beim Atopischen Ekzem-Patienten—Klinische Und Neurophysiologische Untersuchungen. Berlin, Germany: BMV, 1991:145–159.
171. Bernhard JD. Pruritus in skin diseases. New York, NY: McGraw-Hill, 1994:44–48.
172. Goldblum RW, Piper WN. Artificial lichenification produced by a scratching machine. J Invest Dermatol 1954; 22:405–415.
173. Endo K, Sumitsuji H, Fukuzumi T, et al. Evaluation of scratch movements by a new scratch-monitor to analyze nocturnal itching in atopic dermatitis. Acta Derm Venereol Suppl (Stockh) 1997; 77:432–435.
174. Ebata T, Aizawa H, Kamide R, et al. The characteristics of nocturnal scratching in adults with atopic dermatitis. Br J Dermatol 1999; 141:82–86.
175. Aoki T, Kushimoto H, Kobayashi E, et al. Computer analysis of nocturnal scratch in atopic dermatitis. Acta Derm Venereol Suppl (Stockh) 1980; 92(suppl.):33–37.
176. Heubeck B, Schonberger A, Hornstein OP. Sind Verschiebungen des zirkadianen Cortisolrhytmus ein endokrines Symptom des atopischen Ekzems? Hautarzt 1988; 39:12–17.
177. Schwarz W, Birau N, Hornstein OP, et al. Alterations of melantonin secretion in atopic dermatitis. Acta Derm Venereol Suppl (Stockh) 1988; 68:224–229.
178. Felix R, Shuster S. A new method for the measurement of itch and the response to treatment. Br J Dermatol 1975; 93:303–311.
179. Jordan JM, Whitlock FA. Emotinons and the skin: The conditioning of scratch responses in cases of atopic dermatitis. Br J Dermatol 1972; 86:574–585.
180. Ginsburg IH, Prystowsky JH, Kornfeld DS, et al. Role of emotional factors in adults with atopic dermatits. Int J Dermatol 1993; 32:656–660.
181. Musaph H. Itching and Scratching: Psychodynamics in Dermatology. Philadelphia, PA: FA Davis Co, 1964.
182. Charleswoth EN. Practical approaches to the treatment of atopic dermatitis. Allergy Proc 1994; 15:269–274.
183. Bueller HA, Bernhard JD. Review of pruritus therapy. Dermatol Nurs 1998; 10:101–107.
184. van der Schaar WW, Lamberts H. Scratching for the itch in eczema; a psychodermatologic approach. Ned Tijdschr Geneeskd 1997; 141:2049–2051.
185. Melin L, Frederiksen T, Norén P, et al. Behavioural treatment of scratching in patients with atopic dermatitis. Br J Dermatol 1986; 115:467–474.
186. Hornstein OP, Gall K, Salzer B, et al. Controlled physical exercise in patients with chronic neurodermitis. Dtsch Zeitschr f Sportmed 1998; 49:39–45.
187. Fruhstorfer H, Hermanns M, Latzke L. The effects of thermal stimulation on clinical and experimental itch. Pain 1986; 24:259–269.
188. Vieluf D, Matthias C, Ring J. Trockene juckende Haut—ihre Behandlung mit einer neuen Polidocanol-Harnstoff-Zubereitung. Dermatological 1992; 169:53–59.
189. Weishaar E, Foster C, Dotzer M, et al. Experimentally induced pruritus and cutaneous reactions with topical antihistamine and local analgetics in atopic eczema. Skin Pharmacol 1997; 10:183–190.
190. Lundeberg T, Bondesson L, Thomas M. Effect of acupuncture on experimental induced itch. Br J Dermatol 1987; 117:771–777.
191. Bjorna H, Kaada B. Succesful treatment of itching and atopic eczema by transcutaneous nerve stimulation. Acupunct Electrother Res 1987; 12:101–112.
192. Nilsson HJ, Levinsson A, Schouenborg J. Cutaneous fiels stimulation (CFS): A new powerful method to combat itch. Pain 1997; 71:49–55.
193. Thoda C, Sugahara H, Kuraishi Y, et al. Inhibitory effect of Byakko-ka-ninjin-to on itch in a mouse model of atopic dermatitis. Phytother Res 2000; 14:192–194.
194. Onda H. The treatment of atopic dermatitis by Kampo medicines. J Tradit Med 1997; 14:245–251.
195. Hanifin JM, Ling MR, Langley R, et al. Tacrolimus ointment for the treatment of atopic dermatitis in adult patients. Part I, efficacy. J Am Acad Dermatol 2001; 44:S28–S38.
196. Jekler J, Larkö O. Combined UVA-UVB versus UVB phototherapy for atopic dermatitis: A paired-comparison study. J Am Acad Dermatol 1990; 22:49–53.
197. Luger T, van Leent EJM, Graeber M, et al. SDZ ASM 981: An emerging safe and effective treatment for atopic dermatitis. Br J Dermatol 2001; 44:788–794.

198. Hoare C, Li Wan Po A, Williams H. Systemic review of treatment for atopic eczema. Health Technol Assess (Rockv) 2000; 4:1–191.
199. Aliaga A, Rodriguez M, Armijo M, et al. Double-blind study of prednicarbate versus flucortin butyl ester in atopic dermatitis. Int J Dermatol 1996; 35:131–132.
200. Maloney JM, Morman MR, Stewart DM, et al. Clobetasol propionate emollient 0.05% in the treatment of atopic dermatitis. Int J Dermatol 1998; 37:128–144.
201. Yosipovitch G, Szolar C, Hui XY,et al. High-potency topical corticosteroid rapidly dereases histamine-induced itch but not thermal sensation and pain in human beeings. J Am Acad Dermatol 1996; 35:118–120.
202. Wahlgren CF. Itch and atopic dermatitis: Clinical and experimental studies. Acta Derm Venereol Suppl (Stockh) 1991, 165:1–53.
203. DeRie MA, Meinardi MM, Bos JD. Lack of efficacy of topical cyclosporin A in atopic dermatitis and allergic contact dermatitis. Acta Derm Venereol Suppl (Stockh) 1991; 71:452–454.
204. Lauerma AI, Maibach HI, Granlund H, et al. Inhibition of contact allergy reactions by topical FK 506. Lancet 1992; 340:556.
205. Fleischer AB. Treatment of atopic dermatitis: Role of tacrolimus ointment as a topical noncorticosteroidal therapy. J Allergy Clin Immunol 1999; 104:S126–S130.
206. Paller A, Eichenfield LF, Leung DY, et al. A 12-week study of tacrolimus ointment for the treatment of atopic dermatitis in pediatric patients. J Am Acad Dermatol 2001; 44:S47–S57.
207. Kang S, Lcuky AW, Pariser D, et al. Long-term safety and efficacy of tacrolimus ointment for the treatment of atopic dermatitis in children. J Am Acad Dermatol 2001; 44:S58–S64.
208. Boguniewicz M, Fiedler VC, Raimer S, et al. A randomized, vesicle-controlled trial of tacrolimus ointment for treatment of atopic dermatitis in children. Pediatric Tacrolimus Study Group. J Allergy Clin Immunol 1998; 102:637–644.
209. Ruzicka T, Bieber T, Schöpf E, et al. A short-term trial of tracolimus ointment for atopic dermatitis. N Engl J Med 1997; 337:816–821.
210. Grassberger M, Baumruker T, Enz A, et al. A novel anti-inflammatory drug, SDZ ASM 981, for the treatment of skin diseases: In vitro pharmacology. Br J Dermatol 1999; 141:264–273.
211. Van Leent EJ, Graber M, Thurston M, et al. Effectiveness of the ascomycin macrolactam SDZ ASM 981 in the topical treatment of atopic dermatitis. Arch Dermatol 1998; 134:805–809.
212. Grundmann-Kollmann M, Korting HC, Behrens S, et al. Successful treatment of severe refractory atopic dermatits with mycophenolate mofetil. Br J Dermatol 1999; 141: 175–176.
213. Neuber K, Schwartz I, Itschert G, et al. Treatment of atopic eczema with oral mycophenolate mofetil. Br J Dermatol 2000; 143:385–391.
214. Hansen ER, Buus S, Deleuran M, et al. Treatment of atopic dermatitis with mycophenolate mofetil. Br J Dermatol 2000; 143:1324–1326.
215. Hanifin JM, Schneider LC, Leung DY, et al. Recombinant interferon gamma therapy for atopic dermatitis. J Am Acad Dermatol 1993; 28:189–197.
216. Jang JG, Yang JK, Lee HJ, et al. Clinical improvement and immunohistochemical findings in severe atopic dermatitis treated with interferon gamma. J Am Acad Dermatol 2000; 42:1033–1040.
217. Watanabe T, Kuroda Y. The effect of a newly developed ointment containing eicosapentaenoic acid and docosahexaenoic acid in the treatment of atopic dermatitis. J Med Invest 1999; 46:173–177.
218. Henz BM, Metzenauer P, Keefe EO, et al. Differential effects of new-generation H1-receptor antagonists in pruritic dermatoses. Allergy 1998; 53:180–183.
219. Berth-Jones J, Graham-Brown RAC. Failure of terenadine in relieving the pruritus of atopic dermatitis. Br J Dermatol 1989; 121:635–637.
220. Doherty V, Sylvester DGH, Kennedy CTC, et al. Treatment of itching in atopic eczema with antihistamines with a low sedative profile. Br Med J 1989; 298:96.
221. Hannuksela M, Kalimo K, Lammintausta K, et al. Dose ranging study: Cetirizine in the treatment of atopic dermatitis in adults. Ann Allergy 1993; 70:127–133.

222. Luger TA, Ruzicka T. Therapie juckender Dermatosen. Stuttgart: Georg Thieme Verlag, 1999; 51–72.
223. Klein PA, Clark RAF. An evidence-based review of the efficacy of antihistamines in reliefing pruritus in atopic dermatitis. Arch Dermatol 1999; 135:1522–1525.
224. Ebata T, Izumi H, Aizawa H, et al. Effects of nitrazepam on nocturnal scratching in adults with atopic dermatitis: A double-blind placebo-controlled crossover study. Br J Dermatol 1998; 138:631–634.
225. Sabroe RA, Kennedy CT, Archer CB. The effects of topical doxepin on responses to histamine, substance P, and prostaglandin E2 in human skin. Br J Dermatol 1997; 137:386–390.
226. Drake LA, Millikan LE; and the Doxepin Study Group. The antipruritic effect of 5% doxepin cream in patients with eczematous dermatitis. Arch Dermatol 1995; 131:1403–1408.
227. Shelley WB, Shelley ED, Talanin NY. Self-potentiating allergic contact dermatitis caused by doxepin hydrochloride cream. J Am Acad Dermatol 1996; 34:143–144.
228. Tamaki K. Antipruritic effect of macrolide antibiotics. J Dermatol 2000; 27:66–67.
229. Kimata H. High dose gammaglobin treatment for atopic dermatitis. Arch Dis Child 1998; 70:107–113.
230. Gelfand EW, Landwehr LP, Esterl B, et al. Intravenous immune globulin: An alternative therapy in steroid-dependent allergic diseases. Clin Exp Immunol 1996; 104(suppl.): 61–66.
231. Mills LB, Mordan LJ, Roth HL, et al. Treatment of severe atopic dermatitis by topical immune modulation using dinitrochlorobenzene. J Am Acad Dermatol 2000; 42:687–689.
232. Yoshizawa Y, Matusi H, Izaki S, et al. Topical dinitrochlorobenzene therapy in the treatment of refractory atopic dermatitis: Systemic immunotherapy. J Am Acad Dermatol 2000; 42:258–262.
233. Hanifin JM, Chan SC, Cheng JB, et al. Type 4 phosphodiesterase inhibitors have clinical and in vitro anti-inflammatory effects in atopic dermatitis. J Invest Dermatol 1996; 107:51–56.
234. Dijkstra D, Stark H, Chazot PL, et al. Human inflammatory dendritic epidermal cells express a functional histamine H4 receptor. J Invest Dermatol 2008; 128:1696–1703.
235. Roßbach K, Wendorff S, Sander K, et al. Histamine H(4) receptor antagonism reduces hapten-induced scratching behaviour but not inflammation. Exp Dermatol 2008 [Epub ahead of print].
236. Ikoma A, Steinhoff M, Ständer S, et al. The neurobiology of itch. Nat Rev Neurosci 2006; 7:535–547.
237. Johanek LM, Meyer RA, Hartke T, et al. Psychophysical and physiological evidence for parallel afferent pathways mediating the sensation of itch. J Neurosci 2007; 27:7490–7497.
238. Lonne-Rahm SB, Rickberg H, El-Nour H, et al. Neuroimmune mechanisms in patients with atopic dermatitis during chronic stress. J Eur Acad Dermatol Venereol 2008; 22:11–18.
239. Schneider G, Ständer S, Burgmer M, et al. Significant differences in central imaging of histamine-induced itch between atopic dermatitis and healthy subjects. Eur J Pain 2008; 12:834–841.
240. Wessler I, Reinheimer T, Kilbinger H, et al. Increased acetylcholine levels in skin biopsies of patients with atopic dermatitis. Life Sci 2003; 72:2169–2172.
241. Kindt F, Wiegand S, Niemeier V, et al. Reduced expression of nicotinic alpha subunits 3, 7, 9 and 10 in lesional and nonlesional atopic dermatitis skin but enhanced expression of alpha subunits 3 and 5 in mast cells. Br J Dermatol 2008 Jul 29 [Epub ahead of print].
242. Ikoma A, Rukwied R, Ständer S, et al. Neurophysiology of pruritus: Interaction of itch and pain. Arch Dermatol 2003; 139:1475–1478.
243. Steinhoff M, Neisius U, Ikoma A, et al. Proteinase-activated receptor-2 mediates itch: A novel pathway for pruritus in human skin. J Neurosci 2003; 23:6176–6180.

244. Shpacovitch VM, Brzoska T, Buddenkotte J, et al. Agonists of proteinase-activated receptor 2 induce cytokine release and activation of nuclear transcription factor kappaB in human dermal microvascular endothelial cells. J Invest Dermatol 2002; 118:380–385.
245. Bender BG, Ballard R, Canono B, et al. Disease severity, scratching, and sleep quality in patients with atopic dermatitis. J Am Acad Dermatol 2008; 58:415–420.
246. Takaoka A, Arai I, Sugimoto M, et al. Expression of IL-31 gene transcripts in NC/Nga mice with atopic dermatitis. Eur J Pharmacol 2005; 516:180–181.
247. Takaoka A, Arai I, Sugimoto M, et al. Involvement of IL-31 on scratching behavior in NC/Nga mice with atopic-like dermatitis. Exp Dermatol 2006; 15:161–167.
248. Sonkoly E, Muller A, Lauerma AI, et al. IL-31: A new link between T cells and pruritus in atopic skin inflammation. J Allergy Clin Immunol 2006; 117:411–417.
249. Kanda N, Koike S, Watanabe S. Prostaglandin E2 enhances neurotrophin-4 production via EP3 receptor in human keratinocytes. J Pharmacol Exp Ther 2005; 315:796–804.
250. Groneberg DA, Serowka F, Peckenschneider N, et al. Gene expression and regulation of nerve growth factor in atopic dermatitis mast cells and the human mast cell line-1. J Neuroimmunol 2005; 161:87–92.
251. Solomon A, Aloe L, Pe'er J, et al. Nerve growth factor is preformed in and activates human peripheral blood eosinophils. J Allergy Clin Immunol 1998; 102:454–460.
252. Dou YC, Hagströmer L, Emtestam L, et al. Increased nerve growth factor and its receptors in atopic dermatitis: An immunohistochemical study. Arch Dermatol Res 2006; 298:31–37.
253. Toyoda M, Nakamura M, Makino T, et al. Nerve growth factor and substance P are useful plasma markers of disease activity in atopic dermatitis. Br J Dermatol 2002; 147:71–79.
254. Takano N, Sakurai T, Kurachi M. Effects of anti-nerve growth factor antibody on symptoms in the NC/Nga mouse, an atopic dermatitis model. J Pharmacol Sci 2005; 99:277–286.
255. Tanaka A, Matsuda H. Expression of nerve growth factor in itchy skins of atopic NC/NgaTnd mice. J Vet Med Sci 2005; 67:915–919.
256. Johansson O, Liang Y, Marcusson JA, et al. Eosinophil cationic protein- and eosinophil-derived neurotoxin/eosinophil protein X-immunoreactive eosinophils in prurigo nodularis. Arch Dermatol Res 2000; 292:371–378.
257. Raap U, Goltz C, Deneka N, et al. Brain-derived neurotrophic factor is increased in atopic dermatitis and modulates eosinophil functions compared with that seen in nonatopic subjects. J Allergy Clin Immunol 2005; 115:1268–1275.
258. Siepmann D, Luger TA, Ständer S. Antipruritic effect of cyclosporine microemulsion in prurigo nodularis: Results of a case series. JDDG 2008; 6:94–96.
259. Senba E, Katanosaka K, Yajima H, et al. The immunosuppressant FK506 activates capsaicin- and bradykinin-sensitive DRG neurons and cutaneous C-fibers. Neurosci Res 2004; 50:257–262.
260. Ständer S, Ständer H, Seeliger S, et al. Topical pimecrolimus (SDZ ASM 981) and tacrolimus (FK 506) transiently induces neuropeptide release and mast cell degranulation in murine skin. Br J Dermatol 2007; 156:1020–1026.
261. Ständer S, Schmelz M, Metze D, et al. Distribution of cannabinoid receptor 1 (CB1) and 2 (CB2) on sensory nerve fibers and adnexal structures in human skin. J Dermatol Sci 2005; 38:177–188.
262. Farquhar-Smith WP, Rice AS. A novel neuroimmune mechanism in cannabinoid-mediated attenuation of nerve growth factor-induced hyperalgesia. Anesthesiology 2003; 99:1391–1401.
263. Eberlein B, Eicke C, Reinhardt HW, et al. Adjuvant treatment of atopic eczema: assessment of an emollient containing N-palmitoylethanolamine (ATOPA study). J Eur Acad Dermatol Venereol 2008; 22:73–82.

12 Role of Aeroallergens in Atopic Eczema: Diagnostic Relevance of the Atopy Patch Test

Ulf Darsow and Johannes Ring

Department of Dermatology and Allergy Biederstein, Technische Universität München and Division of Environmental Dermatology and Allergy Helmholtz Center/TUM, München, Germany

ROLE OF AEROALLERGENS

Atopic eczema (AE, atopic dermatitis, eczema) is characterized by a combination of clinical features including pruritus and a typically age-related distribution and skin morphology (1,2). Patients with AE in the meaning of the World Allergy Organization (WAO) definition (3), formerly called "extrinsic" type, all have evidence for elevated levels of total and/or allergen-specific immunoglobulin E (IgE), frequently directed against aeroallergens (e.g., house dust mite) and food allergens. These allergens produce flares in some patients with AE, but not in all sensitized individuals. Apart from the long-standing clinical reports and experience on single cases, flares can be experimentally induced, as has been shown with bronchial house dust mite exposure (4). Although the percentage of aeroallergen-responsive eczema cases in the total eczema population is not known, a recent German population–based panel study established a significant association of eczema severity and the regional grass pollen count in a subgroup of 46% of children with eczema investigated for seasonal changes (5). The association was stronger in children sensitized to grass pollen.

Parallels of AE with bronchial asthma (extrinsic) and allergic rhinoconjunctivitis in the role of atopy, laboratory analyses, and epidemiology suggest a pathophysiologic significance of aeroallergens also in AE patients. Correlation of AE disease activity with total IgE serum levels has been described repeatedly (6–8). In a cross-sectional study of 2200 children in East Germany by Schäfer et al. (9), the prevalence of sensitization to grass pollen, birch pollen, Cladosporium, *Dermatophagoides pteronyssinus*, and cat was higher in AE than that in controls (OR 2.9–8.8). Linear correlation of AE severity and sensitization was most pronounced for indoor allergens.

Aeroallergen avoidance, especially with regard to house dust mites, can result in marked improvement of skin lesions (10–13). Studies in this field are difficult due to the influence of remarkable placebo effects and interfering other allergens like animal dander or food. Consequently, a close look on the investigated population and inclusion criteria applied is mandatory to interpret seemingly contradictory outcomes (14,15).

Therapeutical consequences of the diagnosis of allergy in AE are currently based upon avoidance strategies, thus the relevance of (often multiple) IgE-mediated sensitizations in patients with AE for the skin disease has to be evaluated. Despite these clinical aspects, the role of allergy in eliciting and maintaining the

TABLE 1   Atopy Patch Test Methods, According to Various Methodological Studies

Selection of allergens: allergen-specific individual history, eczema pattern, and routine diagnosis skin-prick test and specific IgE
Patients should be in remission phase of eczema
Lyophilized aeroallergens (house dust mite, cat dander, grass, and birch pollen) are used
Allergen doses: 5000–7000 PNU/g or 200 IR/g as a result of dose-finding trials
As vehicle, petrolatum in Large Finn Chambers gave best results
Application for 48 hr on clinically uninvolved, not pretreated back skin (no tape stripping)
Evaluation is done after 48 and 72 hr and documented according to ICDRG guidelines or ETFAD key[a]

[a]See Table 4.
Sources: Adapted from Refs. 26–28.

eczematous skin lesions has been discussed (14), partially due to a lack of specificity of the classic tests for IgE-mediated hypersensitivity, skin-prick test, and measurement of specific serum-IgE. On the other hand, the most recent encouraging results of specific immunotherapy studies in AE patients with IgE-mediated allergies represent another line of evidence for the role of aeroallergens in AE. These aspects are discussed elsewhere in this volume.

CLINICAL EVIDENCE AND DIAGNOSIS USING ATOPY PATCH TESTS

An epicutaneous patch test with allergens known to elicit IgE-mediated reactions, and the evaluation of eczematous skin lesions after 24 to 72 hours is called atopy patch test (APT) (16). This test was developed as a diagnostic tool for characterizing patients with aeroallergen-triggered AE.

Early studies describing experimental patch testing with aeroallergens were published in 1937 by Rostenberg and Sulzberger (17) and in 1982 by Mitchell et al. (18); since then the methods and results have shown wide variations. Potentially irritating procedures like skin abrasion (19,20), tape stripping (21,22), and sodium lauryl sulfate application (23) were used to enhance allergen penetration. No clearcut correlations to skin-prick test or specific IgE measurements were obtained, and the sensitivity and specificity of experimental APTs with regard to clinical history remained unclear. For better standardization we performed APT on nonlesional, nonabraded, untreated skin during remission (16,24). The results were compared for vehicle and dose of allergen in the preparations used. It was shown that healthy controls and patients with respiratory atopy without a history of eczema do not react in the APT (24) or with a lower frequency and intensity of APT reactions to whole body mite extract compared to patients with AE (25).

APT Methods

Table 1 summarizes the methods for APT as published in methodological studies (26–28): APT with significant correlations to clinical parameters like allergen-specific IgE or patients history are today performed with a very similar technique to conventional patch tests for the diagnosis of classical contact allergy. Exclusion criteria (use of antihistamines, systemic, and in loco topical steroids: one week, UV radiation three weeks, acute eczema flare) and the possibility of contact urticaria should be considered. Epicutaneous tests with lyophilized allergens, for example, from house dust mite (*D. pteronyssinus*), cat dander, and grass pollen are performed

TABLE 2 Results of APT Methodology Studies

Controls: no positive reaction (nonatopic/rhinoconjunctivitis only)
Vehicle: petrolatum better than hydrogel
Allergen concentration >1000 PNU/g; 7000 PNU/g gave "optimal results" in adults
Biologically standardized allergens: 200 IR/g
Atopic eczema in uncovered skin areas: associated with higher frequency of positive APT
Seasonal eczema flares: positive grass pollen-APT
APT correlates with clinical history

Sources: Adapted from Refs. 26–28.

with a petrolatum vehicle (including a vehicle control). Patients should be in a state of remission of their eczema; the patch test is applied in large Finn Chambers for 48 hours on their back on nonabraded and uninvolved skin. Any potentially irritating methods of skin barrier disruption like tape stripping of the skin should be avoided.

In several studies, nonatopic volunteers and patients suffering from allergic rhinoconjunctivitis only presented no positive APT reactions with the methods described in Table 1. The reproducibility of different APT methods is high, if the test is performed on the back. Allergens in petrolatum elicited twice as many APT reactions as allergens in a hydrophilic vehicle (24). High allergen-specific IgE in serum is not a prerequisite for a positive APT, but 62% of patients with *D. pteronyssinus*–positive APT showed a corresponding positive skin-prick test and 77% of patients showed a corresponding elevated specific IgE. In other allergens, the concordance was even higher. Allergen concentrations of 500, 3000, 5000, and 10,000 PNU (protein nitrogen units)/g in petrolatum were comparatively used in 57 patients (27). It was shown that the "percentage of patients with clear-cut positive reactions was significantly higher in patients with eczematous skin lesions in air-exposed areas (69%) as compared to patients without this predictive pattern (39%; $p = 0.02$)." In the first group, the maximum reactivity was nearly reached with 5000 PNU/g. The data from a randomized, double-blind multicenter trial, involving 253 adult patients and 30 children with AE, were used to calculate a suitable APT allergen dosage (26,29). The optimal allergen doses were in the range of 5000 to 7000 PNU/g. For children, lower allergen concentrations seem possible (29). Simultaneously tested, the allergen doses of 7000 PNU/g and 200 IR/g (biological unit; Index réactif) of the most important aeroallergens in Europe showed comparable concordance with the patients' history suggesting clinical relevance in another study in 50 patients with AE. An example of a positive APT reaction to a biologically standardized allergen preparation is shown in Figure 1. The clinical outcome of the methodological studies is summarized in Table 2.

The standardization of aeroallergen APT is currently more advanced than food patch testing; in Europe, the efforts are coordinated in the European Task Force on Atopic Dermatitis (ETFAD), a subspeciality society of the European Academy of Dermatology and Venereology (EADV). A recent ETFAD study in six European countries ($n = 314$) showed again that house dust mite (*D. pteronyssinus*) most often elicited positive APT reactions, followed by pollen allergens (Table 3) (30).

Usually, APT reactions are read after 48 and 72 hours. In patients with contact urticaria, a wheal and flare reaction may be seen after 30 minutes. Most reactions are visible and palpable at 48 hours, sometimes with decrescendo to 72 hours.

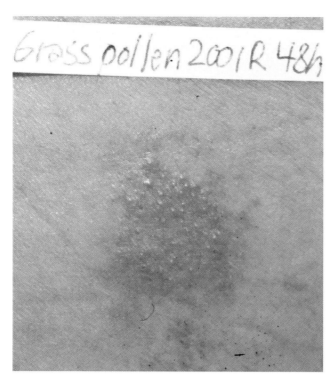

FIGURE 1 APT reaction to grass pollen allergens after removal of Finn Chamber after 48 hours. Clear-cut eczematous appearance with infiltration and spreading papules, partially with a follicular pattern.

After tape stripping followed by allergen application, there are more early reactions visible. Clear-cut positive reactions should be distinguished from negative or questionable ones understanding the fact that only reactions showing papules or at least some degree of infiltration were correlated with clinical relevance. Consensus meetings of most groups performing APT for clinical use in Europe were held in Munich in 1997 and 1998 and a consensus APT reading key for describing the intensity of APT reactions was developed and published (31). Following its use

TABLE 3 Clinical Relevance and Different Test Methods in Patients with AE

Aeroallergens	SPT (%)	sIgE (%)	APT (%)	History (%)	Hx-concordance (%)
D. pteronyssinus	56	56	39	34	57
Birch pollen	49	53	17	20	61
Grass pollen	57	59	15	31	64
Cat dander	44	46	10	30	62

Frequency of positive APT reactions is lower than of positive IgE-mediated sensitizations. Patients allergen-specific history of eczema flares after allergen exposure was obtained prospectively. $N = 314$, 24% children ≤10 years.
Abbreviations: SPT, skin-prick test ≥3 mm; sIgE, specific IgE ≥0.35 kU/L; APT, atopy patch test ≥+; Hx-concordance, allergen-specific concordance of APT result and clinical history
Source: Adapted from Ref. 30.

TABLE 4 ETFAD Key for the Grading of Positive APT Reactions

−	Negative
?	Only erythema, questionable
+	Erythema, infiltration
++	Erythema, few papules
+++	Erythema, many or spreading papules
++++	Erythema, vesicles

Abbreviations: ETFAD, European Task Force on Atopic Dermatitis.
Source: Adapted from Ref. 31.

in a multicenter trial in six European countries, ETFAD proposed in 2003 a simplified version given in Table 4. However, clinically meaningful APT results were also obtained with the ICDRG key for conventional patch testing (24,26). Problems like irrelevant positive or spreading APT reactions may occur in patients undergoing APT during an eczema flare, or if methods of abrasion of the stratum corneum are used. The issue of pharmacologic influence on APT still holds many unanswered questions. As the standardization of the high-molecular-weight allergens holds some specific problems, a commercial provider of test substances with reproducible quality and major allergen content is desirable. However, to date such allergen preparations are not easily available. Even more problems with allergen standardization are known for food APT. The current state of APT is summarized in a recent ETFAD/EAACI position paper (32).

Predictors and Consequences of APT

As long as no "gold standard" of provocation for aeroallergen allergy in AE exists, the history of allergen-specific exacerbation is used as a parameter for clinical relevance. A study compared outcome of the APT with a seasonal history of "summer eruption" of AE in 79 patients (28). Significantly higher frequencies of positive grass pollen APT reactions (with two methods used) occurred in patients with a corresponding history of exacerbation of skin lesions during the grass pollen season of the previous year (75% with positive APT). Patients without this history showed significantly lower APT reactivity (16% with positive APT; $p < 0.001$).

In two multicenter studies with up to five aeroallergens, the predictors of a positive APT reaction were investigated (Table 5) (26,30). Sensitivity and specificity of the APT in these studies are also shown in Table 6. It has to be kept in mind that

TABLE 5 Logistic Regression Model: Predictors of a Positive APT Reaction

Positive APT reactions are associated with
Increased corresponding specific serum IgE
Positive corresponding skin prick test reaction
Aeroallergen-specific corresponding history
Increased total IgE
Long eczema duration
Rhinoconjunctivitis (grass pollen)

IgE-mediated sensitization and allergen-specific positive history of eczema flares are the most important predictors of a positive APT reaction.
Source: Adapted from Ref. 26.

TABLE 6 Sensitivity and Specificity of Different Test Procedures With Regard to Clinical History

Test	Sensitivity[a] (%)	Specificity[a] (%)
Different grass pollen preparations, $n = 79$		
Skin prick	100	33
sIgE	92	33
APT	75	84
European multicenter study, $n = 314$, 4 aeroallergens		
Skin prick	68–80	50–71
sIgE	72–84	52–69
APT	14–45	64–91
German multicenter study, $n = 253$, 3 aeroallergens		
Skin prick	69–82	44–53
sIgE	65–94	42–64
APT	42–56	69–92

The APT shows a higher specificity than classical tests for IgE-mediated hypersensitivity with regard to the allergen-specific history. Studies used different allergen standardizations.
[a]Depending on allergen, with regard to a clinical history with eczema flares in pollen season or after direct contact with allergen.
Sources: Adapted from Refs. 26, 28, 30.

at least for a nonseasonal aeroallergen, the history may be unreliable, thus limiting the precision of such calculations like the one shown in Table 6. For most allergens, a significant association of APT and specific IgE could be demonstrated.

The APT does not replace the classical methods of diagnosis of IgE-mediated allergy, but adds specificity to allergy diagnosis starting with the screening tests. Appropriate allergen specific avoidance strategies are recommended in patients showing positive APT reactions (33).

APT and "Intrinsic Type" Atopic Eczema

A sensitization detected by APT, which is supposedly T-cell mediated, may be even more relevant for the clinical course of AE than the demonstration of an IgE-mediated sensitization. Interestingly, 7% of the tested patients who would be labeled as "intrinsic type" of AE, according to Schmid-Grendelmeier's and B. Wüthrich's definition (34), show a sensitization in the APT. A similar finding of positive APT reactions in subjects without sIgE to *Dermatophagoides* was described by Seidenari et al. and Manzini et al. (35,36). Recently also 8 out of 12 "intrinsic" AE patients were reported to react to a partially purified whole mite APT preparation (37). Similar results have been obtained by APT with *Malassezia sympodialis* antigen (38). House-dust-mite–specific antibodies of the IgG4 subtype as well as a rapid influx of inflammatory dendritic epidermal cell (IDEC) in the APT lesions has recently been reported in two otherwise "intrinsic" AE patients (39). However, the mechanism of these "intrinsic" APT reactions remains hypothetical to date, but a T-cell–mediated mechanism without specific IgE involvement seems probable.

Questions remain open concerning the clinical relevance of positive APT results in patients with a negative history and discordant negative skin-prick tests or radioallergosorbent test (RAST), since no gold standard exists for the provocation of eczematous skin lesions in aeroallergen-triggered AE. These questions may only be answered by controlled studies using specific provocation and elimination procedures in patients with positive and negative APT results.

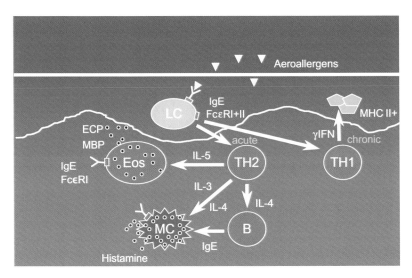

FIGURE 2 Proposed simplified pathophysiology of aeroallergen-triggered atopic eczema. *Abbreviations*: LC, Langerhans cell; FcεRI, IgE receptor; Eos, eosinophil granulocyte; TH, T-cell populations; B, B cell; MC, mast cell.

IMMUNOPATHOLOGY OF AEROALLERGEN REACTIONS IN AE SKIN

Mite allergen in the epidermis of patients with AE under natural conditions (40) as well as in APT sites (19,23) has been demonstrated in proximity to Langerhans cells. Langerhans cells in the skin express IgE receptors of three different classes (41–43). In addition, a Birbeck granule negative, non-Langerhans cell population with an even higher IgE-receptor expression than the Langerhans cell, the so-called IDEC (44), has been found in freshly induced APT lesions, a phenomenon which occurred in both "intrinsic" and "extrinsic" patients (45). This might explain IgE-associated activation of allergen-specific T cells, finally leading to eczematous skin lesions in the APT (Fig. 2) (46,47). Basophils and eosinophils are involved in APT reactions (18,22). According to the results of Langeveld-Wildschut et al., the positive APT reaction requires the presence of epidermal IgE$^+$ CD1a$^+$ cells (48). From APT biopsies, allergen specific T cells have been cloned (46). These T cells showed a characteristic TH2 secretion pattern initially, whereas after 48 hours a TH1 pattern was predominant. This same pattern is also found in chronic lesions of AE. In addition, positive APT reactions to house dust mite, cat dander, and grass pollen are intraindividually associated with allergen-specific T-cell proliferation responses (49). This can be interpreted as indirect evidence for the relevance of these allergens.

FACTORS INFLUENCING AEROALLERGEN REACTIONS IN AE SKIN

Due to the defined time course of eczematous APT reactions, this model has repeatedly been used to study AE (see section, immunopathology of aeroallergen reactions in AE skin) and AE symptoms (50). Moreover, the influence of therapy and environmental factors was also investigated. An effect of pretreatment with 1% pimecrolimus cream on the APT was seen in a randomized, controlled, double-blind study enrolling 20 patients with AE and positive APT screening reaction to house dust mite *D. pteronyssinus*, cat dander, grass, or birch pollen (51). For two weeks, patients applied twice daily pimecrolimus and vehicle control to marked fields on their backs and forearms. Then, APT was performed on both fields on the back. Including only patients with different readings ($n = 13$), stronger APT suppression of at least 1 ETFAD grade in the pimecrolimus area versus intraindividual control was observed in 10 of these patients after 48 and 72 hours ($p < 0.05$; 90% CI 50.5, 93.4). Including all 20 subjects still showed a borderline significance compared with vehicle ($p = 0.0564$). Immunohistochemical analysis in two patients revealed an induction of interferon-γ in pimecrolimus-pretreated skin.

It was concluded that pimecrolimus treatment has a potential to suppress the development of lesions induced by aeroallergen exposure in patients with AE.

Recently, volatile organic compounds (VOCs) in ambient air have been shown to increase APT reactivity, and transepidermal water loss, probably by changes in epidermal barrier function (52). Compared to intraindividual crossover controls, six out of seven patients showed enhanced APT reactions to *D. pteronyssinus* allergen after previous exposure to a mixture of 22 VOCs ($5 \, \text{mg}/\text{m}^3$) in a total body exposure chamber for four hours. These findings suggest that exposure to VOCs at concentrations commonly found in indoor environments can enhance the adverse effect of house dust mite allergen on sensitized subjects with AE.

SUMMARY AND CONCLUSIONS

Aeroallergens are relevant trigger factors of AE flares. Due to possibility of several different trigger factors in the same patient, the diagnosis of such cases remains difficult. Following extensive analysis of patient's history, skin-prick tests and allergen-specific serum IgE measurement [regional standard panels (53)] remain necessary with critical allergologic interpretation. The APT, an epicutaneous patch test with allergens known to elicit IgE-mediated reactions, and the evaluation of eczematous skin lesions after 24 to 72 hours, was developed as diagnostic tool for characterizing patients with aeroallergen-triggered AE. Positive APT reactions are associated with allergen-specific T-cell responses. The APT specificity exceeded the specificity of the classic tests of IgE-mediated hypersensitivity, which was only 0.33 for skin-prick test and RAST. The APT with aeroallergens may provide an important diagnostic tool as has been shown in two patient subgroups: In patients with an air-exposed eczema distribution pattern, positive APT reactions occurred at lower allergen doses compared with other patients with AE. Patients with an aeroallergen-specific history had significantly more positive APT reactions. The APT does not replace the classical methods of diagnosis of IgE-mediated allergy, but adds specificity to allergy diagnosis starting with the screening tests. Appropriate allergen-specific avoidance strategies are recommended in patients showing positive APT reactions (33). The diagnostic validity of APT in routine diagnosis of aeroallergen-triggered AE is investigated in further controlled studies.

REFERENCES

1. Ring J, Przybilla B, Ruzicka T, eds. Handbook of Atopic Eczema, 2nd ed. Berlin, Germany: Springer, 2006.
2. Rajka G. Essential Aspects of Atopic Dermatitis. Berlin, Germany: Springer, 1989.
3. Johansson SGO, Bieber T, Dahl R, et al. Revised nomenclature for allergy for global use: Report of the Nomenclature Review Committee of the World Allergy Organization, October 2003. J Allergy Clin Immunol 2004; 113:832–836.

4. Tupker R, DeMonchy J, Coenraads P, et al. Induction of atopic dermatitis by inhalation of house dust mite. J Allergy Clin Immunol 1996; 97:1064–1070.
5. Krämer U, Weidinger S, Darsow U, et al. Seasonality in symptom severity influenced by temperature or grass pollen: Results of a panel study in children with eczema. J Invest Dermatol 2005; 124:514–523.
6. Meneghini CL, Bonifazi E. Correlation between clinical and immunological findings in atopic dermatitis. Acta Derm Venereol (Stockh) 1985; 114:140–142.
7. Barnetson RSC, MacFarlane HAF, Benton EC. House dust mite allergy and atopic eczema: A case report. Br J Dermatol 1987; 116:857–860.
8. Jones HE, Inouye JC, McGerity JL, et al. Atopic disease and serum immunoglobulin-E. Br J Dermatol 1975; 92:17–25.
9. Schäfer T, Heinrich J, Wijst M, et al. Association between severity of atopic eczema and degree of sensitization to aeroallergens in schoolchildren. J Allergy Clin Immunol 1999; 104:1280–1284.
10. Tan B, Weald D, Strickland I, et al. Double-blind controlled trial of effect of housedust-mite allergen avoidance on atopic dermatitis. Lancet 1996; 347:15–18.
11. Lau S, Ehnert B, Cremer B, et al. Häusliche Milbenallergenreduktion bei spezifisch sensibilisierten Patienten mit atopischem Ekzem. Allergo J 1995; 4:432–435.
12. Fukuda H, Imayama S, Okada T. Mite-free room (MFR) for the management of atopic dermatitis. Jpn J Allergol 1991; 40:626–632.
13. Sanda T, Yasue T, Oohashi M, et al. Effectiveness of house-dust mite allergen avoidance through clean room therapy in patients with atopic dermatitis. J Allergy Clin Immunol 1992; 89:653–657.
14. Oosting AJ, de Bruin-Weller MS, Terreehorst I, et al. Effect of mattress encasings on atopic dermatitis outcome measures in a double-blind, placebo-controlled study: The Dutch mite avoidance study. J Allergy Clin Immunol 2002; 110:500–506.
15. Holm L, Ohman S, Bengtsson A, et al. Effectiveness of occlusive bedding in the treatment of atopic dermatitis—a placebo-controlled trial of 12 months' duration. Allergy 2001; 56:152–158.
16. Ring J, Kunz B, Bieber T, et al. The "atopy patch test" with aeroallergens in atopic eczema. J Allergy Clin Immunol 1989; 82:195.
17. Rostenberg A, Sulzberger MD. Some results of patch tests. Arch Dermatol 1937; 35:433–454.
18. Mitchell E, Chapman M, Pope F, et al. Basophils in allergen-induced patch test sites in atopic dermatitis. Lancet 1982; I:127–130.
19. Gondo A, Saeki N, Tokuda Y. Challenge reactions in atopic dermatitis after percutaneous entry of mite antigen. Br J Dermatol 1986; 115:485–493.
20. Norris P, Schofield O, Camp R. A study of the role of house dust mite in atopic dermatitis. Br J Dermatol 1988; 118:435–440.
21. van Voorst Vader PC, Lier JG, Woest TE, et al. Patch tests with house dust mite antigens in atopic dermatitis patients: Methodological problems. Acta Derm Venereol (Stockh) 1991; 71:301–305.
22. Bruijnzeel-Koomen C, van Wichen D, Spry C, et al. Active participation of eosinophils in patch test reactions to inhalant allergens in patients with atopic dermatitis. Br J Dermatol 1988; 118:229–238.
23. Tanaka Y, Anan S, Yoshida H. Immunohistochemical studies in mite antigen-induced patch test sites in atopic dermatitis. J Derm Science 1990; 1:361–368.
24. Darsow U, Vieluf D, Ring J. Atopy patch test with different vehicles and allergen concentrations—an approach to standardization. J Allergy Clin Immunol 1995; 95:677–684.
25. Seidenari S, Giusti F, Pellacani G, et al. Frequency and intensity of responses to mite patch tests are lower in non atopic subjects in respect to patients with atopic dermatitis. Allergy 2003; 58:426–429.
26. Darsow U, Vieluf D, Ring J; for the APT Study Group. Evaluating the relevance of aeroallergen sensitization in atopic eczema with the atopy patch test: A randomized, double-blind multicenter study. J Am Acad Dermatol 1999; 40:187–193.

27. Darsow U, Vieluf D, Ring J. The atopy patch test: An increased rate of reactivity in patients who have an air-exposed pattern of atopic eczema. Br J Dermatol 1996; 135:182–186.
28. Darsow U, Behrendt H, Ring J. Gramineae pollen as trigger factors of atopic eczema—evaluation of diagnostic measures using the atopy patch test. Br J Dermatol 1997; 137:201–207.
29. Darsow U, Vieluf D, Berg B, et al. Dose response study of atopy patch test in children with atopic eczema. Pediatr Asthma Allergy Immunol 1999; 13:115–122.
30. Darsow U, Laifaoui J, Bolhaar S, et al. Atopy patch test with aeroallergens and food allergens in petrolatum: A European multicenter study. Allergy 2004; 59:1318–1325.
31. Darsow U, Ring J. Airborne and dietary allergens in atopic eczema: A comprehensive review of diagnostic tests. Clin Exp Dermatol 2000; 25:544–551.
32. Turjanmaa K, Darsow U, Niggemann B, et al. EAACI/GA2LEN Position Paper: Present status of the atopy patch test—Position paper of the Section on Dermatology and the Section on Pediatrics of the EAACI. Allergy 2006; 61:1377–1384.
33. Darsow U, Lübbe J, Taïeb A, et al.; for the European Task Force on Atopic Dermatitis. Position paper on diagnosis and treatment of atopic dermatitis. J Europ Acad Dermatol 2005; 19:286–295.
34. Schmid-Grendelmeier P, Simon D, Simon HU, et al. Epidemiology, clinical features, and immunology of the "intrinsic" (non-IgE-mediated) type of atopic dermatitis (constitutional dermatitis). Allergy 2001; 56:841–849.
35. Seidenari S, Manzini BM, Danese P, et al. Positive patch tests to whole mite culture and purified mite extracts in patients with atopic dermatitis, asthma, and rhinitis. Ann Allergy 1992; 69:201–206.
36. Manzini BM, Motolese A, Donini M, et al. Contact allergy to *Dermatophagoides* in atopic dermatitis patients and healthy subjects. Contact Dermatitis 1995; 33:243–246.
37. Ingordo V, D'Andria G, D'Andria C, et al. Results of atopy patch tests with house dust mites in adults with "intrinsic" and "extrinsic" atopic dermatitis. J Eur Acad Dermatol Venereol 2002; 16:450–454.
38. Johansson C, Sandstrom MH, Bartosik J, et al. Atopy patch test reactions to *Malassezia* allergens differentiate subgroups of atopic dermatitis patients. Br J Dermatol 2003; 148:479–488.
39. Kerschenlohr K, Decard S, Darsow U, et al. Clinical and immunologic reactivity to aeroallergens in 'intrinsic' atopic dermatitis patients. J Allergy Clin Immunol 2003; 111:195–197.
40. Maeda K, Yamamoto K, Tanaka Y, et al. House dust mite (HDM) antigen in naturally occurring lesions of atopic dermatitis (AD): The relationship between HDM antigen in the skin and HDM antigen-specific IgE antibody. J Derm Science 1992; 3:73–77.
41. Bieber T, Rieger A, Neuchrist C, et al. Induction of FCeR2/CD23 on human epidermal Langerhans-cells by human recombinant IL4 and IFN. J Exp Med 1989; 170:309–314.
42. Bieber T, de la Salle H, Wollenberg A, et al. Human epidermal Langerhans cells express the high affinity receptor for immunoglobulin E (Fc epsilon RI). J Exp Med 1992; 175:1285–1290.
43. Wollenberg A, de la Salle H, Hanau D, et al. Human keratinocytes release the endogenous β-galactoside-binding soluble lectin εBP which binds to Langerhans cells where it modulates their binding capacity for IgE glycoforms. J Exp Med 1993; 178:777–785.
44. Wollenberg A, Kraft S, Hanau D, et al. Immunomorphological and ultrastructural characterization of Langerhans cells and a novel, inflammatory dendritic epidermal cell (IDEC) population in lesional skin of atopic eczema. J Invest Dermatol 1996; 106:446–453.
45. Kerschenlohr K, Decard S, Przybilla B, et al. Atopy patch test reactions show a rapid influx of inflammatory dendritic epidermal cells (IDEC) in extrinsic and intrinsic atopic dermatitis patients. J Allergy Clin Immunol 2003; 111:869–874.
46. van Reijsen FC, Bruijnzeel-Koomen CAFM, Kalthoff FS. Skin-derived aeroallergen-specific T-cell clones of Th2 phenotype in patients with atopic dermatitis. J Allergy Clin Immunol 1992; 90:184–192.

47. Sager N, Feldmann A, Schilling G, et al. House dust mite-specific T cells in the skin of subjects with atopic dermatitis: Frequency and lymphokine profile in the allergen patch test. J Allergy Clin Immunol 1992; 89:801–810.
48. Langeveld-Wildschut EG, Bruijnzeel PLB, Mudde GC, et al. Clinical and immunologic variables in skin of patients with atopic eczema and either positive or negative atopy patch test reactions. J Allergy Clin Immunol 2000; 105:1008–1016.
49. Wistokat-Wülfing A, Schmidt P, Darsow U, et al. Atopy patch test reactions are associated with T lymphocyte-mediated allergen-specific immune responses in atopic dermatitis. Clin Exp Allergy 1999; 29:513–521.
50. Weissenbacher S, Bacon T, Targett D, et al. Atopy patch test—Reproducibility and elicitation of itch in different application sites. Acta Derm Venereol 2005; 85:147–151.
51. Weissenbacher S, Traidl-Hoffmann C, Eyerich K, et al. Modulation of atopy patch test and skin prick test by pretreatment with 1% pimecrolimus cream. Int Arch Allergy Immunol 2006; 140:239–244.
52. Huss-Marp J, Eberlein-König B, Breuer K, et al. Influence of short term exposure to airborne Der p 1 and volatile organic compounds on skin barrier function and dermal blood flow in patients with atopic eczema and healthy individuals. Clin Exp Allergy 2006; 36:338–345.
53. Heinzerling L, Frew AJ, Bindslev-Jensen C, et al. Standard skin prick testing and sensitization to inhalant allergens across Europe—A survey from the GA2LEN network. Allergy 2005; 60:1287–1300.

13 Food Allergens and Atopic Dermatitis

Julie Wang and Hugh A. Sampson

Department of Pediatrics, Jaffe Food Allergy Research Institute, Mount Sinai School of Medicine, New York, U.S.A.

Atopic dermatitis (AD) is a chronically relapsing skin disorder that is associated with severe pruritus and a typical distribution. It is a common condition in children, affecting approximately 10% of children in the United States and 14.7% of children worldwide (1). Symptoms present in the first year of life in nearly one-half of patients, and in 80% by five years of age. The distribution of eczematous lesions varies by age. The cheeks and extensor surfaces of the arms and legs are generally affected in young infants, whereas the flexor surfaces, hands, and feet are more commonly affected in teenagers and young adults (2).

Several observations have supported the notion that IgE-mediated mechanisms play a significant role in at least a subset of individuals suffering from AD. Over 80% of children with AD have elevated serum total IgE levels (3), and approximately 80% of children with AD have positive skin prick tests (SPT) and serum specific IgE antibodies to foods and aeroallergens (4). These findings suggest that at least two forms of AD likely exist: an extrinsic form associated with IgE-mediated sensitization and an intrinsic form affecting 20% to 30% of patients without IgE-mediated sensitization (5). Both forms have been found to be associated with eosinophilia. In a recent review of 12 population-based studies, the authors found that IgE sensitization in AD patients may not be as high as previously reported (6). Up to 50% of patients with AD in a hospital setting did not have allergic sensitization, and an even higher percentage of patients with AD in the community were not sensitized to allergens.

In addition, children with AD have higher rates of other atopic disorders such as allergic rhinitis and asthma. Studies have found that approximately one-third of children with AD will later develop asthma (7,8), and nearly half will develop allergic rhinitis (7,9).

EPIDEMIOLOGY

Several epidemiologic studies demonstrated the presence of elevated serum-specific IgE antibodies to foods in AD patients. The Melbourne Atopy Cohort consisted of 487 infants with a positive family history of atopy who were recruited at birth and followed until 12 months of age (10). Skin prick testing (SPT) was performed at 6 and 12 months to three foods (milk, egg, and peanut) in addition to aeroallergens. SPT wheal diameters greater than twice the wheal size of the histamine control were considered to be indicative of food hypersensitivity (FH), based on prior studies correlating wheal sizes to positive open food challenges in children less than two years of age in the same patient population. Data was also correlated with reported adverse reactions to foods. Among children with severe AD ($n = 35$), 69% had IgE-mediated FH. The relative risk (RR) of an infant with AD having associated IgE-mediated FH was 5.9 for the most severe AD group compared to the group without AD.

Hill et al. (11) conducted a study of 2184 young children (mean age 17.6 months, range 11.8–25.4; 1246 males) with active AD from atopic families from 94 centers in 12 countries. The authors found that 64% of children with early onset severe AD (<3 months of age) had food specific IgE levels (ImmunoCAP, Phadia) above the 95% positive predictive values (PPV) for clinical reactivity to foods. There was no association between AD severity and high food specific IgE in children with AD onset after 12 months of age.

Several limitations to these studies included the lack of oral food challenges to confirm clinical reactivity to foods and testing limited to three foods (egg, milk, and peanut). These limitations may underestimate children with real FH who had SPT or food-specific IgE levels below the predictive cutoffs. Moreover, information regarding AD treatment was not collected, and diet history/avoidance of foods and non-IgE–mediated FH were not evaluated.

Several epidemiologic studies recruiting subjects from dermatology clinics have provided similar results. Of 63 children with moderate-to-severe AD (median 2.8 years, median SCORAD 41.1), 37% had evidence of FH (six foods tested) based on 95% PPV levels and double-blind, placebo-controlled oral food challenges (DBPCFC) (12). In another study of 51 infants with AD, ages 6 to 12 months referred from dermatologists, 90% had FH based on either predictive SPT results or serum specific IgE levels (13). SPT and food specific-IgE levels were performed to three foods (milk, egg, and peanut). Wheal sizes or specific IgE levels that had 95% PPV for clinical reactivity were used to define food allergy. Of note, since this study included infants under one year of age, most of the children in this study were too young to have ever ingested these foods, so the majority of the children had no clinical history of reactivity to these foods and therefore the certainty of clinical reactivity was not established.

LABORATORY INVESTIGATIONS

The histology of AD lesions suggests a type IV cell-mediated hypersensitivity, whereas FH is often thought of as a type I IgE-mediated hypersensitivity (14). However, a classical division between type I and type IV hypersensitivities has been challenged; studies have shown that the terminal stages of IgE-mediated reactions (type I) are characterized by monocyte and lymphocyte infiltration, which is similar to that found in type IV hypersensitivity (15). In fact, acute AD lesions are characterized by spongiosis of the epidermis and a marked perivenular infiltrate primarily with lymphocytes and occasional monocytes in the dermis. Furthermore, cytokine mRNA expression by lymphocytes obtained from skin biopsies in patients with acute AD is primarily Th2 (IL-4, IL-5, and IL-13) (16, 17), not the classic type IV cellular response in which the Th1 cytokine IFN-γ is predominant (18).

In chronic AD, there is tissue remodeling due to chronic inflammation and increased numbers of IgE-bearing Langerhans cells and inflammatory dendritic epidermal cells, with macrophages dominating the dermal mononuclear cell infiltrate. Eosinophils and T cells are also present, but in fewer numbers than acute AD. There are increased IL-5, GM-CSF, IL-12, and IFN-γ mRNA expressing cells as compared to acute AD (19).

Recently, a strong association between AD and filaggrin null mutations has been found. Filaggrin mutations result in defective gene expression of this skin barrier protein and are highly associated with allergen sensitization (20–22). Howell et al. (23) found significantly decreased filaggrin expression in acute AD skin as compared with normal skin. Furthermore, keratinocytes differentiated in the presence of IL-4 and IL-13 exhibited significantly reduced filaggrin gene expression compared with media alone. These results indicate that allergic inflammation leads to downregulation of filaggrin expression, which further impairs barrier function, potentially creating a vicious cycle.

Several studies have demonstrated the involvement of mast cells, basophils, and eosinophils in IgE-mediated food allergic reactions in patients with AD. Children with AD who developed symptoms during oral food challenges have evidence of plasma eosinophil activation (24). In a study of 33 AD patients with a total of 35 positive food challenges, 31 of which had cutaneous symptoms, positive challenges were associated with increased plasma histamine. These findings confirm the involvement of mast cell and/or basophil mediators in the pathogenesis of FH, and suggest a role in cutaneous changes in these AD patients as well (25). Increased eosinophil cationic protein (ECP) was found in 17 of 28 cow milk allergic patients who had a positive oral food challenge to milk with skin manifestations, but not in those demonstrating gastrointestinal symptoms alone (11/28 patients) (26).

T cells have also been found to have a role in the pathogenesis of AD. Food allergen–specific T cells have been cloned from the skin lesions of patients with AD, providing evidence that foods may contribute to skin inflammation (27–30). In one study, peripheral blood mononuclear cells were isolated from seven milk allergic children with a history of AD when exposed to milk (28). All patients had a positive SPT and DBPCFC to milk. Ten children with either allergic eosinophilic gastroenteritis or milk-induced enterocolitis and eight nonatopic adults served as controls. After casein stimulation, allergic patients with milk-induced skin disease had an expanded population of CLA^+ T cells, as compared with nonatopic individuals or allergic patients without skin involvement. Kondo et al. (31) demonstrated that T cells and monocytes in children with food-sensitive AD proliferated well to ovalbumin or bovine serum albumin (BSA), compared with T cells from healthy children and children with immediate allergic symptoms who were sensitive to hen's egg or cow's milk. The responding cells were shown to be predominantly $CD4^+$ T lymphocytes. IL-2 activity and IFN-γ concentrations in culture supernatants of ovalbumin-stimulated peripheral blood mononuclear cells (PBMCs) from patients with AD who were egg allergic were significantly higher than those of healthy children and patients with immediate allergic symptoms with egg exposure. Therefore, the authors concluded that cell-mediated immunity likely occurs in addition to IgE-mediated hypersensitivity in patients with food-sensitive AD.

ANIMAL MODELS

Several mouse models have been used to investigate the immunopathogenic mechanisms of AD. In a study using mice orally sensitized to cow's milk or peanut with a cholera toxin adjuvant, low-grade allergen exposure resulted in an eczematous eruption in approximately one-third of mice (32). Peripheral blood eosinophilia and elevated serum IgE levels were found in these mice. Histologic examination of the lesional skin revealed spongiosis and a cellular infiltrate consisting of $CD4^+$ lymphocytes, eosinophils, and mast cells. IL-5 and IL-13 mRNA expression was elevated only in the skin of mice with the eczematous eruption. Treatment of the eruption with topical corticosteroids led to decreased pruritus and resolution of the cutaneous eruption.

Another group used a murine model of AD elicited by epicutaneous sensitization with ovalbumin (OVA) in mice with targeted deletions of the IL-4, IL-5, and IFN-γ cytokine genes (33). OVA-sensitized skin from IL-5(−/−) mice had no detectable eosinophils and exhibited decreased epidermal and dermal thickening. Sensitized skin from IL-4(−/−) mice displayed normal thickening of the skin layers, but had a drastic reduction in eosinophils and a significant increase in infiltrating T cells. Sensitized skin from IFN-γ(−/−) mice was characterized by reduced dermal thickening. From this data, the authors concluded that both the Th2 cytokines IL-4 and IL-5 and the Th1 cytokine IFN-γ play important roles in the inflammation and hypertrophy of the skin in AD.

Recently, Prescott et al. (34) also used a mouse model of AD to demonstrate that oral consumption of food can lead to exacerbations of cutaneous allergic inflammation. Food challenges in their mice resulted in early- and late-phase skin reactions. The early-phase reaction was associated with mast cell degranulation, while the late-phase response was characterized by lymphoid and eosinophilic infiltration, indicating that food allergy can predispose to cutaneous inflammatory reactions.

CLINICAL STUDIES

The role of IgE-mediated mechanisms in the pathogenesis of AD has long been debated. Although several studies show that children with AD have elevated allergen-specific IgE levels, whether there is a causal relationship between IgE-mediated allergies and the manifestation of AD lesions has been questioned.

Several authors believe that AD and FH can occur simultaneously in a patient, but remain unrelated, without a causal relationship. A recent study by Rowlands et al. (35) concluded that foods rarely cause flares in AD. The authors report only one positive eczematous food response in 17 children (age 1–16 years) with AD in a dermatology clinic who were on food restriction diets. However, these patients were presumed to have food allergy, but were never appropriately evaluated (i.e., SPT, allergen-specific IgE levels). Another three children had convincing histories of food-induced IgE-mediated reactions and were not challenged. In addition, several of the foods challenged are not typically considered to be responsible for food allergic reactions, including banana, wine, coffee, ketchup, and chocolate.

Several well-controlled clinical studies have demonstrated that IgE-mediated food allergy contributes to exacerbations of AD lesions. A number of studies examined how elimination of offending food allergens affected the severity of AD. While early studies reported mixed results regarding elimination diets for the treatment of AD, most of these did not control for other trigger factors, placebo effect, or observer bias (14). Atherton et al. (36) reported that two-thirds of children with AD had improvement during a double-blind cross-over trial of egg and milk exclusion. This study was limited by the high dropout rate and lack of control for other AD trigger factors. In a similarly designed study, of 40 patients who completed the crossover trial, 10 appeared to benefit from the diet and were advised to continue egg and milk avoidance (37). However, the response rate to the diet was not statistically significant. In a prospective follow-up study of 34 children with AD, children with FH who went on allergen elimination diets experienced a significantly greater improvement in AD at one to two years and three to four years follow-up as compared to 12 similar patients who did not have food allergy and five children who had FH but did not adhere to the elimination diet (38). Lever et al. (39) performed a randomized, controlled trial evaluating the effect of egg exclusion from the diet of young children with AD and evidence of IgE antibodies to eggs. Following a prolonged period on aggressive, standardized skin care, 55 children were randomized either to receive specific advice from a dietician about an egg exclusion diet (diet group) or to a control group in which only general AD advice was provided. Both groups continued topical AD treatment. The mean reduction in surface area affected by eczema was significantly greater ($P = 0.02$) in the diet group (from 19.6% to 10.9% area affected) as compared to the control group (from 21.9% to 18.9%). There was also a significant improvement in severity score ($P = 0.04$) for the diet group. The authors concluded that elimination of eggs is useful as part of the overall management of young children with AD and sensitivity to eggs.

Many studies have also shown that food allergens can have a role in inciting eczematous lesions. Placebo-controlled food challenge studies have shown that foods can induce eczematoid skin rashes in nearly 40% of children with moderate-to-severe AD (12,40). Bock et al. (41) reported that 4 of 7 children with eczematous reactions to foods developed rash within two hours of double-blind, placebo-controlled food challenges. In a study of 113 children with AD, in which 63 (56%) of the children had 101 positive food challenges (42), skin symptoms developed during 85 (84%) challenges, gastrointestinal symptoms in 53 (52%), and respiratory symptoms in 32 (32%). When patients were given appropriate restrictive diets based on oral food challenge results, approximately 40% of the 40 patients re-evaluated lost their hypersensitivity after one or two years, and most showed significant improvement in their clinical course compared to patients in whom no food allergy was documented. Therefore, the authors concluded that FH plays a pathogenic role in some children with AD and that appropriate diagnosis and exclusionary diets can lead to significant improvement in their skin symptoms. In a retrospective analysis of 106 double-blind placebo-controlled food challenges to milk, egg, wheat, and soy in 64 children with AD (median age two years), 45% of the positive challenges were associated with late eczematous responses, which followed immediate-type reactions (43).

Early experiments demonstrated that ingested food antigens can penetrate the gastrointestinal barrier and are transported to IgE bearing mast cells in the skin. This was demonstrated in 65 normal adults who were first passively sensitized by intracutaneous injection of serum from a fish-allergic patient and a normal control (44). The next day, the participants ingested fish, and 61 subjects developed a local wheal and flare reaction within 90 minutes at the sensitized site, but not at the control site. Similar results were found in a series of experiments conducted in 66 normal children with serum from an egg-allergic subject (44). Subsequent experiments have shown that patients with AD have increased intestinal permeability due to an impaired gut mucosal barrier (45, 46), which may facilitate sensitization to food allergens.

Because AD is characterized by a dry and damaged skin barrier, increased allergen absorption can occur through the skin and lead to allergen sensitization as well (47). This has been demonstrated in murine models where skin barrier dysfunction has been shown to lead to systemic sensitization to allergens, including foods (48). In addition, Lack et al. (49) have found that in children with AD, the use of topical creams that contain peanut oil is associated with an increased risk for the development of peanut allergy.

TABLE 1 Studies Supporting a Role of Food Hypersensitivity in Patients with Atopic Dermatitis

Laboratory studies
1. Increased total and food-specific IgE levels in AD patients
2. Elevated plasma histamine levels in AD patients following positive oral food challenge
3. Increased activation of eosinophils and eosinophil products in AD patients after positive oral food challenge
4. Food-specific T cells cloned from active AD skin lesions
5. Casein-stimulated elevated expression of cutaneous lymphocyte antigen on T cells from AD patients with milk allergy
6. Murine models of food-induced atopic dermatitis

Clinical studies
1. Dietary elimination of food allergens leads to improvement in AD
2. Positive oral food challenges lead to worsening of AD symptoms
3. Breast-feeding and use of hypoallergenic infant formulas decrease the prevalence of AD in infants at high risk for atopic disease

Together, these studies suggest that AD and food allergies can play a role in the development and exacerbation of each other. A birth cohort of over 600 infants was investigated to determine whether FH precedes and predicts the development of AD or whether the converse was true (50). Infants with large SPT (>6 mm wheal) to at least one of three common food allergens (milk, egg, and/or peanut) at six months of age had a higher risk of developing AD (instantaneous RR, 2.28; 95% CI, 1.34–3.87) compared to infants without sensitization. The risk increased with sensitization to a greater number of foods. Excluding infants who already had allergic sensitization at six months, AD before six months was associated with an increased risk of having new sensitizations at one year (RR, 2.26; 95% CI, 1.34–3.82) when most new sensitizations were due to foods. Although this study was limited by the lack of oral food challenges to confirm food allergy, and AD was defined either as physician-diagnosed or any rash that was treated with corticosteroids, it does suggest a reciprocal pathogenic relationship between FH and AD.

Table 1 summarizes the findings from many of the studies discussed thus far.

PREVENTION OF AD AND FOOD ALLERGY IN INFANCY

Studies have also examined whether dietary modification can prevent the development of FH and AD. Nearly 80 years ago, Grulee and Sanford (51) reported that breast-feeding could reduce the development of AD. In addition to many health benefits of breast-feeding, several studies have demonstrated a protective effect on the development of various allergic disorders. A 17-year prospective study of 150 children by Saarinen and Kajosaari (52) supported breast-feeding as a preventative measure for the development of allergy. Children who had little or no breast-feeding (<1 month) had the highest prevalence of AD, food allergy, and respiratory allergy.

Several studies add further support for the protective effect of breast-feeding. A meta-analysis by Gdalevich et al. (53) found that of 18 prospective studies, the summary odds ratio (OR) for the protective effect of breast-feeding was 0.68 (95% CI, 0.52–0.88). This protective effect was more significant for children with a family history of atopy. For this population, exclusive breast-feeding during the first three months of life was associated with a decreased incidence of AD during childhood. These and many other studies conclude that breast-feeding is protective for allergic disease, mostly for high-risk children with an atopic family history.

However, the degree of benefit of breast-feeding for the prevention of allergic disease has been debated. A Cochrane review by Kramer and Kakuma (54) reported no significant reduction in the risk of AD, asthma, or other atopic diseases in breast-feeding studies from Finland, Australia, and Belarus. Many factors may contribute to these conflicting results, including differences in study designs, study populations, and duration of breast-feeding. In a 2006 Cochrane review (55), the authors concluded that dietary avoidance of allergenic foods by lactating mothers of infants with AD may reduce the severity of the eczema, however, larger trials are needed to confirm this.

The German Infant Nutritional Intervention (GINI) Study investigated the allergy preventive effect of three hydrolyzed infant formulas compared with cow's milk formula in a randomized, double-blind trial. In a study of 3903 infants, the investigators found that exclusive breast-feeding for the first four months of life was associated with a significant protective effect on AD if compared with conventional cow's milk formula [OR (adj), 0.64; 95% CI, 0.45–0.90] (56), and that the risk for AD can be reduced by supplementing with certain cow's milk hydrolysate formulas in high-risk infants when breast-feeding is insufficient (57). After three years, there was a significant reduction in the incidence of AD in high-risk infants supplemented with the extensively hydrolyzed casein formula in the intention-to-treat (ITT; $n = 1363$) and per protocol (PP; $n = 904$) analyses (ITT: population odds ratio [95% CI], 0.67 [0.45–0.99]; PP: adjusted odds ratio [OR(adj)], 0.53 [0.32–0.88]), and with the partially hydrolyzed whey formula in the PP analysis (ITT: population odds ratio, 0.76 [0.52–1.11]; PP: adjusted OR, 0.60 [0.37–0.97]). Interestingly, there was no significant difference in the incidence of AD for infants unselected for a history of atopy, whether they were exclusively breastfed for four months, fed cow's milk formula with or without breast-feeding, or fed hydrolyzed formula with or without breast-feeding (56).

Another area of interest for nutritional modification entails the timing of solid food introduction to infants. Kajosaari and Saarinen (58) reported that exclusive breast-feeding for the first six months of life led to decreased AD at one year of age as compared to introducing solids at three months of age. However, there was no difference in the prevalence of AD in a five-year follow-up study (59). In addition to timing, the diversity of foods that are introduced appeared to have some correlation with the development of allergy. Fergusson et al. (60) reported that increased rates of AD correlated with the introduction of increasing numbers of solid foods in the first four months of life.

In contrast, Zutavern et al. (61) reported that delayed introduction of solid foods is not protective against the development of asthma and allergy. They demonstrated that delayed introduction of egg and milk was associated with an increased risk of AD. Also, the GINI study reported that neither delaying introduction of solids beyond the 4th month nor delaying introduction of the most allergenic foods beyond the 6th month had a protective effect for the development of AD (62). Based on these conflicting findings, further studies are necessary before making specific conclusions or recommendations regarding the timing of solid food introduction and the development of AD.

TABLE 2   Approach to Food Hypersensitivity in Patients with Atopic Dermatitis

1. Consider evaluation if patient has
   (a) Moderate-to-severe atopic dermatitis
   (b) Need for constant topical steroids or calcineurin inhibitors to control skin symptoms
   (c) Worsening symptoms with particular foods
   (d) Known history of food hypersensitivity
   (e) Atopic history

2. Diagnostic work up
   (a) History and physical examination, including dietary history
   (b) Skin prick testing
   (c) Specific IgE testing
   (d) Oral food challenge for specific foods (unless history of severe reaction)
   (e) Periodic repeat testing/challenge to monitor for resolution of food hypersensitivity

DIAGNOSIS OF FH IN AD PATIENTS

The general approach for the diagnosis of FH begins with a complete history (Table 2). Details regarding immediate reactions to foods, including type of food, symptoms, and treatment required should be obtained. A dietary history is important, and in particular a three-day diet record can be very useful. For breast-feeding infants, the maternal diet history should be recorded because food allergen exposures can occur through breast milk (63). Based on the history, selected foods are evaluated by skin prick testing (SPT) or serum-specific IgE testing.

Although many reports have suggested that children with AD are sensitive to a large number of foods, analysis of data from a subset of patients revealed that most patients (80%) developed symptoms to only 1 to 3 foods when diagnosed by DBPCFC (64). Most children in this subset had positive prick skin tests to several foods (mean 3.5 years, range 0–10 years), although only about one-third of positive skin tests correlated with positive food challenges. Five foods (egg, peanut, milk, wheat, and soy) accounted for approximately 60% of the positive clinical responses.

The pattern of FH in children with AD appears to be stable. The major food allergens (milk, egg, wheat, soy, peanut, tree nuts, and seafood) accounted for 87% of positive food challenges in 1988 to 1989 and 91% of positive food challenges in 1998 to 1999 (Table 3) (65). Eigenmann and Calza (66) also found that egg, milk, and peanuts were most frequently responsible for positive food challenges in 74 Swiss children with AD. In adults, peanuts, tree nuts, fish, and shellfish are more commonly implicated (67, 68).

SPTs and/or serum IgE antibody testing are performed to detect food-specific IgE antibodies. SPT have high negative predictive value (>95%) (69, 70); therefore, a negative test virtually rules out IgE-mediated food allergy. However, the positive predictive value is approximately 30% to 50%; (69, 70) therefore a positive test in isolation may not be clinically relevant. Intradermal skin testing to foods is not indicated because there is a very high false-positive rate and a greater risk for adverse reactions (69).

SPT wheal sizes and food-specific IgE levels have been shown to have predictive value for clinical reactivity and are often relied upon to determine the management of food hypersensitivities (Table 4) (71–74). For example, when an allergen-specific IgE level is above an empirically determined threshold where there is a 95% positive predictive value for clinical reactivity (95 PPV), the specific food should be

TABLE 3 Foods Triggering the Majority of Food-Allergic Reactions

Infants/children	Adolescents/adults
Milk	Peanut
Egg	Tree nuts
Wheat	Fish
Soy	Shellfish
Peanut	
Tree nuts	
Fish	
Shellfish	

considered clinically reactive and strict dietary elimination is recommended. If the IgE level is close to a threshold where there is a 50% positive predictive value for clinical reactivity (50 PPV), an oral food challenge is entertained in the appropriate clinical setting to confirm or rule out clinical reactivity (72). In addition, monitoring IgE levels over time can provide additional prognostic information as shown by Shek et al. (75).

There has been increasing interest in the use of atopy patch testing (APT) to detect the late-onset skin symptoms following ingestion of food allergens. Several groups have demonstrated that eczematous skin lesions can be induced in patients with AD by patch testing with foods, however, the reported sensitivity and specificity of this test have been highly variable (76). In a recent study of over 400 children with suspected FH, patients underwent SPT, serum-specific IgE, APT, and oral food challenges to the suspected food allergens. The authors concluded that the APT only added a small increase in predictive value to the standard SPT and specific-IgE measurements in the diagnostic workup of FH (77). Although the APT shows some promise in identifying foods that may be involved in non-IgE–mediated reactions, there are currently no standardized reagents or methods of application and interpretation. Therefore, the APT remains an investigational tool at this time.

MANAGEMENT AND NATURAL HISTORY OF FH

Currently, there are no proven treatments that can cure or provide long-term remission from food allergy. The mainstay of management consists of avoidance and

TABLE 4 Predictive Values of Specific IgE (sIgE) and Skin Prick Testing (SPT) for Selected Food Allergens

	~50% react (72)	~95% react (71, 72)	~95% react (≤2 yrs of age) (86–88)
Milk	sIgE = 2 kIU/L	sIgE = 15 kIU/L [a]SPT = 8 mm wheal	sIgE = 5 kIU/L SPT = 6 mm wheal
Egg	sIgE = 2 kIU/L	sIgE = 7 kIU/L SPT = 7 mm wheal	sIgE = 2 kIU/L SPT = 5 mm wheal
Peanut	sIgE = 2 kIU/L (convincing history)	sIgE = 14 kIU/L	–
	sIgE = 2 kIU/L (unconvincing history)	SPT = 8 mm wheal	SPT = 4 mm wheal

[a]SPT: dependent upon extracts and technique utilized.

education as well as providing emergency medications for the treatment of allergic reactions. The importance of examining all the ingredients of foods to be consumed cannot be overemphasized, because the majority of fatal food reactions occur in individuals who are aware of their allergy, but unaware that the allergen is contained in commercially prepared foods (78). Recently, new labeling laws went into effect in the United States and Europe that should facilitate this process, as less-complicated terminology is required on all packaging labels (79). In addition, patients should be given guidance for managing their food allergies outside the home, such as in schools or restaurants, since not everyone may be educated about food allergies. Contamination of cookware and serving utensils or hidden ingredients in sauces are often not appreciated by cooking and serving staff and can pose a risk for food-allergic individuals. Despite these preventive measures, accidental exposures to food allergens still occur. Therefore, individuals should be instructed in the use of self-injectable epinephrine, and an individualized emergency plan should be in place.

The persistence of food allergy is variable and depends on the specific food allergen. Approximately 85% of children with cow's milk allergy will become tolerant by 8.6 years of age (80) and about 66% of those with egg allergy will become tolerant by age five years (81). More recent studies suggest that the rates of "outgrowing" food allergy are more prolonged for milk than reported previously (79% by 16 years) (82), and that it also takes longer for children to outgrow their egg allergy (68% outgrow by 16 years) (83). In contrast, only 20% of children with peanut allergy and 9% with tree nut allergy will eventually develop clinical tolerance (84, 85). Currently, there are no reliable predictive biomarkers to determine when and in whom clinical tolerance will occur; hence, periodic follow-up with measurement of serum-specific IgE levels and skin prick testing can help determine when oral food challenges would be appropriate. Predictive values for serum food–specific IgE levels and skin prick testing have been published for the major food allergens (Table 4) (71,72,86–88).

Even for those who are thought to be tolerant by double-blind, placebo-controlled food challenge, recurrence of allergy has been reported to occur in about 8% of peanut allergic individuals (89). This risk may be higher for those who continue to avoid peanut after having negative food challenges (although reverse causation cannot be ruled out), and therefore regular consumption is recommended for these individuals to confirm and maintain a tolerant state.

CLINICAL AND LABORATORY INVESTIGATIONS IN ADULTS
Few studies have examined the role of food allergy in adults with AD. Many adult patients do, however, report food-related worsening of their disease. In a study of 88 adolescent and adult AD patients who reported worsening of symptoms after ingestion of milk products, DBPCFC confirmed that ingestion of milk led to exacerbation of the AD in 22 of the patients (90). These patients had lymphocyte proliferative responses to casein that were significantly higher than those with AD whose milk sensitivity was not confirmed by oral food challenge and controls. Casein-specific IgE was elevated in only 41% of these patients, suggesting that non-IgE–mediated mechanisms may play a role for some.

In a study of 37 adult patients with AD and evidence of sensitization to birch pollen, patients were instructed to avoid birch-pollen associated foods (i.e., carrot, celery, hazelnut, apple, etc.) for a four-week period and then underwent DBPCFC to these foods (91). Seventeen patients had worsening of AD (with a median increase of 21 SCORAD points) within 48 hours of the challenge. In addition, sera from those who had positive challenges had a significantly higher proportion of their lymphocytes expressing cutaneous lymphocyte antigen (CLA$^+$) after incubation with birch pollen antigens as compared to lymphocytes from those who were nonresponsive to foods. Skin-derived T-cell lines also showed significantly greater degrees of stimulation after exposure to birch pollen antigen. Another study demonstrated that in patients who have birch allergy and AD, worsening of skin lesions without oral symptoms can also be observed when eating cooked versions of birch-related fruits and vegetables (i.e., apple, carrot, and celery) (92). These authors suggest that eating birch-related foods outside the birch season can lead to pollen-specific T-cell activation (high IL-4 and thus elevated IgE) and maintenance of the allergic immune response perennially.

A recent study compared 40 adults with poorly controlled severe AD despite the use of topical and oral corticosteroids, topical calcineurin inhibitors, antibiotics, and antihistamines with adults who had quiescent AD or moderate AD (treatment responsive) (93). The severe AD group had significantly higher total IgE levels and higher rates of sensitization to environmental and food allergens by skin testing as compared to the other groups. The most common foods that tested positive on skin testing were peanut, egg, shellfish, soy, and milk. Further prospective controlled studies are needed to determine whether food elimination diets would be effective for this group of adults.

CONCLUSIONS

There are clear and convincing data that FH plays a significant role in the symptomatology of AD in a subgroup of children with moderate-to-severe disease. Evaluations of skin biopsy and serologic specimens from children with AD, as well as from murine models of food-induced AD, have demonstrated the importance of IgE-mediated mechanisms. Clinical studies using double-blind, placebo-controlled food challenges and food elimination diets provide proof that clinical symptoms are directly affected by the ingestion or avoidance of certain food allergens in this subpopulation. This association is becoming better recognized by physicians as evidenced by recent increased referrals for food allergy evaluation in children with AD. For adults with AD, more studies need to be performed in order to determine the role of food allergens as trigger factors.

REFERENCES

1. Williams H, Stewart A, von Mutius E, et al. International study of asthma and allergies in childhood phase one and three study groups. Is eczema really on the increase worldwide? J Allergy Clin Immunol 2007; 121:947–54.
2. Hanifin JM, Rajka G. Diagnostic features of atopic dermatitis. Acta Derm Venereol Suppl (Stockh) 1980; 92:44,45–47.
3. Johnson EE, Irons JS, Patterson R, et al. Serum IgE concentration in atopic dermatitis. Relationship to severity of disease and presence of atopic respiratory disease. J Allergy Clin Immunol 1974; 54(2):94–99.
4. Sampson HA. Atopic dermatitis. Ann Allergy 1992; 69(6):469–479.
5. Novak N, Bieber T. Allergic and nonallergic forms of atopic diseases. J Allergy Clin Immunol 2003; 112(2):252–262.

6. Williams H, Flohr C. How epidemiology has challenged 3 prevailing concepts about atopic dermatitis. J Allergy Clin Immunol 2006; 118(1):209–213.
7. Ricci G, Patrizi A, Baldi E, et al. Long-term follow-up of atopic dermatitis: Retrospective analysis of related risk factors and association with concomitant allergic diseases. J Am Acad Dermatol 2006; 55(5):765–771.
8. Van Der Hulst AE, Klip H, Brand PL. Risk of developing asthma in young children with atopic eczema: A systematic review. J Allergy Clin Immunol 2007; 120(3): 565–569.
9. Gustafsson D, Sjoberg O, Foucard T. Development of allergies and asthma in infants and young children with atopic dermatitis—A prospective follow-up to 7 years of age. Allergy 2000; 55(3):240–245.
10. Hill DJ, Hosking CS. Food allergy and atopic dermatitis in infancy: An epidemiologic study. Pediatr Allergy Immunol 2004; 15(5):421–427.
11. Hill DJ, Hosking CS, de Benedictis FM, et al. Confirmation of the association between high levels of immunoglobulin E food sensitization and eczema in infancy: An International Study. Clin Exp Allergy 2007; 38(1):161–168.
12. Eigenmann PA, Sicherer SH, Borkowski TA, et al. Prevalence of IgE-mediated food allergy among children with atopic dermatitis. Pediatrics 1998; 101(3):E8.
13. Hill DJ, Heine RG, Hosking CS, et al. IgE food sensitization in infants with eczema attending a dermatology department. J Pediatr 2007; 151(4):359–363.
14. Sicherer SH, Sampson HA. Food hypersensitivity and atopic dermatitis: Pathophysiology, epidemiology, diagnosis, and management. J Allergy Clin Immunol 1999; 104 (3 Pt 2):S114–S122.
15. Solley GO, Gleich GJ, Jordon RE, et al. The late phase of the immediate wheal and flare skin reaction. Its dependence upon IgE antibodies. J Clin Invest 1976; 58(2):408–420.
16. Hamid Q, Boguniewicz M, Leung DY. Differential in situ cytokine gene expression in acute versus chronic atopic dermatitis. J Clin Invest 1994; 94(2):870–876.
17. Hamid Q, Naseer T, Minshall EM, et al. In vivo expression of IL-12 and IL-13 in atopic dermatitis. J Allergy Clin Immunol 1996; 98(1):225–231.
18. Tsicopoulos A, Hamid Q, Varney V, et al. Preferential messenger RNA expression of Th1-type cells (IFN-gamma$^+$, IL-2+) in classical delayed-type (tuberculin) hypersensitivity reactions in human skin. J Immunol 1992; 148(7):2058–2061.
19. Boguniewicz M, Leung DY. Atopic dermatitis. J Allergy Clin Immunol 2006; 117(2 Suppl Mini-Primer):S475–S480.
20. Palmer CN, Irvine AD, Terron-Kwiatkowski A, et al. Common loss-of-function variants of the epidermal barrier protein filaggrin are a major predisposing factor for atopic dermatitis. Nat Genet 2006; 38(4):441–446.
21. Weidinger S, Illig T, Baurecht H, et al. Loss-of-function variations within the filaggrin gene predispose for atopic dermatitis with allergic sensitizations. J Allergy Clin Immunol 2006; 118(1):214–219.
22. Baurecht H, Irvine AD, Novak N, et al. Toward a major risk factor for atopic eczema: Meta-analysis of filaggrin polymorphism data. J Allergy Clin Immunol 2007; 120(6): 1406–1412.
23. Howell MD, Kim BE, Gao P, et al. Cytokine modulation of atopic dermatitis filaggrin skin expression. J Allergy Clin Immunol 2007; 120(1):150–155.
24. Magnarin M, Knowles A, Ventura A, et al. A role for eosinophils in the pathogenesis of skin lesions in patients with food-sensitive atopic dermatitis. J Allergy Clin Immunol 1995; 96(2):200–208.
25. Sampson HA, Jolie PL. Increased plasma histamine concentrations after food challenges in children with atopic dermatitis. N Engl J Med 1984; 311(6):372–376.
26. Suomalainen H, Soppi E, Isolauri E. Evidence for eosinophil activation in cow's milk allergy. Pediatr Allergy Immunol 1994; 5(1):27–31.
27. Leung DY, Boguniewicz M, Howell MD, et al. New insights into atopic dermatitis. J Clin Invest 2004; 113(5):651–657.
28. Abernathy-Carver KJ, Sampson HA, Picker LJ, et al. Milk-induced eczema is associated with the expansion of T cells expressing cutaneous lymphocyte antigen. J Clin Invest 1995; 95(2):913–918.

29. Reekers R, Beyer K, Niggemann B, et al. The role of circulating food antigen-specific lymphocytes in food allergic children with atopic dermatitis. Br J Dermatol 1996; 135(6):935–941.
30. van Reijsen FC, Felius A, Wauters EA, et al. T-cell reactivity for a peanut-derived epitope in the skin of a young infant with atopic dermatitis. J Allergy Clin Immunol 1998; 101 (2 Pt 1):207–209.
31. Kondo N, Fukutomi O, Agata H, et al. The role of T lymphocytes in patients with food-sensitive atopic dermatitis. J Allergy Clin Immunol 1993; 91(2):658–668.
32. Li XM, Kleiner G, Huang CK, et al. Murine model of atopic dermatitis associated with food hypersensitivity. J Allergy Clin Immunol 2001; 107(4):693–702.
33. Spergel JM, Mizoguchi E, Oettgen H, et al. Roles of TH1 and TH2 cytokines in a murine model of allergic dermatitis. J Clin Invest 1999; 103(8):1103–1111.
34. Prescott VE, Forbes E, Foster PS, et al. Mechanistic analysis of experimental food allergen-induced cutaneous reactions. J Leukoc Biol 2006; 80(2):258–266.
35. Rowlands D, Tofte SJ, Hanifin JM. Does food allergy cause atopic dermatitis? Food challenge testing to dissociate eczematous from immediate reactions. Dermatol Ther 2006; 19(2):97–103.
36. Atherton DJ, Sewell M, Soothill JF, et al. A double-blind controlled crossover trial of an antigen-avoidance diet in atopic eczema. Lancet 1978; 1(8061):401–403.
37. Neild VS, Marsden RA, Bailes JA, et al. Egg and milk exclusion diets in atopic eczema. Br J Dermatol 1986; 114(1):117–123.
38. Sampson HA, Scanlon SM. Natural history of food hypersensitivity in children with atopic dermatitis. J Pediatr 1989; 115(1):23–27.
39. Lever R, MacDonald C, Waugh P, et al. Randomised controlled trial of advice on an egg exclusion diet in young children with atopic eczema and sensitivity to eggs. Pediatr Allergy Immunol 1998; 9(1):13–19.
40. Burks AW, Mallory SB, Williams LW, et al. Atopic dermatitis: Clinical relevance of food hypersensitivity reactions. J Pediatr 1988; 113(3):447–451.
41. Bock SA, Lee WY, Remigio LK, et al. Studies of hypersensitivity reactions to foods in infants and children. J Allergy Clin Immunol 1978; 62(6):327–334.
42. Sampson HA, McCaskill CC. Food hypersensitivity and atopic dermatitis: Evaluation of 113 patients. J Pediatr 1985; 107(5):669–675.
43. Breuer K, Heratizadeh A, Wulf A, et al. Late eczematous reactions to food in children with atopic dermatitis. Clin Exp Allergy 2004; 34(5):817–824.
44. Brunner M, Walzer M. Absorption of undigested proteins in human beings: The absorption of unaltered fish protein in adults. Arch Intern Med 1928; 42:173–179.
45. Pike MG, Heddle RJ, Boulton P, et al. Increased intestinal permeability in atopic eczema. J Invest Dermatol 1986; 86(2):101–104.
46. Majamaa H, Isolauri E. Evaluation of the gut mucosal barrier: Evidence for increased antigen transfer in children with atopic eczema. J Allergy Clin Immunol 1996; 97(4):985–990.
47. Leung DY. Atopic dermatitis: New insights and opportunities for therapeutic intervention. J Allergy Clin Immunol 2000; 105(5):860–876.
48. Strid J, Strobel S. Skin barrier dysfunction and systemic sensitization to allergens through the skin. Curr Drug Targets Inflamm Allergy 2005; 4(5):531–541.
49. Lack G, Fox D, Northstone K, et al. Avon Longitudinal Study of Parents and Children Study Team. Factors associated with the development of peanut allergy in childhood. N Engl J Med 2003; 348(11):977–985.
50. Lowe AJ, Abramson MJ, Hosking CS, et al. The temporal sequence of allergic sensitization and onset of infantile eczema. Clin Exp Allergy 2007; 37(4):536–542.
51. Grulee CG, Sanford HN. The influence of breast and artificial feeding on infantile eczema. J Pediatr 1930; 9:223–225.
52. Saarinen UM, Kajosaari M. Breastfeeding as prophylaxis against atopic disease: Prospective follow-up study until 17 years old. Lancet 1995; 346(8982):1065–1069.
53. Gdalevich M, Mimouni D, David M, et al. Breast-feeding and the onset of atopic dermatitis in childhood: A systematic review and meta-analysis of prospective studies. J Am Acad Dermatol 2001; 45(4):520–527.

54. Kramer MS, Kakuma R. The optimal duration of exclusive breastfeeding: A systematic review. Adv Exp Med Biol 2004; 554:63–77.
55. Kramer MS, Kakuma R. Maternal dietary antigen avoidance during pregnancy or lactation, or both, for preventing or treating atopic disease in the child. Cochrane Database Syst Rev 2006; 3:CD000133.
56. Laubereau B, Brockow I, Zirngibl A, et al. Effect of breast-feeding on the development of atopic dermatitis during the first 3 years of life—Results from the GINI-birth cohort study. J Pediatr 2004; 144(5):602–607.
57. von Berg A, Koletzko S, Filipiak-Pittroff B, et al. Certain hydrolyzed formulas reduce the incidence of atopic dermatitis but not that of asthma: Three-year results of the German infant nutritional intervention study. J Allergy Clin Immunol 2007; 119(3):718–725.
58. Kajosaari M, Saarinen UM. Prophylaxis of atopic disease by six months' total solid food elimination. Evaluation of 135 exclusively breast-fed infants of atopic families. Acta Paediatr Scand 1983; 72(3):411–414.
59. Kajosaari M. Atopy prophylaxis in high-risk infants. Prospective 5-year follow-up study of children with six months exclusive breastfeeding and solid food elimination. Adv Exp Med Biol 1991; 310:453–458.
60. Fergusson DM, Horwood LJ, Beautrais AL, et al. Eczema and infant diet. Clin Allergy 1981; 11(4):325–331.
61. Zutavern A, von Mutius E, Harris J, et al. The introduction of solids in relation to asthma and eczema. Arch Dis Child 2004; 89(4):303–308.
62. Filipiak B, Zutavern A, Koletzko S, et al. Solid food introduction in relation to eczema: Results from a four-year prospective birth cohort study. J Pediatr 2007; 151(4):352–358.
63. Sorva R, Makinen-Kiljunen S, Juntunen-Backman K. Beta-lactoglobulin secretion in human milk varies widely after cow's milk ingestion in mothers of infants with cow's milk allergy. J Allergy Clin Immunol 1994; 93(4):787–792.
64. Sampson HA, Ho DG. Relationship between food-specific IgE concentrations and the risk of positive food challenges in children and adolescents. J Allergy Clin Immunol 1997; 100(4):444–451.
65. Ellman LK, Chatchatee P, Sicherer SH, et al. Food hypersensitivity in two groups of children and young adults with atopic dermatitis evaluated a decade apart. Pediatr Allergy Immunol 2002; 13(4):295–298.
66. Eigenmann PA, Calza AM. Diagnosis of IgE-mediated food allergy among Swiss children with atopic dermatitis. Pediatr Allergy Immunol 2000; 11(2):95–100.
67. Bock SA, Atkins FM. The natural history of peanut allergy. J Allergy Clin Immunol 1989; 83(5):900–904.
68. Yunginger JW, Sweeney KG, Sturner WQ, et al. Fatal food-induced anaphylaxis. JAMA 1988; 260(10):1450–1452.
69. Bock SA, Buckley J, Holst A, et al. Proper use of skin tests with food extracts in diagnosis of hypersensitivity to food in children. Clin Allergy 1977; 7(4):375–383.
70. Sampson HA, Albergo R. Comparison of results of skin tests, RAST, and double-blind, placebo-controlled food challenges in children with atopic dermatitis. J Allergy Clin Immunol 1984; 74(1):26–33.
71. Sampson HA. Utility of food-specific IgE concentrations in predicting symptomatic food allergy. J Allergy Clin Immunol 2001; 107(5):891–896.
72. Perry TT, Matsui EC, Kay Conover-Walker M, et al. The relationship of allergen-specific IgE levels and oral food challenge outcome. J Allergy Clin Immunol 2004; 114(1):144–149.
73. Garcia-Ara MC, Boyano-Martinez MT, Diaz-Pena JM, et al. Cow's milk-specific immunoglobulin E levels as predictors of clinical reactivity in the follow-up of the cow's milk allergy infants. Clin Exp Allergy 2004; 34(6):866–870.
74. Celik-Bilgili S, Mehl A, Verstege A, et al. The predictive value of specific immunoglobulin E levels in serum for the outcome of oral food challenges. Clin Exp Allergy 2005; 35(3):268–273.
75. Shek LP, Soderstrom L, Ahlstedt S, et al. Determination of food specific IgE levels over time can predict the development of tolerance in cow's milk and hen's egg allergy. J Allergy Clin Immunol 2004; 114(2):387–391.

76. Turjanmaa K, Darsow U, Niggemann B, et al. EAACI/GA2LEN position paper: Present status of the atopy patch test. Allergy 2006; 61(12):1377–1384.
77. Mehl A, Rolinck-Werninghaus C, Staden U, et al. The atopy patch test in the diagnostic workup of suspected food-related symptoms in children. J Allergy Clin Immunol 2006; 118(4):923–929.
78. Pumphrey R. Anaphylaxis: Can we tell who is at risk of a fatal reaction? Curr Opin Allergy Clin Immunol 2004; 4(4):285–290.
79. Simons E, Weiss CC, Furlong TJ, et al. Impact of ingredient labeling practices on food allergic consumers. Ann Allergy Asthma Immunol 2005; 95(5):426–428.
80. Saarinen KM, Pelkonen AS, Makela MJ, et al. Clinical course and prognosis of cow's milk allergy are dependent on milk-specific IgE status. J Allergy Clin Immunol 2005; 116(4):869–875.
81. Boyano-Martinez T, Garcia-Ara C, Diaz-Pena JM, et al. Prediction of tolerance on the basis of quantification of egg white-specific IgE antibodies in children with egg allergy. J Allergy Clin Immunol 2002; 110(2):304–309.
82. Skripak JM, Matsui EC, Mudd K, et al. The natural history of IgE-mediated cow's milk allergy. J Allergy Clin Immunol 2007; 120(5):1172–1177.
83. Savage JH, Matsui EC, Skripak JM, et al. The natural history of egg allergy. J Allergy Clin Immunol 2007; 120(6):1413–1417.
84. Skolnick HS, Conover-Walker MK, Koerner CB, et al. The natural history of peanut allergy. J Allergy Clin Immunol 2001; 107(2):367–374.
85. Fleischer DM, Conover-Walker MK, Matsui EC, et al. The natural history of tree nut allergy. J Allergy Clin Immunol 2005; 116(5):1087–1093.
86. Garcia-Ara C, Boyano-Martinez T, Diaz-Pena JM, et al. Specific IgE levels in the diagnosis of immediate hypersensitivity to cows' milk protein in the infant. J Allergy Clin Immunol 2001; 107(1):185–190.
87. Boyano Martinez T, Garcia-Ara C, Diaz-Pena JM, et al. Validity of specific IgE antibodies in children with egg allergy. Clin Exp Allergy 2001; 31(9):1464–1469.
88. Hill DJ, Heine RG, Hosking CS. The diagnostic value of skin prick testing in children with food allergy. Pediatr Allergy Immunol 2004; 15(5):435–441.
89. Fleischer DM, Conover-Walker MK, Christie L, et al. Peanut allergy: Recurrence and its management. J Allergy Clin Immunol 2004; 114(5):1195–1201.
90. Werfel T, Ahlers G, Schmidt P, et al. Milk-responsive atopic dermatitis is associated with a casein-specific lymphocyte response in adolescent and adult patients. J Allergy Clin Immunol 1997; 99(1 Pt 1):124–133.
91. Reekers R, Busche M, Wittmann M, et al. Birch pollen-related foods trigger atopic dermatitis in patients with specific cutaneous T-cell responses to birch pollen antigens. J Allergy Clin Immunol 1999; 104(2 Pt 1):466–472.
92. Bohle B, Zwolfer B, Heratizadeh A, et al. Cooking birch pollen-related food: Divergent consequences for IgE- and T cell-mediated reactivity in vitro and in vivo. J Allergy Clin Immunol 2006; 118(1):242–249.
93. Salt BH, Boguniewicz M, Leung DY. Severe refractory atopic dermatitis in adults is highly atopic. J Allergy Clin Immunol 2007; 119(2):508–509.

14 Fungi in Atopic Dermatitis

Peter Schmid-Grendelmeier

Allergy Unit, Department of Dermatology, University Hospital, Gloriastr, Zuerich, Switzerland

Sabine Zeller and Reto Crameri

Swiss Institute for Allergy and Asthma Research SIAF, Davos, Switzerland

INTRODUCTION

Atopic dermatitis (AD) is a relapsing, high-purity skin inflammation. AD has a worldwide prevalence of 10% to 20% in children and of 1% to 3% in adults (1–3). During the past few years, an increased prevalence has been recognized in not only highly but also in some less-industrialized countries, particularly in upper social classes and urban regions (4). The manifestations of AD result from a complex interaction between environmental factors, pharmacologic abnormalities, skin barrier dysfunction, susceptibility genes, and immunologic phenomena, which have been confirmed in numerous experimental and epidemiologic studies and discussed in the other chapters of this book (5).

Among several contributing factors, cutaneous hyperactivity and inappropriate immune responses to various microorganisms such as bacteria or fungi as well as secondary infections appear to play an important role not only in the underlying pathology but also as factors responsible for sustained disease activity (6). Bacterial influences are a well-recognized and important contributing factor in the pathogenesis of AD interacting with inflammatory processes in this disease (7,8). Also the so-called hygiene hypothesis explaining a rise of inhalant allergic disease due to lacking microbial stimulation does not seem to apply to AD (9).

Since years there is also a strong debate whether and what role may fungi play in AD (10–13). In this chapter the currently available data on fungi and their possible role in AD are reviewed and critically discussed.

FUNGAL COLONIZATION IN AD

Fungal colonization can not only occur on healthy and affected atopic skin as normal part of the skin flora but can also cause actual infections such as *Tinea corporis*, *Tinea pedis*, or *Pityriasis versicolor*. Mainly Basidiomyceta and yeasts such as *Candida* and *Malassezia* spp. have been described in relation with AD—all of them able to colonize the skin (14–19).

Culture of nonpathogenic fungal species is not widely established and sometimes difficult, but it is well known that such species can also induce immunologic responses and therefore act as possible pathogens in AD. There is still somehow limited data about the composition and quantity of fungal colonization in AD in comparison with individuals with healthy skin. Some important progress in differentiation between various fungal species has taken place within the last decade by fungal detection based on PCR, allowing a more sensitive detection of various species.

Conflicting results have been reported on the role of intestinal or skin colonization with *Candida albicans* in AD. Candida species, especially *C. albicans* have been cultured more frequently from patients with AD, preferentially from the gastrointestinal tract, than from healthy donors, but reports about any correlation between disease severity and fungal colonization are rare (19).

Basidiomycetous yeasts such as *Cryptococcus diffluens* and *Cryptococcus liquefaciens* have been identified by PCR in 42% (15/36) and 33% (12/36) of patients, and for healthy subjects these two yeasts are identified in 20% (6/30) and 20% (6/30), respectively (20).

THE SPECIAL ROLE OF COLONIZATION WITH *MALASSEZIA* SPP.

The yeast *Malassezia*, formerly known as *Pityrosporum*, belongs to the normal cutaneous microflora. *Malassezia* species are lipophilic yeasts commonly found on the body surface in humans and warm-blooded animals, typically predominating seborrhoic skin sites, such as head and neck, because of their defect in the synthesis of fatty acids and their need for nutritive requirement of exogenous fatty acids.

Malassezia is usually a harmless organism, but under certain conditions it may act as an opportunistic pathogen causing skin infections, such as *Pityriasis versicolor* and *Pityrosporum folliculitis*, and has been described besides AD in relation with seborrhoic dermatitis (21,22).

Today, 11 different *Malassezia* species are known. Of these *M. furfur*, *M. globosa*, *M. restricta*, *M. slooffiae*, *M. obtus*, *M. yamatoensis*, and *M. sympodialis* have been investigated in relation with human skin diseases (23,24). Another species, *M. pachydermatis* plays in important role in veterinarian skin diseases such as canine AD (see below) (25).

M. sympodialis has been reported as the most frequent species in both AD patients and healthy individuals in various studies when analyzed by fungal cultures (26).

Preferentially not only *M. sympodialis*, but also *M. globosa* and *M. restricta* occur in up to 90% of the AD patients as well as in 34% of normal cutaneous flora (27) on the grounds that it colonizes sebum-rich skin. In AD positive cultures are found more common in nonlesional than in lesional skin (44% vs. 28%; $P < 0.05$) (27). This is different in seborrhoic dermatitis, where positive cultures are found in up to 75% of both lesional and nonlesional skin of patients.

Based on PCR analysis, mostly *M. globosa* and *M. restricta* were found to form 80% of the colonization by *Malassezia*, in AD. PCR analysis also shows that *M. sympodialis* is found to be more common in healthy skin than in AD patients (28). In own measurements based on PCR-REA and sequencing (BLAST), it was found that *Malassezia* spp. were also as common on healthy skin as on AD patients. In addition the fungi were more commonly detected on unaffected than on affected skin. *M. globosa* (pos. in 32 of 66 patients) and *M. restricta* (30 of 66 patients) were also more common than *M. sympodialis* (8 of 66 patients.) (29).

Malassezia Colonization in Other Inflammatory Skin Diseases

Malassezia was also investigated in other skin diseases than in AD. Strains of *M. restricta* occur in the lesional skin of patients with seborrhoic dermatitis (30). It was recently shown that dandruff (31) can be mediated by *Malassezia* metabolites resulting in increased levels of scalp free fatty acids, specifically irritating free fatty acids released from sebaceous triglycerides. In Japan also the so-called Akatsuki disease (pomade crust) has been reported to be related with *Malassezia* (32).

Also in psoriatic skin the overall detection rates by PCR in lesional and non-lesional skin of *M. restricta, M. globosa*, and *M. sympodialis* are high (being 96%, 82%, and 64%, respectively) (33). Also there seems to be no difference between lesional and nonlesional skin area.

Measuring genetic polymorphism of *Malassezia* spp. in patients suffering from various skin diseases such as AD, *Pityriasis versicolor*, seborrhoic dermatitis, and seborrhoic dermatitis associated with HIV dermatitis as well as from healthy individuals, *M. furfur, M. globosa, M. restricta, M. slooffiae*, and *M. obtusa* were observed in homogenous strains, whereas *M. sympodialis* showed the greatest homogeneity (23). The skin microflora of AD patients seems to show greater diversity than that of healthy subjects.

In summary, colonization with *Malassezia* spp., especially *M. sympodialis* does not seem to be more common in AD than in healthy controls or other skin diseases and is at least as frequent in nonaffected skin compared to lesional skin.

Variation in Fungal Colonization During Lifetime

There are substantial variations between fungal colonization and especially *Malassezia* flora during age. Both *Candida* and *Malassezia* can be found in neonates (34). *Malassezia* colonization increases after the first week of life. The correlation between neonatal cephalic pustulosis and *Malassezia* is controversially discussed (35). However, *M. restricta* seems to be the predominant species in the children with AD, while both *M. restricta* and *M. globosa* are predominated in the adults. Skin infections, especially in tropical areas are also caused by *Malassezia* spp. such as *P. versicolor* and are quite common in infants (36,37).

INNATE AND HUMORAL IMMUNE RESPONSE TO FUNGI IN AD

Innate Immune Response
Skin Barrier Dysfunction and Antimicrobial Proteins and Their Impact on Fungal Colonization

Patients with AD present an altered skin structure, which is characterized by the following features:

Deficient skin barrier due to a lack of barrier proteins such as filaggrin (38,39)
Changed, less optimal lipid layer
Predominantly alkaline skin pH
Decreased expression and synthesis of antimicrobial peptides (8,40).

Skin barrier dysfunction together with immunologic deficiency favors colonization both of lesional skin and unaffected skin by different microorganisms, including fungal species.

Human antimicrobial proteins such as defensins are able to kill *Candida* spp. and also *Malassezia* (41). Synthetic or human cathelicidins such as cathelicidin LL-37 also play a role in skin defence against dermatophytes and *M. furfur* (42). On the other hand, *M. sympodialis* can also trigger the innate immune response differently in patients with AE and healthy individuals by enhanced LL-37 secretion from monocyte-derived dendritic cells (43). Another important linking element between *Malassezia* colonization and AD is the decreased expression of β-defensin-2 (HBD-2) in keratinocytes. Usually, HBD-2–expression is upregulated after *Malassezia* uptake in human keratinocytes which limits the uptake of further *Malassezia* cells from the extracellular environment and reflects regulated innate host defence (44). This immunmodulatory ability is not present in AD and allows uncontrolled penetration of *Malassezia* spp. into keratinocytes.

Skin pH

Also the "acid mantle" of the stratum corneum is important for both permeability barrier formation and cutaneous antimicrobial defence (45). The pH of the skin follows a sharp gradient across the stratum corneum, which is suspected to be important in controlling enzymatic activities and skin renewal. The skin pH is affected by a great number of endogenous factors, for example, skin moisture, sweat, sebum, anatomic site, genetic predisposition, and age. In addition, exogenous factors like detergents, cosmetic products, occlusive dressings as well as topical antibiotics influence the skin pH.

Such changes in the pH are also involved in the fungal colonization in AD— especially for yeasts such as *Malassezia* colonizing the upper layer of the stratum corneum. Because both lipid organization and lipid metabolism in the stratum corneum require an acidic pH, these changes might additionally contribute to the disturbance of skin barrier function observed in AD. An impaired release of proton donors to the stratum corneum in AD is also the result of reductions in filaggrin proteolysis and sweat secretion (46). In addition, the release of allergens of *Malassezia* spp. is increased with the higher skin pH found in AD (47).

Thus, there might be a mutual influence of the disrupted skin barrier in AD allowing *Malassezia* allergens to penetrate on one hand and favoring the increased expression of its allergens on the other hand.

ADAPTIVE IMMUNE RESPONSE

Cellular and Humoral Immune Response to Fungi in AD

It is nowadays well accepted that both cellular and humoral immunity play a role in the defense against fungal elements. Already in older studies a strikingly weaker cellular response to fungi was found in AD patients compared to healthy individuals, while the total and specific IgE synthesis was increased (14,15).

IgE-Mediated Sensitization Against *Malassezia*

The first description of a specific immunglobuline response against *P. ovale* reports an IgG response and dates from 1982 (48). Faergemann et al. found IgG against these species in individuals independently whether they were healthy or had AD. In patients suffering from pityrosporum folliculitis with detectable IgG response, no IgE-mediated hypersensitivity as investigated by skin-prick tests with the fungal extracts was found (49). IgE-mediated sensitizations against *Malassezia* were for the first time observed only when patients with AD were finally investigated by intradermal skin tests and IgE determination (50). Subsequently many studies confirmed specific IgE against *Malassezia* in AD and a pathogenetic role of the lyophilic yeast in the disease has been postulated (10,11,17,51–62).

Later, it has been shown that only AD patients but not healthy controls are sensitized to *M. sympodialis*, demonstrated by either positive skin-prick test, positive atopy patch test, or specific IgE antibodies to *Malassezia* (63). Also in other studies, specific IgE was detected almost or exclusively in AD patients but not in patients with other atopic diseases, or other inflammatory skin conditions, and never in healthy subjects (10). We investigated 706 individuals by ImmunoCAPm70 and skin-prick tests with a crude *M. sympodialis* extract and found in 52/97 AD patients specific IgE against *M. sympodialis*, but only in 4 out of 609 other patients sensitization to *M. sympodialis* was detectable (62).

Humoral Sensitization Against Other Fungi

There is a strong variation in the prevalence of patients with AD and positive skin-prick test to *C. albicans* extract and positive specific IgE. In vitro *C. albicans* induces high secretion of IL-4 and macrophage-derived chemokines and only low levels of IFN-γ, which indicates a Th2-type immune response and a possible sensitization to this yeast (64). However, IgE-sensitization against *Candida* can occur in variety of allergic diseases compared to sensitization against *Malassezia*, which is almost exclusively restricted to AD patients.

A further ubiquitous Basidiomycetous species, *Coprinus comatus*, was also investigated for its capacity to induce eczematous reactions in sensitized patients and was able to induce positive skin-prick tests (in 20 of 38 patients) and positive atopy-patch-test reactions in 12 out of 38 AD patients (65,66).

Cellular Immune Response

Although IgE-mediated sensitization mainly against *Malassezia* is largely documented, the mechanisms of the allergic responses are not fully understood, possibly due to the large number of allergens contained in fungi (67). T-cell reactivity and PBMC response to fungal allergens in AD differ markedly in their response to *Malassezia* antigen stimulation (68–73); stimulation of PBMC can lead to increased production of various cytokines such as IL2, IL-4, IL-10, or IFN-γ (72,74). In general, *Malassezia* seems to induce more Th2-dominated cytokine profile from PBMC (70,71).

In addition, *Malassezia* spp. are also able to induce cytokine production by keratinocytes such as IL-1 (73,75). However, this cytokine production needs the presence of *Malassezia*, and there are differences in ability to induce cytokine production by human keratinocytes among *Malassezia* yeasts. Such differences may also reflect the different inflammatory responses in *Malassezia*-associated dermatoses, resulting in different clinical and pathologic manifestations. Unlike in *Staphylococci* (76,77), no superantigen activity of *Malassezia* could be demonstrated till now (68).

Only recently, interactions between dendritic cells and *Malassezia* have been investigated in detail. *Malassezia* allergens adhere to antigen-presenting cells (APC's) via different receptors (mannose receptors, etc.) or pinocytosis. Among these, Langerhans cells, usually increased in number in atopic affected skin and expressing MHC class II on their cell surface, and AD-specific inflammatory dendritic epidermal cells (IDECs) (78) play the key role in first sensitization phase. This process is associated with the release of proinflammatory and immunoregulatory cytokines from activated APCs (TNF-α, IL-1β, IL-16, and IL-18) and surrounding

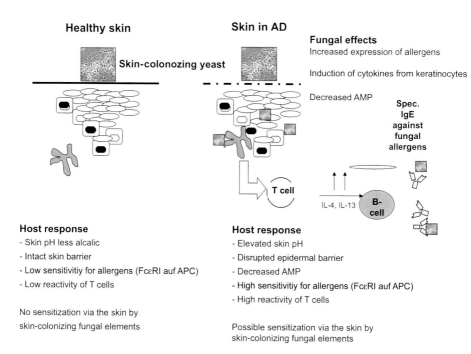

Healthy skin

Skin-colonozing yeast

Host response
- Skin pH less alcalic
- Intact skin barrier
- Low sensitivitiy for allergens (FcɛRI auf APC)
- Low reactivity of T cells

No sensitization via the skin by
skin-colonizing fungal elements

Skin in AD

Fungal effects
Increased expression of allergens

Induction of cytokines from keratinocytes

Decreased AMP

Spec. IgE against fungal allergens

T cell

IL-4, IL-13   B-cell

Host response
- Elevated skin pH
- Disrupted epidermal barrier
- Decreased AMP
- High sensitivitiy for allergens (FcɛRI auf APC)
- High reactivity of T cells

Possible sensitization via the skin by
skin-colonizing fungal elements

FIGURE 1 Various factors leading to IgE-mediated sensitization against skin colonizing yeasts such as Malassezia in AD in comparison with normal skin.

keratinocytes [human thymic stromal lymphopoietin (TSLP)], which act as migratory signals for Th2-type cells and therefore Th2-type immune response (79). Sensitization of AD patients to *M. furfur* can be mediated by immature dendritic cells in the skin as shown by Buentke et al. (80,81). *Malassezia* also enhances natural killer cell–induced maturation of dendritic cell maturation (82). Also monocyte-derived dendritic cells from AD patients show an increased trafficking and stimulatory capacity in response to *M. sympodialis* than healthy subjects resulting in a stronger inflammatory response to this agent (83).

IgE-mediated sensitization against *Malassezia* is a common and quite specific phenomenon for AD. This might be due to a combination of various factors, including both innate and adaptive immunity: a decreased epidermal barrier, elevated skin pH, and reduced antimicrobial peptides allowing this yeast to penetrate the skin and even to produce more allergens than in healthy subjects—and the atopic skin condition formed by APC with increased stimulatory capacity and T cells and increased tendency to produce Th2-directect cytokine patterns including increased IgE production (Fig. 1). *Malassezia* spp. itself are able to upregulate this inflammatory response by stimulation of APC and both cytokine and chemokine production in keratinocytes.

THE PREVALENCE AND CLINICAL FEATURES OF FUNGAL SENSITIZATION IN AD

Sensitization rates vary from 31% to 68% in adult AD patients based on *Malassezia*-specific serum IgE and approximately 30% to 80% using positive SPT with

Malassezia extracts (54). Thus, sensitization against *Malassezia* is a quite common phenomenon, especially among adult AD patients.

Fungal Sensitization During Lifetime

Although large epidemiologic or genetic studies are lacking, it can be stated that there are substantial variations between fungal sensitization, especially to *Malassezia* spp. during age. IgE antibodies against *Malassezia* spp. seem to be less prevalent in children, varying between 13% and 21% (53,84). In our own study including 369 children aged from 3 months to 12 years, we compared sensitization against *Malassezia* adults with those in children. Adults showed an increased colonization and sensitization rates in comparison with children of 19% in terms of anti–*Malassezia*-specific IgE (measured by ImmunoCAP m223) responses in the sera (85).

On the other hand, sensitization rates of 67% to *Malassezia* were found in elderly adult patients with AD (mean age 52 years) (86). Interestingly, in these patients IgE antibodies to *Malassezia* (m70) were more common in patients with ongoing AD, while positive *Malassezia* culture was seen mainly in patients without ongoing AD. Also these conflicting findings point out that a possible pathogenetic role of *Malassezia* in AD seems to be rather due to the very individual immune response of some AD patients than to a simple result of colonization.

Clinical Features in *Malassezia*-Associated AD

A preferential observation of *Malassezia*-specific IgE in the head and neck type of AD has been observed in many studies (11,56,58,60,87–89). Although IgE formation against *Malassezia* is not at all restricted to this subgroup of AD (62), these patients show the highest prevalence rate reaching up to 81% in some studies.

An increased incidence of *Malassezia*-specific IgE with elevated disease activity has been found in several studies. On the other hand, no correlation between a positive PCR and detectable IgE sensitization against *Malassezia* or disease activity was observed (29). Thus, when there is a pathogenetic role of *Malassezia* in AD, it seems to be rather due to the allergens secreted or due to direct influences of the yeast on skin barrier than to the colonization of the skin itself.

IgE- and T-cell–mediated reactivity against *M. sympodialis* was also found in patients with the nonallergic (non-IgE–mediated or intrinsic) form of AD (62,90,91). Thus, microbial agents such as *Staphylococci* and *Malassezia* may play a trigger role in this form of AD hitherto undiscovered by a usual diagnostic workup with common inhalant or food allergens (92).

Geographic Distribution

Fungal sensitization in AD has been described worldwide; by far the most of the reports are coming not only from Europe (11,60,89) and Asia, especially Far East, namely, Japan and Korea (52,93), but also from the Middle East (94). However, the occurrence of sensitization against *Malassezia* has also been reported in North and Latin America (24,57,95), East Africa (37), and Australia (96), although the prevalence of *Malassezia*-related IgE in AD is less investigated in these areas. As especially studies looking routinely for sensitization rates in large AD populations are still lacking, it is unclear whether possible geographic differences in the sensitization rate to *Malassezia* and its importance are due to real climatic, ethnic, or sociocultural differences or are just a consequence of the lack of the according detection of fungal specific IgE in some areas.

DIAGNOSTIC TOOLS TO DETERMINE FUNGAL SENSITIZATION

As in all fungal allergies, the testable allergen panel is limited in regard to specificity and sensitivity also in the diagnosis of AD (67)

Diagnosis of *Malassezia* sensitization can be done by detecting specific serum IgE or skin tests. Serum IgE against *M. sympodialis* extract can be measured using a commercial kit (ImmunoCAP® m70 by Phadia) based on *M. sympodialis* extract obtained from the American Type Culture Collection strain no. 42132. Recently, a new kit containing several species of *Malassezia* has also been introduced (m227), leading to a slightly increased sensitivity according to our experience.

Skin test extracts for *Malassezia* are not yet commercially available. For study purposes extracts made of the same strain as used for measurement of serum IgE have been used with good specificity and sensitivity in skin-prick tests and also in atopy patch tests (21,97,98).

Atopy patch tests are also an additional tool to define T-cell–mediated sensitization against *Malassezia* species (21,62,87,97,98). Using paper discs in Finn chambers (12 mm; Epitest Ltd., Hermal, Germany) and 30 µL *M. sympodialis* extract at a concentration of 5 mg/mL, added to skin that has been tape-stripped 10 times with scotch tape, allows to detect a specific and sensitive response that can be read after 48 and 72 hours.

Because the storage of extracts of fungal allergens is limited to as little as about a month even when stored at 4°C, there is still only limited use of such delicate allergen extracts in daily practice (99).

RECOMBINANT ALLERGENS OF *MALASSEZIA* SPECIES

The use of single recombinant allergens might substantially improve the specificity of diagnosis of *Malassezia* sensitization (21,98).

To date three genes encoding allergens from *M. furfur* (100,101) and 10 from *M. sympodialis* have been cloned and used to produce the corresponding recombinant allergens (102) (Table 1). The recombinant proteins span a molecular weight ranging from 12 to 86 kDa and belong to different families of proteins.

Mala s 1 is a component of the cell wall of the yeast and represents a protein without any relevant sequence homology to known proteins (103). It is a major *M. sympodialis* allergen which is exquisitely species-specific and, therefore, of high diagnostic value.

Mala f 2 and Mala s 3 from *M. furfur* as well as Mala s 5 from *M. sympodialis* belong to the class of peroxisomal proteins, highly cross-reactive allergens occurring in many fungal species (104,105).

Mala s 6, Mala s 10, Mala s 11, and Mala s 13 are members of phylogenetically highly conserved proteins showing also sequence homology to the corresponding human self-antigens (discussed below in more detail) (106).

Mala f 4 is a malate dehydrogenase and Mala s 12 is a member of the glucose–methanol–choline oxidoreductase family (107). The allergen repertoire of *M. sympodialis* is far to be completed as shown by high throughput screening of a cDNA library displayed on phage surface which delivered at least 27 different allergen-encoding sequences (108). However, the allergens, which are available so far have been proven to be of high diagnostic value (62).

A panel composed of Mala s 1 as a highly *Malassezia*-specific allergen added by Mala s 2, 3, 5, and 9 would be a useful tool to detect most cases of sensitization to these yeast. The allergens Mala s 6, Mala s 10, Mala s 11, and Mala s 13 are of special

TABLE 1 Cloned IgE-Binding Proteins from *Malassezia furfur* and *Malassezia sympodialis*

Cross-reactivity

Allergen	GenBank acc. no.	PDB ID[a]	Size (kDa)	Function	Skin tests	Cross-reactivity	Ref.
Mala s 1[b]	X96486	2p9 w	36	Unknown, cell wall protein	Yes	—	(103)
Mala f 2[c]	AB011804	—	20	Peroxisomal protein	No	—	(101)
Mala f 3	AB011805	—	21	Peroxisomal protein	No	—	(101)
Mala f 4	AF084828	—	35	Malate dehydrogenase	No	—	(100)
Mala s 5	AJ011955	—	18	Peroxisomal protein	Yes	—	(102)
Mala s 6	AJ011956	2cfe	17	Cyclophilin	Yes	Asp f 11, Hom s CyP A-C	(120)
Mala s 7	AJ011957	—	16	Unknown	Yes	—	(154)
Mala s 8	AJ011958	—	18	Unknown	Yes	—	(154)
Mala s 9	AJ011959	—	14	Unknown	Yes	—	(154)
Mala s 10	AJ428052	—	86	Heat shock protein 70	No	Hom s MnSOD	(155)
Mala s 11	AJ548421	—	22	MnSOD	No	—	(155)
Mala s 12	AJ871960	—	66	Glucose-methanol-choline oxidoreductase	No	—	(107)
Mala s 13	AJ937743	2j23	12	Thioredoxin	Yes	Asp f 28, Asp f 29, Hom s Trx	(117)

Sequence homology

Allergen	GenBank acc. no.	PDB ID[a]	Size (kDa)	Function	Skin tests	Sequence homology	Ref.
Mala s 1b	X96486	2p9 w	36	Unknown, cell wall protein	Yes	Asp f 2, Mala f 3, Mala f 5	(156)
Mala f 2[c]	AB011804	—	20	Peroxisomal protein	No	Asp f 2, Mala f 2, Mala f 5	(101)
Mala f 3	AB011805	—	21	Peroxisomal protein	No	—	(101)
Mala f 4	AF084828	—	35	Malate dehydrogenase	No	—	(100)
Mala s 5	AJ011955	—	18	Peroxisomal protein	Yes	Asp f 2, Mala f 2, Mala f 3	(102)
Mala s 6	AJ011956	2cfe	17	Cyclophilin	Yes	Asp f 11, Asp f 27, Cand a CyP, Sac c Cyp, Hom s CyP A, Hom s CyP B, Hom s CyP C	(102)
Mala s 7	AJ011957	—	16	Unknown	Yes	—	(154)
Mala s 8	AJ011958	—	18	Unknown	Yes	—	(154)
Mala s 9	AJ011959	—	14	Unknown	Yes	—	(154)
Mala s 10	AJ428052	—	86	Heat shock protein 70	No	Hom s Hsp-105, *Neurospora crassa* hsp-88, *Schizosaccharomyces pombe* hsp homolog pss1	(155)
Mala s 11	AJ548421	—	22	MnSOD	No	Asp f 6, Hev b 10, Pis v 4, Sac c MnSOD, Dro m MnSOD, Hom s MnSOD	(155)
Mala s 12	AJ871960	—	66	Glucose-methanol-choline oxidoreductase	No	—	(107)
Mala s 13	AJ937743	2j23	12	Thioredoxin	Yes	Asp f 28, Asp f 29, Cop c 2, Hom s Trx	(117)

a Protein Data Bank identification of crystal structure.
b *Malassezia sympodialis* strain ATCC 42132.
c *Malassezia furfur* strain TIMM 2782.

use if highly conserved proteins being candidates for autoreactive phenomenons are investigated.

According to our experience, recombinant single allergens can be used for skin-prick tests and also APT at a concentration of 100 mg/mL, the later needing additional skin tape stripping. IgE measurement can be based on ELISA or Immuno-CAP. To date, recombinant allergens of *Malassezia* or *Candida* are not yet commercially available neither for measuring specific serum IgE nor for skin test use.

AUTOREACTIVITY TO FUNGAL ALLERGENS DUE TO MOLECULAR MIMICRY

Autoreactivity to human proteins has been postulated as a decisive pathogenetic factor for AD patients based on the detection of IgE directed against various proteins (109–113).

Immunologic studies have shown that various fungal proteins can also act as cross-reacting allergens with human proteins: manganese superoxide dismutase (MnSOD) (114,115), cyclophilins (116), and thioredoxins (117,118) are highly relevant, cross-reactive fungal allergens (119). As clearly demonstrated, all these human proteins are also able to bind serum IgE from AD patients sensitized to the corresponding environmental allergen, to stimulate T-cell proliferation in vitro, and to elicit positive SPT in vivo.

STRUCTURAL ANALYSIS OF POTENTIAL SELF-ALLERGENS HOMOLOGOUS TO FUNGAL ALLERGENS

To elucidate the molecular basis of self-reactivity at molecular level, we have concentrated our efforts in solving the 3D structures of Mala s 6 (cyclophilin) (120) and Mala s 13 (thioredoxin) (117). Both proteins are, together with Mala s 11 (MnSOD), phylogenetically highly conserved and stress inducible. This applies not only for the fungal allergens, but also to the structurally related human self-antigens.

The solved crystal structures of Asp f 6, the MnSOD of *A. fumigatus* (121,122), Mala s 6 (120), and Mala s 13 (123) offer a rational explanation for the observed phenomena. In all three cases the crystal structures of the corresponding human proteins are available. This allows a direct comparison of the shared structural features. Although the sequence identity between the environmental allergens and the corresponding human proteins at amino acid level is high (45–71%), only a very limited number of identical amino acids are exposed to the solvent in the correctly folded protein pairs.

However, only those residues that are identical in pairs of allergens and at least partly exposed to the solvent can contribute to the binding of cross-reactive IgE antibodies in native proteins. Because the environmental allergens and the corresponding human self-antigens show cross-reactivity in Western blot, ELISA, and skin tests, they must share common IgE-binding epitopes.

In all these cases, the conserved surface-exposed residues are scattered over the whole sequences of the molecules and are thus likely to define the typical discontinuous structures found in B-cell epitopes. In fact in the pairwise superimposition of the solved 3D crystal structures, these amino acids are clustered over the surfaces forming patches covering solvent-accessible surface areas involving 15 to 22 identical amino acid residues located in different surface loops defining buried surfaces compatible with the structure of B-cell epitopes (124) (Fig. 2).

Perhaps the most impressive indication for the involvement of such B-cell epitopes in the pathogenesis of AD derives from APT performed with human

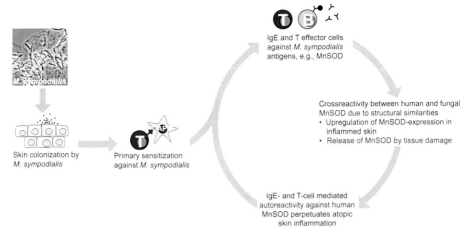

FIGURE 2   Mechanism leading to autoreactivity against fungal allergens such as MnSOD due to cross-reactivity and molecular mimicry with human proteins.

recombinant MnSOD in AD patients sensitized to fungal MnSOD (97). Simple application of human MnSOD for APT on the skin of these patients was sufficient to elicit an eczematous reaction clearly showing a role of cross-reactive MnSOD-specific IgE antibodies in the exacerbation of AD.

According to the allergenicity of cyclophilin, thioredoxin, and other IgE-binding human autoallergens, which has been demonstrated in vitro and in SPT, it can be assumed that also these human proteins could be able to contribute to the development of eczematous reactions. However, the repertoire of IgE-binding self-antigens is far to be completed as demonstrated by high throughput screening of human cDNA libraries displayed on phage surface with serum IgE of AD patients, which yielded more than 140 sequences of human proteins potentially representing autoallergens.

Based on these results and findings from Valenta et al. (109–113) nowadays a role of self-reactivity in the pathogenesis of AD can clearly be postulated (106). Sensitization might be most likely induced primarily by exposure to environmental fungal proteins such as MnSOD, cyclophilin, or thioredoxin of *M. sympodialis* leading than by molecular mimicry to secondary autoreactivity to its human counterpart (Fig. 2). Autoreactivity might therefore be of pivotal importance for the perpetuation of AD in the absence of external exposure, especially at later stages of AD with longstanding inflammatory damage (125).

THE ROLE OF FUNGAL ELELMENTS IN CANINE AD

AD is a common skin problem in dogs, especially affecting some breeds such as Beagles or West Highland White Terriers (126). *Malassezia* plays an important role not only in seborrhoic dermatitis and otitis externa, but also in canine AD (25). Skin colonization is mainly due to *M. pachydermatis* (127), which is also capable of inducing positive intradermal reactions or specific IgE in dogs with an AD phenotype (128,129). IgE-mediated sensitization against *M. pachydermatis* is specific for dogs suffering from AD, but does not occur in healthy dogs or in nonatopic dogs with simple colonization to *Malassezia* related to dermatitis or otitis (129,130). Also in

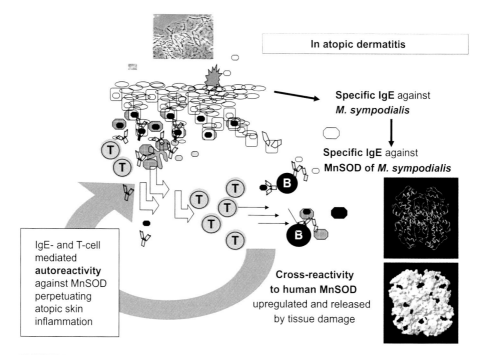

FIGURE 3 Molecular mimicry with allergens of skin-colonizing yeasts leading to autoreactivity with human tissue proteins such as MnSOD in AD.

dogs, unaffected skin areas are often as much colonized as apparently affected skin areas (131). Due to this similarity, canine AD might represent a useful model for the study of mechanism of sensitization and also for the pathogenetic role of fungal colonization in human AD (132).

Epidermal hyperplasia as seen in *Malassezia* dermatitis does not seem to be caused by fungal products acting on keratinocytes directly by secretion of products from the organism (133). Patch tests with extracts of *M. pachydermatis* also showed conflicting results as being positive in some healthy dogs after two to eight days (134). So far no circulating skin-specific autoreactive IgE-antibodies could be found in canine AD (135).

Malassezia dermatitis, but not canine AD is principally managed by antifungals (136). Immunotherapy with *M. pachydermatis* extracts is sometimes performed in *Malassezia*-sensitized dogs with AD but sometimes additional antifungals for extended control of recurrent yeast infections is needed (128,137).

THE USE OF ANTIFUNGALS AS A TREATMENT OPTION IN AD
The standard for AD patients is based on skin care to reconstitute skin barrier, identification, and elimination of trigger factors and anti-inflammatory treatment. However, antifungal therapy has been shown to be efficient in a subgroup of AD patients in various studies (138–142).

The local application of antifungals such as ketokonazole in AD namely of the face is commonly used by many clinicians with effects possibly due to a partial overlap with seborrhoic dermatitis in some cases. However, a placebo-controlled study with topical miconazole-hydrocsortisone cream and ketokonazole shampoo in AD of the head and neck type did not show any difference to treatment with hydrocortisone alone (51). In contrast, oral ketokonazole was efficient in patients with head- and neck-type AD and positive skin test to *Malassezia* extract (138). Application of 2% ketokonazole cream topical or systemic itroconazole together with tacrolimus has an additional effect on the reduction of fungal colonization measured and also reduces disease activity in AD (143,144). The combination of itroconazole 100 mg/day for one week followed by 200 mg/day weekly was found as the minimal effective dose (145).

A dosage of 200 mg/day for a week in combination with ketokonazole shampoo seems to be ideal. An eventual effect can usually be seen within the first two weeks of initiation of antifungal treatment (142).

A correlation between response to antifungals and levels of fungal-specific IgE is mostly observed (138–142). However, the use of oral itraconazole in a randomized, double-blind, placebo-controlled trials in patients suffering from head and neck dermatitis showed a significant reduction of the Scoring Atopic Dermatitis Index, but irrespectively of the presence of detectable IgE sensitization (142).

From all these findings it seems that removal of *Malassezia* results in an improvement in the clinical condition of AD patients. Mostly patients with AD from the head and neck type and high titers of specific IgE against *Malassezia* species may have a remarkable improvement of AD under antifungal treatment, ideally by systemic itraconazole. However, controlled studies to assess the real benefit of antifungal therapy in AD are definitely needed not only to define the real potential of these drugs, but also to recruit the ideal candidates and optimal treatment regimens.

Also it is still unclear whether the reduction of fungal colonization or reduced proinflammatory activity of fungal elements paired with the anti-inflammatory activity of some antifungals (146) is more important for such an improvement.

Future therapeutic approach might be based not only on the use of antimicrobial peptides (AMP) (147) that may play an important role in several infectious and inflammatory diseases such as AD (148), but also on other chronic inflammatory diseases such as cystic fibrosis and Crohn's disease. Another therapeutic approach to AD is based on the use of coated textiles (149,150). It still needs to be determined to what extent such coated textiles are also useful against fungal elements and thus might have an additional effect in AD by the reduction of fungal colonization.

Nasal vaccination strategies have been described in the murine system able to improve intestinal colonization with *Candida* and favoring possible vaccination approaches (151). Specific immunotherapy with fungal extracts, as being successfully described with house dust mite extracts in AD (152,153), has not yet been investigated.

CONCLUSIONS

Sensitizations against fungal allergens mainly from *Malassezia* spp. is a commonly found phenomenon in AD patients ranging from 15% up to 80% according to age, population, and diagnostic test used. Not only *M. sympodialis* but also *M. globosa* and *M. restricta* are commonly found in both AD patients and healthy individuals.

The pathogenetic role of fungal elements in AD still remains partly unclear. Unlike with bacteria, colonization with *Malassezia* does not seem to be increased in AD, but a mutual influence between fungi and the host local immune response may cause an eventual disease exacerbation. Also IgE-mediated sensitization against *Malassezia* is a specific phenomenon for AD not occurring in other atopic diseases.

This might be due to a decreased epidermal barrier, elevated skin pH, and reduced antimicrobial proteins allowing this yeast to penetrate the skin, favoring an immune response in AD patients leading to increased IgE production. *Malassezia* spp. itself are able to upregulate this inflammatory response by stimulation of APC and both cytokine and chemokine production in keratinocytes and express higher amount of allergens than in healthy subjects in the atopic skin milieu.

Autoreactivity with human self-antigens due to molecular mimicry with fungal elements might be of pivotal importance for the perpetuation of AD at later stages with longstanding inflammatory damage.

Measuring specific serum IgE using the commercial ImmunoCAP kit might be sufficient to detect any relevant form of sensitization against *Malassezia*. The future use of recombinant fungal allergens should allow an improved diagnosis and possibly also the detection of disease- and prognosis-specific reactivity patterns in AD.

Currently, a subpopulation of AD patients mostly with head and neck type and elevated IgE against *Malassezia* seems to benefit ideally from systemic antifungal treatment. However, larger clinical studies are required to evaluate the benefits of antifungal treatments in preventing exacerbation of AD and to select the adequate patients.

REFERENCES

1. Harris JM, Williams HC, White C, et al. Early allergen exposure and atopic eczema. Br J Dermatol 2007; 156(4):698–704.
2. Leung AK, Hon KL, Robson WL. Atopic dermatitis. Adv Pediatr 2007; 54:241–273.
3. Laughter D, Istvan JA, Tofte SJ, et al. The prevalence of atopic dermatitis in Oregon schoolchildren. J Am Acad Dermatol 2000; 43(4):649–655.
4. Flohr C, Weiland SK, Weinmayr G, et al. The role of atopic sensitization in flexural eczema: Findings from the International Study of Asthma and Allergies in Childhood Phase Two. J Allergy Clin Immunol 2008; 121(1):141–147 e4.
5. Bieber T. Atopic dermatitis. N Engl J Med 2008; 358(14):1483–1494.
6. Leung AD, Schiltz AM, Hall CF, et al. Severe atopic dermatitis is associated with a high burden of environmental *Staphylococcus aureus*. Clin Exp Allergy 2008; 38(5):789–793.
7. Howell MD, Novak N, Bieber T, et al. Interleukin-10 downregulates anti-microbial peptide expression in atopic dermatitis. J Invest Dermatol 2005; 125(4):738–745.
8. Ong PY, Ohtake T, Brandt C, et al. Endogenous antimicrobial peptides and skin infections in atopic dermatitis. N Engl J Med 2002; 347(15):1151–1160.
9. Flohr C, Pascoe D, Williams HC. Atopic dermatitis and the 'hygiene hypothesis': Too clean to be true? Br J Dermatol 2005; 152(2):202–216.
10. Ring J, Abeck D, Neuber K. Atopic eczema: Role of microorganisms on the skin surface. Allergy 1992; 47(4 Pt 1):265–269.
11. Jensen-Jarolim E, Poulsen LK, With H, et al. Atopic dermatitis of the face, scalp, and neck: Type I reaction to the yeast *Pityrosporum ovale*? J Allergy Clin Immunol 1992; 89(1 Pt 1):44–51.
12. Svejgaard E. The role of microorganisms in atopic dermatitis. Semin Dermatol 1990; 9(4):255–261.
13. Marcon MJ, Powell DA. Epidemiology, diagnosis, and management of *Malassezia furfur* systemic infection. Diagn Microbiol Infect Dis 1987; 7(3):161–175.
14. McGeady SJ, Buckley RH. Depression of cell-mediated immunity in atopic eczema. J Allergy Clin Immunol 1975; 56(5):393–406.

15. Elliott ST, Hanifin JM. Delayed cutaneous hypersensitivity and lymphocyte transformation: Dissociation in atopic dermatitis. Arch Dermatol 1979; 115(1):36–39.
16. Wierenga EA, Snoek M, de Groot C, et al. Evidence for compartmentalization of functional subsets of CD2+ T lymphocytes in atopic patients. J Immunol 1990; 144(12):4651–4656.
17. Wessels MW, Doekes G, Van Ieperen-Van Kijk AG, et al. IgE antibodies to *Pityrosporum ovale* in atopic dermatitis. Br J Dermatol 1991; 125(3):227–232.
18. Nordvall SL, Scheynius A. *Pityrosporum orbiculare* and atopic eczema. Allergy 1993; 48(6):391–393.
19. Savolainen J, Lammintausta K, Kalimo K, et al. *Candida albicans* and atopic dermatitis. Clin Exp Allergy 1993; 23(4):332–339.
20. Sugita T, Saito M, Ito T, et al. The basidiomycetous yeasts *Cryptococcus diffluens* and *C. liquefaciens* colonize the skin of patients with atopic dermatitis. Microbiol Immunol 2003; 47(12):945–950.
21. Johansson C, Eshaghi H, Linder MT, et al. Positive atopy patch test reaction to *Malassezia furfur* in atopic dermatitis correlates with a T helper 2-like peripheral blood mononuclear cells response. J Invest Dermatol 2002; 118(6):1044–1051.
22. Faergemann J. *Pityrosporum* species as a cause of allergy and infection. Allergy 1999; 54(5):413–419.
23. Celis AM, Cepero de Garcia MC. Genetic polymorphism of *Malassezia* spp. yeast isolates from individuals with and without dermatological lesions. Biomedical 2005; 25(4):481–487.
24. Gupta AK, Batra R, Bluhm R, et al. Skin diseases associated with *Malassezia* species. J Am Acad Dermatol 2004; 51(5):785–798.
25. Akerstedt J, Vollset I. *Malassezia pachydermatis* with special reference to canine skin disease. Br Vet J 1996; 152(3):269–281.
26. Sandstrom Falk MH, Tengvall Linder M, Johansson C, et al. The prevalence of *Malassezia* yeasts in patients with atopic dermatitis, seborrhoeic dermatitis and healthy controls. Acta Derm Venereol 2005; 85(1):17–23.
27. Sugita T, Suto H, Unno T, et al. Molecular analysis of malassezia microflora on the skin of atopic dermatitis patients and healthy subjects. Nihon Ishinkin Gakkai zasshi 2001; 42(4):217–218.
28. Sugita T, Tajima M, Tsubuku H, et al. Quantitative analysis of cutaneous malassezia in atopic dermatitis patients using real-time PCR. Microbiol Immunol 2006; 50(7):549–552.
29. Taieb A, Hanifin J, Cooper K, et al. Proceedings of the 4th Georg Rajka International Symposium on Atopic Dermatitis, Arcachon, France, September 15–17, 2005. J Allergy Clin Immunol 2006; 117(2):378–390.
30. Tajima M, Sugita T, Nishikawa A, et al. Molecular analysis of *Malassezia microflora* in seborrheic dermatitis patients: Comparison with other diseases and healthy subjects. J Invest Dermatol 2008; 128(2):345–351.
31. DeAngelis YM, Gemmer CM, Kaczvinsky JR, et al. Three etiologic facets of dandruff and seborrheic dermatitis: *Malassezia* fungi, sebaceous lipids, and individual sensitivity. J Investig Dermatol Symp Proc 2005; 10(3):295–297.
32. Tajima M, Amaya M, Sugita T, et al. Molecular analysis of *Malassezia* species isolated from three cases of Akatsuki disease (pomade crust). Nihon Ishinkin Gakkai zasshi 2005; 46(3):193–196.
33. Amaya M, Tajima M, Okubo Y, et al. Molecular analysis of *Malassezia microflora* in the lesional skin of psoriasis patients. J Dermatol 2007; 34(9):619–624.
34. Smolinski KN, Shah SS, Honig PJ, et al. Neonatal cutaneous fungal infections. Curr Opin Pediatr 2005; 17(4):486–493.
35. Ayhan M, Sancak B, Karaduman A, et al. Colonization of neonate skin by *Malassezia* species: Relationship with neonatal cephalic pustulosis. J Am Acad Dermatol 2007; 57(6):1012–1018.
36. Jena DK, Sengupta S, Dwari BC, et al. *Pityriasis versicolor* in the pediatric age group. Indian J Dermatol, Venereol Leprol 2005; 71(4):259–261.

37. Dinkela A, Ferie J, Mbata M, et al. Efficacy of triclosan soap against superficial dermatomycoses: A double-blind clinical trial in 224 primary school-children in Kilombero District, Morogoro Region, Tanzania. Int J Dermatol 2007; 46(suppl. 2):23–28.

38. Weidinger S, Illig T, Baurecht H, et al. Loss-of-function variations within the filaggrin gene predispose for atopic dermatitis with allergic sensitizations. J Allergy Clin Immunol 2006; 118(1):214–219.

39. Palmer CN, Irvine AD, Terron-Kwiatkowski A, et al. Common loss-of-function variants of the epidermal barrier protein filaggrin are a major predisposing factor for atopic dermatitis. Nat Genet 2006; 38(4):441–446.

40. Howell MD. The role of human beta defensins and cathelicidins in atopic dermatitis. Curr Opin Allergy Clin Immunol 2007; 7(5):413–417.

41. Vylkova S, Nayyar N, Li W, et al. Human beta-defensins kill *Candida albicans* in an energy-dependent and salt-sensitive manner without causing membrane disruption. Antimicrob Agents Chemother 2007; 51(1):154–161.

42. Lopez-Garcia B, Lee PH, Gallo RL. Expression and potential function of cathelicidin antimicrobial peptides in dermatophytosis and *Tinea versicolor*. J Antimicrob Chemother 2006; 57(5):877–882.

43. Agerberth B, Buentke E, Bergman P, et al. *Malassezia sympodialis* differently affects the expression of LL-37 in dendritic cells from atopic eczema patients and healthy individuals. Allergy 2006; 61(4):422–430.

44. Donnarumma G, Paoletti I, Buommino E, et al. *Malassezia furfur* induces the expression of beta-defensin-2 in human keratinocytes in a protein kinase C-dependent manner. Arch Dermatol Res 2004; 295(11):474–481.

45. Schmid-Wendtner MH, Korting HC. The pH of the skin surface and its impact on the barrier function. Skin Pharmacol Physiol 2006; 19(6):296–302.

46. Rippke F, Schreiner V, Doering T, et al. Stratum corneum pH in atopic dermatitis: Impact on skin barrier function and colonization with *Staphylococcus aureus*. Am J Clin Dermatol 2004; 5(4):217–223.

47. Selander C, Zargari A, Mollby R, et al. Higher pH level, corresponding to that on the skin of patients with atopic eczema, stimulates the release of *Malassezia sympodialis* allergens. Allergy 2006; 61(8):1002–1008.

48. Faergemann J, Tjernlund U, Scheynius A, et al. Antigenic similarities and differences in genus Pityrosporum. J Invest Dermatol 1982; 78(1):28–31.

49. Faergemann J, Johansson S, Back O, et al. An immunologic and cultural study of *Pityrosporum folliculitis*. J Am Acad Dermatol 1986; 14(3):429–433.

50. Young E, Koers WJ, Berrens L. Intracutaneous tests with pityrosporon extract in atopic dermatitis. Acta Derm Venereol Suppl (Stockh) 1989; 144:122–124.

51. Broberg A. *Pityrosporum ovale* in healthy children, infantile seborrhoeic dermatitis and atopic dermatitis. Acta Derm Venereol Suppl (Stockh) 1995; 191:1–47.

52. Kawano S, Nakagawa H. The correlation between the levels of anti-*Malassezia furfur* IgE antibodies and severities of face and neck dermatitis of patients with atopic dermatitis. Arerugi = [Allergy] 1995; 44(3 Pt 1):128–133.

53. Lindgren L, Wahlgren CF, Johansson SG, et al. Occurrence and clinical features of sensitization to *Pityrosporum orbiculare* and other allergens in children with atopic dermatitis. Acta Derm Venereol 1995; 75(4):300–304.

54. Lintu P, Savolainen J, Kalimo K. IgE antibodies to protein and mannan antigens of *Pityrosporum ovale* in atopic dermatitis patients. Clin Exp Allergy 1997; 27(1):87–95.

55. Nissen D, Petersen LJ, Esch R, et al. IgE-sensitization to cellular and culture filtrates of fungal extracts in patients with atopic dermatitis. Ann Allergy Asthma Immunol 1998; 81(3):247–255.

56. Kim TY, Jang IG, Park YM, et al. Head and neck dermatitis: The role of *Malassezia furfur*, topical steroid use and environmental factors in its causation. Clin Exp Dermatol 1999; 24(3):226–231.

57. Scalabrin DM, Bavbek S, Perzanowski MS, et al. Use of specific IgE in assessing the relevance of fungal and dust mite allergens to atopic dermatitis: A comparison with

asthmatic and nonasthmatic control subjects. J Allergy Clin Immunol 1999; 104(6):1273–1279.

58. Devos SA, van der Valk PG. The relevance of skin prick tests for *Pityrosporum ovale* in patients with head and neck dermatitis. Allergy 2000; 55(11):1056–1058.
59. Mayser P, Gross A. IgE antibodies to *Malassezia furfur, M. sympodialis* and *Pityrosporum orbiculare* in patients with atopic dermatitis, seborrheic eczema or *Pityriasis versicolor*, and identification of respective allergens. Acta Derm Venereol 2000; 80(5):357–361.
60. Arzumanyan VG, Serdyuk OA, Kozlova NN, et al. IgE and IgG antibodies to *Malassezia* spp. yeast extract in patients with atopic dermatitis. Bull Exp Biol Med 2003; 135(5):460–463.
61. Zargari A, Midgley G, Back O, et al. IgE-reactivity to seven *Malassezia* species. Allergy 2003; 58(4):306–311.
62. Fischer Casagande B, Fluckiger S, Linder MT, Johansson C, et al. Sensitization to the yeast *Malassezia sympodialis* is specific for extrinsic and intrinsic atopic eczema. J Invest Dermatol 2006; 126(11):2414–2421.
63. Johansson C, Tengvall Linder M, Aalberse RC, et al. Elevated levels of IgG and IgG4 to *Malassezia* allergens in atopic eczema patients with IgE reactivity to *Malassezia*. Int Arch Allergy Immunol 2004; 135(2):93–100.
64. Kosonen J, Lintu P, Kortekangas-Savolainen O, et al. Immediate hypersensitivity to *Malassezia furfur* and *Candida albicans* mannans in vivo and in vitro. Allergy 2005; 60(2):238–242.
65. Fischer B, Yawalkar N, Brander KA, et al. *Coprinus comatus* (shaggy cap) is a potential source of aeroallergen that may provoke atopic dermatitis. J Allergy Clin Immunol 1999; 104(4 Pt 1):836–841.
66. Brander KA, Borbely P, Crameri R, et al. IgE-binding proliferative responses and skin test reactivity to Cop c 1, the first recombinant allergen from the basidiomycete *Coprinus comatus*. J Allergy Clin Immunol 1999; 104(3 Pt 1):630–636.
67. Crameri R, Weichel M, Fluckiger S, et al. Fungal allergies: A yet unsolved problem. Chem Immunol Allergy 2006; 91:121–133.
68. Johansson C, Jeddi-Tehrani M, Grunewald J, et al. Peripheral blood T-cell receptor beta-chain V-repertoire in atopic dermatitis patients after in vitro exposure to *Pityrosporum orbiculare* extract. Scand J Immunol 1999; 49(3):293–301.
69. Tengvall Linder M, Johansson C, Bengtsson A, et al. *Pityrosporum orbiculare*-reactive T-cell lines in atopic dermatitis patients and healthy individuals. Scand J Immunol 1998; 47(2):152–158.
70. Kanda N, Tani K, Enomoto U, et al. The skin fungus-induced Th1- and Th2-related cytokine, chemokine and prostaglandin E2 production in peripheral blood mononuclear cells from patients with atopic dermatitis and psoriasis vulgaris. Clin Exp Allergy 2002; 32(8):1243–1250.
71. Savolainen J, Lintu P, Kosonen J, et al. *Pityrosporum* and *Candida* specific and non-specific humoral, cellular and cytokine responses in atopic dermatitis patients. Clin Exp Allergy 2001; 31(1):125–134.
72. Neuber K, Kroger S, Gruseck E, et al. Effects of *Pityrosporum ovale* on proliferation, immunoglobulin (IgA, G, M) synthesis and cytokine (IL-2, IL-10, IFN gamma) production of peripheral blood mononuclear cells from patients with seborrhoeic dermatitis. Arch Dermatol Res 1996; 288(9):532–536.
73. Walters CE, Ingham E, Eady EA, et al. In vitro modulation of keratinocyte-derived interleukin-1 alpha (IL-1 alpha) and peripheral blood mononuclear cell-derived IL-1 beta release in response to cutaneous commensal microorganisms. Infect Immun 1995; 63(4):1223–1228.
74. Kroger S, Neuber K, Gruseck E, et al. *Pityrosporum ovale* extracts increase interleukin-4, interleukin-10 and IgE synthesis in patients with atopic eczema. Acta Derm Venereol 1995; 75(5):357–360.
75. Watanabe S, Kano R, Sato H, et al. The effects of *Malassezia* yeasts on cytokine production by human keratinocytes. J Invest Dermatol 2001; 116(5):769–773.

76. Ou LS, Goleva E, Hall C, et al. T regulatory cells in atopic dermatitis and subversion of their activity by superantigens. J Allergy Clin Immunol 2004; 113(4):756–763.

77. Skov L, Olsen JV, Giorno R, et al. Application of Staphylococcal enterotoxin B on normal and atopic skin induces up-regulation of T cells by a superantigen-mediated mechanism. J Allergy Clin Immunol 2000; 105(4):820–826.

78. Wollenberg A, Kraft S, Hanau D, et al. Immunomorphological and ultrastructural characterization of Langerhans cells and a novel, inflammatory dendritic epidermal cell (IDEC) population in lesional skin of atopic eczema. J Invest Dermatol 1996; 106(3):446–453.

79. Reich K, Hugo S, Middel P, et al. Evidence for a role of Langerhans cell-derived IL-16 in atopic dermatitis. J Allergy Clin Immunol 2002; 109(4):681–687.

80. Buentke E, Heffler LC, Wallin RP, et al. The allergenic yeast *Malassezia furfur* induces maturation of human dendritic cells. Clin Exp Allergy 2001; 31(10):1583–1593.

81. Buentke E, Zargari A, Heffler LC, et al. Uptake of the yeast *Malassezia furfur* and its allergenic components by human immature CD1 a+ dendritic cells. Clin Exp Allergy 2000; 30(12):1759–1770.

82. Buentke E, D'Amato M, Scheynius A. *Malassezia* enhances natural killer cell-induced dendritic cell maturation. Scand J Immunol 2004; 59(5):511–516.

83. Gabrielsson S, Buentke E, Lieden A, et al. *Malassezia sympodialis* stimulation differently affects gene expression in dendritic cells from atopic dermatitis patients and healthy individuals. Acta Derm Venereol 2004; 84(5):339–345.

84. Lange L, Alter N, Keller T, et al. Sensitization to *Malassezia* in infants and children with atopic dermatitis: Prevalence and clinical characteristics. Allergy 2008; 63(4):486–487.

85. Takahata Y, Sugita T, Kato H, et al. Cutaneous Malassezia flora in atopic dermatitis differs between adults and children. Br J Dermatol 2007; 157(6):1178–1182.

86. Sandstrom Falk MH, Faergemann J. Atopic dermatitis in adults: Does it disappear with age? Acta Derm Venereol 2006; 86(2):135–139.

87. Ramirez de Knott HM, McCormick TS, Kalka K, et al. Cutaneous hypersensitivity to *Malassezia sympodialis* and dust mite in adult atopic dermatitis with a textile pattern. Contact Dermatitis 2006; 54(2):92–99.

88. Bayrou O, Pecquet C, Flahault A, et al. Head and neck atopic dermatitis and *Malassezia-furfur*-specific IgE antibodies. Dermatology (Basel, Switzerland) 2005; 211(2):107–113.

89. Faergemann J. Atopic dermatitis and fungi. Clin Microbiol Rev 2002; 15(4):545–563.

90. Schmid-Grendelmeier P, Simon D, Simon HU, et al. Epidemiology, clinical features, and immunology of the "intrinsic" (non-IgE-mediated) type of atopic dermatitis (constitutional dermatitis). Allergy 2001; 56(9):841–849.

91. Johansson C, Sandstrom MH, Bartosik J, et al. Atopy patch test reactions to *Malassezia* allergens differentiate subgroups of atopic dermatitis patients. Br J Dermatol 2003; 148(3):479–488.

92. Novak N, Allam JP, Bieber T. Allergic hyperreactivity to microbial components: A trigger factor of "intrinsic" atopic dermatitis? J Allergy Clin Immunol 2003; 112(1):215–216.

93. Koyama T, Kanbe T, Ishiguro A, et al. Antigenic components of *Malassezia* species for immunoglobulin E antibodies in sera of patients with atopic dermatitis. J Dermatol Sci 2001; 26(3):201–208.

94. Khosravi AR, Hedayati MT, Mansouri P, et al. Immediate hypersensitivity to *Malassezia furfur* in patients with atopic dermatitis. Mycoses 2007; 50(4):297–301.

95. Canteros CE, Soria M, Rivas C, et al. *Malassezia* species isolated from skin diseases in a care center in the city of Buenos Aires, Argentina. Rev Argent Microbiol 2003; 35(3):156–161.

96. Montealegre F, Villa J, Vargas W, et al. Risk factors for atopic dermatitis in southern Puerto Rico. P R Health Sci J 2007; 26(2):109–118.

97. Schmid-Grendelmeier P, Fluckiger S, Disch R, et al. IgE-mediated and T cell-mediated autoimmunity against manganese superoxide dismutase in atopic dermatitis. J Allergy Clin Immunol 2005; 115(5):1068–1075.

98. Tengvall Linder M, Johansson C, Scheynius A, et al. Positive atopy patch test reactions to *Pityrosporum orbiculare* in atopic dermatitis patients. Clin Exp Allergy 2000; 30(1):122–131.

99. Lintu P, Savolainen J, Kalimo K, et al. Stability of *Pityrosporum ovale* allergens during storage. Clin Exp Allergy 1998; 28(4):486–490.

100. Onishi Y, Kuroda M, Yasueda H, et al. Two-dimensional electrophoresis of *Malassezia* allergens for atopic dermatitis and isolation of Mal f 4 homologs with mitochondrial malate dehydrogenase. Eur J Biochem/FEBS 1999; 261(1):148–154.

101. Yasueda H, Hashida-Okado T, Saito A, et al. Identification and cloning of two novel allergens from the lipophilic yeast, *Malassezia furfur*. Biochem Biophys Res Commun 1998; 248(2):240–244.

102. Lindborg M, Magnusson CG, Zargari A, et al. Selective cloning of allergens from the skin colonizing yeast *Malassezia furfur* by phage surface display technology. J Invest Dermatol 1999; 113(2):156–161.

103. Vilhelmsson M, Zargari A, Crameri R, et al. Crystal structure of the major *Malassezia sympodialis* allergen Mala s 1 reveals a beta-propeller fold: A novel fold among allergens. J Mol Biol 2007; 369(4):1079–1086.

104. Hemmann S, Blaser K, Crameri R. Allergens of *Aspergillus fumigatus* and *Candida boidinii* share IgE-binding epitopes. Am J Respir Crit Care Med 1997; 156(6):1956–1962.

105. Simon-Nobbe B, Denk U, Poll V, et al. The spectrum of fungal allergy. Int Arch Allergy Immunol 2008; 145(1):58–86.

106. Zeller S, Glaser AG, Vilhelmsson M, et al. Immunoglobulin-E-mediated reactivity to self antigens: A controversial issue. Int Arch Allergy Immunol 2008; 145(2):87–93.

107. Zargari A, Selander C, Rasool O, et al. Mala s 12 is a major allergen in patients with atopic eczema and has sequence similarities to the GMC oxidoreductase family. Allergy 2007; 62(6):695–703.

108. Crameri R, Kodzius R, Konthur Z, et al. Tapping allergen repertoires by advanced cloning technologies. Int Arch Allergy Immunol 2001; 124(1–3):43–47.

109. Altrichter S, Kriehuber E, Moser J, et al. Serum IgE autoantibodies target keratinocytes in patients with atopic dermatitis. J Invest Dermatol 2008; 128:2232–2239.

110. Valenta R, Seiberler S, Natter S, et al. Autoallergy: A pathogenetic factor in atopic dermatitis? J Allergy Clin Immunol 2000; 105(3):432–437.

111. Seiberler S, Bugajska-Schretter A, Hufnagl P, et al. Characterization of IgE-reactive autoantigens in atopic dermatitis. 1. Subcellular distribution and tissue-specific expression. Int Arch Allergy Immunol 1999; 120(2):108–116.

112. Natter S, Seiberler S, Hufnagl P, et al. Isolation of cDNA clones coding for IgE autoantigens with serum IgE from atopic dermatitis patients. FASEB J 1998; 12(14):1559–1569.

113. Valenta R, Maurer D, Steiner R, et al. Immunoglobulin E response to human proteins in atopic patients. J Invest Dermatol 1996; 107(2):203–208.

114. Crameri R, Faith A, Hemmann S, et al. Humoral and cell-mediated autoimmunity in allergy to *Aspergillus fumigatus*. J Exp Med 1996; 184(1):265–270.

115. Schmid-Grendelmeier P, Crameri R. Recombinant allergens for skin testing. Int Arch Allergy Immunol 2001; 125(2):96–111.

116. Fluckiger S, Fijten H, Whitley P, et al. Cyclophilins, a new family of cross-reactive allergens. Eur J Immunol 2002; 32(1):10–17.

117. Limacher A, Glaser AG, Meier C, et al. Cross-reactivity and 1.4-A crystal structure of *Malassezia sympodialis* thioredoxin (Mala s 13), a member of a new pan-allergen family. J Immunol 2007; 178(1):389–396.

118. Glaser AG, Menz G, Kirsch A, et al. Auto- and cross-reactivity to thioredoxin allergens in allergic bronchopulmonary aspergillosis. Allergy 2008; 63(12):1617–1623.

119. Crameri R, Zeller S, Glaser A, et al. Cross-reactivity among fungal allergens: A clinically relevant phenomenon? Mycoses 2008; 18:1443–1451.

120. Glaser AG, Limacher A, Fluckiger S, et al. Analysis of the cross-reactivity and of the 1.5 A crystal structure of the *Malassezia sympodialis* Mala s 6 allergen, a member of the cyclophilin pan-allergen family. Biochem J 2006; 396(1):41–49.

121. Fluckiger S, Mittl PR, Scapozza L, et al. Comparison of the crystal structures of the human manganese superoxide dismutase and the homologous *Aspergillus fumigatus* allergen at 2-A resolution. J Immunol 2002; 168(3):1267–1272.
122. Fluckiger S, Scapozza L, Mayer C, et al. Immunological and structural analysis of IgE-mediated cross-reactivity between manganese superoxide dismutases. Int Arch Allergy Immunol 2002; 128(4):292–303.
123. Limacher A, Kloer DP, Fluckiger S, et al. The crystal structure of *Aspergillus fumigatus* cyclophilin reveals 3D domain swapping of a central element. Structure 2006; 14(2):185–195.
124. Laver WG AG, Webster RG, Smith-Gill SJ. Epitopes on protein antigens: Misconceptions and realities. Cell 1990; 61:553–556.
125. Mothes N, Niggemann B, Jenneck C, et al. The cradle of IgE autoreactivity in atopic eczema lies in early infancy. J Allergy Clin Immunol 2005; 116(3):706–709.
126. Nett CS, Reichler I, Grest P, et al. Epidermal dysplasia and *Malassezia* infection in two West Highland White Terrier siblings: An inherited skin disorder or reaction to severe *Malassezia* infection? Vet Dermatol 2001; 12(5):285–290.
127. Nardoni S, Dini M, Taccini F, et al. Occurrence, distribution and population size of *Malassezia pachydermatis* on skin and mucosae of atopic dogs. Vet Microbiol 2007; 122(1–2):172–177.
128. Morris DO, Olivier NB, Rosser EJ. Type-1 hypersensitivity reactions to *Malassezia pachydermatis* extracts in atopic dogs. Am J Vet Res 1998; 59(7):836–841.
129. Nuttall TJ, Halliwell RE. Serum antibodies to *Malassezia* yeasts in canine atopic dermatitis. Vet Dermatol 2001; 12(6):327–332.
130. Chen TA, Halliwell RE, Pemberton AD, et al. Identification of major allergens of *Malassezia pachydermatis* in dogs with atopic dermatitis and *Malassezia* overgrowth. Vet Dermatol 2002; 13(3):141–150.
131. DeBoer DJ, Marsella R. The ACVD task force on canine atopic dermatitis (XII): The relationship of cutaneous infections to the pathogenesis and clinical course of canine atopic dermatitis. Vet Immunol Immunopathol 2001; 81(3–4):239–249.
132. Olivry T, Dean GA, Tompkins MB, et al. Toward a canine model of atopic dermatitis: Amplification of cytokine-gene transcripts in the skin of atopic dogs. Exp Dermatol 1999; 8(3):204–211.
133. Chen TA, Halliwell RE, Hill PB. Failure of extracts from *Malassezia pachydermatis* to stimulate canine keratinocyte proliferation in vitro. Vet Dermatol 2002; 13(6):323–329.
134. Bond R, Habibah A, Patterson-Kane JC, et al. Patch test responses to *Malassezia pachydermatis* in healthy dogs. Med Mycol 2006; 44(2):175–184.
135. Olivry T, Dunston SM, Pluchino K, et al. Lack of detection of circulating skin-specific IgE autoantibodies in dogs with moderate or severe atopic dermatitis. Vet Immunol Immunopathol 2008; 122(1–2):182–187.
136. Olivry T, Mueller RS. Evidence-based veterinary dermatology: A systematic review of the pharmacotherapy of canine atopic dermatitis. Vet Dermatol 2003; 14(3):121–146.
137. Colombo S, Hill PB, Shaw DJ, et al. Requirement for additional treatment for dogs with atopic dermatitis undergoing allergen-specific immunotherapy. Vet Rec 2007; 160(25):861–864.
138. Back O, Scheynius A, Johansson SG. Ketoconazole in atopic dermatitis: Therapeutic response is correlated with decrease in serum IgE. Arch Dermatol Res 1995; 287(5):448–451.
139. Back O, Bartosik J. Systemic ketoconazole for yeast allergic patients with atopic dermatitis. J Eur Acad Dermatol Venereol 2001; 15(1):34–38.
140. Lintu P, Savolainen J, Kortekangas-Savolainen O, et al. Systemic ketoconazole is an effective treatment of atopic dermatitis with IgE-mediated hypersensitivity to yeasts. Allergy 2001; 56(6):512–517.
141. Ikezawa Z, Kondo M, Okajima M, et al. Clinical usefulness of oral itraconazole, an antimycotic drug, for refractory atopic dermatitis. Eur J Dermatol 2004; 14(6):400–406.

142. Svejgaard E, Larsen PO, Deleuran M, et al. Treatment of head and neck dermatitis comparing itraconazole 200 mg and 400 mg daily for 1 week with placebo. J Eur Acad Dermatol Venereol 2004; 18(4):445–449.

143. Sugita T, Tajima M, Ito T, et al. Antifungal activities of tacrolimus and azole agents against the eleven currently accepted *Malassezia* species. J Clini Microbiol 2005; 43(6):2824–2829.

144. Takechi M. Minimum effective dosage in the treatment of chronic atopic dermatitis with itraconazole. J Int Med Res 2005; 33(3):273–283.

145. Aspres N, Anderson C. Malassezia yeasts in the pathogenesis of atopic dermatitis. Australas J Dermatol 2004; 45(4):199–205 [quiz 6–7].

146. Kanda N, Watanabe S. Ketoconazole suppresses interleukin-4 plus anti-CD40-induced IgE class switching in surface IgE negative B cells from patients with atopic dermatitis. J Invest Dermatol 2002; 119(3):590–599.

147. Harder J, Glaser R, Schroder JM. The role and potential therapeutical applications of antimicrobial proteins in infectious and inflammatory diseases. Endocr Metab Immune Disord Drug Targets 2007; 7(2):75–82.

148. Izadpanah A, Gallo RL. Antimicrobial peptides. J Am Acad Dermatol 2005; 52(3 Pt 1):381–390 [quiz 91–92].

149. Ricci G, Patrizi A, Bellini F, et al. Use of textiles in atopic dermatitis: Care of atopic dermatitis. Curr Probl Dermatol 2006; 33:127–143.

150. Haug S, Roll A, Schmid-Grendelmeier P, et al. Coated textiles in the treatment of atopic dermatitis. Curr Probl Dermatol 2006; 33:144–151.

151. Suenobu N, Kweon MN, Kiyono H. Nasal vaccination induces the ability to eliminate *Candida* colonization without influencing the pre-existing antigen-specific IgE Abs: A possibility for the control of *Candida*-related atopic dermatitis. Vaccine 2002; 20(23–24):2972–2980.

152. Bussmann C, Maintz L, Hart J, et al. Clinical improvement and immunological changes in atopic dermatitis patients undergoing subcutaneous immunotherapy with a house dust mite allergoid: A pilot study. Clin Exp Allergy 2007; 37(9):1277–1285.

153. Werfel T, Breuer K, Rueff F, et al. Usefulness of specific immunotherapy in patients with atopic dermatitis and allergic sensitization to house dust mites: A multi-centre, randomized, dose–response study. Allergy 2006; 61(2):202–205.

154. Rasool O, Zargari A, Almqvist J, et al. Cloning, characterization and expression of complete coding sequences of three IgE binding *Malassezia furfur* allergens, Mal f 7, Mal f 8 and Mal f 9. Eur J Biochem 2000; 267:4355–4361.

155. Andersson A, Rasool O, Schmidt M, et al. Cloning, expression and characterization of two new IgE-binding proteins from the yeast *Malassezia sympodialis* with sequence similarities to heat shock proteins and manganese superoxide dismutase. Eur J Biochem 2004; 271:1885–1894.

156. Schmidt M, Zargari A, Holt P, et al. The complete cDNA sequence and expression of the first major allergenic protein of *Malassezia furfur*, Mal f 1. Eur J Biochem 1997; 246:181–185.

Role of *Staphylococcus aureus* in Atopic Dermatitis

Peck Y. Ong

Division of Clinical Immunology and Allergy, Children's Hospital Los Angeles, and Department of Pediatrics, University of Southern California Keck School of Medicine, Los Angeles, California, U.S.A.

Donald Y. M. Leung

Division of Pediatric Allergy-Immunology, National Jewish Health, and Department of Pediatrics, University of Colorado Denver Health Sciences Center, Denver, Colorado, U.S.A.

INTRODUCTION

Atopic dermatitis (AD) is a pruritic skin condition that is characterized by skin barrier defects, *Staphylococcus aureus* (*S. aureus*) colonization, and a waxing and waning course of inflammation that leads to disturbances in sleep, work and activities. The inflammation of AD is the result of complex interactions between dendritic cells, T cells, mast cells, keratinocytes, eosinophils, and a combination of mediators including inflammatory cytokines and chemokines (1). Although recent data indicate that the genetic basis of skin barrier defects plays a crucial role in the pathogenesis of AD (2), the trigger of inflammation in AD remains poorly understood. A number of known triggers for AD include changes in irritants, stress, food allergens, aeroallergens, and infection. Evidence for the latter as a trigger of AD has been particularly compelling. This is particularly true for *S. aureus*, which colonizes almost all AD patients. A key piece of evidence that supports *S. aureus* as a trigger for AD has come from the observation that AD improves when patients are treated with anti-staphylococcal antibiotics (3,4).

S. aureus produces a number of virulence factors that may induce cutaneous inflammation. The inherited barrier defects of AD may facilitate the entry of these virulence factors, which then interact with the cutaneous immune system to induce inflammation. These virulence factors include staphylococcal superantigens, alpha-toxin, and bacterial cell wall components. The current review will examine why AD is susceptible to *S. aureus* colonization, and how various staphylococcal virulence factors lead to skin inflammation in AD. An understanding of these mechanisms may lead to new approaches in the management and treatment of AD.

PREVALENCE OF *STAPHYLOCOCCUS AUREUS* IN ATOPIC DERMATITIS

S. aureus is found on the skin of over 90% of patients with AD (5). The density of *S. aureus* colonization on AD lesions correlates with the severity of dermatitis. In addition, the rate of *S. aureus* colonization is significantly higher in AD patients with extrinsic features (i.e., elevated total serum IgE and/or the presence of specific IgE

TABLE 1 Mechanisms for Increased *S. aureus* Colonization and Infection in AD

1. Skin barrier defects.
2. Mediation of *S. aureus* attachment to atopic skin by Th2 cytokines.
3. Suppression of antimicrobial peptides (HBD-2, HBD-3, LL-37) by Th2 cytokines.
4. Decreased expression of sweat dermcidin.
5. Decreased expression of cutaneous antimicrobial lipids (sphingosine and hexadecenoic acid).

sensitization), as compared to intrinsic AD patients (i.e., patients with normal total serum IgE and without any specific IgE sensitization) (6), suggesting a role for atopic inflammation in the colonization of *S. aureus* in AD (discussed in the section, mechanism(s) for enhanced *Staphylococcus aureus* colonization in AD). The high prevalence of *S. aureus* colonization in AD patients is also contributed by various environmental factors. In AD patients with more severe disease, a higher level of *S. aureus* is found in their home environment (7). A high percentage (65%) of parents of AD children also carry *S. aureus*, increasing the potential risk of recolonization of these children (8). Topical anti-inflammatory medications may also be a source for the recolonization of *S. aureus* in AD, as these medications have been found to be contaminated by *S. aureus* (9). In addition to environmental factors, intrinsic factors in the cutaneous immune system of AD patients may also predispose these patients to increased colonization by *S. aureus*.

MECHANISM(S) FOR ENHANCED *STAPHYLOCOCCUS AUREUS* COLONIZATION IN AD

The mechanism(s) leading to increased *S. aureus* colonization in AD is not fully understood, but likely involve skin barrier defects, atopic inflammation, and decreased cutaneous innate immunity (Table 1). The initial adherence of *S. aureus* to AD skin may be facilitated by the binding of the bacteria to plasma proteins including fibronectin and fibrinogen through skin barrier disruption. This is supported by the observations that isogenic mutants of *S. aureus* that were selectively deficient in fibronectin- or fibrinogen-binding proteins, as compared to their corresponding wild-type parent strains, demonstrated reduced binding to allergen-sensitized/challenged Th2, but not Th1, skin reactions in mice (10). In addition, *S. aureus* mutants deficient in fibronectin- or fibrinogen-binding proteins demonstrated reduced binding to human AD skin but not psoriatic skin or normal skin (11). The prototypic Th2 cytokine, IL-4, but not the Th1 cytokine, interferon-γ, was found to increase the binding of *S. aureus* to normal mouse skin explants (10). The mechanism(s) of this observation is not fully understood, but likely related to Th2 cytokine induction of fibronectin production in skin fibroblasts and monocytes (10,12,13).

In addition to their potential role in enhancing the binding of *S. aureus* to AD skin, Th2 cytokines are also capable of suppressing local cutaneous innate immunity, leading to increased colonization of *S. aureus* in AD. Antimicrobial peptides (AMPs) are important effector molecules of the innate immune system. These molecules including HBD-2, HBD-3, and LL-37 are capable of killing *S. aureus* alone or in combination (14,15). Among these three AMPs, HBD-3 has been found to be the most potent anti-staphylococcal AMP (16). The bactericidal concentration, $BC_{99.9}$ (i.e., concentrations of AMP needed to kill 99.9% of *S. aureus* in two hours), for HBD-3 was 10.70 ± 5.75 μM, followed by LL-37 (43.68 ± 18.39 μM) and HBD-2

(483.03 $\pm$ 43.22 μM) (16). When *S. aureus* was exposed to cultures of differentiated keratinocyes, it was found that the amount of AMP that came in contact with *S. aureus* on keratinocytes was 120.9 μM for HBD-2, 34 μM for HBD-3, and 13.8 μM for LL37. The amount of HBD-3 that was deposited on the *S. aureus* in contact with the keratinocytes was well above its $BC_{99.9}$, as compared to that of HBD-2 and LL-37. Similar results were obtained when *S. aureus* was incubated with human skin explants (16). Using specific blocking antibodies against AMPs, it was shown that the killing effect of HBD-2 and HBD-3 on *S. aureus* incubated with cultured keratinocyes was reduced by 75% and 25%, respectively (16). On the other hand, specific blocking antibody against LL-37 did not have significant effect on the killing ability of the keratinocytes. It was concluded that the ability of keratinocytes to kill cell-associated *S. aureus* was dependent mainly on HBD-3 (16).

Both IL-4 and IL-13 have been shown to suppress the production of HBD-2 and HBD-3 in keratinocytes (14,15). More recent data from our laboratory have shown that incubating epidermal keratinocytes from normal skin with fluorescently labeled *S. aureus* for one hour resulted in only 1% survival of *S. aureus*, as compared to 16.3% survival of *S. aureus* after incubation with epidermal keratinocytes from the skin biopsies of AD patients (17). The amount of HBD-3 that was mobilized onto *S. aureus* bound to keratinocytes in normal skin was found to be 34.3 $\pm$ 2.4 μmol/L, which was significantly higher that the level (10.7 μmol/L) that was required to kill *S. aureus*. In contrast, the amount of HBD-2 that was mobilized from the keratinocytes of AD skin onto *S. aureus* was found to be only 12.2 $\pm$ 3.0 μmol/L (17). When cultured human keratinocytes was incubated with *S. aureus* and the combination of IL-4 and IL-13, it was found that the percentage of *S. aureus* that was killed after contacting with the keratinocytes decreased by twofold (17). In the same study, IL-4 and IL-13 were shown to decrease the amount of HBD-3 on *S. aureus* via the inhibition of HBD-3 mobilization within cultured keratinocytes, rather than the synthesis or accumulation of this AMP in keratinocyte cytoplasm (17). Because IL-10 has also been shown to suppress AMP expression in keratinocytes (18), the effects of blocking antibodies against IL-4, IL-10, and IL-13 on the expression of HBD-3 surrounding *S. aureus* bound to the epidermal keratinocytes of AD skin were examined (17). It was found that antibodies to IL-4, IL-13, and IL-10 caused a threefold increase in the amount of HBD-3 deposited onto the surface of *S. aureus* by the keratinocytes of AD skin, whereas there was no significant increase in the amount of HBD-3 expressed in the normal control skin samples (17). In summary, AMPs, particularly HBD-3, play an important role in the killing of *S. aureus* by keratinocytes. The high levels of Th2 cytokines (IL-4, IL-10, and IL-13) in AD skin are responsible for suppression of these AMPs in AD skin, contributing to the increased colonization of *S. aureus* in AD patients.

Other factors that may contribute to the decreased cutaneous innate immunity and increased *S. aureus* colonization in AD include reduced expression of sweat dermcidin–derived AMP (19), sphingosine (20), hexadecenoic acid (21), and changes in stratum corneum pH, which may affect AMP activity (22).

STAPHYLOCOCCAL VIRULENCE FACTORS

Superantigens

The best-studied mechanism by which *S. aureus* induces skin inflammation in AD is via staphylococcal superantigens, which include staphylococcal enterotoxin (SE) A, SEB, SEC, SED, and toxic shock syndrome toxin-1 (TSST-1) (Table 2). About

TABLE 2   Mechanisms by Which *S. aureus* Triggers AD

1. Polyclonal activation of T cells by staphylococcal superantigens.
2. Induction of staphylococcal superantigen-specific IgE.
3. Modulation of proinflammatory chemokines and cytokines via Toll-like receptors.
4. Subversion of T regulatory cell functions by staphylococcal superantigens.
5. Induction of steroid–resistance in T cells by staphylococcal superantigens.
6. Enhancement of house dust mite sensitization by staphylococcal superantigens.
7. Induction of keratinocyte cytotoxicity by alpha-toxin.

44% to 57% of *S. aureus* isolated from AD patients secrete superantigens (23–25). In addition, clinical severity of AD correlates with superantigen production by *S. aureus* isolated from AD patients (25,26). A more recent study showed that *S. aureus* strains isolated from patients with steroid-resistant AD, a subgroup of patients with the most severe AD, were capable of producing more superantigens per organisms as compared to a general population of AD patients (27). The superantigens produced by *S. aureus* of steroid-resistant AD patients include classical staphylococcal superantigens SEA, SEB, and SED, as well as non-classical superantigens including staphylococcal enterotoxin–like (SEl) H, J, and K, etc. Superantigens activate T cells via the stimulation of variable β (vβ) chain of T-cell receptor, resulting in a polyclonal T-cell activation. Variable β repertoire of T cells in the skin lesions and systemic circulation of AD patients have been shown to correspond to the staphylococcal superantigens found on their skin (24,28). In addition, the skewing of vβ repertoire was found to be among the circulating T cells that are positive for cutaneous lymphocyte–associated antigen (CLA), the skin-homing receptor, rather than in the CLA-population [reviewed in Ref. (29)]. Topically applied superantigen in murine model and human skin consistently produce T-cells inflammation consisting of vβ repertoire that reflects the corresponding superantigen stimulation (30–32).

Superantigens may modulate Th1 cytokines, chemokines [reviewed in Ref. (33)] and Th2 cytokines. The latter include IL-4 (31,34), IL-13 (32,35), and a more recently described Th2 cytokine, IL-31, which induces severe pruritus (36). The action of Th2 cytokines leads to the production of IgE molecules, which may include superantigen-specific IgE. These IgE molecules have been shown to trigger basophil degranulation, leading to the release of histamine or other inflammatory mediators that may cause persistent itch–scratch cycle of AD patients (37). Up to 80% of children with AD that include those with severe skin disease was found to produce specific IgE against superantigens (38). The presence of these specific IgE molecules correlates with the severity of AD (38,39). Particularly, the presence of SEB-specific IgE was significantly associated with younger children who have severe AD, as compared to those with mild-to-moderate AD (38). More recently, a high prevalence of superantigen-specific IgE has also been found in young children with mild (38%)–to-moderate (63%) AD (40). In addition, the presence of SEA- and SED-specific IgE was significantly associated with moderate AD, as compared to mild AD in these young children. It has been hypothesized that microbial allergens including staphylococcal superantigens may play a role in the pathogenesis intrinsic AD (i.e., AD patients with total serum IgE <150 IU/mL and no food or inhalant allergic sensitization) (41). However, more recent data showed a lack of specific association between allergic sensitization to microbial allergens including superantigens and patients with intrinsic AD (40–43). However, since allergic sensitization to microbial allergens is found in 10% to 20% of AD patients with low total serum IgE (i.e., <150 IU/mL, but with or without specific allergic sensitization to food or inhalant allergens) (40,42), staphylococcal superantigen IgE may still play a role in the disease process of these patients.

In addition to their direct effects on T-cell activation and the production of specific IgE by B cells, superantigens may also subvert the suppressive function of T regulatory cells, resulting in increased activity of T effector cells and AD inflammation (44). The presence of superantigens in the skin of AD patients may also enhance the sensitization of other environmental allergens including house dust mites (33,45). Other indirect effects of superantigens include the induction of corticosteroid- or calcineurin inhibitor–resistance in the T cells of AD patients (46,47).

Nonsuperantigenic Virulence Factors

Toll-like receptors (TLR) are the best-studied pattern-recognition receptors in the innate immune system that differentiate "self" from "microbial nonself" (48). Increasing data suggest that TLR polymorphisms may play a role in the innate immune responses of AD patients (49–51). Staphylococcal cell wall components, peptidoglycan (PGN) and lipoteichoic acid (LTA), are known agonists for TLR-2. The monocytes of AD patients with TLR-2 polymorphism R753Q were found to express significantly higher levels of the proinflammatory cytokine, IL-6, when incubated with PGN or LTA, as compared to healthy individuals or AD patients with wild-type TLR-2 (50). PGN has also been found to increase keratinocyte production of granulocyte-monocyte colony-stimulating factor (GM-CSF) (52), which inhibits monocyte apoptosis and leads to persistent inflammatory state in AD (53). In murine model of AD, LTA may induce Th2 cytokines that include IL-4 and IL-5 (54). The induction of Th2 response by LTA may lead to enhanced allergen-specific IgE production (55). PGN and protein A, another staphylococcocal product, are capable of inducing the expression of IL-18 (56,57), which leads to the development of a subtype of T cells with both Th1 and Th2 features, and murine dermatitis (57). SEB has also been found to have nonsuperantigenic activity that signal through TLR2 on monocytes (58). Monocytes from AD patients were found to be hyporesponsive to in vitro stimulation by SEB. The authors speculated that in vivo activation of AD monocytes by SEB (via TLR2) could render them refractory to in vitro restimulation. Alpha-toxin–producing *S. aureus* is found in 34% of AD patients (59). It was previously shown that alpha-toxin from *S. aureus* was capable of inducing profound keratinocyte cytotoxicity in a time- and dose-dependent manner (60). The morphologic and functional characteristics of cell death induced by alpha-toxin were consistent with cell necrosis, not apoptosis. Additionally, alpha-toxin induced the release of tumor necrosis factor-alpha from keratinocytes within 30 minutes of addition to cultures. Alpha-toxin may also play an important role in the development of Th1 cells and chronic AD (59).

THERAPEUTIC IMPLICATIONS

In addition to its role in triggering the exacerbation of AD (61), multiple reports have documented the role *S. aureus* in causing invasive infections in AD patients. These infections include bacteremia, endocarditis, osteomyelitis, and septic arthritis [reviewed in Ref. (62)]. Therefore, prompt treatment of AD patients who have signs and symptoms of infection is crucial. These include fever, purulent discharge, pustules, crusting, and a widespread weeping discharge. Empirical anti-staphylococcal antibiotics should be started because most secondarily infected AD lesions are caused by *S. aureus* (63). A wound culture and sensitivity prior to treatment is recommended due to increasing prevalence of methicillin-resistant *S. aureus* (MRSA). Antibiotics, used in conjunction with topical corticosteroids, can be useful in the treatment of localized impetiginized skin lesions (64,65) colonized with *S. aureus*, where *S. aureus* is thought to be triggering the eczematoid reaction.

Due to the increased risk of bacterial resistance accompanying frequent use of antibiotics, it is important to combine antimicrobial therapy with effective skin care and timely use of topical anti-inflammatory medications. Improved skin hydration has been shown to be associated with improved barrier function and decreased *S. aureus* colonization in AD (66). This may be accomplished by a soaking bath or shower for 10 to 20 minutes, followed by application of an emollient or topical anti-inflammatory medications (67). Both topical corticosteroids (TCS) and topical calcineurin inhibitors (TCI) have been shown to decrease *S. aureus* colonization in AD when applied to affected areas (68–73). In addition, the use of TCS also leads to the improvement of barrier function (66,74), potentially decreasing further trigger by *S. aureus*. However, TCS has been noted to be a source of *S. aureus* contamination and recolonization of AD patients (9), therefore patients should be instructed on the hygiene of topical medication use such as using a clean hand or tongue blade to scoop out the TCI from the container.

Nonantibiotic Approaches for Control of *Staphylococcus aureus*
Antimicrobial Fabrics
There have been multiple studies on the treatment of *S. aureus* colonization in AD using antimicrobial fabrics. Silver-coated textiles were found to improve both objective and subjective symptoms of AD patients in a multicenter, double-blind, placebo-controlled trial (75). In addition, these textiles were found to have steroid-sparing effects in AD patients (76). The efficacy of silver-coated textiles in AD was attributed to their antimicrobial effects on *S. aureus* (77). Silk fabrics coated with an antimicrobial substance, AEGIS AEM 5772/5, have also been noted to improve the severity of AD, as compared to another group of AD patients wearing cotton clothing (78). Although there was a decrease in *S. aureus* colonization after treatment with these fabrics in AD patients, the difference in *S. aureus* colonization before and after treatment was not significant (79). In a more recent study comparing silk fabrics coated with AEGIS AEM 5772/5 versus silk fabrics without AEGIS AEM 5772/5, the investigators found the former had a greater efficacy in improving AD severity, as compared to the latter (80). They speculated that this difference in efficacy is likely due to the small, but statistically insignificant, reduction of *S. aureus* colonization in the former group. Further studies are needed to confirm these observations.

Anti-infectives
Multiple studies have documented the use of antiseptics in treating *S. aureus* colonization in AD patients. These antiseptics include antibacterial cleansers (55), gentian-violet (81), 10% povidone-iodine solution (82), and 1.5% triclocarban antibacterial soap (83). Triclosan, another antiseptic with similar structure to triclocarban, also has anti-staphylococcal activity (84). A recent study using a

combination of low-dose triclosan and chlorhexidine, another antiseptic with known anti-staphylococcal activity, showed equal efficacy in reducing *S. aureus* colonization and in improving AD, as compared to monotherapy with triclosan at a five-time higher concentration (85). Of note, all these anti-infective strategies may be limiting, as they can be too irritating for the inflamed skin of AD patients.

CONCLUSIONS

S. aureus contributes to the severity of AD via the production of proinflammatory molecules including staphylococcal superantigens, alpha-toxin, and cell wall components (protein A, LTA, and PGN). The allergic inflammation is further enhanced by host production of superantigen-specific IgE. In addition, secondary infection of AD by *S. aureus*, particularly MRSA, may lead to invasive infections including bacteremia, endocarditis, osteomyelitis, and septic arthritis. Appropriate use of antibiotics for superinfected AD, together with intensive hydration and topical antiinflammatory medications, can lead to a decrease in *S. aureus* level and improvement of AD. Antiseptic and antimicrobial fabrics may be beneficial in treating *S. aureus* colonization. Enhancement of cutaneous innate immunity, such as replacement of AMPs or antimicrobial lipids, represents a potential future treatment modality. Because Th2 cytokines are crucial for the attachment of *S. aureus* to AD skin, and the suppression of AMP in AD lesions, targeting these cytokines also constitutes another novel approach in controlling *S. aureus* colonization in AD.

REFERENCES

1. Ong PY, Leung DYM. Immune dysregulation in atopic dermatitis. Curr Allergy Asthma Rep 2006; 6:384–389.
2. Baurecht H, Irvine AD, Novak N, et al. Toward a major risk factor for atopic eczema: Meta-analysis of filaggrin polymorphism data. J Allergy Clin Immunol 2007; 120:1406–1412.
3. Nilsson EJ, Henning CG, Magnusson J. Topical corticosteroids and *Staphylococcus aureus* in atopic dermatitis. J Am Acad Dermatol 1992; 27:29–34.
4. Breuer K, Haussler S, Kapp A, et al. *Staphylococcus aureus*: Colonizing features and influence of an antibacterial treatment in adults with atopic dermatitis. Br J Dermatol 2002; 147:55–61.
5. Leyden JJ, Marples RR, Kligman AM. *Staphylococcal aureus* in the lesions of atopic dermatitis. Br J Dermatol 1974; 90:525–530.
6. Ricci G, Patrizi A, Neri I, et al. Frequency and clinical role of *Staphylococcus aureus* overinfection in atopic dermatitis in children. Pediatr Dermatol 2003; 20:389–392.
7. Leung AD, Schiltz AM, Hall CF, et al. Severe atopic dermatitis is associated with a high burden of environmental *Staphylococcus aureus*. Clin Exp Allergy 2008; 38:789–793.
8. Bonness S, Szekat C, Novak N, et al. Pulsed-field gel electrophoresis of *Staphylococcus aureus* isolates from atopic patients revealing presence of similar strains in isolates from children and their parents. J Clin Microbiol 2008; 46:456–461.
9. Gilani SJ, Gonzalez M, Hussain I, et al. *Staphylococcus aureus* re-colonization in atopic dermatitis: Beyond the skin. Clin Exp Dermatol 2005; 30:10–13.
10. Cho SH, Strickland I, Tomkinson A, et al. Preferential binding of *Staphylococcus aureus* to skin sites of Th2-mediated inflammation in a murine model. J Invest Dermatol 2001; 116:658–663.
11. Strickland I, Cho SH, Boguniewicz M, et al. Fibronectin contributes to the enhanced binding of *Staphylococcus aureus* to atopic skin. J Allergy Clin Immunol 2001; 107:778A.

12. Postlethwaite AE, Holness MA, Katai H, et al. Human fibroblasts synthesize elevated levels of extracellular matrix proteins in response to interleukin 4. J Clin Invest 1992; 90:1479–1485.

13. Chaitidis P, O'Donnell V, Kuban RJ, et al. Gene expression alterations of human peripheral blood monocytes induced by medium-term treatment with the TH2-cytokines interleukin-4 and -13. Cytokine 2005; 30:366–377.

14. Ong PY, Ohtake T, Brandt C, et al. Endogenous antimicrobial peptides and skin infections in atopic dermatitis. N Engl J Med 2002; 347:1151–1160.

15. Nomura I, Goleva E, Howell MD, et al. Cytokine milieu of atopic dermatitis, as compared to psoriasis, skin prevents induction of innate immune response genes. J Immunol 2003; 171:3262–3269.

16. Kisich KO, Howell MD, Boguniewicz M, et al. The constitutive capacity of human keratinocytes to kill *Staphylococcus aureus* is dependent on beta-defensin 3. J Invest Dermatol 2007; 127:2368–2380.

17. Kisich KO, Carspecken CW, Fieve S, et al. Defective killing of *Staphylococcus aureus* in atopic dermatitis is associated with reduced mobilization of human beta-defensin-3. J Allergy Clin Immunol 2008; 122:62–68.

18. Howell MD, Novak N, Bieber T, et al. Interleukin-10 downregulates anti-microbial peptide expression in atopic dermatitis. J Invest Dermatol 2005; 125:738–745.

19. Rieg S, Steffen H, Seeber S, et al. Deficiency of dermcidin-derived antimicrobial peptides in sweat of patients with atopic dermatitis correlates with an impaired innate defense of human skin in vivo. J Immunol 2005; 174:8003–8010.

20. Arikawa J, Ishibashi M, Kawashima M, et al. Decreased levels of sphingosine, a natural antimicrobial agent, may be associated with vulnerability of the stratum corneum from patients with atopic dermatitis to colonization by *Staphylococcus aureus*. J Invest Dermatol 2002; 119:433–439.

21. Takigawa H, Nakagawa H, Kuzukawa M, et al. Deficient production of hexadecenoic acid in the skin is associated in part with the vulnerability of atopic dermatitis patients to colonization by *Staphylococcus aureus*. Dermatology 2005; 211:240–248.

22. Rippke F, Schreiner V, Doering T, et al. Stratum corneum pH in atopic dermatitis: Impact on skin barrier function and colonization with *Staphylococcus aureus*. Am J Clin Dermatol 2004; 5:217–223.

23. Nomura I, Tanaka K, Tomita H, et al. Evaluation of the staphylococcal exotoxins and their specific IgE in childhood atopic dermatitis. J Allergy Clin Immunol 1999; 104:441–446.

24. Bunikowski R, Mielke ME, Skarabis H, et al. Evidence for a disease-promoting effect of *Staphylococcus aureus*-derived exotoxins in atopic dermatitis. J Allergy Clin Immunol 2000; 105:814–819.

25. Tomi NS, Kranke B. Aberer: Staphylococcal toxins in patients with psoriasis, atopic dermatitis, and erythroderma, and in healthy control subjects. J Am Acad Dermatol 2005; 53:67–72.

26. Zollner TM, Wichelhaus TA, Hartung A, et al. Colonization with superantigen-producing *Staphylococcus aureus* is associated with increased severity of atopic dermatitis. Clin Exp Allergy 2000; 30:994–1000.

27. Schlievert PM, Case LC, Strandberg KL, et al. Superantigen profile of *Staphylococcus aureus* isolates from patients with steroid-resistant atopic dermatitis. Clin Infect Dis 2008; 46:1562–1567.

28. Strickland I, Hauk PJ, Trumble AE, et al. Evidence for superantigen involvement in skin homing of T cells in atopic dermatitis. J Invest Dermatol 1999; 112:249–253.

29. Santamaria-Babi LF. CLA(+) T cells in cutaneous diseases. Eur J Dermatol 2004; 14:13–18.

30. Skov L, Olsen JV, Giorno R, et al. Application of staphylococcal enterotoxin B on normal and atopic skin induces up-regulation of T cells by a superantigen-mediated mechanism. J Allergy Clin Immunol 2000; 105:820–826.

31. Laouini D, Kawamoto S, Yalcindag A, et al. Epicutaneous sensitization with superantigen induces allergic skin inflammation. J Allergy Clin Immunol 2003; 112:981–987.

32. Savinko T, Lauerma A, Lehtimaki S, et al. Topical superantigen exposure induces epidermal accumulation of CD8+ T cells, a mixed Th1/Th2-type dermatitis and vigorous

production of IgE antibodies in the murine model of atopic dermatitis. J Immunol 2005; 175:8320–8326.

33. Homey B, Meller S, Savinko T, et al. Modulation of chemokines by staphylococcal super-antigen in atopic dermatitis. Chem Immunol Allergy 2007; 93:181–194.
34. Ardern-Jones MR, Black AP, Bateman EA, et al. Bacterial superantigen facilitates epithe-lial presentation of allergen to T helper 2 cells. Proc Natl Acad Sci USA 2007; 104:5557–5562.
35. Lehmann HS, Heaton T, Mallon D, et al. Staphylococcal enterotoxin-B-mediated stimula-tion of interleukin-13 production as a potential aetiologic factor in eczema in infants. Int Arch Allergy Immunol 2004; 135:306–312.
36. Sonkoly E, Muller A, Lauerma AI, et al. IL-31: A new link between T cells and pruritus in atopic skin inflammation. J Allergy Clin Immunol 2006; 117:411–417.
37. Leung DYM, Harbeck R, Bina P, et al. Presence of IgE antibodies to staphylococcal exotox-ins on the skin of patients with atopic dermatitis. Evidence for a new group of allergens. J Clin Invest 1993; 92:1374–1380.
38. Nomura I, Tanaka K, Tomita H, et al. Evaluation of the staphylococcal exotoxins and their specific IgE in childhood atopic dermatitis. J Allergy Clin Immunol 1999; 104: 441–446.
39. Bunikowski R, Mielke M, Skarabis H, et al. Prevalence and role of serum IgE antibodies to the *Staphylococcus aureus*-derived superantigens SEA and SEB in children with atopic dermatitis. J Allergy Clin Immunol 1999; 103:119–124.
40. Ong PY, Patel M, Ferdman RM, et al. Association of staphylococcal superantigen-specific immunoglobulin E with mild and moderate atopic dermatitis. J Pediatr 2008 [Epub ahead of print].
41. Novak N, Allam JP, Bieber T. Allergic hyperreactivity to microbial components: A trigger factor of "intrinsic" atopic dermatitis? J Allergy Clin Immunol 2003; 112:215–216.
42. Reefer AJ, Satinover SM, Wilson BB, et al. The relevance of microbial allergens to the IgE antibody repertoire in atopic and nonatopic eczema. J Allergy Clin Immunol 2007; 120:156–163.
43. Schnopp C, Grosch J, Ring J, et al. Microbial allergen-specific IgE is not suitable to identify the intrinsic form of atopic eczema in children. J Allergy Clin Immunol 2008; 121:267–268.e1.
44. Ou LS, Goleva E, Hall C, et al. T regulatory cells in atopic dermatitis and subversion of their activity by superantigens. J Allergy Clin Immunol 2004; 113:756–763.
45. Langer K, Breuer K, Kapp A, et al. *Staphylococcus aureus*-derived enterotoxins enhance house dust mite-induced patch test reactions in atopic dermatitis. Exp Dermatol 2007; 16:124–129.
46. Hauk PJ, Hamid QA, Chrousos GP, et al. Induction of corticosteroid insensitivity in human PBMCs by microbial superantigens. J Allergy Clin Immunol 2000; 105:782–787.
47. Fukushima H, Hirano T, Shibayama N, et al. The role of immune response to *Staphylococ-cus aureus* superantigens and disease severity in relation to the sensitivity to tacrolimus in atopic dermatitis. Int Arch Allergy Immunol 2006; 141:281–289.
48. Medzhitov R, Janeway CA Jr. Decoding the patterns of self and nonself by the innate immune system. Science 2002; 296:298–300.
49. Ahmad-Nejad P, Mrabet-Dahbi S, Breuer K, et al. The toll-like receptor 2 R753Q polymor-phism defines a subgroup of patients with atopic dermatitis having severe phenotype. J Allergy Clin Immunol 2004; 113:565–567.
50. Mrabet-Dahbi S, Dalpke AH, Niebuhr M, et al. The Toll-like receptor 2 R753Q muta-tion modifies cytokine production and Toll-like receptor expression in atopic dermatitis. J Allergy Clin Immunol 2008; 121:1013–1019.
51. Niebuhr M, Langnickel J, Draing C, et al. Dysregulation of toll-like receptor-2 (TLR-2)-induced effects in monocytes from patients with atopic dermatitis: Impact of the TLR-2 R753Q polymorphism. Allergy 2008; 63:728–734.
52. Matsubara M, Harada D, Manabe H, et al. *Staphylococcus aureus* peptidoglycan stimulates granulocyte macrophage colony-stimulating factor production from human epidermal keratinocytes via mitogen-activated protein kinases. FEBS Lett 2004; 566:195–200.

53. Bratton DL, Hamid Q, Boguniewicz M, et al. Granulocyte macrophage colony-stimulating factor contributes to enhanced monocyte survival in chronic atopic dermatitis. J Clin Invest 1995; 95:211–218.

54. Matsui K, Nishikawa A. Lipoteichoic acid from *Staphylococcus aureus* induces Th2-prone dermatitis in mice sensitized percutaneously with an allergen. Clin Exp Allergy 2002; 32:783–788.

55. Matsui K, Nishikawa A. Lipoteichoic acid from *Staphylococcus aureus* enhances allergen-specific immunoglobulin E production in mice. Clin Exp Allergy 2003; 33:842–848.

56. Matsui K, Wirotesangthong M, Nishkawa A. Peptidoglycan from *Staphylococcus aureus* induces IL-4 production from murine spleen cells via an IL-18-dependent mechanism. Int Arch Allergy Immunol 2008; 146:262–266.

57. Terada M, Tsutsui H, Imai Y, et al. Contribution of IL-18 to atopic-dermatitis-like skin inflammation induced by *Staphylococcus aureus* product in mice. Proc Natl Acad Sci USA 2006; 103:8816–8821.

58. Mandron M, Aries MF, Boralevi F, et al. Age-related differences in sensitivity of peripheral blood monocytes to lipopolysaccharide and *Staphylococcus aureus* toxin B in atopic dermatitis. J Invest Dermatol 2008; 128:882–889.

59. Breuer K, Wittmann M, Kempe K, et al. Alpha-toxin is produced by skin colonizing *Staphylococcus aureus* and induces a T helper type 1 response in atopic dermatitis. Clin Exp Allergy 2005; 35:1088–1095.

60. Ezepchuk YV, Leung DYM, Middleton MH, et al. Staphylococcal toxins and protein A differentially induce cytotoxicity and release of tumor necrosis factor-alpha from human keratinocytes. J Invest Dermatol 1996; 107:603–609.

61. David TJ, Cambridge GC. Bacterial infection and atopic eczema. Arch Dis Child 1986; 61:20–23.

62. Benenson S, Zimhony O, Dahan D, et al. Atopic dermatitis—A risk factor for invasive *Staphylococcus aureus* infections: Two cases and review. Am J Med 2005; 118:1048–1051.

63. Brook I. Secondary bacterial infections complicating skin lesions. J Med Microbiol 2002; 51:808–812.

64. Lever R, Hadley K, Downey D, et al. Staphylococcal colonization in atopic dermatitis and the effect of topical mupirocin therapy. Br J Dermatol 1988; 119:189–198.

65. Parish LC, Jorizzo JL, Bretton JJ, et al; SB275833/032 Study Team: Topical retapamulin ointment (1%, wt/wt) twice daily for 5 days versus oral cephalexin twice daily for 10 days in the treatment of secondarily infected dermatitis: Results of a randomized controlled trial. J Am Acad Dermatol 2006; 55:1003–1013.

66. Schnopp C, Holtmann C, Stock S, et al. Topical steroids under wet-wrap dressings in atopic dermatitis—A vehicle-controlled trial. Dermatology 2002; 204:56–59.

67. Gutman AB, Kligman AM, Sciacca J, et al. Soak and smear: A standard technique revisited. Arch Dermatol 2005; 141:1556–1559.

68. Hung SH, Lin YT, Chu CY, et al. Staphylococcus colonization in atopic dermatitis treated with fluticasone or tacrolimus with or without antibiotics. Ann Allergy Asthma Immunol 2007; 98:51–56.

69. Xhauflaire-Uhoda E, Thirion L, Pierard-Franchimont C, et al. Comparative effect of tacrolimus and betamethasone valerate on the passive sustainable hydration of the stratum corneum in atopic dermatitis. Dermatology 2007; 214:328–332.

70. Gong JQ, Lin L, Lin T, et al. Skin colonization by *Staphylococcus aureus* in patients with eczema and atopic dermatitis and relevant combined topical therapy: A double-blind multicentre randomized controlled trial. Br J Dermatol 2006; 155:680–687.

71. Remitz A, Kyllönen H, Granlund H, et al. Tacrolimus ointment reduces staphylococcal colonization of atopic dermatitis lesions. J Allergy Clin Immunol 2001;107:196.

72. Nilsson EJ, Henning CG, Magnusson J. Topical corticosteroids and *Staphylococcus aureus* in atopic dermatitis. J Am Acad Dermatol 1992; 27:29–34.

73. Ramsay CA, Savoie LM, Gilbert M. The treatment of atopic dermatitis with topical fusidic acid and hydrocortisone acetate. J Eur Acad Dermatol Venerol 1996; 7:S15–22.

74. Aalto-Korte K. Improvement of skin barrier function during treatment of atopic dermatitis. J Am Acad Dermatol 1995; 33:969–972.

75. Gauger A, Fischer S, Mempel M, et al. Efficacy and functionality of silver-coated textiles in patients with atopic eczema. J Eur Acad Dermatol Venereol 2006; 20:534–541.

76. Juenger M, Ladwig A, Staecker S, et al. Efficacy and safety of silver textile in the treatment of atopic dermatitis (AD). Curr Med Res Opin 2006; 22:739–750.

77. Gauger A, Mempel M, Schekatz A, et al. Silver-coated textiles reduce *Staphylococcus aureus* colonization in patients with atopic eczema. Dermatology 2003; 207:15–21.

78. Ricci G, Patrizi A, Bendandi B, et al. Clinical effectiveness of a silk fabric in the treatment of atopic dermatitis. Br J Dermatol 2004; 150:127–131.

79. Ricci G, Patrizi A, Mandrioli P, et al. Evaluation of the antibacterial activity of a special silk textile in the treatment of atopic dermatitis. Dermatology 2006; 213:224–227.

80. Stinco G, Piccirillo F, Valent F. A randomized double-blind study to investigate the clinical efficacy of adding a non-migrating antimicrobial to a special silk fabric in the treatment of atopic dermatitis. Dermatology 2008; 217:191–195.

81. Brockow K, Grabenhorst P, Traupe B. Gentian violet for the treatment of atopic eczema antibacterial and clinical efficacy. J Invest Dermatol 1997; 109:463.

82. Akiyama H, Tada J, Toi J, et al. Changes in *Staphylococcus aureus* density and lesion severity after topical application of povidone-iodine in cases of atopic dermatitis. J Dermatol Sci 1997; 16:23–30.

83. Breneman DL, Hanifin JM, Berge CA, et al. The effect of antibacterial soap with 1.5% triclocarban on *Staphylococcus aureus* in patients with atopic dermatitis. Cutis 2000; 66:296–300.

84. Bamber AI, Neal TJ. An assessment of triclosan susceptibility in methicillin-resistant and methicillin-sensitive *Staphylococcus aureus*. J Hosp Infect 1999; 41:107–109.

85. Wohlrab J, Jost G, Abeck D. Antiseptic efficacy of a low-dosed topical triclosan/chlorhexidine combination therapy in atopic dermatitis. Skin Pharmacol Physiol 2007; 20:71–76.

16 Virus Infections in Atopic Dermatitis

Natalija Novak
Department of Dermatology and Allergy, University of Bonn, Bonn, Germany

Donald Y. M. Leung
Division of Pediatric Allergy-Immunology, National Jewish Health, and Department of Pediatrics, University of Colorado Denver Health Sciences Center, Denver, Colorado, U.S.A.

INTRODUCTION AND BACKGROUND

Atopic dermatitis (AD) in childhood as well as in adulthood can be complicated by localized or widespread cutaneous infections, which are specific for the disease; although nearly one-third of patients with AD suffer from microbial skin infections, cutaneous skin infections are only detectable in 6% to 7% of patients with other chronic inflammatory skin diseases such as psoriasis (1). Virus infections observable in AD patients are most often caused by Herpes simplex virus, Human papilloma virus, or Molluscipox virus (Table 1). It is assumed that skin barrier impairment as well as AD specific deficiencies on the level of the innate and the adaptive immune system, in particular the excessive supply of Th2 cytokines, as opposed to relatively low amounts of Th1 cytokines, promotes these infections (Table 2) (2).

Eczema Molluscatum

Eczema molluscatum occurs frequently in children with AD and is caused by Molluscipox (Molluscum contagiosum) virus, which contains a large, double-stranded DNA genome and replicates in the cytoplasm of infected cells leading to cell hyperplasia. Clinically, the lesions are often grouped or disseminated and represent as skin-colored, centrally umbilicated, dome-shaped papules which include a white, expressible core (3). The lesions are asymptomatic or accompanied by pruritus and in most of the cases surrounded by eczematous reactions. The characteristic appearance of the lesions, sometimes combined with a biopsy and histologic analysis, form the basis for the diagnosis. Lesions can heal spontaneously. Recurrence of the lesions or rapid spreading of new lesions caused by autoinoculation is frequently observable (3). Therapeutic removal is conducted mechanically with curettage or liquid nitrogen or podophyllotoxin application.

Verrucae Vulgares

Although subclinical infections with human papilloma virus are very common, they often become manifest as verrucae vulgares in particular in children with AD and are localized at the extremities. Clinically, they present as rough, scaly papules or nodules on the skin surfaces and are often grouped. Histologically, these lesions consist of papillomatosis and acanthotic epidermis, hyper- and parakeratosis, and elongated rete ridges. Removal of warts can be achieved mechanically or by

TABLE 1 Overview of the Different Virus Infection of the Skin, Which Might Complicate the Course of Atopic Dermatitis

Virus	Molluscipox	Human papilloma	Herpes simplex	Vaccinia
Skin manifestation	Eczema molluscatum	Verruae vulgares	Eczema herpeticatum	Eczema vaccinatum
Clinical picture	Skin colored, centrally umbilicated, dome-shaped papules; grouped or disseminated, surrounded by eczema	Rough, scaly, skin colored papules or nodules, often grouped	Papulovesicles, which develop into widespread erosions and punched-out crusts, disseminated over large body sites, impairment of the general condition	Blisters and pustules, disseminated over the entire body, impairment of the general condition
Primary treatment	Mechanical/ chemical removal	Mechanical/ chemical removal	Antiviral treatment (aciclovir, valaciclovir), local antiseptic lotions, topical or systemic antibiotics if required	Vaccinia immunglobulin

TABLE 2 Factors Associated with or Suspected to be Causative for the Higher Susceptibility of AD Patients to Virus Infections

Clinical factors	Early onset of AD Predilection in the head and neck area High total serum IgE High number of allergen specific IgE
Skin barrier	Inherited and acquired impairment of the skin barrier function Irregular use of emollients Local immunosuppression by topical steroids or calcineurin inhibitors
Innate immunity	Low amount of cathelicidins and human beta defensins in the skin
Adaptive immunity	Th2 overbalance in the skin and blood Diminished induction of Th1 immune responses Deficiency of plasmacytoid DC Low MIP-3α level in the skin Low number of NK cells in the blood

application of various agents, which mainly induce localized inflammation and subsequent clearance of the virus infected cells. Spontaneous remission of the warts is very common.

Eczema Vaccinatum

Vaccination against smallpox, caused by variola virus is done with live vaccinia virus. The rate of adverse events observed during smallpox vaccination is one of the highest among all vaccination types. Effective 30 years ago, widespread routine vaccination against smallpox infection has been stopped due to its eradication and is now limited to military personnel or individuals with specific risk for infection (3,4). Patients with immunodeficiencies and patients with active AD or AD in their history are excluded from this form of vaccination due to high risk for the development of eczema vaccinatum. Eczema vaccinatum develops as disseminated blisters and pustules over the entire body which go along with severe, life-threatening impairment of the general condition (3,4). Both, vaccination itself or accidental vaccinia inoculation by contact with vaccinated individuals can cause eczema vaccinatum. The latest case of eczema vaccinatum reported in the literature was a 28-month-old child with AD exposed to his smallpox vaccinated father in 2008 (5). Administration of vaccinia immunoglobulin at the earliest time point possible is important for the efficacy and prognosis of the disease.

Eczema Herpeticum

Severe viral superinfection with Herpes simplex virus (HSV), designated as Eczema herpeticum (EH), occurs as one or more episodes in about 10% to 20% of AD patients. HSV belongs to the double-stranded DNA virus family; it is 100 nm large and surrounded by an envelop of different glycoproteins (gG) and spikes (gD, gB). After primary infection, which typically involves mucocutaneous locations and occurs in most of the cases subclinically during childhood, HSV persists for the whole lifetime in the ganglia of the nervous system. This enables HSV to cause secondary infections after latency. Reactivation of HSV infections can be favored by stress, UV light, transient or manifest immunodeficiency, mechanical trauma, and a lot of other exogenous and endogenous factors. Seroprevalence of HSV 1 is about 90% in some regions, while seroprevalence of HSV 2 is below 20% (6). The high seroprevalence represents besides the capability of HSV to be easily reactivated another cofactor, which forwards the relatively frequent complications of AD by cutaneous HSV infections. Both types of HSV, 1 and 2 can cause EH as a primary or secondary infection. In one study from Japan, a particular genotype of HSV1, F35 has been linked to EH infections in Japanese AD patients (7). HSV enters the cells via nectin-1 and nectin-2 (8), the herpes virus entry mediator (HVEM) and specific sites in heparin sulfates (9,10). Eosinophilic nuclear inclusion and marginal nuclear chromatin as well as multinucleated clusters of giant cells are characteristic features of HSV-infected cells. Degenerating infected cells elicit intracellular edema and swelling.

The initial lesions of EH represent dome-shaped papulovesicles. Later on, these papulovesicles develop into pustules, excoriations, and crusts, which spread in severe cases over the entire body. Spreading of the virus occurs from cell to cell and via the blood and lymphatic system. Predilection of EH is the head, neck, and thoracal region. Impairment of the general condition, fever, lymphadenopathy, pruritus, and malaise are symptoms accompanying EH (3). Due to the high colonization rate of the skin of AD patients with *Staphylococcus aureus*, bacterial superinfections might complicate the course of EH.

Clinically, adult patients with one or more episodes of EH have a predilection of AD in the head and neck area and higher total as well as allergen specific IgE levels (11,12). An early onset of AD as well as chronic course seems to be other cofactors leading to the manifestation of EH in 10% to 20% of AD patients (11). However, strong epidemiologic data on large cohorts as well as detailed information about cofactors, which abet EH in adults versus infants with AD, are still missing.

Viral proof for HSV can be done by light microscopy using the Tzank test, by viral culture, immunofluorescence staining, electron microscopy, and PCR. Samples for virus testing should be taken before onset of any treatment. Serum IgM titers increase usually during a primary infection and may be within normal ranges during reinfections with HSV, which often cause EH.

Anti-viral therapy should be applied as early as possible during the initial phase of EH. Clinical efficacy of aciclovir has been proven in a double-blind placebo-controlled study with significant differences in terms of the duration of EH and healing results (13). Aciclovir is recommended for intravenous treatment over a time period of seven days, while valaciclovir has a better oral bioavailability. The question, whether any benefit of prophylactic treatment with oral aciclovir or valaciclovir in patients with recurrent episodes of EH exists, needs to be ruled out in additional studies. For bacterial superinfection of EH, local antiseptic lotions or topical antibiotics and in severe cases systemic antibiotic treatment is recommended. Topical and systemic glucocorticoids as well as calcineurin inhibitors, UV treatment, and immunosuppressants such as cyclosporin A should be avoided in the initial phase of EH due to unwanted immunosuppression, which might promote rapid viral spreading (3).

PUTATIVE RISK FACTORS FOR THE DEVELOPMENT OF VIRUS INFECTIONS IN AD

Contribution of the Impaired Skin Barrier Function

As compared to other chronic inflammatory skin diseases, AD appears to be more often complicated by cutaneous virus infections, which implies that specific predisposing factors in the pathophysiologic puzzle of AD contribute to this phenomenon. Without any doubt, the deficient skin barrier function, which has been shown to be in part genetically predetermined for instance by loss-of-functions mutations in the filaggrin gene (14), or modifications in gene regions encoding serine protease inhibitors such as the lymphoepithelial kazal type 5 serine inhibitor (15), the stratum corneum chymotryptic enzyme gene (16), or a novel kollagenase (17) contribute to this. Besides these inherited factors, Th2 cytokines in the micromilieu of the AD skin might secondarily impair the skin barrier function by reducing the amount of filaggrin (18), loricrin (19), involucrin (19), or S100 proteins (20) in the upper layers of the skin. This might explain in part, why though deficient skin barrier represents a rather general feature of AD, especially the subgroup of AD patients with accentuated Th2 overbalance, mirrored by high number of allergen sensitizations and IgE serum levels (11,21) are much more prone to virus infections. In addition, the frequency and type of topical treatment might influence the skin barrier function and explain partially the increased propensity of AD patients to viral skin infections. Noncompliance in regard to continuous topical treatment with emollients as well as local immunosuppression induced by glucocorticosteroids or topical immunomodulators are currently discussed as additional factors contributing to the susceptibility to cutaneous virus infections in AD. In a small study, mutations in the promoter region of the *IL18* gene have been associated with eruption of EH during treatment with tacrolimus (22). However, data underlining the hypothesis of a direct link between specific skin barrier deficiencies and sensitivity to virus infections are still missing.

Innate Immunity and Virus Infections in AD

Important and effective defensive elements against microbial infections derive from the innate immune system. Antimicrobial peptides, released in the skin by different cell types, are integral components of this sophisticated defense network (23). Next to the clinical observation of a high rate of cutaneous virus infections in AD, experiments with skin explants from various skin diseases revealed a faster HSV replication on explants from AD skin (24). Besides yet unidentified factors of the skin micromilieu such as increased expression of viral entry structures or respective adhesion molecules, which might benefit both, infection of cells with the virus and spreading of the virus from cell to cell, these observations imply that mechanisms on the level of innate immunity might be deficient in AD. There is strong evidence that two types of antimicrobial peptides, namely, human β-defensins and cathelicidins are expressed in low amount in AD skin (25). While HBD-1 is expressed constitutively, the other HBDs and cathelicidins are upregulated in inflamed skin or after skin damage (26). Within the AD patients, less expression of the cathelicidin LL37 in inflamed skin has been shown in particular in AD patients with EH (27). Interestingly, an inverse relationship between serum IgE levels and expression of LL37 in the skin has been observed (27). Selective killing of vaccinia virus by this cathelicidin has been shown in an impressive series of experiments (28). As a consequence, vaccinia replication rate is much higher in explants from AD skin than from other skin diseases such as psoriasis.

Expression of antimicrobial peptides seems to be controlled by the amount of cytokines in the micromilieu. Th2 cytokines interleukin (IL)-4 and IL-13 as well as IL-10, detectable in AD skin have been shown to reduce the amount of human beta defensin (HBD)-3 produced by keratinocytes, which revealed antiviral activity against vaccinia virus in viral plaque assays (25,29,30). Therefore, low LL37 and HBD-3 skin levels combined with a specific cytokine micromilieu (31) might represent a risk factor for EH as well as eczema vaccinatum.

Adaptive Immunity

Other factors, which are associated with increased risk for HSV infections, are higher levels of total IgE and Th2 cytokines in the blood and periphery such as the skin and are mirrored partially by higher allergen-specific IgE serum levels (11,32). After stimulation with inactivated HSV, peripheral blood mononuclear cells (PBMC) from AD patients with a history for EH as opposed to AD patients without a history of EH revealed lower interferon (IFN)-α producing capacity of PBMC in the subgroup of AD patients at risk for EH (11), implying lack of induction of defensive Th1 immune responses in these patients. Further on, results from murine models reveal that local allergic inflammation seems to impair Th1 immune responses necessary for the defense of virus and thereby benefits viral spreading (33). Locally in the skin, a reduced number of plasmacytoid DC (PDC) in the epidermis in AD compared to other inflammatory skin diseases such as contact dermatitis, psoriasis, or lupus erythematodes might contribute to a lower cellular defense reaction toward HSV to counteract and limit viral spreading (34). Without any doubt, Th2 cytokines in AD skin play a crucial role in this context, since IL-4 and IL-10 induce rapid cell death of PDC in vitro (35). In contrast, increase of PDC in the peripheral blood of AD patients during the acute phase of EH has been observed (36). PDC bridge innate and adaptive immunity and are capable to produce type I interferons.

Pattern recognition receptors help them to sense the environment for viral antigens. Toll-like receptor (TLR) 9, which is expressed by PDC (37) has been shown to be involved in the recognition of HSV antigens. Further, PDC express the high affinity receptor for IgE (FcεRI), and the expression of this receptor correlates with IgE serum levels (38). A counter-regulation of FcεRI and TLR9 (39) might explain, why preactivation of PDC via FcεRI lowers their capacity to produce IFNα/β, which is crucial for the defense against virus infections (38). Since PDC of patients with AD are frequently activated via FcεRI, this might be one reason for a lower cellular capacity in AD patients to produce soluble factors which are necessary for viral defense (38). Further on, a lower number of circulating CD56+ natural killer cells and IL-2R expression on peripheral blood cells has been observed in children with EH (40) and might contribute to the higher susceptibility to HSV infections, too. Antiviral activity of macrophage inflammatory protein (MIP)-3α has been proven with the help of plaque assays with vaccinia virus, since virus replication in keratinocytes was low in the presence of high concentrations of MIP-3α in the microenvironment (41). Therefore, reduced amounts of MIP-3α in the skin of AD patients most likely elicited by the Th2 prone micromilieu are assumed to contribute in addition to the susceptibility to virus infections (41).

CONCLUSION

In summary, recent insights into both innate and adaptive immune mechanisms, in general, as well as specific deficiencies on the different levels of the pathophysiologic network of AD contribute to viral skin infections in this common skin disease. New insights into the barrier dysfunction of AD will help to improve our knowledge required to develop novel prophylactic as well as therapeutic strategies for the treatment of viral complications in AD.

REFERENCES

1. Christophers E, Henseler T. Contrasting disease patterns in psoriasis and atopic dermatitis. Arch Dermatol Res 1987; 279(suppl):S48–S51.
2. Leung DY, Bieber T. Atopic dermatitis. Lancet 2003; 361(9352):151–160.
3. Wollenberg A, Wetzel S, Burgdorf WH, et al. Viral infections in atopic dermatitis: Pathogenic aspects and clinical management. J Allergy Clin Immunol 2003; 112(4):667–674.
4. Parrino J, Graham BS. Smallpox vaccines: Past, present, and future. J Allergy Clin Immunol 2006; 118(6):1320–1326.
5. Vora S, Damon I, Fulginiti V, et al. Severe eczema vaccinatum in a household contact of a smallpox vaccine. Clin Infect Dis 2008; 46(10):1555–1561.
6. Wutzler P, Doerr HW, Farber I, et al. Seroprevalence of herpes simplex virus type 1 and type 2 in selected German populations-relevance for the incidence of genital herpes. J Med Virol 2000; 61(2):201–207.
7. Yoshida M, Umene K. Close association of predominant genotype of herpes simplex virus type 1 with eczema herpeticum analyzed using restriction fragment length polymorphism of polymerase chain reaction. J Virol Methods 2003; 109(1):11–16.
8. Sakisaka T, Taniguchi T, Nakanishi H, et al. Requirement of interaction of nectin-1alpha/HveC with afadin for efficient cell–cell spread of herpes simplex virus type 1. J Virol 2001; 75(10):4734–4743.
9. Campadelli-Fiume G, Amasio M, Avitabile E, et al. The multipartite system that mediates entry of herpes simplex virus into the cell. Rev Med Virol 2007; 17(5):313–326.

10. Novak N, Peng W. Dancing with the enemy: The interplay of herpes simplex virus with dendritic cells. Clin Exp Immunol 2005; 142(3):405–410.
11. Peng WM, Jenneck C, Bussmann C, et al. Risk factors of atopic dermatitis patients for eczema herpeticum. J Invest Dermatol 2007; 127(5):1261–1263.
12. Bussmann C, Bockenhoff A, Henke H, et al. Does allergen-specific immunotherapy represent a therapeutic option for patients with atopic dermatitis? J Allergy Clin Immunol 2006; 118(6):1292–1298.
13. Sanderson IR, Brueton LA, Savage MO, et al. Eczema herpeticum: A potentially fatal disease. Br Med J (Clin Res Ed) 1987; 294(6573):693–694.
14. Baurecht H, Irvine AD, Novak N, et al. Toward a major risk factor for atopic eczema: Meta-analysis of filaggrin polymorphism data. J Allergy Clin Immunol 2007; 120(6):1406–1412.
15. Walley AJ, Chavanas S, Moffatt MF, et al. Gene polymorphism in Netherton and common atopic disease. Nat Genet 2001; 29(2):175–178.
16. Vasilopoulos Y, Cork MJ, Murphy R, et al. Genetic association between an AACC insertion in the 3′UTR of the stratum corneum chymotryptic enzyme gene and atopic dermatitis. J Invest Dermatol 2004; 123(1):62–66.
17. Soderhall C, Marenholz I, Kerscher T, et al. Variants in a novel epidermal collagen gene (COL29A1) are associated with atopic dermatitis. PLoS Biol 2007; 5(9):e242.
18. Howell MD, Kim BE, Gao P, et al. Cytokine modulation of atopic dermatitis filaggrin skin expression. J Allergy Clin Immunol 2007; 120(1):150–155.
19. Kim BE, Leung DY, Boguniewicz M, et al. Loricrin and involucrin expression is downregulated by Th2 cytokines through STAT-6. Clin Immunol 2008; 126(3):332–337.
20. Howell MD, Fairchild HR, Kim BE, et al. Th2 Cytokines Act on S100/A11 to downregulate keratinocyte differentiation. J Invest Dermatol 2008; 128(9):2248–2258.
21. Wollenberg A, Zoch C, Wetzel S, et al. Predisposing factors and clinical features of eczema herpeticum: A retrospective analysis of 100 cases. J Am Acad Dermatol 2003; 49(2):198–205.
22. Osawa K, Etoh T, Ariyoshi N, et al. Relationship between Kaposi's varicelliform eruption in Japanese patients with atopic dermatitis treated with tacrolimus ointment and genetic polymorphisms in the IL-18 gene promoter region. J Dermatol 2007; 34(8):531–536.
23. Bardan A, Nizet V, Gallo RL. Antimicrobial peptides and the skin. Expert Opin Biol Ther 2004; 4(4):543–549.
24. Goodyear HM, Davies JA, McLeish P, et al. Growth of herpes simplex type 1 on skin explants of atopic eczema. Clin Exp Dermatol 1996; 21(3):185–189.
25. Howell MD, Boguniewicz M, Pastore S, et al. Mechanism of HBD-3 deficiency in atopic dermatitis. Clin Immunol 2006; 121(3):332–338.
26. Howell MD. The role of human beta defensins and cathelicidins in atopic dermatitis. Curr Opin Allergy Clin Immunol 2007; 7(5):413–417.
27. Howell MD, Wollenberg A, Gallo RL, et al. Cathelicidin deficiency predisposes to eczema herpeticum. J Allergy Clin Immunol 2006; 117(4):836–841.
28. Howell MD, Jones JF, Kisich KO, et al. Selective killing of vaccinia virus by LL-37: Implications for eczema vaccinatum. J Immunol 2004; 172(3):1763–1767.
29. Howell MD, Novak N, Bieber T, et al. Interleukin-10 downregulates anti-microbial peptide expression in atopic dermatitis. J Invest Dermatol 2005; 125(4):738–745.
30. Howell MD, Streib JE, Leung DY. Antiviral activity of human beta-defensin 3 against vaccinia virus. J Allergy Clin Immunol 2007; 119(4):1022–1025.
31. Howell MD, Gallo RL, Boguniewicz M, et al. Cytokine milieu of atopic dermatitis skin subverts the innate immune response to vaccinia virus. Immunity 2006; 24(3):341–348.
32. Wollenberg A, Zoch C, Wetzel S, et al. Predisposing factors and clinical features of eczema herpeticum: A retrospective analysis of 100 cases. J Am Acad Dermatol 2003; 49(2):198–205.
33. Scott JE, ElKhal A, Freyschmidt EJ, et al. Impaired immune response to vaccinia virus inoculated at the site of cutaneous allergic inflammation. J Allergy Clin Immunol 2007; 120(6):1382–1388.

34. Wollenberg A, Wagner M, Gunther S, et al. Plasmacytoid dendritic cells: A new cutaneous dendritic cell subset with distinct role in inflammatory skin diseases. J Invest Dermatol 2002; 119(5):1096–1102.
35. Rissoan MC, Soumelis V, Kadowaki N, et al. Reciprocal control of T helper cell and dendritic cell differentiation. Science 1999; 283(5405):1183–1186.
36. Kabashima K, Sugita K, Tokura Y. Increment of circulating plasmacytoid dendritic cells in a patient with Kaposi's varicelliform eruption. J Eur Acad Dermatol Venereol 2008; 22(2):239–241.
37. Hochrein H, Schlatter B, O'Keeffe M, et al. Herpes simplex virus type-1 induces IFN-alpha production via Toll-like receptor 9-dependent and -independent pathways. Proc Natl Acad Sci U S A 2004; 101(31):11416–11421.
38. Novak N, Allam JP, Hagemann T, et al. Characterization of FcepsilonRI-bearing CD123 blood dendritic cell antigen-2 plasmacytoid dendritic cells in atopic dermatitis. J Allergy Clin Immunol 2004; 114(2):364–370.
39. Schroeder JT, Bieneman AP, Xiao H, et al. TLR9- and FcepsilonRI-mediated responses oppose one another in plasmacytoid dendritic cells by down-regulating receptor expression. J Immunol 2005; 175(9):5724–5731.
40. Goodyear HM, McLeish P, Randall S, et al. Immunological studies of herpes simplex virus infection in children with atopic eczema. Br J Dermatol 1996; 134(1):85–93.
41. Kim BE, Leung DY, Streib JE, et al. Macrophage inflammatory protein 3 alpha deficiency in atopic dermatitis skin and role in innate immune response to vaccinia virus. J Allergy Clin Immunol 2007; 119(2):457–463.

17

Psychoimmunology and Evaluation of Therapeutic Approaches

Uwe Gieler, Volker Niemeier, and Burkhard Brosig
Department of Psychosomatic Medicine, Justus Liebig University Giessen, Giessen, Germany

Bruce G. Bender
National Jewish Health, Denver, Colorado, U.S.A.

HISTORY

Awareness of the psychologic correlates of atopic dermatitis is longstanding. Emerging as early as 1850 with the statement that "the primary cause [of eczema] is disorders of the nervous system, like emotions, especially of a depressive nature," (1) reference to a psychosomatic relationship between psychologic stress and atopic dermatitis were increasingly frequent in the second half of the 19th century. Hiller (2) expressed the conviction that "nervous excitement may lead to urticaria, shock is known as a cause of eczema, and fear turns the hair white." At that time, nothing was known of parallel studies or of the detailed relationships within the nervous system, the function of which was elucidated only after development of embryology and the horrible revelations presented on brain damage related to injuries during the First World War. Late in the 19th century, Brocq and Jacquet (3) coined the term "neurodermatitis," which they considered to be weakness of the nerves and which has remained unchanged, especially among patients, to the present day.

STRESS AND ATOPIC DERMATITIS

Psychologic factors seem to be important in atopic dermatitis as significant modulators of the disease. Stress increases atopic dermatitis symptoms depending on the severity of stress.

In a very large population of 1457 patients questioned after the Japanese earthquake in Hanshin in 1995, Kodama et al. (4) showed that 38% of patients with atopic dermatitis in the most severely hit region and 34% in a moderately hit region reported exacerbation, compared to only 7% in a control group without earthquake stress. However, 9% and 5% in the respective earthquake regions and only 1% in the control region reported a marked improvement in atopic dermatitis. In a multiple regression analysis, subjective stress was the best indicator predicting exacerbation compared to genetic and treatment-related factors. The results of this study show that stress apparently has an immunologic effect, which can, though to a slighter extent, exert an opposite inflammatory effect.

Similar influencing factors had already been described by Brown and Bettley (5). In a prospective controlled study of children with asthma, it could also be demonstrated that psychosocial stress had the greatest influence in eliciting an asthma attack (6).

The relationship between stress and atopic dermatitis is underlined by studies showing that daily hassles could be associated with symptom severity. Using a diary technique for severity and emotional state, King and Wilson (7) demonstrated a significant positive relationship between interpersonal stress on a given day and skin condition 24 hours later. This study as well as further time-series analyses (8,9) indicated the influence of daily hassles on the exacerbation of atopic dermatitis.

NEUROANATOMY

Atopy-relevant effector cells, such as mast cells and Langerhans cells, form a close anatomical relationship with nerve fibers staining positive for a number of neuroactive substances, for instance substance P, vasoactive peptide, or nerve growth factor (NGF) (10). Regarding this close anatomical relationship of nerve terminals and effector cells in atopic dermatitis, it seems possible that stress-induced stimulation of nerve fibers induces secretion of neuroactive substances. There are a growing number of studies indicating that atopic dermatitis patients show disturbances in the cyclic adenosine monophosphate (cAMP) system, suggesting an altered catecholamine responsiveness. This concept was introduced by Szentivany (11), who reported reduced responsiveness of β-adrenergic receptors in atopic dermatitis patients, and has been confirmed by Niemeier et al. (12).

PSYCHONEUROENDOCRINOLOGY

Functional changes in the hypothalamus–pituitary–adrenal cortex axis are under discussion (13,14). Buske-Kirschbaum et al. (15) compiled an overview of the psychobiologic aspects of neurodermatitis and confirmed by means of hypotheses the various endocrine, immunologic, and psychophysiologic influences on atopic dermatitis.

Pathophysiologic studies follow the behavioral approach and address the pathophysiologic reactibility of neurodermatitis patients and conditioning as a means of influence. The following are among the parameters used: heart rate, electrical skin resistance, electromyographic activity, and skin temperature under defined stress situations. In addition, psychometric data such as scores for anxiety and hostility and depressivity are measured.

Jordan and Whitlock (16,17) compared neurodermatitis patients with a control group of neurologic and internal medicine patients with no atopic-type diseases either themselves or in any family member. In the first phase, psychometric data (Cattel Personality Inventory, Esenck Personality Inventory, Buss-Durkee Hostility Inventory, Depression and Anxiety Scales of the Minnesota Multiphasic Personality Inventory) were recorded, and in the second phase, the authors examined the scratching reaction and changes in skin resistance in eliciting by both an unconditioned stimulus (itching via electrodes) and a conditioned stimulus (bell tone). The neurodermatitis patients had significantly higher values in the scales Neuroticism (EPI), Anxiety (MMPI), and Suppressed Hostility (BDHI). No correlation could be demonstrated between emotional alteration (elevated scores for Neuroticism, Anxiety, Hostility) and vasomotor reactivity in the sense of Eysenecks "autonomic reactivity."

A study by Faulstich et al. (18) compared 10 neurodermatitis patients with a conception of autonomic reactivity to a control group with regard to measured values of heart rate, electromyography, peripheral vasomotor response, skin temperature, and skin resistance. The patients were subjected to emotional (intelligence test) and physical stress. The neurodermatitis patients reacted remarkably only with elevation of heart rate and of muscle tone under provocation by placing the hand in ice water ("cold-pressor test"). The neurodermatitis subjects attained significantly high values in the scores for anxiety in the Symptom Checklist 90 (SCL-90R). However, no other connection to pathophysiologic data could be made.

In a similar study, Münzel and Schandry (19) compared 18 atopic dermatitis patients with a healthy-skin control group. In this study, heart rate, skin resistance, axial skin temperature, and pulse volume amplitude were also measured under emotional stress in the form of mental arithmetic and social (expressing an opinion on a topic in front of a group). The patients reported their feelings with respect to tension, annoyance, and restlessness using constant scales (0–100) during the breaks.

All physiologic parameters of the neurodermatitis patients, as well as the feeling of tension, were significantly higher than in the control group. The skin temperature also increased in the neurodermatitis patients and decreased in the control group. The authors divided the neurodermatitis patient group with respect to subjective malaise due to itching; the values of the subgroup of patients suffering greatly from itching were responsible for the statistical increase in skin temperature in the entire group. The assumption was that there is a relationship between emotional stress and the course of the disease, especially in patients with sustained high levels of activation.

By contrast, Köhler and Weber (20) found absolutely no evidence of a general hyperreactivity in relation to the skin system of neurodermatitis patients in a study of similar design.

These results demonstrate that a general hyperreactivity in neurodermatitis patients can apparently not be assumed.

The influence of serious events in life and of stressors of various degrees on the immune system is known. The autonomic nervous system acts as the connector between feelings and subsequent somatic response. Lymph nodes contain sympathic afferents; adrenergic and cholinergic fibers are found in the thymus, the lymphocytes also have adrenergic and cholinergic receptors (21).

In a study of 75 students in the phase preceding final examinations, Kiecolt-Glaser et al. (22) found considerably reduced activity of the natural killer (NK) cells. These cells play a special role in carcinogenesis and virus defense. The study group was subdivided on the basis of psychometric tests (Brief Symptom Inventory, Symptom Checklist 90, Social Readjustment Rating Scale, UCLA Loneliness Scale), which revealed a correlation between loneliness and feeling of distress due to stressors and a reduced NK cell activity. Moreover, the tested students had an elevated serum IgA level. In additional studies with similar conditions and populations (23), reduced interferon levels were found, as was a correlation between the extent of relaxation exercises and the number of T-helper cells. Moreover, Kiecolt-Glaser et al. (22) found evidence of influence by stressors in DNA repair of lymphocytes.

Baker (21) emphasizes that the altered reactivity of defense cells is decisive, rather than the fluctuations in their counts. He also points out the significantly higher incidence of neurodermatitis in depressive patients compared to schizophrenic patients. A large number of studies have demonstrated a reduced T-cell count as well as an increase in eosinophils, B lymphocytes, and serum IgE in neurodermatitis patients (24). Eosinophils and IgE correlate with the degree of skin eruptions in eczema (25). Stone et al. (26) registered a reduction in the IgE levels when the eczema abated in half of the neurodermatitis patients they examined. Wüthrich (27) ascribed a prognostic value to the eosinophil count in eczema therapy.

Kupfer (9) examined the interaction between the severity of skin symptoms, the expression of individual emotions, and the excretion of salivary cortisol and salivary IgA. Aggression, depression, and anxiety were found to be emotions particularly related to skin symptoms.

McGeady and Buckley (25) found a limited cellular defense. Buske-Kirschbaum et al. (14) examined neurodermatitis patients by applying intracutan-*Candida-Candida albi-cans* antigen and streptokinase-streptodornase. A pronounced energy was found, which correlated with the severity of the eczema. It is a fact that neurodermatitis patients more frequently suffer sometimes generalized viral infections (herpes-, coxsackie-, and other viruses) and bacterial superinfections (27,28).

Ring (88) has delineated the central immunoetiologic role of vasoactive mediators such as histamine and ECF-A (eosinophil-chemotactic factor of anaphylaxis) in neurodermatitis patients. He cites the following factors as the decisive influence of this mediator liberation: Increased readiness of the basophiles to excrete histamines, so-called "leaky" mast cells, a β2-adrenergic control defect among other things at the level of the intracellular cAMP system, increased sensitivity to α-adrenergic and cholinergic stimuli demonstrated in vivo and in vitro, and elevated IgE levels. The histamine effect, besides its effect on the capillary–bronchial system, lies in a limitation of T-suppressor activity with consecutive IgE elevation. Increased sensitivity to histamine was found in nearly all atopics at the T-cell level.

STUDIES OF ANXIETY, HOSTILITY, AND DEPRESSION

Developments in research recognize atopic dermatitis as a psychosomatic illness (29–31). Psychosomatic causes are considered important eliciting factors. Numerous studies on the personality of the neurodermatitis patient have shown, however, that there is no "specific neurodermaitis personality." According to studies by Pürschel (32) up to 40% of patients themselves cite emotional factors as eliciting neurodermatitis, while Griesemer and Nadelsohn (33) report up to 70%.

Anxiety was studied by Jordan and Whitlock (17) as one partial aspect of the etiologic discussion in neurodermatitis patients. The results showed elevated anxiety values among neurodermatitis patients compared to a control group with other types of disease; the MMPI additional scale was used to measure anxiety. Garrie et al. (34) arrived at similar results in their studies. Faulstich et al. (18) performed a pathophysiologic study in which elevated anxiety could be demonstrated in neurodermatitis patients.

In a study by Gieler et al. (35) using the HESTIBAR test procedure, the neurodermatitis patients also recorded considerably elevated anxiety values. In this study, cluster analysis showed subgroups, some of which presented extremely high anxiety values and others in which values were in the normal range. It can be assumed that the elevated anxiety values of neurodermatitis patients are not a component of a "neurodermatitis personality," but that they do influence the course of the disease and the patient's coping with the disease.

Suppressed hostility is frequently cited as one characteristic of the supposed "neurodermatitis personality." The study by Jordan and Whitlock (17) using the Buss-Durkee Hostility Inventory Test determined that neurodermatitis patients had elevated values with respect to felt but not outwardly expressed hostility compared to the control group. However, no differences were measured with respect to openly expressed hostility. Other authors like Borelli (36), Cleveland and Fischer (17,37–41), also reported on studies using projective procedures in which elevated hostility parameters were measured.

Garrie et al. (34) found elevated neuroticism values in their emotionally remarkable subgroup of neurodermatitis patients, already mentioned above. Elevated values toward depressive moods were also remarkable in this group.

It appears as if personal aspects like suppressed hostility and anxiety, as well as depression, are frequently confirmed in neurodermatitis patients in these studies, but these aspects might also be interpreted as a consequence of the disease.

PSYCHOTHERAPY IN ATOPIC DERMATITIS

Suggested therapies in the literature refer mainly to behavioral therapeutic and in-depth psychologic forms of therapy. In addition, there are numerous suggestions for combined therapy (for example, with relaxation training, dermatologic training) (42). According to the in-depth psychology concept, psychotherapy can be performed with individual patients, with families, or even in groups. The treatment technique does not differ in these groups. The basis of psychoanalytic-psychotherapeutic treatment is the creation of a viable therapeutic relationship via acceptance. On this basis, latent conflicts can be made accessible and conscious during the course of treatment. Correspondingly arising inner resistance and defense processes can be made accessible in order to be dealt with and overcome. This usually results in stabilization of the emotional balance and improved coping with the actual disease episodes. Supportive interventions alternate with revelatory interventions.

In in-depth psychologic psychotherapy, special attention is paid to the affects (sadness, rage, etc.) and fantasies that arise during treatment. Making these affects and fantasies conscious should help the patient to obtain better insight into his own world and thus to attain altered coping ability in experiencing his disease.

An analytically oriented psychotherapeutic treatment may be indicated, especially in conjunction with chronic skin diseases, since stable and supportive family relationships appear to considerably improve the coping with disease in chronically ill patients.

BEHAVIORAL THERAPY

Treatment begins initially with behavior analysis, which records certain behaviors that are elicited by certain situations (stimulus constellations or specific stimuli) or promoted by certain situations (controlling stimuli, which precede the problem, and stimuli that follow as a consequence of expressed behavior). In this connection, it is also interesting to note the importance of the patient's person of reference, especially how this person reacts to the patient's problems. From a behavioral-therapeutic point of view, it is important that the patient see the causes of his disorder, that is, attribute them. At the end of the session, considerations are addressed concerning which therapeutic procedures could be applied. An important treatment procedure is thus based on rational development of new coping strategies in dealing with "stress situations," that is, the patient is taught to expand his behavioral repertoire (43). In behavioral therapy, behavior analysis always serves targeted therapeutic planning for the individual patient, whereby the controlling momentary stimulus conditions (operant, classical, conditional, and cognitive aspects) in the maintenance of a disease are isolated, which are then further documented in parallel to the individual phases in the course of treatment. Changes in the goal of therapy and the use of new treatment methods may occur during treatment. The active participation of the patient by means of so-called homework or documentation of strategies, which the patient uses or which are suggested by the therapist, is in any case part of treatment. Operant "conditioning" with application of so-called positive rewards plays an important role in the differentiated psychotherapy program of the behavioral therapist. Operant reward models are more effective if certain aspects are taken into account:

1. Self-confidence training or social training seeks to attain improvement in the possibility of realizing one's own wishes and needs in face of the environment. This is made possible by role-playing, training, and social confrontations, taking nonverbal aspects of behavior into account.
2. In learning models in role-playing, the patient observes therapeutically desirable behaviors in other persons and the positive consequences that result from their behavior. Certain characteristics of these persons (sex, age, social attractiveness) may promote or limit this learning model.
3. Many behavior-therapeutic interventions are carried out in complex or chronic behavioral problems that do not immediately offer a chance to attain completely different (desired) behavior within a short time. Various therapeutic steps may lead ultimately to a desired therapy modification (shaping). Parts of behavioral patterns are analyzed and influenced, especially in individual steps. These steps are related to one another and potentiate the patient's willingness to change.
4. In biofeedback, the patient cognitively registers physiologic parameters, and support in changing these parameters is given a particular direction by means of light and sound signals. Additional techniques are counterconditioning (e.g., in overcoming anxiety), aversion techniques, operant deleting, and exposition therapy—especially in phobic states, confrontation with the situation that elicits the fear.

To complete the picture, the behavioral-therapeutic approach in itching should be mentioned (44). In a presentation of the dynamics of the scratch reaction, they reveal the unconscious aspect of this process. Diffuse distress, and not the visual or haptic perception of a scratch site, precedes the scratching reaction typical of neurodermatitis.

At the start of the scratching phase, the need to scratch increases, only to decrease rapidly again when pain and bleeding have begun. The curve of circadian scratching rate recorded on a large patient collective is a mirror image of the daily activity curve. This makes it apparent that wakefulness and nonwakefulness exert a control function and are one criterion of scratching.

The vicious circle of scratching begins when a frustrating, fear-eliciting stimulus (S) meets an organism (O) with a characteristic behavioral deficit (deficit in recognition, permissiveness, and dealing with one's own emotions). These patients tend, according to the authors' observations, to reject a psychologic interpretation of the scratching symptoms. The authors attribute this attitude to the fact that "the organ skin in our culture is the one which most readily permits expression of emotional distress, without being unmasked by the patient or his environment" (44). The tension reduction (C1) appears more spontaneously under reaction (R) in the form of scratching when S meets O than the negative consequences (C2) like pain and exacerbation of the skin condition.

The therapy concept of Böddecker and Böddecker (44) is based on positive reinforcement of not scratching, punishment preceding reward (tension reduction) (e.g., by protocolling before scratching), and withdrawal of reinforcement (e.g., armbands with alarm devices).

ANALYTICAL AND PSYCHODYNAMIC-ORIENTED SINGLE, FAMILY, AND GROUP THERAPY

At the center of the psychoanalytic treatment method is making the patient aware of unrecognized meanings in respect to his own life situation. This is made without behavioral instructions from the therapist (104) (45). The treatment techniques consist essentially of "elucidation," "confrontation," "interpretation," especially perception of "transfer" and "countertransfer." The individual terms are explained briefly below.

Elucidation proceeds via examination of experience and behavior patterns in dealing with others in the patient's personal environment. Important interaction and experience patterns are to be worked out in connection with the patient's internalized importance.

In confrontation, blocked and denied modes of behavior and experience and their effect on others are made clear, whereby the therapeutic situation is also made clear by using everyday situations.

Interpretations are intended to significantly reveal unrecognized relationships of the experience and behavioral patterns among others. Past experiences, such as in childhood, which are blocked and denied, are addressed.

The aspect of transfer and countertransfer plays a special role in analytically oriented psychotherapeutic treatment. It is based on the idea that working through emotions and relationship fantasies in connection with behavior represents a particular psychodynamic configuration and is understood as a mutual process of therapist and patient, or as a therapeutic process. Within the therapeutic framework, wishes for independence and the fear of consequences and reaching a compromise between wishes and fears are understood and their defense mechanisms with resultant modes of behavior dissipated. Psychotherapeutic treatment is considered successful when the patient is able to work out more satisfying possibilities in his personal life.

Analytic in-depth psychology-oriented psychotherapeutic group therapy enables a therapeutic relationship constellation in which patients have the possibility of experiencing and working out neuroticizing or pathologic relationships within the group, where a multiple transfer resource arises between the group leader and group participants, with the possibility of working out personal conflicts as well as conflicts with one another. Psychotherapeutic treatment procedures are relatively effective for neurodermatitis patients (46).

FAMILY ASPECTS

Some studies take special notice of the family situation of neurodermatitis patients. It appears that the family environment is co-responsible to a high degree for the course of the disease. Essentially, the studies concentrate on the mother–child relationship.

Gieler and Effendy (47) reported on disrupted communication between infants and their environment, elicited by neurodermititis skin disease. In their view, no delineated body image can crystallize because of the early disruption of communication, which leads to impairment in the child's overall emotional development with a tendency to withdrawal to the organ skin. Adult atopic dermatitis patients engaged in a problem discussion with their mothers or with their partners showed less acceptance, less self-disclosure, and more justification than a nonatopic control group (48).

Rechenberger (1993) also sees an altered body image of patients with neurodermatitis as essential. The neurodermatitis patient is incapable of experiencing his skin as a protective, enveloping shell.

Pürschel (32) is of the opinion that a child with skin disease experiences marked limitations in respect to his relationship to his environment, which results in a persistent impairment of contact to that environment.

It was remarkable in the study by Ring et al. (49) that children with neurodermatitis displayed more aggression toward their parents and reported more separation events in their lives to that point. The mothers in these studies were also seen to be rather cool and to show little emotion; they were sparing in their praise of their children, which they limited essentially to performance. Bräutigam et al. (50) are of the opinion that mothers of neurodermitic children feel stressed by the outward appearance of the child with skin disease and from the experience that the child apparently desire physical contact, which they are unable to accept. It is assumed that the distancing posture of the mothers is elicited mostly by the child's disease. By contrast, Pürschel (32) points out that parents react with overprotection toward their skin-diseased child and thus inhibit the child's development.

Generally, the particular stress for the child with neurodermatitis, as well as for the other family members in early-onset and chronic course of the disease, appears to give the skin a special value as an "organ of limitation" in these families and complicated neuroticizing interactions may result.

AFFECTIVE AREA AND NEUROTIC SYMPTOMS

According to the study by Kuypers (51), psychosocial factors coupled with emotional conflicts have a marked influence on the onset or exacerbation of neurodermatitis. The tensions caused by certain emotional states and their resolution are accompanied in many cases by a reduction in skin symptoms. The importance of emotions and the experience of related conflicts are variously experienced by neurodermatitis patients. Decisive for elicitation of skin reactions is probably not the conflict itself, but rather the emotional quality ascribed to the conflict.

In a study with 448 neurodermatitis patients, Pürschel (32) found that 57.5% had problems in private areas, with women reporting difficulties more often (76.1%) than men (29%). Stress situations were viewed as a central theme with regard to onset of neurodermatitis episodes. Of the 448 patients, 187 (41%) ascribed the exacerbation to problems at work and especially in interpersonal relationships. The skin reactions in the sense of neurodermatitis were also reported in connection with examinations, engagements, and weddings. Apparently, general stress situations are decisive; according to Pürschel (32), the individual tolerance limits are lower than that among healthy individuals. Rechardt (52) found that feelings of dependence and hopelessness occurred more often during episodes of the disease but did not occur in an episode-free interval nine years later. He attributed the emotional disturbances to stress caused by the skin disease. Likewise, according to Bosse (53), neurodermatitis episodes occur in connection with actual conflict situations. These conflict situations are age-related threshold situations, which may lead to a subsequent exacerbation of the skin condition. In children, he typically observed the absence or lack of one or both parents, tensions in the parents' marriage or within the family, job situations, change of schools, move, periods of looking for a job, looking for a partner, or examinations. In adults, weddings, interpersonal problems, death, or temporary emotional or physical overload led to recurrent exacerbation of the skin condition.

STRESS IN CONNECTION WITH LIFE EVENTS

King and Wilson (7) examined 50 neurodermatitis patients over a period of 14 days. In a subsequent meta-analysis, the calculated correlation coefficients revealed that the skin condition cross-correlated synchronously with values for anxiety/tension, interpersonal stress, depression, frustration, feelings of aggression, expressed aggression, and suppressed aggression (in that order). The authors showed that stress on the previous day correlated with the actual skin condition, and the actual skin condition led to increased stress and elevated depression values on the following day.

Hospitalized neurodermatitis patients were examined in a pilot study by Hünecke et al. (54). An attempt was made to discover certain events that elicited the episodes. It was found that demonstrable psychosocial events (weekends, visits, discharge) were coupled significantly frequently with disease exacerbation. Schubert (55) was also able to demonstrate a number of cross-correlations between stress events and disease outbreak, as well as between emotional well-being and skin symptoms in a timed series study of six neurodermatitis patients. Conversely, it was not possible to predict the skin condition on the subsequent day from the occurrence of stress events or any particular mood.

SLEEP DISTURBANCE AND DAYTIME FUNCTIONING

Adults (56) and children (57) with atopic dermatitis are more restless in their sleep, awaken more often, spend less minutes in sleep, and report more daytime fatigue than those without atopic dermatitis. Sleep disruption in turn can bring significant daytime consequences. Poor sleep has a well-documented deleterious effect on mood, cognition, and motor performance (58). Further, individuals deprived of sufficient sleep are at markedly increased risk of causing a motor-vehicle accident. Crashes or near-crashes are increased among truck drivers (59), airline pilots (60), shift workers (61), and medical residents (62) all of whom are exposed to irregular and reduced sleep. Although sleep science has long recognized the dramatic changes in human performance that accompany multiple nights of total sleep deprivation (63), more recent research has provided insight into the consequences of partial sleep deprivation, or the "poor night's sleep" often accompanying not only atopic and respiratory diseases but also commonly associated with the stress and demands of daily life. Even as little as four nights of partial sleep restriction resulting in less than seven hours of sleep causes measurable increases in daytime sleepiness and impaired cognitive performance (64,65). In a comprehensive study of sleep deprivation, two weeks of sleep restricted to four hours created deficits in attention and memory equivalent to two nights of total sleep deprivation (66). A systematic review of intermittent hypoxia in children concluded that even at mild levels of desaturation, children with sleep-disordered breathing demonstrate lower levels of performance on tests of attention and verbal intelligence (67).

The causes of poor sleep in patients with atopic dermatitis may not be as obvious as they first appear. The discomforts experienced by patients with skin diseases are recognized and their implications for sleep seem more than evident. Yet the origins of disordered sleep in these patients may also be traced to altered inflammatory processes. Seventy-two percent of patients with rheumatologic diseases have sleep disturbances (68). Studies of individuals with diseases causing systemic inflammation (69) and healthy volunteers in sleep deprivation studies (70,71) reveal that a variety of cytokines are implicated in sleep regulation. For example, IL-4 and IL-1β, both of which are elevated in allergic patients, are associated with increased latency to rapid eye movement sleep and lower overall quality of sleep (72). The causal pathway may be that cytokine changes resulting from these diseases contribute to sleep changes by affecting the role of these substances in the brain neurochemistry of sleep regulation. Equally plausible is the possibility that sleep disturbance resulting from the discomfort of allergic rhinitis or atopic dermatitis promotes further changes in cytokines, hormones, or other neuropeptides, which in turn influence the course of the disease. A growing body of electrophysiologic, biochemical, and genetic evidence indicates that IL-1 and TNF-α play a role in supporting sleep (73,74). When injected into animals peripherally, or microinjected directly into the brain, IL-1 and TNF-α increase nonrapid eye movement (NREM) sleep, while suppressing rapid eye movement (REM) sleep (75–77). Daytime sleepiness is decreased in sleep apnea patients given intravenous TNF-α receptor antagonist (78). In healthy volunteers, injection of IL-1 or TNF-α alters REM sleep (73). Patients successfully treated for sleep apnea demonstrated improved sleep and a reduction in TNF-α and IL-6. Cytokine changes after surgical treatment of obstructive sleep apnea syndrome (79).

Regardless of the cause, disturbed sleep can have many negative consequences, including impaired motor and cognitive function, and changes in mood, sleep, and quality of life (80,81).

Given the negative effects of disturbed sleep for patients with AD, providing an effective therapy for sleep disturbances and nocturnal scratching is important, although not always addressed. A comprehensive approach to the management of atopic dermatitis should evaluate triggers and response to treatment, address-confounding factors including sleep disruption, and educate patients and caregivers (82). Disease, inflammation, and sleep are thus linked in a complex set of relationships. The possibilities are intriguing and the continuing task of teasing apart the causal sequences promises important discoveries. Treatments for asthma, allergic rhinitis, and atopic dermatitis should slow or stop the interaction between disease and sleep while improving both. For example, a group of children with atopic dermatitis treated with pimecrolimus cream demonstrated improvement in their skin that in turn was correlated with the improvement in sleep (83). As Sutherland notes, understanding the circadian cycles of inflammation and symptoms may direct choice and timing of specific treatments. In the case of asthma, this includes dosing strategies to optimize therapeutic effects during periods of nocturnal worsening. The role of sleep-promoting medications for these groups of patients is unclear and should be approached cautiously. In the case of atopic dermatitis, the possibility of treating sleep with such medications as a way to interrupt the itch–scratch–itch cycle is a strategy that warrants further exploration.

STATUS OF RESEARCH INTO THERAPEUTIC EFFECTIVENESS
Research into the effectiveness of psychotherapy in skin diseases, especially neurodermatitis, is still largely in the beginning phase. To date, differential aspects in

adult neurodermatitis patients have only limited value with respect to prognostically relevant indication criteria, since the studies thus far refer usually to individual cases or very small numbers of patients. In general, clinical dermatology does not appear to have paid sufficient attention to psychologic factors and psychotherapeutic possibilities.

A high level of motivation for therapy is considered prognostically positive (55), while early onset of disease and other additional atopical diseases are viewed as prognostically unfavorable (84).

Another study was performed at the request of the Institute for Social Medicine Epidemiology and Health Systems Research (ISEG Study) to evaluate therapeutic measures in neurodermatitis (46). In cooperation with the Gmünder Ersatzkasse health insurance group, it could be demonstrated that, among other forms of therapy, psychotherapy was rated by the patients as having the most positive long-term effect.

In a meta-analysis (85), various psychotherapeutic procedures were examined with respect to skin condition and subjective well-being. It was found that the psychotherapeutic procedures were clearly more effective than somatic-medical standard measures. The neurodermatitis personality postulated in this study could not be confirmed, but the characteristics of anxiety, depression, and neuroticism were significantly high. A total of 865 subjects were examined: 553 adult neurodermatitis patients and 129 children. The effects of various combined psychotherapeutic interventions were examined. The skin symptoms improved significantly with all measures in the patients receiving psychotherapy. Their medication consumption and scratching frequency were also reduced.

Kaschel (86) studied various methods and developed a training program, especially for neurodermatitis patients, taking psychotherapeutic aspects into account. Positive affects were also described by Klein (87), Walsh and Kierland (88), Williams (89), and Thomä (104) (45). Since skin diseases may be caused, according to psychoanalytic theory, by disruptions in early childhood development, other psychologic therapy forms, like gestalt therapy or client-centered conversation (defined by Rogers) may be effective. However, no results with respect to neurodermatitis have yet been published.

Neurodermatitis has considerable influence on a patient's quality of life. Satisfaction with life is of central importance in experiencing and coping with disease (90). A number of stresses with corresponding psychosocial consequences make high demands on coping resources (91). It can therefore be assumed that various aspects of the disease will elicit various coping reactions, and they, in turn, may differ from the coping reactions in other stress situations (92). Chronic skin diseases like neurodermatitis may lead to serious limitations in emotional well-being and are frequently coupled with social problems. It can be demonstrated that these stressing effects are underestimated in relation to other chronic diseases. Dermatologic diseases like neurodermatitis are particularly likely to be of considerable detriment to self-image and social relationships, since the symptoms are so visible. It happens frequently that persons with skin diseases experience negative social reactions from other persons, starting with ambivalent reserve to distancing and on to open rejection (93). Occasionally, fear of contagion makes social contact more difficult (94). Expectation of rejection and avoidance, for example, in public, leads to a consistent coping strategy of avoidance, which in turn leads to generalization and exacerbation of the symptoms (95).

Itching is one skin symptom of neurodermitis. The intensive need to scratch is a serious limitation of well-being. Because itching can be elicited by external and internal stimuli, like heat, skin dryness, or simply imagining such sensations (96), it is a particularly stressful symptom. Likewise, the itching threshold can be lowered by "stress" (97,98). The scratching impulse to itching stimuli is a reflex that can be inhibited spinal by cortical structures (96). Scratching irritates the pain receptors. For a time, this reduces the sensation of itching, accompanied by a feeling of relief. With a slight delay, the itching threshold is reduced, which brings increased sensation of itching and in turn increased scratching. When the skin is finally bleeding, it hardly itches (99). Pain takes precedence over itching. In this constantly widening vicious circle, new skin damage arises, neurodermatitis becomes chronic with the known symptoms of thickening of the afflicted epidermis and coarsening of the skin structures. It was demonstrated (17) that even slight diffuse tensions or malaise can elicit scratching. According to Bosse and Hünecke (30), helplessness in the face of this vicious circle and guilt feelings of having failed in self-control give rise to additional emotional stress for the patients, which in turn can maintain the itching–scratching cycle. The ever-recurrent sequence of recurrences and freedom from episodes are also often accompanied by feelings of helplessness, of being thrown to the wolves, and by anxious-depressive moods (100). The stress of constant itching is also frequently underestimated. Sleep deficits and reduced ability to concentrate during episodes of the disease are frequent symptoms (101).

Due to disease-related habits like constant scratching or the experienced limitation of attractiveness, the negative effects on communication increase (48). This, in turn, leads to additional unsolved problems in social relationships. The resultant increase in tension and aggression is expressed by more scratching and contributes to further exacerbation of the disease.

MEASURES TO INFLUENCE THE ITCHING–SCRATCHING CYCLE

Reduction of Physiologic Stress Reactions

There is a wealth of experience concerning the reduction of the physiologic excitation level. The following relaxation methods are practiced: autogenic training (AT), EMG-feedback training, cue-controlled relaxation, and the progressive muscle relaxation according to Jacobson.

Horne et al. (102), Kaschel et al. (103), and Niebel (104) were successful in combination therapies with progressive muscle relaxation. The balancing of vegetative and immunologic dysfunction as well as improved body perception and an active conviction concerning physical reactions (105), are considered as effective factors in muscle relaxation and autogenic training.

The technique of so-called cue-controlled relaxation, that is, the flexible deployment of relaxation techniques following an exciting cue (e.g., scratching impulse), has been proven successful by Horne et al. (86,102,104). Another effective method for the reduction of stress, EMG-feedback training, was demonstrated in eight patients (106). The extent to which the ability to relax led to an improvement of her skin state (over 30 months) is, however, unclear, for an improved ability to relax could not be proven (107).

In an EMG-biofeedback study with progressive muscle relaxation, McMenamy et al. (108) were able to achieve a complete remission of symptoms, which persisted in three patients during a two-year follow-up. Unfortunately, this study, like many others, had no control group without therapy (placebo effect).

Kämmerer (109) and Cole et al. (110) employed AT in combination with other behavioral therapies, for example, self-observation, self-control following a scratching impulse, and the alteration of stress-evoking basic convictions. Following therapy a significantly improved skin condition was diagnosed. In the study by Cole et al. (110), the problem of the control group was solved by using the patients during the three-month period before the begin of the therapy as "controls." Unfortunately, the follow-up period amounted to only one month. But even in this study (as in many other studies), the problem remains that AT was employed only in combination with other behavioral therapies. Therefore, it is not clear which therapy was responsible for the positive results. In a prospective randomized study of 125 atopic eczema patients treated with different therapies, Stangier and Gieler (111) showed that AT was unexpectedly effective. Besides the therapy studies (unfortunately executed in combination) investigations with other aims showed positive effects of AT on skin reaction. Through AT the extent of skin reactions to standardized allergy testing could be reduced (112). Ely and Henry (113) found that inflammatory reactions of the skin following allergen contact rose if anxiety and stress were artificially produced by experimental conditions. According to Kämmerer (109) AT can lead to a reduction of affective tension provoking itch and to an improved perception of one's body. In addition, AT can contribute to an alteration of the perception of itching and to a lowering of the elevated psychophysiologic excitation level. The effects of suggestive procedures like hypnosis depend on previous experience, expectations, and, above all, on the inclination of the person to be hypnotized; of great importance is imaginative capability.

For the alteration of the itching perception there are several approaches: Schubert (114) transformed some suggestion techniques of hypnosis studies into an imagination training, and Luthe and Schultz (115) used imagination techniques (imagination of coolness) [see also Refs. (102,107)]. Suggestive techniques like hypnotherapy were used successfully in some studies (116–119). Hajek et al. (120) reported long-lasting positive effects in the sense of raising of the itching threshold. These results suggest that imaginative methods can be effective because of the relationship between perceptions, (auto-)suggestive reaction expectations, and physiologic skin functions in skin diseases.

Strategies for Scratching Avoidance

Bar and Kuypers (121) reported their work with children whose scratching behavior was simply ignored, while abstaining from scratching was rewarded. During the 18-month follow-up, the children remained symptom-free. The technique, based on a better perception of an automated procedure and the learning of alternative behavior incompatible with scratching (pinching, muscle tension), has proved a success (122,123).

Melin and coworkers (122) and Noren and Melin (124) compared the effect of behavior-oriented and medical treatment with that of medical treatment (corticosteroids) alone. The interventions carried out with control groups, but unfortunately without long-time follow-up, included several habit-reversal techniques. Following the early perception of the scratch impulse and its accompanying conditions, the patients reacted with two kinds of behavior incompatible with scratching. The marked reduction of scratching and the improvement of symptoms correlated highly, leading to the conclusion that these were the results of scratching-avoidance strategies.

Rosenbaum and Ayllon (123) were able to obtain long-term success (six months follow-up) with such habit-reversal techniques in four patients. Scratching, eliciting risk situations, and consequences were described in detail by the patients, a signal was installed for the interruption of the time course, then an alternative behavior, for example, pinching, was learned, and this course sequence practiced repeatedly.

Niebel (104,125) also applied training with specific scratch-control and stress-control techniques (habit-reversal, "scratching-blocks" replacing skin). Similar to the comparison group, which was more directed to coping with stress, a reduction of the scratching frequency and severity of symptoms was observed during the six-month follow-up ($n = 15$). However, there were no significant differences between the groups, which is not surprising given the minimal therapeutic differences between the groups.

METHODS TO REDUCE NEGATIVE EFFECTS ON SOCIAL RELATIONSHIPS BY ATOPIC ECZEMA PREVENTION PROGRAMS

Development of behavioral competence for improved coping with stress and improved coping with the illness-specific mental stress have received little attention in studies so far. Training for attaining social competence with the aim of improved coping with situations stressing atopic eczema patients was practiced successfully by Kaschel et al. (103) and Niebel (104,125) in combination with relaxation exercises.

Schubert et al. (55) found significant differences when comparing a group with unspecific discussion therapy and a behavioral therapy group (reduction of scratching, stress-coping techniques). In five case studies, Kaschel et al. (103) noted essentially short-term success concerning the reduction of scratching and medication. Great individual differences were pointed out.

The attempt to improve the control over the disease (self-therapeutic competence) by acquiring knowledge in the framework of dermatologic teaching has been neglected in the studies published. However, the various psychotherapeutic approaches have obviously stood the test.

STATUS OF EMPIRICAL RESEARCH WITH ATOPIC ECZEMA PREVENTION PROGRAMS

The effect of different combined psychotherapeutic interventions was investigated in 12 studies (55,104,106,110,117,120,122,125–129). Melin et al. (122) and Cole et al. (110) studied the effects of medical treatment on skin symptoms. Melin et al. (122) compared a hydrocortisone therapy alone with concomitant self-control strategies for the reduction of scratching, and Cole et al. (110) investigated different topical applications including systemic steroids in comparison to a combined psychotherapy. The skin symptoms improved following all the methods, but significantly more so in patients with psychotherapy. The use of drugs decreased and systemic steroids were no longer used, even at one-month follow-up (122). The paper of Cole et al. (110) had no follow-up.

In four methodically well-controlled studies (55,104,125,126), the effects of different forms of therapy were compared. Dermatologic symptoms and scratching frequency were reduced by all the evaluated therapies studies (55,104,125,126) better by combined behavior therapy and scratching control techniques (19,130) and in tendency better by behavior therapy compared with dermatologic education and school medical therapy (126). No significant differences were obtained in one study (55). In a further study, the scratching frequency declined in one group, while another group yielded better results with regard to itching, skin symptoms, and scratching frequency; in the first group, the psychologic variables "depressions," "fear of failure," "restrictions through atopic eczema," and "lack of self-assurance and attractiveness" were reduced; dermatologic state and itching improved only in individual cases (104,125).

In a subsequent study (125), the psychologic variables improved, especially following combined behavioral therapy and least in the control group. The fear tendency was most effectively reduced in the group with relaxation training and the combined behavior therapy group (126). The variable "anxiety" was in one study improved by dermatologic teaching and combination therapy, but not significantly. The follow-up after 6 and 12 months showed that psychotherapeutical interventions had more positive long-term effects on the course of the disease. The skin improved further following all psychologic interventions (126). Eleven out of 15 patients in the study of Niebel (125) stopped using cortisone, and the skin remained improved in all groups and the positive effects of the behavior therapy persisted in contrast to those of the dermatologic standard therapy (55). The combination of behavioral therapy and education (126) and the combined behavior therapy (125) yielded marginally better results than the other forms of psychotherapy.

There are also studies concerning the effectivity of therapies in children with atopic eczema or their parents. In one study with children (129), a complex dermatologic therapy in a rehabilitation clinic was compared with an additional behavior therapy of seven hours per week. At the end of the treatment the skin was similarly improved in both atopic eczema groups. Broberg et al. (131), Allen and Harris (132), Köhnlein et al. (133), and Gieler et al. demonstrated that parent education is effective.

In two recent controlled studies, it was shown that educational measures were superior to routine therapy. Niebel (130) observed similar effects in two groups, one of which underwent direct training devised to change behavior, while the other was schooled by video tapes. In a randomized study with 204 families, Kehrt et al. (134) showed that the quality of life of the mothers had improved significantly in the intervention groups compared to the control group.

REFERENCES

1. Wilson E. Diseases of the Skin. London, UK: Churchill, 1867.
2. Hiller T. Handbook of Skin Disease. London, UK: Walton & Maberly, 1865.
3. Brocq L, Jackquet L. Notes pour servir a l'histoire des neurodermatitis. Ann Dermatol Venerol 1891; 97:193–195.
4. Kodama A, Horikawa T, Suzuki T, et al. Effects of stress on atopic dermatitis: Investigations in patients after the great Hanshin earthquake. J Allergy Clin Immunol 1999; 104:173–176.
5. Brown D, Bettley F. Psychiatric treatment of eczema: A controlled trial. Br Med J 1971; 2:729–734.
6. Sandberg S, et al. The role of acute and chronic stress in asthma attacks in children. Lancet 2000; 356:982–987.
7. King R, Wilson G. Use of a diary technique to investigate psychosomatic relations in atopic dermatitis. J Psychosom Res 1991; 35:697–706.
8. Helmbold P, Gaisbaure G, Kupfer J, et al. Longitudinal case analysis in atopic dermatitis. Acta Derm Venereol 2000; 80:348–352.

9. Kupfer J. Psychoimmunologische Verlaufsstudie bei Patientinnen mit atopischer Dermatitis. Dissertation, Gieen, Germany, 1994.
10. Sugiura H, Maeda T, Uehara M. Mast cell invasion of peripheral nerve in skin lesions of atopic dermatitis. Acta Derm Venereol 1992; 90:613–622.
11. Szentivany A. The beta adrenergic theory of the atopic abnormality in bronchial asthma. J Allergy 1968; 42.
12. Niemeier V, Gieler U, Barwald C, et al. Decreased density of adrenergic receptors on peripheral blood mononuclear cells in patients with atopic dermatitis. Eur J Dermatol 1996; 6:377–380.
13. Arnetz B, Fjellner B, Eneroth P, et al. Endocrine and dermatological concomitants of mental stress. Acta Derm Venereol Suppl (Stockh) 1991; 156:9–12.
14. Buske-Kirschbaum A, Jobst S, Wustmans A, et al. Attenuated free cortisol to psychosocial stress in children with atopic dermatitis. Psychosom Med 1997; 59:419–426.
15. Buske-Kirschbaum A, Geiben A, Hellhammer D. Psychobiological aspects of atopic dermatitis: An overview. Psychother Psychosom 2001; 70:6–16.
16. Jordan J, Whitlock F. Atopic dermatitis, anxiety and conditioned scratch responses. J Psychosom Res 1974; 18:297–299.
17. Jordan J, Whitlock F. The conditioning of scratch responses in the cases of atopic dermatitis. Br J Dermatol 1972; 86:574–585.
18. Faulstich M, Williamson D, Duchman E, et al. Psychophysiological analysis of atopic dermatitis. J Psychosom Res 1985; 29:415–417.
19. Munzel K, Schandry R. Atopisches Ekzem. Pathophysiologische Reaktivitat unter standardisierter Belastung. Hautarzt 1990; 41:606–611.
20. Kohler T, Weber D. Psychophysical reactions of patients with atopic dermatitis. J Psychosom Res 1992; 36:391–394.
21. Baker G. Psychological factors and immunity. P Psychosom 1987; 31:1–10.
22. Kiecolt-Glaser J, Garner W, Speicher C. Psychosocial modifiers of immunocompetence in medical students. Psychosom Med 1984; 46:7–14.
23. Kiecolt-Glaser J, Glaser R. Psychological influences on immunity. Psychosom Med 1986; 27:621–624.
24. Byrom N, Timlin D. Immune status in atopic eczema. A survey. Br J Dermatol 1979; 100:491–498.
25. McGeady S, Buckley R. Depression of cell-mediated immunity in atopic eczema. J Allergy Clin Immunol 1975; 56:393–406.
26. Stone S, Gleich G, Muller S. Atopic dermatitis and IgE. Arch Dermatol 1976; 112:1254–1255.
27. Wuthrich B. Immunologische Befunde bei endogenem Ekzem. Dermatologie in Praxis und Klinik, vol 2. Stuttgart: Thieme, 1980.
28. Braun-Falco O, Ring J. Zur Therapie des Atopischen Ekzems. Hautarzt 1984; 35:447–454.
29. Alexander F. Psychosomatische Medizin. Berlin: Verlag De Gruyter, 1971.
30. Bosse K, Hunecke P. Der Juckreiz des endogenen Ekzematikers. Munch Med Wochenschr 1981; 123:1013–1016.
31. Koblenzer C, Koblenzer P. Chronic intractable atopic eczema. Its occurrence as a physical sign of impaired parent–child relationships and psychologic developmental arrest: Improvement through parent insight and education. Arch Dermatol 1988; 11:1673–1677.
32. Pürschel W. Neurodermititis und Psyche. Zeitschr Psychosom Med Psychoanal 1976; 22:62–70.
33. Griesemer R, Nadelsohn T. Emotional aspects of cutaneous disease. In: Fitzpatrick T, et al., eds. Dermatology in General Medicine. New York, NY: McGraw-Hill, 1979.
34. Garrie E, Garrie S, Mote T. Anxiety and atopic dermatitis. J Consutl Clin Psychol 1974; 42:742–748.
35. Gieler U, Ehlers A, Hohler T, et al. Die psychosoziale Situation der Patienten mit endogenem Ekzem. Der Hautarzt 1990; 41:416–423.
36. Borelli S. Untersuchungen zur Psychosomatik des Neurodermitikers. Hautarzt 1950; 1:250–256.

37. Cleveland S, Fischer S. Psychological factors in the neurodermatoses. Psychosom Med 1956; 18:209–220.
38. Fiske C, Obermayer M. Personality and emotional factors in chronic disseminated neurodermatitis. Arch Dermatol Syphilol 1954; 70:261–267.
39. Levy R. The Rorschach pattern of neurodermatitis. Psychosom Med 1952; 14:41–49.
40. McLaughlin J, Shoemaker R, Guy W. Personality factors in adult atopic eczema. Arch Dermatol Syphilol 1953; 68:506–516.
41. Ott G, Schonberger A, Langenstein B. Psychologisch-psychosomatische Befunde bei einer Gruppe von Patienten mit endogenem Ekzem. Aktuel Dermataol 1986; 12:209–213.
42. Gieler U, Stangier U, Ernst R. Psychosomatische Behandlung im Rahmen der klinischen Therapie von Hautkrankheiten. In: K Bosse UG, ed. Seelische Faktoren bei Haukrankheiten. Bern: Huber, 1985:154–160.
43. Meichenbaum D. Kognitiv-behavioral Modifikation. New York, NY: Plenum Press, 1977.
44. Boddecker K, Boddecker M. Verhaltenstherapeutische Ansatze bei der Behandlung des endogenen Ekzems unter besonderer Berucksichtigung des zwanghaften Kratzens. Z Psychosom Med Psychoanal 1976; 21:61–101.
45. Thomä H. Uber die Unspezifitat psychosomatischer Erkrankungen am Beispiel einer Neurodermitis mit zwanzigjahriger Katamnese. Psychedelic 1980; 7:589–624.
46. Bitzer E, Grobe T, Dorning H. Die Bewertung therapeutischer Manahmen bei atopischer Dermatitis und Psoriasis aus der Perspektive der Patienten unter Beruck-sichtigung komplementar medizinischer Verfahren. ISEG studie Endbericht, 1997.
47. Gieler U, Effendy I. Psychosomatische Aspekte in der Dermatologie. Akt Dermatol 1984; 10:103–106.
48. Wenninger K, Ehlers A, Gieler U. Kommunikation von Neurodermitis-Patienten mit ihrer Bezugsperson. Eine empirische Analyse. Z Klin Psychol 1991; 20:251–264.
49. Ring J, Palos E, Zimmermann F. Psychosomatische Aspekte der Eltern-Kind-Beziehung bei atopischem Ekzem im Kindesalter. Erziehungsstil Familiensituation im Zeichentest and strukturierten Interview. Hautarzt 1986; 1(37):560–567.
50. Bräutigam W, Christian P, Rad M. Psychosomatische Medizin, vol 5th ed. Stuttgart: Thieme Verlag, 1992.
51. Kuypers B. Atopic dermatitis. Some observations from a psychologoical viewpoint. Dermatologica 1967; 136:387–394.
52. Rechardt E. An investigation in the psychosomatic aspects of prurigo Besnier. Monographs of the Psychiatric Clinic Helsinki. University-Central Hospital, Helsinki, 1970.
53. Bosse K. Psychosomatische Gesichtspunkte bei der Betreuung atopischer Ekzematiker. Zeitschr Hautkr 1990; 65:543–545.
54. Hunecke P, Bosse K, Finckh H. Krankheitsverlauf und psychosoziale Ereignisse wahrend der stationaren Behandlung atopischer Ekematiker Pilostudie. Zeitschr Hautkr 1990; 65:428–434.
55. Schubert H. Evaluation of effects of psychosocial interventions in the treatment of atopic eczema. Psychossoziale Faktoren bei Hauterkrankungen. Gottingen: Vandenhoeck & Ruprecht, 1989:158–215.
56. Bender B, Leung S, Leung D. Actigraphy assessment of sleep disturbance in patients with atopic dermatitis: An objective life quality measure. J Allergy Clin Immunol 2003; 111(3):598–602.
57. Reuveni H, Chaonick G, Tal A. Sleep fragmentation in children with atopic dermatitis. Arch Ped Adoles Med 1999; 153:249–253.
58. Kelsay K. Management of sleep disturbance associated with atopic dermatitis. J Allergy Clin Immunol 2006; 118(1):198–201.
59. McCartt A, Rohrbaugh J, Hammer M, et al. Factors associated with falling asleep at the wheel among long-distance truck drivers. Accid Anal Prev 2000; 32:493–504.
60. Bourgeois-Bougrine S, Casrbon P, Gounelle C, et al. Perceived fatigue for short and long haul flights: A survey of 739 airline pilots. Aviat Space Environ Med 2003; 74:1072–1077.
61. Folkard S, Monk T. Shiftwork and performance. Hum Factors 1979; 21:483–492.

62. Steele M, Ma O, Watson W, et al. The occupational risk of motor vehicle collisions for emergency medicine resdients. Acad Emerg Med 1999; 6:1050–1053.
63. Kleitman N. Sleep and wakefulness. Chicago, IL: The University of Chicago Press, 1963.
64. Drake C, Roehrs T, Burduvali E, et al. Effects of rapid versus slow accumulation of eight hours of sleep loss. Psychophysiology 2001; 38:979–987.
65. Belenky G, Wesensten N, Thorne D. Patterns of performance degradation and restoration during sleep restriction and subsequent recovery: A sleep dose–response study. J Sleep Res 2003; 12:1–12.
66. Van Dongen H, Maislin G, Mullington J. The cumulative cost of additional wakefulness: Dose–response effects on neurobehavioral functions and sleep physiology from chronic sleep restriction and total sleep deprivation. Sleep 2003; 26(2):117–126.
67. Bass J, Corwin M, Gozal Dea. The effect of chronic or intermittent hypoxia on cognition in childhood: A review of evidence. Pediatrics 2004; 114(3):805–816.
68. Abad V, Sarinas P, Guilleminault C. Sleep and rheumatologic disorders. Sleep Med Rev 2008; 12(3):211–228.
69. Majde J, Krueger J. Neuroimmunology of sleep. Textbook of Biological Psychiatry. London, UK: John Wiley & Sons, Ltd., 2002:1247–1257.
70. Redwin L, Hauger R, Christian G, et al. Effects of sleep and sleep deprivation on interleukin-6, growth hormone, cortisol, and melatonin levels in humans. J Clin Endocrinol Metab 2000; 85(10):3597–3603.
71. Sutherland E, Ellison M, Kraft M, et al. Elevated serum metalonin is associated with nocturnal worsening of asthma. J Alelrgy Clin Immunol 2003; 112:513–517.
72. Krouse H, Davis J, Krouse J. Immune mediators in allergic rhinitis and sleep. Otolaryngol Hed Neck Surg 2002; 126:607–613.
73. Krueger J, Ferenc O, Fang J. The role of cytokines in physiological sleep regulation. Acad Sci 2001; 933:211–221.
74. Opp M. Cytokines and sleep. Sleep Med Rev 2005; 9:355–364.
75. Manfridi A, Grambilla D, Bianchi S, et al. Interleukin enhances non-rapid eye movement sleep when microinjected into the dorsal raphe nucleus and inhibits serotonergic neurons in vitro. Eur J Neurosci 2003; 18(5):1041–1049.
76. Kubota T, Li N, Guan Z, et al. Intrapreoptic microinjection of TNF-α enhances non-REM sleep in rats. Brain Res 2002; 932(1–2):37–44.
77. Alam M, McGinty D, Bashir T, et al. Interleukin-modulates state-dependent discharge activity of preoptic area and basal forebrain neurons: Role in sleep regulation. Eur J Neurosci 2004; 20(1):207–216.
78. Vgontzad A, Zoumakis E, Llin H, et al. Marked decrease in sleepiness in patients with sleep apnea by etanercept, a tumor necrosis factor-{alpha} antagonist. J Clin Endocrinol Metab 2004; 89(9):4409–4413.
79. Constantinidis J, Ereliadis S, Angouridakis N, et al. Cytokine changes after surgical treatment of obstructive sleep apnea syndrome. Eur Arch Otorhinolaryngol 2008 [Epub].
80. Bender B, Leung D. Sleep disorder in patients with asthma, atopic dermatitis, and allergic rhinitis. J Allergy Clin Immunol 2005; 116(6):1200–1201.
81. Bender B, Ballard R, Canono B, et al. Disease severity, scratching, and sleep quality in patients with atopic dermatitis. J Am Acad Dermatol 2008; 58(3):415–420.
82. Boguniewicz M, Nicol N, Kelsay K, et al. A multidisciplinary approach to evaluation and treatment of atopic dermatitis. Semin Curtan Med Surg 2008; 27(2):115–127.
83. Leo H, Bender B, Leung S, et al. Effect of pimecrolimus cream 1% on skin condition and sleep disturbance in children with atopic dermatitis. J Allergy Clin Immunol 2004; 114(3):691–693.
84. Korting G, Laux B, Niemoller M. Das endogene Ekzem. Persisenz und Wandel wahrend der vergangenen Jahrezehnte. Dtsch Arztebl 1987; 84:224–229.
85. Al Abesie S. Atopische Ermatitis und Psyche. Dissertation des Fachbereichs Human Medizin, Giessen, 2000.
86. Kaschel R. Neurodermitis in den Griff bekommen. Heidelberg: Verlag fur Medizin, 1990.

87. Klein H. Psychogenic factors in dermatitis and their treatment by group therapy. Br J Med Psychol 1949; 22:32–45.
88. Walsh M, Kierland R. Psychotherapy in the treatment of neurodermatitis. Proc May Clin 1947; 22:578–583.
89. Williams D. Management of atopic dermatitis in children; control of the maternal rejection factor. Arch Dermatol Syphilol Children; 1951(63):545–556.
90. Augustin M, Zschocke I, Lange S, et al. Lebensqualitat bei Hauterkrankungen: Vergleich verschiedener Lebensqualitats-Fragebogen bei Psoriasis und atopischer Dermatitis. Hautarzt 1999; 50:715–722.
91. Cohen F, Lazarus R. Coping with the stresses of illness. In: Stone NAG, Cohen F, eds. Health Psychology. San Francisco: Jossey-Bass, 1979:217–254.
92. Beutel J. Bewaltigungsprozesse bei chronischen Erkrankungen. Berlin: Springer; 1988.
93. Bosse K, Fassheber P, Hunecke P, et al. Zur sozialen Situation des Hautkranken als Phanomen interpersoneller Wahrnehmung. Psycho Med Psychoanal 1976; 21(3): 6–1.
94. Hornstein O, Bruckner G, Graf V. Uber die soziale Bewertung von Hautkrankheiten in der Bevolkerung. Hautarzt 1973; 24:230–235.
95. Liebowitz M, Gormann H, Fyer A, et al. Social phobia: Review of a neglected anxiety disorder. Arch Gen Psychiatry 1985; 12:729–736.
96. Stuttgen G. Physiologie und Pathophysiologie des Juckreizes. Junch Med Wochenschr 1981; 123:987–991.
97. Cormia F. Experimental histamine pruritus. Influence of physical and psychological factors on threshold reactivity. J Invest Dermatol 1952; 19:21–29.
98. Graham D, Wolf S. Pathogenesis of urticaria. JAMA 1950; 143:1396–1402.
99. Munzel K. Atopische Dermatitis Ergebnisse und Fragen aus verhaltensmedizinischer Sicht. Verhaltensmodif Verhaltensmed 1988; 9:169–193.
100. Stangier U, Kirn U, Ehlers A. Ein ambulantes psychologisches Gruppenprogramm bei Neurodermitis. Prakis der klinischen verhaltens medizin und rehabilitation 1993; 6:103–113.
101. Hofmann S, Ehlers A, Stangier U, et al. Zusammenhang von Juckreiz und Kratzverhalten mit Befindlichkeit und Aufmerksamkeit bei Neurodermitis Unveroff. Vortrag Dtsch Kolleg. Paper presented at: Psychosomatische Medizin, 1989.
102. Horne D, White A, Varigos G. A preliminary study of psychological therapy in the management of atopic eczema. Br J Med Psychol 1989; 62:241–248.
103. Kaschel R, Miltner H, Egenrieder H, et al. Verhaltenstherapie bei atopischem Ekzem: Ein Traingsprogramm fur ambulante und stationare Patienten. Aktuel Dermatol 1990; 15:275–280.
104. Niebel G. Verhaltensmedizinisches Gruppentraining fur Patienten mit atopischer Dermatitis in Erganzung zur dermatologischen Behandlung: Pilotstudie zur Erprobung von Selbsthifestrategien. Verhaltenmodif Verhaltensmed 1990; 11:24–44.
105. Bernstein D, Borkovec I. Entspannungstraining. Munich: Pfeiffer; 1078.
106. Haynes S, Wilson C, Jaffe F, et al. Biofeedback treatment of atopic dermatitis: Controlled case studies of eight cases. Biofeedback Self Regul 1979; 4:195–209.
107. Gray S, Lawlis G. A case study of pruritic eczema treated by relaxation and imagery. Psychol Rep 1982; 51:627–633.
108. McMeanamy C, Katz R, Gipson M. Treatment of eczema by EMG biofeedback and relaxation training: A multiple baseline analysis. J Behav Ther Exp Psychiatry 1988; 19:221–227.
109. Kammerer W. Die psychosomatische Erganzungstherapie der Neurodermitis Atopica. Autogenes Training und andere Manahmen. Allergologie 1987; 10:536–541.
110. Cole W, Roth H, Lewis BS, et al. Group psychotherapy as an aid in the medical treatment of eczema. J Am Acad Dermatol 1988; 18:286–291.
111. Stangier U, Gieler U. Autogenes Training bei Neurodermitis. Z Allgemeinmed 1992; 68:392–400.
112. Teshmia I. Psychosomatic aspects of skin disease from the standpoint of immunology. Psychother Psychosom 1982; 37:165–175.

113. Ely D, Henry J. Ethological and physiological theories. In: Kutash IL, Schlesinger LB, et al. eds. Handbook on Stress and Anxiety. San Francisco: Jossey-Bass, 1980.
114. Schubert H, ed. Psychosoziale Faktoren bei Hauterkrankungen. Gottingen: Vandenhoek & Ruprecht, 1988.
115. Luthe W, Schultz J. Autogenic Therapy, vol II: Medical Applications. New York, NY: Grune and Stratton, 1969.
116. Kline M. Neurodermatitis and hypnotherapy: The acceptance of resistance in the treatment of a long-standing neurodermatitis with a sensory imagery techniques. J Clin Exp Hypnosis 1854; 2:313–322.
117. Sokel B, Christie D, Kent A, et al. A comparison of hypnotherapy and biofeedback in the treatment of childhood atopic eczema. Contemp Hypnosis 1993; 10:145–154.
118. Stewart A, Thomas S. Hypnotherapy as a treatment of atopic dermatitis in adults and children. Br J Dermatol 1995; 132(5):778–783.
119. Twerski A, Naar R. Hypnotherapy in a case of refractory dermatitis. Am J Clin Hypnosis 1974; 16:202–205.
120. Hajek P, Jakoubek B, Radil T. Gradual increase in cutaneous threshold induced by repeated hypnosis of healthy individual and patients with atopic eczema. Percept Mot Skills 1990; 70(2):549–550.
121. Bar L, Kuypers BRM. Behaviour therapy in dermatological practice. Br J Dermatol 1973; 88:591–598.
122. Melin L, Fredericksen T, Noren P, et al. Behavioral treatment of scratching in patients with atopic dermatitis. Br J Dermatol 1986; 115:467–474.
123. Rosenbaum M, Ayllon T. The behavioral treatment of neurodermitis through habit reversal. Behav Res Ther 1981; 19:313–318.
124. Noren P, Melin L. The effect of combined topical steroids and habit-reversal treatment in patients with atopic dermatitis. Br J Dermatol 1989; 121:359–366.
125. Niebel G. Entwicklung verhaltensorientierter Gruppentrainingsprogramme fur AD-Patienten—eine experimentelle Studie. In: Niebel G, ed. Behavior Medicine of Chronical Dermatological Disorders-Interdisciplinary Perspectives on Atopic Dermatitis and its Treatment. Bern: Huber, 1990:420–525.
126. Ehlers A, Stangier U, Gieler U. Treatment of atopic dermatitis: A comparison of psychological and dermatological approaches to relapse prevention. J Consult Clin Psychol 1995; 63(4):624–635.
127. Lowenberg H, Peters M. Psychosomatic dermatology: Results of an intergrated inpatient treatment approach from the patients perspective. Prax Psychother Psychosom 1992; 37:138–148.
128. Lowenberg H, Peters M. Evaluation of inpatient psychotherapeutic and dermatological treatment in atopic dermatitis. Atopic Psychother Psychosom Med Psychol 1994; 44(8):267–272.
129. Warschburger P. Psychologie der atopischen Dermatitis im Kindes-und Jugendalter. Munich: Quintessenz MMV Medizin Verlag GmbH; 1996.
130. Niebel G. Direkte versus videovermittelte Elternschulung bei atopischen Ekem im Kindsalter als Erganzung facharztlicher Behandlung. Hautarzt 2000; 51:401–411.
131. Broberg A, Kalimo K, Lindblad B, et al. Parental education in the treatment of childhood atopic eczema. Acta Derm Venereol 1990; 70:495–499.
132. Allen K, Harris E. Elimination of a child's excessive scratching by the training of the mother in reinforcement procedures. Behav Res Ther 1966; 4:79–84.
133. Köhnlein B, Stangier U, Freiling G, et al. Elternberatung von Neurodermitiskindern. In: Gieler U, Stangier U, Brahler E, eds. Hautkrankheiten in psychologischer Sicht; Jahrbuch fur Medizinische Psychologie Bd 9. Gottingen: Hofgrefe-Verlag, 1993.
134. Kehrt R, von Ruden U, Wenninger K, et al. Schulung von 204 Eltern von neurodermitiskranken Kindern. Poster 21. Tagung der Deutschen Gesellschaft fur Allergologie und klinische Immunologie. Munchen, 1999.

18

Conventional Topical Treatment of Atopic Dermatitis

Mark Boguniewicz

National Jewish Health and University of Colorado School of Medicine, Denver, Colorado, U.S.A.

INTRODUCTION AND GENERAL MEASURES

Since the first edition of this textbook, a number of new insights into genetic and immune abnormalities in atopic dermatitis (AD), discussed in earlier chapters, suggest that more specific, targeted therapy should lead to better outcomes in this disease. While "outside-inside" versus "inside-outside" hypothesis continue to be debated (1,2), patients and caregivers need practical measures to manage their AD. At present, avoidance of irritants and proven allergens, hydration, and moisturization as well as topical anti-inflammatory therapy remain the key components of step-care in AD. Many of the topical treatments were recently addressed in a stepwise approach to management in comprehensive PRACTALL review devoted to AD (3). Education of patients and caregivers is a critical component of successful management of AD (4). Having a realistic understanding of the course of the disease and exacerbating factors is important in dealing with a chronic, relapsing illness. Adequate time and teaching materials are necessary to provide effective education. Most patients or caregivers will forget or confuse the skin care recommendations given to them without written instructions. For many patients, a written step-care treatment plan will lead to improved outcomes (4). Patients and caregivers should demonstrate an appropriate level of understanding of the recommendations, and these should be reviewed and adjusted at follow-up visits. Educational brochures and videos can be obtained from the National Eczema Association (800–818–7546 or *www.eczema-assn.org*) or the Lung Line (800 222-LUNG or *www.njc.org*). Patient-oriented support groups and updates on progress in AD research may also benefit patients.

IDENTIFICATION AND ELIMINATION OF EXACERBATING FACTORS

Irritants

Identifying and avoiding irritants is integral to the successful management of this disease, as patients with AD have a lowered threshold of irritant responsiveness (5). An abnormal stratum corneum is present even in noninvolved AD skin and is associated with increased diffusional water loss seven days after application of a topical irritant, confirming a functional abnormality (6). Furthermore, the irritant was shown to induce inflammatory changes including spongiosis, perivenular mononuclear infiltrate, along with activated eosinophils. Thus, in AD, similar to the other atopic diseases, both specific and nonspecific triggers may contribute to chronic inflammation. These studies also support the important concept that normal-appearing skin in AD is in fact abnormal (7). Cleansers, rather than soaps should be used sparingly and have minimal defatting activity and a neutral pH. Of note, soaps and detergents can increase the pH of the skin, leading to increased activity of endogenous proteases, which together with exogenous proteases from dust mites or *Staphylococcus (S.) aureus* can also contribute to epithelial damage (1). Mild cleansers available in sensitive skin formulations should be used. A double-blind study looked at whether daily bathing with an antibacterial soap would reduce the number of *S. aureus* on the skin and result in clinical improvement of AD (8). Over a period of nine weeks, 50 patients with moderately severe AD bathed daily with either an antimicrobial soap containing 1.5% triclocarban or a placebo soap. The antimicrobial soap regimen caused significantly greater improvement in the severity and extent of skin lesions than that in the placebo soap regimen, which correlated with reductions both in *S. aureus* in patients with positive cultures at baseline and in total aerobic organisms. Overall, daily bathing with an antibacterial soap was well tolerated, provided clinical improvement, and reduced levels of skin microorganisms. While antibacterial cleansers may reduce staphylococcal colonization, they may be too irritating for some patients with AD. In a different study looking at the effects of syndet bars containing synthetic detergents or surfactants, 50 subjects with mild AD on a stable treatment regimen were asked to use 1 of 2 syndet bars as part of their normal shower routine for 28 days (9). The severity of eczematous lesions, skin dryness, erythema, texture, and hydration was evaluated at baseline and after 28 days of syndet application by investigators and subjects. Use of syndet bar reduced the severity of eczematous lesions, improved skin condition, and maintained hydration, suggesting that syndet formulations are compatible with therapy of AD, although this study was done in patients with mild disease.

Alcohol and astringents found in skin care products can be drying, and exposure to them should be minimized. New clothing should be laundered prior to wearing to remove formaldehyde and other chemicals. Residual laundry detergent in clothing may be irritating, and using a liquid rather than powder detergent and adding a second rinse cycle to facilitate removal of the detergent may be helpful. Occlusive clothing should be avoided, and open-weave, loose-fitting cotton, or cotton blend garments substituted. The effectiveness of a special silk fabric (MICROAIR DermaSilk) for acute AD lesions was evaluated in 46 children with a mean age of two years (10). Thirty-one children received special silk clothes (group A), which they were instructed to wear for a week; the other 15 served as a control group (group B) and wore cotton clothing. Topical moisturizing creams were the only topical treatment prescribed in both groups. The overall severity of the disease was evaluated using the SCORAD index. In addition, the local score of an area covered by the silk clothes was compared with the local score of an uncovered area in the same child. All patients were evaluated at baseline and seven days after the initial examination. At the end of the study, a significant decrease in AD severity was observed in the children of group A (mean SCORAD decrease from 43 to 30; $p = 0.003$). At the same time, the improvement in the mean local score of the covered area (from 32 to 18.6; $p = 0.001$) was significantly greater than that of the uncovered area (from 31 to 26; $p = 0.112$). The authors concluded that the use of special silk clothes may be useful in the management of AD in children. In a multicenter, double-blind, placebo-controlled trial investigating the clinical efficacy and functionality of silver-coated textiles in AD, patients were instructed to wear either silver-coated or cotton garments directly on the skin for two weeks (11). Only basic skin care and ongoing therapy with topical steroids or oral antihistamines was permitted. In the silver-coated textile group, eczema improved significantly after one week with further improvement at the end of study ($p = 0.03$ and $p < 0.001$). Pruritus and self-assigned skin condition improved significantly more than with cotton garments ($p < 0.001$ and $p = 0.003$). In addition, the silver-coated textiles showed wearing comfort and functionality comparable to cotton.

Temperature in the home and work environments should be temperate with moderate humidity to minimize sweating. Patients generally do better in an air-conditioned environment. Swimming is usually well tolerated; however, since pools typically are treated with chlorine or bromine, patients should shower and use a cleanser to help remove these drying chemicals afterwards, then apply a moisturizer. Sun exposure can lead to evaporation or overheating and sweating, both of which can be irritating. While ultraviolet rays in sunlight may be beneficial to some patients, photodamage can occur. Sunscreens should be used to protect the skin, and sensitive skin preparations or those made specifically for use on the face are often best tolerated by patients with AD.

Allergens

Clinical studies support the role of contact with aeroallergens causing exacerbations of AD (discussed in chap. 12). Epicutaneous application of aeroallergens to uninvolved skin by patch test techniques results in eczematous reactions in approximately 50% of aeroallergen-sensitized patients with AD (12,13). Positive reactions have been described with a number of allergens including house dust mite, pollens, animal danders, and molds. Corroborating laboratory data include the finding of specific IgE antibodies to inhalant allergens in most patients with AD. Ninety-five percent of sera from AD patients had IgE to house dust mite allergen compared with 42% of asthmatic subjects (14). The degree of sensitization to aeroallergens has been shown to correlate directly with the severity of AD (15). The isolation from AD skin lesions and allergen patch test sites of T cells that recognize *Dermatophagoides pteronyssimus* (Der p1) and other aeroallergens provide further evidence that the inflammatory response in AD can be elicited by inhalant allergens (16).

Environmental control measures aimed at decreasing dust mite load have also been shown in a double-blind controlled trial to improve AD in those patients who demonstrate specific IgE to dust mite allergen (17). Dust mite control measures include the use of dust mite–proof encasings on pillows, mattresses, and box springs; washing bedding in hot water weekly; removal of bedroom carpeting; and decreasing indoor humidity levels with air conditioning. HEPA (high efficiency particulate air) filters are not particularly effective in reducing dust mite allergen levels and in addition have not been shown to improve clinical signs in pet-associated asthma and allergic rhinitis (18). The use of polyurethane-coated cotton encasings was compared to cotton encasings in a 12-month study of adults with AD (19). Eczema severity decreased in both groups but was more pronounced in patients using the treated covers. Both house dust mite exposure and specific IgE decreased significantly in the active treatment group. Of note, patients not sensitized to house dust mite benefited from the use of the allergy-proof covers as much as the sensitized patients. The authors speculated that impermeable covers may reduce exposure to other allergens (such as furred animals or yeast), irritants, or possibly microbial toxins. Because patients with AD make specific IgE directed at staphylococcal toxins found on their skin, it is of interest that in a recent study patients with severe AD (geometric mean: 14.67 pg/mg dust) had significantly more *S. aureus* DNA in their bed dust than those with moderate (0.41 pg/mg dust, $p < 0.0001$), mild (1.42 pg/mg dust, $p = 0.0051$), and no AD [0.09 pg/mg dust, $p < 0.0001$ (t-test)] (20). Similar patterns were observed for dust from the bedroom floors and vacuum bags. *S. aureus* DNA was the highest in dust from beds as compared with dust from the bedroom floors or vacuum bags (medians: 1.51, 0.69, 0.21 pg/mg dust, respectively; $p = 0.007$). Eczema Area and Severity Index scores correlated with *S. aureus* DNA from the bed (Spearman's $r = 0.7263$; $p = 0.0004$) and floor (0.6846; $p = 0.0002$) dust, but not with the vacuum bag dust (0.3783; 0.0684). Thus, higher levels of *S. aureus* in the home environment, especially the bedroom, may contribute to disease severity and persistence in AD patients.

HYDRATION AND MOISTURIZERS
The benefits of fundamental skin care including hydration and moisturizers to help restore and maintain normal barrier function cannot be overemphasized. Research in this important area has been comprehensively reviewed (21). The dry skin of patients with AD shows an enhanced transepidermal water loss (TEWL), denoting an impaired water permeability barrier function (22,23). The water permeability barrier is formed by intercellular lipid lamellae located between the horny cells of stratum corneum (24). The stratum corneum has been shown to have reduced water-binding capacity (25). In addition, TEWL is increased from both involved and normal-appearing atopic skin, and water content is decreased. The decreased ceramide levels in skin of patients with AD may contribute to reduced water-binding capacity, higher TEWL, and decreased water content (26). Recently, reduced levels of Natural Moisturizing Factor (NMF) were demonstrated in the stratum corneum of patients with loss-of-function mutations in the filaggrin gene (27). Filaggrin is the precursor protein for the amino acid–derived components of the NMF, although NMF content is dependent on several factors other than the FLG genotype (28). The breakdown of filaggrin is under the control of proteolytic enzymes and is influenced by the hydration gradient across the skin that is dependent on the external humidity and TEWL. The latter factor, in turn, is influenced by the quality of the skin barrier, primarily by the composition and structure of the lipid bilayers. There are also other possible genetic modifiers of the effect of FLG mutations, which are possibly involved in controlling filaggrin processing, including SPINK5 and SCCE (29). In addition, filaggrin expression in the skin can be modulated by Th2-type cytokines such as IL-4 and IL-13 that are overexpressed in AD (30).

Bathing may also remove allergens from the skin surface and reduce colonization by *S. aureus*. Despite a drying or irritating effect, swimming in chlorinated pools results in clinical improvement in some patients with AD. Balneotherapy in acidic hot springs has been shown to help some patients with refractory AD (31). Manganese and iodide ions in the latter have been shown to have a bactericidal effect on *S. aureus* (32). Of note, a recent study of extracts prepared from silica mud and two different microalgae species derived from a specific geothermal biotope in Iceland known to be beneficial for patients with AD have shown them to be capable of inducing involucrin, loricrin, transglutaminase-1, and filaggrin gene expression in primary human epidermal keratinocytes (33). These extracts also affect primary human dermal fibroblasts, inhibiting UVA radiation–induced upregulation of matrix metalloproteinase-1 expression and inducing collagen 1A1 and 1A2 gene expression in this cell type. Topical treatment of healthy human skin with a formulation containing all three extracts induced identical gene regulatory effects in vivo, associated with a significant reduction of TEWL.

Hydration, therefore, is an important component of successful therapy in AD (4). This can be accomplished by bathing or soaking the affected area for 10 to 15 minutes in warm water. Hydration of the face or neck can be achieved by applying a wet washcloth or towel to the involved area. A wet washcloth may be better tolerated when eye and mouth holes are cut out, allowing the patient to read or engage in other bath-appropriate activities. Isolated hand or foot dermatitis can be treated with soaks in basins. Baths may need to be taken on a long-term daily basis and may even need to be increased to two or three times daily during flares of AD. On the other hand, showers may be appropriate for patients with mild disease. Addition of substances such as oatmeal or baking soda to the bath water may be soothing to certain patients but does not promote increased water absorption. Bath oils, on the other hand, may give the patient a false sense of lubrication and can make the bathtub slippery. Recently, some dermatologists have been advocating addition of bleach (sodium hypochlorite) to bath water, especially for patients with methicillin resistant *S. aureus* (34). However, the amount of bleach per volume of water (e. g., 1/8–1/2 cup per tub of water) and frequency (e. g., 1–3 times weekly) of such treatment has not been well studied and bleach baths may cause significant skin irritation. A recent review on management of AD describes bleach bath technique in detail (35).

After hydrating the skin, patients should gently pat away excess water with a soft towel and *immediately* apply an occlusive preparation. Since wet skin is more permeable to water, it is essential that the skin be covered within the first few minutes to prevent evaporation. Appropriate use of hydration together with occlusives or moisturizers will help reestablish and maintain the skin's barrier function (36). It is critical for patients and caregivers to understand the concept of proper hydration and moisturization in order to achieve optimal control of their disease. Effective moisturizers consist of ingredients with properties of humectants to attract and hold water in the skin such as glycerol, occlusives such as petrolatum to retard evaporation, and emollients such as lanolin to lubricate the stratum corneum (21). Daily moisturizer therapy has been shown to substantially increase high-frequency conductance, a parameter for the hydration state of the skin surface (37). This approach allows for ranking the efficacy of moisturizers according to either the duration of the lasting effects or the magnitude of an increase in the hydration levels of the stratum corneum. Regular use of moisturizers has been shown to decrease the need for topical corticosteroids (38,39).

Moisturizers are available in the form of lotions, oils, creams, and ointments. In general, ointments have the fewest additives and are the most occlusive, although in a hot, humid environment their use may lead to trapping of sweat with associated irritation of the skin. Lotions and creams may be irritating due to added preservatives, solubilizers, and fragrances. Lotions contain more water than creams and may be drying due to an evaporative effect. Oils are also less-effective moisturizers. Moisturizers should be obtained in the largest size available because they usually need to be applied several times each day on a long-term basis. Vegetable shortening (Crisco®) can be used as an inexpensive moisturizer. An occlusive such as petroleum jelly (Vaseline®) can be used as a sealer after hydrating the skin; however, it should be noted that petroleum jelly is not a moisturizer and is most effective when used in conjunction with hydration.

Urea-containing preparations have been used in AD primarily to treat the associated xerosis, as application on open, excoriated areas results in burning and discomfort. In a study of a urea-containing moisturizer on the barrier properties of atopic skin with a twice-daily protocol, skin capacitance and TEWL were measured at the start of the study and after 10 and 20 days (40). On day 21, the skin was exposed to sodium lauryl sulfate (SLS), and on day 22, the irritant reaction was measured noninvasively. Skin capacitance was significantly increased by the treatment, indicating increased skin hydration. The water barrier function, as reflected by TEWL values, tended to improve ($p = 0.07$), and the skin susceptibility to SLS was significantly reduced, as measured by TEWL and superficial skin blood flow ($p < 0.05$). This suggests that certain moisturizers could improve skin barrier function in AD and reduce skin susceptibility to irritants. In a double-blind, randomized study in AD, the combination of urea and sodium chloride applied in a topical moisturizing cream was found to be superior to the identical cream with urea alone with respect to ability to reverse impedance indices of atopic skin towards normal, an effect ascribed mainly to changes in hydration of the stratum corneum (41).

Alpha-hydroxy acids impact keratinization at the lowest levels of the stratum corneum, where they affect corneocyte cohesion and new stratum corneum formation. In addition, they increase dermal mucopolysaccharides and collagen formation. The efficacy and safety of 12% ammonium lactate emulsion has been assessed by clinical criteria and by noninvasive methods including electrical capacitance of stratum corneum, skin surface lipids, TEWL, skin surface topography, as well as the biomechanical properties of the skin (42). All patients tested showed a significant increase in electrical capacitance, skin surface lipids, extensibility and firmness of the skin, and an improvement in the skin barrier function and skin surface topography. Of potential clinical importance in AD, 12% ammonium lactate was shown to mitigate epidermal and dermal atrophy from a topically applied potent corticosteroid (43).

A number of studies suggest that AD is associated with decreased levels of ceramides, contributing not only to a damaged permeability barrier, but also making the stratum corneum susceptible to colonization by *S. aureus* (44). The activities of epidermal ceramidase, sphingomyelin deacylase, and glucosylceramide deacylase are increased in AD, while sphingolipid activator protein levels are decreased [reviewed in Ref. (45)]. In one study, direct enzymatic measurements demonstrated that stratum corneum from lesional skin of AD patients has an extremely high sphingomyelin deacylase activity that is at least five times higher than that in the stratum corneum of normal controls (46). In stratum corneum from nonlesional AD skin, sphingomyelin deacylase activity was still at least three times higher than that in normal controls, another example of normal appearing skin in AD not being normal. Whether topical lipid supplementation has any impact on ceramide deficiency and leads to clinical benefit in AD remains to be definitively demonstrated. Of potential practical significance, although an equimolar ratio of ceramides, cholesterol, and either the essential fatty acid linoleic acid, or the nonessential fatty acids palmitic and stearic acids allows normal repair of damaged human skin, further acceleration of barrier repair occurs as the ratio of any of these ingredients is increased up to threefold (47). In one study, a ceramide-dominant emollient added to standard therapy in place of moisturizer in children with "stubborn-to-recalcitrant" AD resulted in clinical improvement, although this was not a blinded trial (48). Most recently, a prescription ceramide containing barrier repair formulation (EpiCeram®) showed efficacy comparable to a mid-potency topical steroid in an investigator blinded multicenter trial of pediatric patients with moderate-to-severe

AD (49). Other ceramide-containing creams marketed today as barrier repair creams include Ceratopic®, TriCeram®, and CeraVe®.

In addition, several prescriptions of nonsteroidal creams such as MAS063DP (Atopiclair®) (50,51) and S236 (Mimyx®) (52) have been shown to benefit some patients with AD. While they are indicated primarily for relief of pruritus of dermatoses, they may have barrier repair and steroid-sparing properties. They are not FDA-regulated products and have no restrictions with respect to age or length of use and may be especially attractive to patients and caregivers who have concerns about using topical corticosteroids and calcineurin inhibitors. They are costly and their place in the treatment algorithm for AD remains to be definitively established.

CORTICOSTEROIDS

Topical corticosteroids have been the mainstay of treatment for AD (3,53). They reduce inflammation and pruritus and are useful for both the acute and chronic phases of the disease. Their mechanism of action is both broad and complex, impacting on multiple resident and infiltrating cells primarily through suppression of inflammatory genes (54). The complexity of the response was demonstrated in a study in AD that showed that expression of IL-12 p40 mRNA, which was significantly enhanced in lesional skin, was strongly downregulated after treatment with topical corticosteroids for 9 to 10 days (55). However, IL-12 p35 transcript levels were not affected by this treatment. Thus, the specific targets of corticosteroids in AD remain to be fully elucidated.

A large number of topical corticosteroids are available, ranging from extremely high- to low-potency preparations (Table 1). The vasoconstrictor assay, which measures the ability of a steroid to produce blanching when applied to normal human skin under controlled conditions, remains the gold standard for determining the potency of a topical corticosteroid. Most authors rank topical corticosteroids into seven potency groups (56). The vehicle in which the product is formulated in can alter the potency of the steroid and move it up or down in this classification. Generic formulations of topical steroids are required to have the same active ingredient and the same concentration as the original product. However, many generics do not have the same formulation of the vehicle, and the bioequivalence of the product can vary significantly (57). In general, the same steroid will be most potent in an ointment followed by cream base.

Use of a particular drug should depend on the severity and distribution of the skin lesions. Patients should be informed of the strength of topical corticosteroid they are given and its potential side effects. Patients often make the mistake of assuming that the potency of their prescribed corticosteroid is based solely on the percent noted after the compound name (e. g., believing that hydrocortisone 2.5% is more potent than fluticasone 0.005%) and may thus apply the preparations incorrectly. As a general rule, the lowest-potency corticosteroid that is effective should be used. However, using a topical corticosteroid that is too low in potency may result in persistence or worsening of AD. In such cases, a step-care approach with a mid- or high-potency preparation (although usually not to the face, axillae, or groin) followed by low-potency preparations may be more successful. In addition, patients are often given a high-potency corticosteroid and told to discontinue it after a period of time without being given a lower-potency corticosteroid to step down to that can result in rebound flaring of the AD, similar to that often seen with oral corticosteroid therapy. Occasionally, therapy-resistant lesions may respond to

TABLE 1 Representative Topical Corticosteroid Preparation

Group[a]	Generic name	Brand name	Vehicle
I	Clobetasol propionate	Temovate 0.05% Cormax Scalp Application 0.05%	Ointment/cream/emollient Solution
	Flurandrenolide	Cordan	Tape
	Halobetasol propionate	Ultravate 0.05%	Ointment/cream
	Betamethasone dipropionate	Diprolene 0.05%	Ointment/cream
	Diflorasone diacetate	Psorcon 0.05%	Ointment
II	Amcinonide	Cyclocort 0.1%	Ointment
	Betamethasone dipropionate	Diprosone 0.05%	Ointment
	Mometasone furcate	Elocon 0.1%	Ointment
	Halcinonide	Halog 0.1%	Cream
	Fluocinonide	Lidex 0.05%	Ointment/cream/gel/solution
	Desoximetasone	Topicort 0.25%	Ointment/cream/gel
III	Fluticasone propionate	Cutivate 0.005%	Ointment
	Amcinonide	Cyclocort 0.1%	Cream/lotion
	Betamethasone diproprionate	Diprosone 0.05%	Cream
	Halcinonide	Halog 0.1%	Ointment/solution
	Betamethasone valerate	Luxiq 0.12%	Foam
IV	Mometasone furoate	Elocon 0.1%	Cream/lotion
	Triamcinolone acetonide	Kenalog 0.1%	Ointment/cream
	Fluocinolone acetonide	Synalar 0.025%	Ointment
V	Fluticasone propionate	Cutivate 0.05%	Cream
	Triamcinolone acetonide	Kenalog 0.1%	Lotion
	Fluocinolone acetonide	Synalar 0.025%	Cream
	Betamethasone valerate	Valisone 0.1%	Cream
	Hydrocortisone valerate	Westcort 0.2%	Ointment
VI	Desonide	DesOwen 0.05%	Ointment/cream/lotion/ hydrogel
	Alclometasone dipropionate	Aclovate 0.05%	Ointment/cream
	Triamcinolone acetonide	Kenalog 0.025%	Cream/lotion
	Fluocinolone acetonide	Synalar 0.01% Derma-Smoothe/FS	Cream/solution Oil/shampoo
VII	Hydrocortisone	Hytone 2.5%, 1.0%	Ointment/cream/lotion

[a] Group I (superpotent) through group VII (least potent).
Source: Adapted from Ref. 55.

a potent topical corticosteroid under occlusion, although this approach should be used with caution and reserved primarily for eczema of the hands or feet (58).

Despite their widespread use, side effects are infrequent with appropriately used low- to medium-potency topical corticosteroids, even when applied over extended periods of time (53,59). With the use of potent topical steroids, thinning of the skin is the most common side effect. After many weeks of topical use, collagen and elastin synthesis are decreased, which can result in skin fragility, dermal atrophy, striae, telangiectasia, purpura, and poor wound healing. In addition, hypopigmentation, secondary infections, and acneiform eruptions may occur. Local side effects are most likely to occur on the face and in the intertriginous areas, and only a low-potency corticosteroid should be used in these areas on a routine basis.

Perioral dermatitis is often associated with the use of topical steroids on the face. It is characterized by erythema, scaling, and follicular papules, and pustules that occur around the mouth, alar creases, and sometimes on the upper lateral eyelids. "Steroid addiction" describes an adverse effect primarily on the face of adult women treated with topical steroids who complain of a burning sensation (60). In a large retrospective review of eyelid dermatitis seen over an 18-year period, a subgroup of 100 patients was identified who had, as the basis for their ongoing problem, an "addiction" to the use of topical or systemic corticosteroids (61). Their recalcitrant eyelid or facial dermatitis often resulted in the use of increasing amounts of corticosteroids for longer periods of time, creating a vicious cycle leading to the steroid "addiction." These patients improved with total discontinuation of the corticosteroid therapy. High- and super-high-potency topical corticosteroids, especially if used under occlusion, may cause systemic side effects along with local atrophic changes and should be used cautiously (62).

Topical corticosteroids are available in a variety of bases including ointments, creams, lotions, solutions, gels, sprays, foams, oil, and even steroid-impregnated tape (Table 1). There is, therefore, no need for the pharmacist or patient to compound these medications. In addition, applying an emollient immediately prior to or over a topical corticosteroid preparation may decrease the effectiveness of the latter. Ointments are most occlusive, providing better delivery of the medication and decreasing water loss from the skin with fewest additives. During periods of excessive heat or humidity, creams may be better tolerated than ointments because the increase in occlusion may result in itching or even folliculitis. Lotions, while easier to spread, may be less effective and can contribute to xerosis. Solutions can be used on the scalp or other hirsute areas, although the alcohol in them can be quite irritating when used on inflamed or excoriated lesions, and lotions or even creams or ointment may be preferred vehicles for topical corticosteroids used to treat scalp eczema in a child. Ingredients used to formulate the different bases may be irritating to individual patients and may cause sensitization. In addition, it is worth remembering that rarely the corticosteroid molecule itself can induce allergic contact dermatitis (63). The diagnosis is often difficult to make on clinical grounds because it can present as a chronic or acute eczema, or even an id-like reaction with an erythema multiforme–type rash occurring at sites distant from the contact [reviewed in Ref. (64)]. Patch testing has been done primarily with tixocortol pivalate and budesonide. However, this approach may miss allergic reactions to some corticosteroid compounds (65). A recent review of contact sensitization to topical corticosteroids in children with AD showed that this was a rare phenomenon, despite prolonged use of topical corticosteroids (66). Only 1 of 71 children (1.4%) patch tested reacted to a topical corticosteroid preparation, tixocortol pivalate, hydrocortisone-17-butyrate and Locoidon® cream. This child's clinical history was positive for worsening of AD after use of the topical corticosteroids that she reacted to on patch testing. The authors concluded that although contact sensitization to topical corticosteroids appears to be rare in children with AD, it is useful to perform patch test with these drugs in select cases, as it may be clinically impossible to distinguish an exacerbation of AD from contact allergy to corticosteroids.

Inadequate prescription size often contributes to suboptimally controlled AD, especially when patients have widespread, chronic, or relapsing disease. Patients or caregivers may become frustrated with the need to refill prescriptions frequently, leading to decreased adherence with the prescribed treatment regimen. In addition, dispensing the prescribed medication in larger (e. g., 1 lb/454g) quantities can result in substantial financial savings for the patient. It is worth remembering that approximately 30 g of medication are needed to cover the entire body of an average adult. The fingertip unit (FTU) has been proposed as a measure for applying topical corticosteroids and has been studied in children with AD (67,68). This is the amount of topical medication that extends from the tip to the first joint on the palmar aspect of the index finger. It takes approximately 1 FTU to cover the hand or groin, 2 FTUs for the face or foot, 3 FTUs for an arm, 6 FTUs for the leg, and 14 FTUs for the trunk. Of note, adequate application of topical corticosteroids has been shown to correlate with clinical improvement. In a study of adults with AD given, topical prednicarbate and the corresponding emollient and examined at four different times over 26 weeks, patients who applied the correct amount of the prednicarbate-containing preparation (not less than 90% of $0.5g/dm^2$) to areas of affected skin showed a significant improvement in SCORAD indices across the four measuring times (69).

Patients should be instructed in the appropriate use of topical corticosteroids (68). Application of topical corticosteroids more than twice daily increases the chance of side effects, makes the therapy more costly, and usually does not increase efficacy. As the dermatitis improves, the frequency of use may be decreased or a less potent topical corticosteroid versus other therapy (e. g., topical calcineurin inhibitor) can be substituted. Once-daily treatment has been shown to be effective for certain corticosteroid preparations, including fluticasone propionate, a molecule with an increased binding affinity for the corticosteroid receptor (70,71). It is worth remembering that most topical corticosteroids have not been studied and approved for children. Several of the newer molecules or newer vehicles (e. g., fluticasone 0.05% cream, desonide 0.05% hydrogel) are approved for children as young as three months of age, although typically only for up to four weeks (72). Fluticasone lotion, alclomethasone ointment, and prednicarbate 0.1% cream are approved for ages 12 months and older for three to four weeks. Topical mometasone has also been studied in children with AD and is approved for once-daily use in children two years and older (73). Once-daily application may also help with adherence with the treatment regimen. A comprehensive review looking at the clinical and cost-effectiveness of once-daily use of topical corticosteroids versus more frequent use of same-potency topical corticosteroids in the treatment of AD found that clinical effectiveness of once-daily and more frequent application of potent topical corticosteroids was very similar, but it does not offer a basis for favoring either option (74). The cost-effectiveness of once-daily versus more frequent use will depend on the generalizability of the findings to the specific treatment decision and the relative product prices. The trials included in this review primarily referred to moderate-to-severe AD, whereas most patients will have mild disease, and furthermore most of the included trials reported on use of potent topical corticosteroids (8 of 10 randomized, controlled trials), thus limiting the ability to generalize the findings. Further studies should include patients with milder disease and outcomes should include quality-of-life assessments and measure compliance. A more recent review from this same group did not identify any clear differences in outcomes between once-daily and more frequent application of topical corticosteroids (75). The authors recommended that clinicians consider once-daily topical corticosteroids when making treatment decisions for patients with AD. However, they admit that the literature on clinical effectiveness is limited and a broader understanding of compliance and phobia associated with topical steroids is needed to inform on this issue.

When the inflammatory process resolves, the topical corticosteroid can be discontinued, but hydration and moisturizer therapy need to be continued. However, since even normal-appearing skin in AD is characterized by immunologic abnormalities (7), the use of topical corticosteroids as "maintenance therapy" may be of benefit. Several studies support such a proactive versus traditionally reactive approach. Van Der Meer et al. (76) showed that once control of AD with a daily regimen is achieved, long-term control can be maintained with twice-weekly therapy. During the maintenance phase of the study, the topical therapy was applied to previously involved areas that had clinically healed, resulting in delayed relapses of AD compared with that of placebo therapy. This approach has been confirmed in several other studies of similar design with fluticasone cream or ointment (77,78) and more recently with methylprednisolone aceponate cream (79).

Other therapeutic approaches involving topical corticosteroids include combination therapy with topical calcineurin inhibitors, which makes sense given the independent and possibly synergistic therapeutic effects. In addition, combination therapy could reduce the amount of each drug used compared with monotherapy and potentially lessen side effects, although the data on such an approach is limited (53,80). One study compared the clinical effects of topical corticosteroid/tacrolimus and corticosteroid/emollient combination treatments in 17 patients with AD (81). An intermittent topical betamethasone butyrate propionate/tacrolimus sequential therapy improved lichenification and chronic papules of patients with AD more efficiently than an intermittent topical betamethasone butyrate propionate/emollient sequential therapy after four weeks of treatment. On the other hand, addition of pimecrolimus cream twice daily to fluticasone 0.05% cream did not appear to offer any significant advantage in the treatment of AD flares (82).

In addition to their anti-inflammatory properties, topical corticosteroids may have an effect on bacterial colonization in AD. Nilsson et al. (83) showed that the density of *S. aureus* on the skin could be reduced by topical corticosteroid therapy. Furthermore, in a double-blind, randomized trial the bacteriologic and clinical effects of desonide were compared with its excipient in 40 children with AD (84). Before treatment, no differences in clinical score or *S. aureus* colonization were noted between the two groups. After seven days of once-daily topical treatment, the clinical score improved ($p < 0.001$) in the desonide group, and *S. aureus* density decreased dramatically ($p < 0.001$). In the excipient group, no significant differences in clinical score or *S. aureus* density were noted. A comparison of the two groups demonstrated statistically significant differences with regard to clinical score ($p < 0.001$) and *S. aureus* density ($p < 0.05$). These results show the efficacy of topical corticosteroid treatment alone on *S. aureus* colonization in atopic skin and suggest a role for inflammation in bacterial colonization.

Finally, a number of patients with AD may not respond appropriately to their topical corticosteroid. Reasons for this may include complication by superinfection or inadequate potency of the preparation used, as discussed above. However, as discussed in chapter 7, allergen-induced immune activation can alter the T-cell response to glucocorticoids by inducing cytokine-dependent abnormalities in glucocorticoid receptor–binding affinity. Of note, peripheral blood mononuclear cells from patients with chronic AD also have reduced glucocorticoid receptor–binding affinity, which can be sustained with the combination of IL-2 and IL-4. In addition, corticosteroid unresponsiveness may contribute to treatment failure in some patients (85). Endogenous cortisol levels have been found to control the magnitude of cutaneous allergic inflammatory responses, suggesting that impaired response to steroids could contribute to chronic AD (86). Alternatively, Blotta et al. (87) have suggested that chronic corticosteroid therapy can have deleterious, albeit insidious effects in allergic patients. The results, however, are based on in vitro data and thus may not recreate the complex milieu in allergic inflammation. A much more practical reason for the failure of corticosteroid therapy is nonadherence with the treatment regimen. As with any chronic disease, patients or caregivers often expect a quick and permanent resolution of the problem and become disillusioned by the lack of cure with topical corticosteroids. In a study to determine adherence to topical treatment in patients with AD, 37 children were instructed to use 0.1% triamcinolone ointment twice daily (88). They were told to return in four weeks, at which time they were told to continue treatment for another four weeks. Electronic monitors were used to measure adherence over the entire eight-week study. Patients were not informed of the compliance monitoring until the end of the study. Twenty-six patients completed eight weeks of treatment. Mean adherence from the baseline to the end of the study was 32%. Adherence was higher on or near office visit days and subsequently decreased rapidly. In addition, a significant number of patients or caregivers admit to nonadherence with topical corticosteroids to fear of using this class of medications (89). The International Study of Life with Atopic Eczema (ISO-LATE) looked at the effect of AD on the lives of patients and society, how patients and caregivers manage the condition, and how well patients and caregivers currently believe that AD is controlled (90). Two thousand two patients (>13 years) and caregivers of children (2–13 years) with moderate-to-severe AD randomly selected from eight countries underwent standardized telephone interviews using questions developed in collaboration with national eczema patient groups and physicians. The data collected revealed that during each year, patients spend, on average, 1 of 3 days in flare. The majority of patients receive prescription topical corticosteroids to treat flares; however, 49% of respondents are concerned about using these agents. On average, patients and caregivers delay initiating treatment for seven days after onset of a flare. These findings point to the need for education of both patients and caregivers, as highlighted in a recent paper from the Dermatology Working Group (68), as well as for alternative therapies.

TAR PREPARATIONS

Prior to the advent of topical steroids, crude coal tar extracts were used to reduce skin inflammation. The anti-inflammatory properties of tars are not as pronounced as those of topical corticosteroids, but they are long lasting and side effects are fewer. Tar preparations may be useful in reducing the need for topical corticosteroids in chronic maintenance therapy of AD. In a comparison with a moderate-potency topical corticosteroid, tar therapy was found to be similar in its ability to inhibit the influx of a number of proinflammatory cells as well as in the expression of adhesion molecules in response to epicutaneous allergen challenge (91).

Tars are currently used primarily in shampoo form for scalp inflammation (T/Gel®, Ionil T®) and as bath additives (Balnetar®). Newer coal tar products have been developed, which are better tolerated with respect to odor and staining of clothes. A moisturizer applied over the tar product will decrease the drying effect on the skin. Some patients prefer a tar compounded in an ointment or cream base such as 5% LCD (Liquor Carbonis detergents) in Aquaphor® ointment to avoid need for multiple layers. Tar preparations may be used primarily at bedtime to increase compliance. This regimen allows the patient to remove the preparation by washing in the morning, thus eliminating the concern about odor during the day and limiting staining to a few pairs of pajamas and bed sheets. Tar preparations should not be used on acutely inflamed skin, since this may result in skin irritation. Side effects associated with tars include inflammation of hair follicles and occasionally photosensitivity.

WET-WRAP THERAPY

Wet-wrap therapy acts as a barrier from trauma associated with scratching, reduces pruritus and inflammation by cooling of the skin, and improves penetration of topical therapies (4). Of note, a recent study examined the difference of nonlesional and lesional atopic skin and evaluated changes in epidermal barrier function before and after treatment measuring SCORAD, epidermal water content, TEWL, skin surface lipids, immunohistochemical staining of filaggrin and loricrin, transmission electron microscopic examination, and calcium ion capture cytochemistry in 10 severe AD patients (92). Use of wet-wrap dressing resulted in recovery of the epidermal barrier with clinical improvement associated with the release of lamellar body and restoration of intercellular lipid lamellar structure. Of note, one week after discontinuation of wet-wrap dressings, increased water content and decreased TEWL was still maintained. Wet-wrap therapy has been shown to benefit patients during acute flares of AD (93). In this prospective, randomized, controlled left-right comparison study, the efficacy of topical prednicarbat with and without additional wet-wrap dressing was investigated in 24 adults and children with an acute flare of AD. One arm or leg was randomly treated with the topical corticosteroid prednicarbat plus wet-wrap dressing, while only prednicarbat was applied on the leg or arm of the other side. After 48 to 72 hours of treatment, decrease in the local SCORAD in the topical corticosteroid and in the wet-wrap dressing group was significantly better ($p < 0.011$). This study points to the usefulness of this topical intervention in acute AD flares and suggests that the time for topical corticosteroid application may be shortened. One form of this treatment modality involves using tubular bandages applied over diluted topical corticosteroids. Children with severe AD showed significant clinical improvement after one week of treatment (94). Of note, there was no significant difference noted using several dilutions of the mid-potency topical corticosteroid. This would suggest that clinical benefit can be obtained with this treatment in more severe patients even with the use of lower-potency corticosteroids. Long-term studies with this therapy are lacking, although most of the improvement in the latter study occurred in the first week. An alternative approach used for many years with success at National Jewish Health in Denver employs wet clothing, such as long underwear and cotton socks, applied over an undiluted layer of topical corticosteroids with a dry layer of clothing on top (4,95,96). Alternatively, the face, trunk, or extremities can be covered by wet, followed by dry, gauze and secured in place with a variety of dressings like Spandage®, elastic bandages, or by pieces of tube socks (Fig. 1). Wraps may be removed when they dry out or they may be rewet. However, it is often practical to apply them at bedtime, and most patients are able to sleep with them on. Overuse of wet wraps may result in chilling or maceration of the skin and may be complicated by secondary infection. While use of wet-wrap therapy over topical calcineurin inhibitors is not indicated per current package labeling, this approach is used "off-label" by clinicians. Given the cumbersome nature of this therapy, it is best reserved for acute exacerbations of AD, although

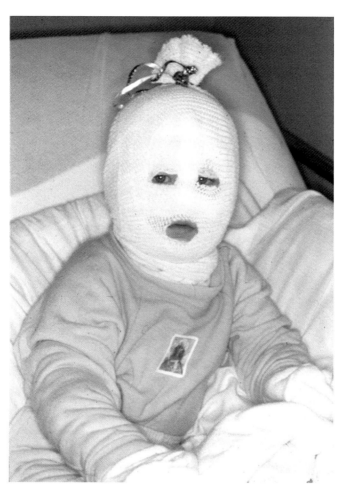

FIGURE 1 Wet-wrap therapy.

it can also be used selectively to limited areas of resistant dermatitis with minimal inconvenience. Maceration of the skin and secondary infections are uncommon in the authors' experience, when wrap therapy is applied properly. In fact, *S. aureus* colonization was found to be decreased in a controlled study of wet-wrap dressings with topical corticosteroid (97). In an evidence-based critical review of the literature, the authors were able to formulate the following conclusions with a grade C of recommendation: (*i*) wet-wrap therapy using cream or ointment and a double layer of cotton bandages, with a moist first layer and a dry second layer, is an efficacious short-term intervention treatment in children with severe and/or refractory AD; (*ii*) the use of wet-wrap dressings with diluted topical corticosteroids is a more efficacious short-term intervention treatment in children with severe and/or refractory AD than wet-wrap dressings with emollients only; (*iii*) the use of wet-wrap dressings with diluted topical corticosteroids for up to 14 days is a safe intervention treatment in children with severe and/or refractory AD, with temporary systemic bioactivity of the corticosteroids as the only reported serious side effect; and (*iv*) lowering the absolute amount of applied topical corticosteroid to once-daily application and further dilution of the product can reduce the risk of systemic bioactivity (98).

ANTI-INFECTIVE THERAPY

Patients with AD have an increased tendency for developing bacterial, viral, and fungal skin infections (see chap. 15). *S. aureus* is found in more than 90% of AD skin lesions. In contrast, only 5% of healthy subjects harbor this organism (99). The density of *S. aureus* on inflamed AD lesions without clinical superinfection can reach up to 10^7 colony-forming units (CFU) per square centimeter on lesional skin. The importance of *S. aureus* is supported by the observation that even AD patients without superinfection show a reduction in severity of skin disease when treated with a combination of antistaphylococcal antibiotics and topical corticosteroids (100,101). Fusidic acid in a topical combination with a corticosteroid has been shown to be effective in AD (102,103). On the other hand, topical anti-inflammatory therapy alone with either a topical corticosteroid or topical calcineurin inhibitor was found to improve skin inflammation in AD and reduce *S. aureus* colonization of the skin (104). The authors concluded that topical antibiotics should be reserved for short-term use in obvious secondary bacterial infection. Similar findings were reported in a different study using mupirocin in combination with a topical corticosteroid (105). Both the antibiotic–corticosteroid combination and corticosteroid alone had good therapeutic effect in AD and both reduced colonization by *S. aureus*. In this study, early combined topical therapy was beneficial to patients with moderate-to-severe AD, while addition of topical antibiotic was unnecessary at later stages of disease or in mild AD. A Cochrane Database analysis of interventions for impetigo found that topical mupirocin and topical fusidic acid are equal to or more effective than oral treatment for patients with limited disease and that fusidic acid and mupirocin are of similar efficacy (106). A newer topical antibiotic, retapamulin ointment 1% used twice daily for five days was as effective as oral cephalexin twice daily for 10 days in treatment of patients with secondarily infected dermatitis and was well tolerated (107). Clinicians should be aware that prolonged or repeated use of topical antibiotics especially when patients self-administer in an "as-needed" fashion can lead to resistant organisms (108,109). In addition, the use of neomycin topically can result in development of allergic contact dermatitis as neomycin is among the most common allergens causing contact dermatitis (110).

Williams et al. (111) showed that a higher rate of *S. aureus* colonization in AD lesions compared to lesions from other skin disorders may be associated with colonization of the nares. In addition, this study pointed to the importance of *S. aureus* carriage on the hands, suggesting that this may be the vector for transmitting these bacteria from the nasal reservoir to lesional skin as well as to close contacts of patients. Of interest, treatment for nasal carriage with an intranasal antibiotic showed a trend for the reduction in *S. aureus* carriage, and hand carriage was significantly reduced in the treated group compared with controls (112). A practical point worth noting is that the source of re-colonization with S. aureus associated with increased AD severity has been shown to be contamination of topical therapies including emollients and topical steroids (113).

Although antibacterial cleansers have been shown to be effective in reducing bacterial skin flora (114), they may be too irritating to use on inflamed skin in AD. The antiseptic gentian violet has been shown to decrease *S. aureus* density significantly in lesional ($p < 0.001$) and uninvolved skin ($p < 0.001$) (115). This treatment also reduced the clinical severity of AD. Use of a 10% povidone-iodine solution also resulted in a 10- to 100-fold decrease in the density of *S. aureus* in patients with an initial density of >1000 CFU/10 cm^2 (116). Erythema and exudation also decreased after povidone-iodine treatment in patients colonized with high levels of *S. aureus*. Of interest, the authors found that *S. aureus* may produce biofilm-like structures in AD patients that may help the organisms colonizing these patients resist the disinfectant therapy. A combination of triclosan and chlorhexidine in low concentrations compared to fusidic acid was shown to be well tolerated in terms of irritancy potential and resulted in pathogen reduction and improvement of AD, although the antimicrobial effect was inferior to the fusidic acid preparation (117). Baths with added sodium hypochlorite (bleach) may also be of benefit to AD patients, especially those with recurrent MRSA as discussed in the section Hydration and Moisturizers, although they can be irritating (34). In addition, as stated above, the nares are an important reservoir of *S. aureus*, so combination therapy with nasal mupirocin may yield better outcomes. Use of antimicrobial clothing is another potential topical therapy for patients with AD. One study compared the efficacy of an antimicrobial silk fabric (DermaSilk) with that of a topical corticosteroid in the treatment of AD (118). Fifteen children wore a dress, where the left side was made of DermaSilk and the right side was made of cotton. The right arm and leg were treated daily with mometasone for seven days. The treatment efficacy was measured with a modified Eczema Area and Severity Index and with an assessment by the patients/parents and by a physician. All patients were evaluated at baseline, as well as 7 and 21 days after the initial examination. All parameters showed that, irrespective of the treatment, there was a significant decrease of eczema after seven days. No significant difference between DermaSilk-treated and corticosteroid-treated skin could be observed. Other studies have shown that silver-impregnated clothing reduced staphylococcal colonization, improved clinical parameters, and reduced topical corticosteroid use in AD (11,119,120). Ultimately, treatment may need to be directed at eliminating or neutralizing the exotoxins secreted by *S. aureus* that contribute to the chronic inflammation and severity of AD (as discussed in chap. 15). Initial attempts at neutralizing staphylococcal enterotoxin B by soluble, high-affinity receptor antagonists appear to be a promising approach (121).

There has also been ongoing interest in the role of fungi, particularly *Malassezia sympodialis* as pathogens in AD (discussed in chap. 14). The potential importance of *M. sympodialis* as well as other dermatophyte infections is supported by the reduction in AD skin severity in patients treated with antifungal agents (122). However, many patients with a head and neck type eczematous dermatitis, even with IgE antibodies to *M. sympodialis*, respond better to topical steroids than to topical antifungal therapy (123).

ANTIHISTAMINES AND ANTIPRURITICS

Pruritus is the hallmark of AD, and an itch–scratch cycle often complicates the course of AD. The pathophysiology of itch in AD is still incompletely understood, although the role of the pruritus-inducing cytokine IL-31 has generated considerable interest and patients with AD have been shown to have CLA$^+$ T cells that produce higher levels of IL-31 (124). In addition, *S. aureus* superantigen has been shown to rapidly induce IL-31 expression in atopic individuals and since patients with AD are heavily colonized with toxin-producing *S. aureus*, this can further contribute to their pruritus (125). Treatment of AD with topical antihistamines and local anesthetics has generally been avoided because of potential sensitization. These drugs can cause cutaneous hypersensitivity reactions, and contact allergy could preclude systemic use of these drugs. However, in a multicenter, double-blind, vehicle-controlled study, treatment with topical 5% doxepin cream resulted in a significant reduction of pruritus (126). In this one-week study, sensitization was not reported, although re-challenge with the drug after the original course of therapy has not been evaluated. In a randomized, double-blind, controlled trial, pruritus relief and lessening of pruritus severity were significantly greater with the use of combination topical doxepin/topical corticosteroid than that of topical doxepin alone (127). In a subsequent study, however, patients with AD treated in a double-blind study with 5% doxepin cream or vehicle ointment had a similar antipruritic response, possibly due to the antipruritic effects of using a moisturizer alone (128). Finally, topical 5% doxepin cream has been associated with marked sedation in patients with AD, which may limit its usefulness (129).

The role of histamine in the pruritus of AD has been called into question. In a study with topically applied capsaicin 0.05% as pretreatment, the pruritogenic and wheal-and-flare reactions to histamine iontophoresis were evaluated in normals and patients with AD (130). In control subjects, but not in AD patients, capsaicin pretreatment significantly reduced the flare area. Compared with control subjects, AD patients showed a lack of alloknesis or significantly smaller areas of alloknesis in pretreated and nonpretreated skin. In control subjects, capsaicin pretreatment significantly reduced itch sensations compared with nonpretreated skin, whereas in AD patients, no differences were seen. Itch sensations in capsaicin-pretreated skin were significantly lower in control subjects than in AD patients. The authors concluded that capsaicin does effectively suppress histamine-induced itching in healthy skin but has less effect in AD. The diminished itch sensations and the absence of alloknesis in atopic individuals suggest that histamine is not the key factor in the pruritus of AD. The importance of other mediators was confirmed in a more recent study using a dermal microdialysis technique (131). Of interest, cutaneous field stimulation is a treatment modality that can mimic beneficial effects of scratching without inducing skin damage and has been shown to be of benefit in patients with AD (132). A placebo-controlled study showed a significant advantage of topically applied opiate receptor antagonist naltrexone over placebo formulation (133). Of note, the placebo formulation also had some antipruritic effects underlining the importance of skin hydration in the treatment of pruritus.

TOPICAL TYPE 4 PHOSPHODIESTERASE INHIBITORS

Monocytes from AD patients have an abnormal increase in PDE (phosphodiesterase) enzyme activity, and PDE inhibitors such as Ro 20–1724 have been shown to decrease IgE synthesis (134) and basophil histamine release in vitro (135). Culture of AD monocytes with Ro 20–1724 also results in significant reduction of abnormal levels of IL-4, IL-10, and PGE_2 (136). In addition, Essayan et al. (137) reported that a PDE inhibitor could inhibit antigen-induced proliferation and cytokine production. In a study of the effects of the PDE4 inhibitor rolipram on toxin-mediated IL-12 production and CLA^+ T-cell induction, the PDE4 inhibitor, but not the PDE3 or PDE5 inhibitors, reduced staphylococcal enterotoxin B–mediated CLA^+ $CD3^+$

induction (138). In addition, they showed that this effect was due to inhibition of IL-12 production and could be reverted by adding exogenous IL-12. Of practical relevance, AD patients treated with CP80633, a potent inhibitor of PDE4 applied topically in a blinded, placebo-controlled paired-lesion study, showed significant clinical improvement with the active drug (136). Results of early clinical trials with cipamfylline, another topically active PDE4 inhibitor demonstrated efficacy in AD (139). In addition, AWD 12–281 (GW 842470) is also under clinical evaluation for topical treatment of AD.

TOPICAL CALCINEURIN INHIBITORS
Since the first edition of this textbook, topical calcineurin inhibitors have become a well-established therapeutic option (3) and are discussed in depth in chapter 22.

OTHER TOPICAL THERAPIES
Herbal treatments are being used with increased frequency to treat dermatologic conditions, including AD [reviewed in Ref. (140)]. Unfortunately, among the most prevalent adulterants in topical herbal preparations are corticosteroids, including potent ones, especially in Chinese herbal creams (141,142). In a study from London, chromatographic analysis showed that 8 of 11 samples of Chinese herbal creams contained dexamethasone in significant concentrations (143). Another study also found that a number of "herbal creams" reported as being effective for the treatment of childhood AD contained corticosteroids including potent or very potent topical steroids (144). Thus, patients and caregivers need to be aware of risks associated with alternative therapies.

Other plant extracts with natural anti-inflammatory properties include flavonoids. A new topical preparation (SK Ato Formula) containing flavonoid mixtures was evaluated in an animal model of chronic skin inflammation (145). When topically applied in this model, this new formulation reduced the inflammatory responses. Furthermore, it inhibited prostaglandin E2 generation and suppressed the expression of proinflammatory genes, cyclooxygenase-2, and interleulin-1β in the skin lesions.

Essential fatty acids are also used in AD in oral as well as topical forms. An ointment containing docosahexaenoic and eicosapentaenoic acids was studied in 64 patients with AD aged two months to 29 years who had a poor response to conventional therapy (146). The authors found significant improvement with the use of these essential fatty acids. In another study, topical oil of evening primrose was studied in two different vehicles (147). The authors concluded that a beneficial effect was seen only with a water-in-oil, not amphiphilic emulsion. Of note, controlled trials with an oral preparation of essential fatty acids have not shown clinical benefit in AD (148).

In a partially double-blind, randomized study carried out as a half-side comparison, Kamillosan® cream containing chamomile extract was tested versus 0.5% hydrocortisone cream and the vehicle cream as placebo in patients with moderate AD (149). After two weeks of treatment, the active chamomile-containing cream showed a mild benefit over the low-potency corticosteroid and vehicle. Unfortunately, topical use of chamomile, as well as a number of other plant and herbal products, has been associated with allergic contact dermatitis (140).

Topical application of nicotinamide, a B vitamin, has been shown to increase ceramide and free fatty acid levels in the stratum corneum and decrease TEWL in dry skin (150). Nicotinamide was shown in vitro to improve the permeability barrier by stimulating de novo synthesis of ceramides with upregulation of serine palmitoyltransferase, the rate-limiting enzyme in sphingolipid synthesis. In addition, nicotinamide increased not only ceramide synthesis but also free fatty acid and cholesterol synthesis. In a left-right comparison study, topical nicotinamide cream 2% was compared with white petrolatum in 28 patients with AD with symmetrical lesions of dry skin on both forearms twice daily over a four- or eight-week treatment period (151). TEWL and stratum corneum hydration were measured by instrumental devices. The desquamation index was determined by an image analyzer. Nicotinamide cream 2% significantly decreased TEWL, while white petrolatum did not show any significant effect. Both nicotinamide and white petrolatum increased stratum corneum hydration, but nicotinamide was significantly more effective than white petrolatum. The desquamation index was positively correlated with stratum corneum hydration at baseline and gradually increased in the nicotinamide group, but not in the white petrolatum group. The authors concluded that nicotinamide cream 2% is a more effective moisturizer than white petrolatum on atopic dry skin, and may be used as a treatment adjunct in AD.

Vitamin B(12) has been reported to be an effective scavenger of nitric oxide (NO). Since experimental application of a NO synthase inhibitor, N omega-nitro-L-arginine, led to decrease in pruritus and erythema in AD, Stücker et al. (152) studied the efficacy and tolerability of a new vitamin B(12) cream as in a prospective, randomized, placebo-controlled phase III multicenter trial involving 49 patients with AD. Patients applied the vitamin B(12)–containing active preparation twice daily to the affected skin areas of one side of the body and a placebo preparation to the contralateral side according to the randomization scheme for eight weeks. On the body side treated with the vitamin B(12) cream, the modified Six Area Six Sign Atopic Dermatitis score dropped to a significantly greater extent than that on the placebo-treated body side (for the investigational drug 55.34 ± 5.74 SEM, for placebo 28.87 ± 4.86 SEM, $p < 0.001$). At the conclusion of the study, the investigator and patients awarded mostly a "good" or "very good" rating to the active drug (58% and 59%, respectively) and a "moderate" or "poor" rating to the placebo (89% and 87%, respectively). The treatment was well tolerated and the authors concluded that topical vitamin B(12) is a new therapeutic approach in AD.

Reduced levels of ceramides have been suggested as one of the abnormalities of the skin of AD patients as discussed above under section Hydration and Moisturizers. An experimental cream containing sonicated *Streptococcus (S.) thermophilus* has been shown to increase skin ceramide levels in the stratum corneum of AD patients (153). A two-week trial of the cream, containing a sonicated preparation of the lactic acid bacterium *S. thermophilus*, applied on the forearms of 11 patients with AD led to a significant and relevant increase of ceramide levels in the skin. The authors suggest that this was due to sphingomyelin hydrolysis through the bacterial sphingomyelinase. In addition, all patients had clinical improvement of their AD. Another bacterial product, OK-432, prepared from the penicillin-treated Su strain of type III Group A *Streptococcus pyogenes*, has been shown to be an effective immunomodulator through IL-12 induction. Treatment with topical OK-432 was found to bring about complete clearance of AD in four adult patients (154). Based on these preliminary results, topical OK-432 may be worth studying in a controlled fashion in a larger AD population.

Systemic administration of suplatast tosilate has been shown to be useful in AD (155). A more recent study showed that topical therapy with suplatast tosilate 3% ointment inhibits the expression of IL-4 and IL-5 and ameliorates skin manifestations in a murine model of AD, suggesting potential usefulness for the treatment of AD (156). In addition, a meta-analysis study showed that suplatast/tacrolimus combination therapy revealed better improvement in skin symptom scores and significantly decreased the dose of tacrolimus compared with topical tacrolimus monotherapy (157). In addition, a significantly greater number of patients could stop using tacrolimus ointment by using the combination with suplatast tosilate than by tacrolimus monotherapy for refractory facial erythema.

Cromolyn in a water-soluble emollient cream in a final concentration of 0.21% was studied in moderate-to-severe AD in a double-blind, placebo-controlled study (158). Treatment with topical cromolyn in the hydrophilic emollient resulted in significant clinical improvement compared to therapy with vehicle alone. More recently, a new aqueous skin lotion of sodium cromoglicate (Altoderm) was com-pared with a placebo control in children with AD with respect to efficacy, safety, and acceptability (159). In this double-blind, controlled trial, children aged 2 to 12 years with a SCORAD score of > or = 25 and < or = 60 at both of two clinic visits 14 days apart were randomized to 12 weeks of treatment with a lotion con-taining 4% sodium cromoglicate (Altoderm) or the lotion base. Subjects continued using existing treatment, which included emollients and topical steroids. The pri-mary outcome was the change in the SCORAD score. The two groups were com-pared for the change in the SCORAD score from the second baseline visit to the visit after 12 weeks of treatment using an analysis of variance. Secondary outcome mea-sures included parents' assessment of symptoms, usage of topical steroids recorded on daily diary cards, and final opinions of treatment by parent and clinician. Par-ents were asked about adverse effects at each clinic visit and the responses were recorded. Fifty-eight children were randomized to Altoderm and 56 to placebo and all were included in the intention-to-treat analysis. The mean $\pm$ SD SCORAD scores at baseline were 41.0 $\pm$ 9.0 (Altoderm) and 40.4 $\pm$ 8.73 (placebo). These scores were reduced after 12 weeks by 13.2 (36%) with Altoderm and by 7.6 (20%) with placebo. The difference of 5.6 (95% confidence interval: 1.0–10.3) was statistically significant ($p = 0.018$). Diary card symptoms improved with both treatments but the improvement was greater in the Altoderm-treated patients. Topical steroid usage was reduced in both groups and was larger in the Altoderm-treated patients. The differences were statistically significant for the mean of all symptoms, the over-all skin condition, and the use of topical steroids. Those for itching and sleep loss were not. Treatment-related adverse events were reported in 11 subjects (Altoderm, seven; placebo, four). Most of these referred to irritation, redness, and burning at the site of application. There were four reports of erythema and pruritus (Altoderm, three; placebo, one), and three reports of application site burning (Altoderm, two; placebo, one). None was reported as severe or very severe. These results suggest a clinical benefit of this sodium cromoglicate lotion in children with moderately severe AD.

Because the NF-κB transcription factor family has been shown to play a cen-tral role in AD, a recent study looked at the possibility of using topical NF-κB decoy as a novel therapeutic agent in experimental AD (160). A high-affinity top-ical NF-κB decoy demonstrated efficient penetration in pigskin, nuclear localiza-tion in keratinocytes and key immune cells, and potent "steroid-like" efficacy in a chronic dust-mite antigen skin inflammation treatment model. NF-κB decoy exerts its anti-inflammatory action through the effective inhibition of essential regula-tors of inflammation and by induction of apoptosis of key immune cells. Unlike betamethasone valerate, long-term NF-κB decoy treatment does not induce skin atrophy. Moreover, topical NF-κB decoy, in contrast to BMV, restores compromised stratum corneum integrity and barrier function. Steroid withdrawal caused rapid rebound of inflammation, while the NF-κB decoy therapeutic benefit was maintained for weeks. A Phase I/IIa human clinical trial using NF-κB decoy oligodeoxynucleotides (ODNs) to treat AD showed that topical application exhibited marked therapeutic effects on the facial skin condition of patients with AD (161).

RDP58 is a novel immunomodulating decapeptide discovered through activity-based screening and computer-aided, rational design. RDP58 disrupts cellular responses signaled through the Toll-like and tumor necrosis factor (TNF) receptor families and occludes important signal transduction pathways involved in inflammation, inhibiting the production of TNF-alpha, interferon-gamma, IL-2, IL-6, and IL-12. These proinflammatory cytokines are thought to be involved in the pathogenesis of several inflammatory and autoimmune diseases, including AD (162). Topical application of RDP58 to the epidermis following TPA treatment resulted in the amelioration of the phorbol ester–induced irritant contact dermatitis. Substantial reductions were observed in skin thickness and tissue weight, neutrophil-mediated myeloperoxidase activity, inflammatory cytokine production, and various histopathologic indicators. RDP58 was also effective in reducing the compounding inflammatory damage brought on by chronic TPA exposure, and was capable of targeting inflammatory mediators specifically in the keratinocyte. These results demonstrate that topically applied RDP58 is an effective anti-inflammatory treatment in the phorbol ester–induced dermatitis model, and suggest that it may have therapeutic potential in a variety of immune-related cutaneous diseases including AD.

Endogenous aliamides are capable of downregulating mastocyte reactivity by their action through the vanilloid (VR1) receptors and keratinocytes and through the CB1 and CB2 cannabinoid receptors linked to G-protein, also expressed by sensitive nerve endings, macrophages, and epithelial cells. Reduction of mast cell degranulation by adelmidrol, as demonstrated by in vitro and in vivo investigations in animals, interferes with the release of various inflammatory mediators, including Nerve Growth Factor. A pilot study assessing the efficacy and safety of twice daily application of a topical emulsion containing adelmidrol 2%, a novel aliamide, in 20 patients (11 male and 9 female, mean age 8, range 3–16 years) with mild AD showed complete resolution with no side effects in 16 (80%) patients after four weeks of treatment, with no relapses at eight-week follow up (163). Six patches in six subjects with multiple lesions that had not been treated and served as controls showed no improvement. Controlled clinical studies in a larger population of patients with AD are warranted to confirm the efficacy of aliamide in this disease.

Massage therapy can be considered a topical adjunct treatment for AD. In one study, young children with AD were treated with standard topical care and massaged by their parents 20 minutes daily for a one-month period, while a control group received standard topical care only (164). The children's affect and activity levels significantly improved, and their parents' anxiety decreased immediately after the massage therapy sessions. Over the one-month period, parents of children in the massaged group reported lower anxiety levels in their children and the children improved significantly on all clinical measures including redness, scaling, lichenification, excoriation, and pruritus. The control group showed significant improvement only in scaling. These data suggest that massage therapy may be a cost-effective adjunct treatment for AD.

CONCLUSIONS

Conventional topical therapy is effective for most patients with AD. Key elements of comprehensive approach to this chronic relapsing disease include patient education, recognition and avoidance of irritants and proven allergens, appropriate use of hydration and moisturizers, and treatment of the inflammatory component with topical corticosteroids and/or topical calcineurin inhibitors (discussed in chap. 22). At present, proactive or early intervention rather than reactive therapy is a promising new direction. Adjunctive therapy includes judicious use of antibiotics, although in topical form these are used primarily to areas of limited involvement or for treatment of *S. aureus* colonization of the nares. Topical antihistamine therapy is of limited value, and as a rule topical antipruritic agents should be avoided due to the possibility of allergic sensitization. New insights into epidermal abnormalities in AD, including gene mutations and immune dysregulation (discussed in chaps. 3,4, and 6), may lead to more specific therapies.

REFERENCES

1. Cork MJ, Robinson DA, Vasilopoulos Y, et al. New perspectives on epidermal barrier dysfunction in atopic dermatitis: Gene–environment interactions. J Allergy Clin Immunol 2006; 118:3–21.
2. Elias PM, Hatano Y, Williams ML. Basis for the barrier abnormality in atopic dermatitis: Outside-inside-outside pathogenic mechanisms. J Allergy Clin Immunol 2008; 121:1337–1343.
3. Akdis CA, Akdis M, Bieber T, et al. Diagnosis and treatment of atopic dermatitis in children and adults: European Academy of Allergology and Clinical Immunology/American Academy of Allergy, Asthma and Immunology/PRACTALL Consensus Report. J Allergy Clin Immunol 2006; 118:152–169.
4. Boguniewicz M, Nicol NH, Kelsay K, et al. A multidisciplinary approach to evaluation and treatment of atopic dermatitis. Semin Cutan Med Surg 2008; 27:117–127.
5. Nassif A, Chan SC, Storrs FJ, et al. Abnormal skin irritancy in atopic dermatitis and in atopy without dermatitis. Arch Dermatol 1994; 130(11):1402–1407.
6. Tabata N, Tagami H, Kligman AM. A twenty-four-hour occlusive exposure to 1% sodium lauryl sulfate induces a unique histopathologic inflammatory response in the xerotic skin of atopic dermatitis patients. Acta Derm Venereol Suppl (Stockh) 1998; 78:244–247.
7. Leung DYM, Boguniewicz M, Howell M, et al. New insights into atopic dermatitis. J Clin Invest 2004; 113:651–657.
8. Breneman DL, Hanifin JM, Berge CA, et al. The effect of antibacterial soap with 1.5% triclocarban on *Staphylococcus aureus* in patients with atopic dermatitis. Cutis 2000; 66(4):296–300.
9. Solodkin G, Chaudhari U, Subramanyan K, et al. Benefits of mild cleansing: Synthetic surfactant based (syndet) bars for patients with atopic dermatitis. Cutis 2006; 77: 317–324.
10. Ricci G, Patrizi A, Bendandi B, et al. Clinical effectiveness of a silk fabric in the treatment of atopic dermatitis. Br J Dermatol 2004; 150:127–131.
11. Gauger A, Fischer S, Mempel M, et al. Efficacy and functionality of silver-coated textiles in patients with atopic eczema. J Eur Acad Dermatol Venereol 2006; 20:534–541.
12. Langeveld-Wildschut EG, Reidl H, Thepen T, et al. Clinical and immunologic variables in skin of patients with atopic eczema and either positive or negative atopy patch test reactions. J Allergy Clin Immunol 2000; 105:1008–1016.

13. Fischer B, Yawalkar N, Brander KA, et al. Coprinus comatus (shaggy cap) is a potential source of aeroallergen that may provoke atopic dermatitis. J Allergy Clin Immunol 1999; 104:836–841.
14. Scalabrin DM, Bavbek S, Perzanowski MS, et al. Use of specific IgE in assessing the relevance of fungal and dust mite allergens to atopic dermatitis: A comparison with asthmatic and nonasthmatic control subjects. J Allergy Clin Immunol 1999; 104:1273–1279.
15. Schafer T, Heinrich J, Wjst M, et al. Association between severity of atopic eczema and degree of sensitization to aeroallergens in schoolchildren. J Allergy Clin Immunol 1999; 104:1280–1284.
16. van Reijsen FC, Bruijnzeel-Koomen CA, Kalthoff FS, et al. Skin-derived aeroallergen-specific T-cell clones of Th2 phenotype in patients with atopic dermatitis. J Allergy Clin Immunol 1992; 90:184–193.
17. Tan BB, Weald D, Strickland I, et al. Double-blind controlled trial of effect of house dust-mite allergen avoidance on atopic dermatitis. Lancet 1996; 347:15–18.
18. Wood RA, Johnson EF, Van Natta ML, et al. A placebo-controlled trial of a HEPA air cleaner in the treatment of cat allergy. Am J Respir Crit Care Med 1998; 158:115–120.
19. Holm L, Ohman S, Bengtsson A, et al. Effectiveness of occlusive bedding in the treatment of atopic dermatitis—A placebo-controlled trial of 12 months' duration. Allergy 2001; 56:152–158.
20. Leung AD, Schiltz AM, Hall CF, et al. Severe atopic dermatitis is associated with a high burden of environmental *Staphylococcus aureus*. Clin Exp Allergy 2008; 38(5):789–793.
21. Johnson AW, ed. Current stratum corneum research: Optimizing barrier function through fundamental skin care. Dermatol Ther 2004; 17(suppl. 1):1–68.
22. Werner Y, Lindberg M. Transepidermal water loss in dry and clinically normal skin in patients with atopic dermatitis. Acta Derm Venereol Suppl (Stockh) 1985; 65:102–105.
23. Werner Y. The water content of the stratum corneum in patients with atopic dermatitis. Acta Derm Venereol Suppl (Stockh) 1986; 66:281–284.
24. Fartasch M, Diepgen T. The barrier function in atopic dry skin. Disturbance of membrane-coating granule exocytosis and formation of epidermal lipids? Acta Derm Venereol Suppl (Stockh) 1992; 176:26–31.
25. Linde Y. Dry skin in atopic dermatitis. Acta Derm Venereol Suppl (Stockh) 1992; 177:9–13.
26. Imokawa G, Abe A, Jin K, et al. Decreased level of ceramides in stratum corneum of atopic dermatitis: An etiologic factor in atopic dry skin? J Invest Dermatol 1991; 96:523–526.
27. Kezic S, Kemperman PM, Koster ES, et al. Loss-of-function mutations in the filaggrin gene lead to reduced level of Natural Moisturizing Factor in the stratum corneum. J Invest Dermatol 2008; 128:2117–2119.
28. Rawlings AV, Matts PJ. Stratum corneum moisturization at the molecular level: An update in relation to dry skin cycle. J Invest Dermatol 2005; 124:1099–1110.
29. Sandilands A, Terron-Kwiatkowski A, Hull PR, et al. Comprehensive analysis of the gene encoding filaggrin uncovers prevalent and rare mutations in ichthyosis vulgaris and atopic eczema. Nat Genet 2007; 39:650–654.
30. Howell MD, Kim BE, Gao P, et al. Cytokine modulation of atopic dermatitis filaggrin skin expression. J Allergy Clin Immunol 2007; 120:150–155.
31. Kubota K, Machida I, Tamura K, et al. Treatment of refractory cases of atopic dermatitis with acidic hot-spring bathing. Acta Derm Venereol 1997; 77:452–454.
32. Inoue T, Inoue S, Kubota K. Bactericidal activity of manganese and iodide ions against *Staphylococcus aureus*: A possible treatment for acute atopic dermatitis. Acta Derm Venereol 1999; 79:360–362.
33. Grether-Beck S, Mühlberg K, Brenden H, et al. Bioactive molecules from the Blue Lagoon: In vitro and in vivo assessment of silica mud and microalgae extracts for their effects on skin barrier function and prevention of skin ageing. Exp Dermatol 2008; 17:771–779.
34. Krakowski AC, Dohil MA. Topical therapy in pediatric atopic dermatitis. Semin Cutan Med Surg 2008; 27:161–167.

35. Krakowski AC, Eichenfield LF, Dohil MA. Management of atopic dermatitis in the pediatric population. Pediatrics 2008; 122: 812–824.
36. Loden M. Biophysical properties of dry atopic and normal skin with special reference to effects of skin care products. Acta Derm Venereol Suppl (Stockh) 1995; 192: 1–48.
37. Tabata N, O'Goshi K, Zhen YX, et al. Biophysical assessment of persistent effects of moisturizers after their daily applications: Evaluation of corneotherapy. Dermatology 2000; 200(4):308–313.
38. Lucky AW, Leach AD, Laskarzewski P, et al. Use of an emollient as a steroid-sparing agent in the treatment of mild-to-moderate atopic dermatitis in children. Pediatr Dermatol 1997; 14(4):321–324.
39. Grimalt R, Mengeaud V, Cambazard F; Study Investigators' Group. The steroid-sparing effect of an emollient therapy in infants with atopic dermatitis: A randomized controlled study. Dermatology 2007; 214:61–67.
40. Loden M, Andersson AC, Lindberg M. Improvement in skin barrier function in patients with atopic dermatitis after treatment with a moisturizing cream (Canoderm). Br J Dermatol 1999; 140(2):264–267.
41. Hagstromer L, Nyren M, Emtestam L. Do urea and sodium chloride together increase the efficacy of moisturisers for atopic dermatitis skin? A comparative, double-blind and randomised study. Skin Pharmacol Appl Skin Physiol 2001; 14(l):27–33.
42. Vilaplana J, Coll J, Trullas C, et al. Clinical and non-invasive evaluation of 12% ammonium lactate emulsion for the treatment of dry skin in atopic and non-atopic subjects. Acta Derm Venereol 1992; 72(l):28–33.
43. Lavker RM, Kaidbey K, Leyden J. Effects of topical ammonium lactate on cutaneous atrophy from a potent topical corticosteroid. J Am Acad Dermatol 1992; 26:535–544.
44. Macheleidt O, Kaiser HW, Sandhoff K. Deficiency of epidermal protein-bound omegahydroxyceramides in atopic dermatitis. J Invest Dermatol 2002; 119:166–173.
45. Choi MJ, Maibach HI. Role of ceramides in barrier function of healthy and diseased skin. Am J Clin Dermatol. 2005; 6(4):215–223.
46. Hara J, Higuchi K, Okamoto R, et al. High-expression of sphingomyelin deacylase is an important determinant of ceramide deficiency leading to barrier disruption in atopic dermatitis. J Invest Dermatol 2000; 115(3):406–413.
47. Man MQ, Feingold KR, Thornfeldt CR, et al. Optimization of physiological lipid mixtures for barrier repair. J Invest Dermatol 1996; 106(5):1096–1101.
48. Chamlin SL, Kao J, Frieden IJ, et al. Ceramide-dominant barrier repair lipids alleviate childhood atopic dermatitis: Changes in barrier function provide a sensitive indicator of disease activity. J Am Acad Dermatol 2002; 47:198–208.
49. Elias PM, Hatano Y, Williams ML. Basis for the barrier abnormality in atopic dermatitis: outside-inside-outside pathogenic mechanisms. J Allergy Clin Immunol 2008; 121:1337–1343.
50. Abramovits W, Boguniewicz M; for the Adult Atopiclair Study Group. A multicenter, randomized, vehicle-controlled clinical study to examine the efficacy and safety of MAS063DP (Atopiclair™) in the management of mild to moderate atopic dermatitis in adults. J Drugs Dermatol 2006; 5:236–244.
51. Boguniewicz M, Zeichner JA, Eichenfield LF, et al. MAS063DP is effective monotherapy for mild to moderate atopic dermatitis in infants and children: A multicenter, randomized, vehicle-controlled study. J Pediatr 2008; 152:854–859.
52. Eberlein B, Eicke C, Reinhardt HW, et al. Adjuvant treatment of atopic eczema: Assessment of an emollient containing N-palmitoylethanolamine (ATOPA study). J Eur Acad Dermatol Venereol 2008; 22:73–82.
53. Del Rosso J, Friedlander SF. Corticosteroids: Options in the era of steroid-sparing therapy. J Am Acad Dermatol 2005; 53(1 suppl. 1):S50–S58.
54. Barnes PJ. New directions in allergic diseases: Mechanism-based anti-inflammatory therapies. J Allergy Clin Immunol 2000; 106(1 Pt 1):5–16.
55. Yawalkar N, Karlen S, Egli F, et al. Down-regulation of IL-12 by topical corticosteroids in chronic atopic dermatitis. J Allergy Clin Immunol 2000; 106(5):941–947.

56. Stoughton RB. Vasoconstrictor assay-specific applications. In: Maibach HI, Surber C, eds. Topical Corticosteroids. Basel: Karger, 1992:42–53.
57. Stoughton RB. The vasoconstrictor assay in bioequivalence testing: Practical concerns and recent developments. Int J Dermatol 1992; 31:26–28.
58. Volden G. Successful treatment of therapy-resistant atopic dermatitis with clobetasol propionate and a hydrocolloid occlusive dressing. Acta Derm Venereol Suppl (Stockh) 1992; 176:126–128.
59. Vernon HJ, Lane AT, Weston W. Comparison of mometasone furoate 0.1% cream and hydrocortisone 1.0% cream in treatment of childhood atopic dermatitis. J Am Acad Dermatol 1991; 24:603–607.
60. Kligman AM, Frosch PJ. Steroid addiction. J Int J Dermatol 1979; 18:23–31.
61. Rapaport MJ, Rapaport V. Eyelid dermatitis to red face syndrome to cure: Clinical experience in 100 cases. J Am Acad Dermatol 1999; 41(3 Pt l):435–442.
62. McLean C, Lobo R, Brazier D. Cataracts, glaucoma, femoral avascular necrosis caused by topical corticosteroid ointment. Lancet 1995; 345:3330.
63. Dooms-Goossens A, Morren M. Results of routine patch testing with corticosteroid series in 2073 patients. Contact Dermatitis 1992; 26:182–191.
64. Matura M, Goossens A. Contact allergy to corticosteroids. Allergy 2000; 55:698–704.
65. Seukeran DC, Wilkinson SM, Beck MH, et al. Patch testing to detect corticosteroid allergy: Is it adequate? Contact Dermatitis 1997; 36:127–130.
66. Foti C, Bonifazi E, Casulli C, et al. Contact allergy to topical corticosteroids in children with atopic dermatitis. Contact Dermatitis 2005; 52:162–163.
67. Long CC, Mills CM, Finlay AY. A practical guide to topical therapy in children. Br J Dermatol 1998; 138(2):293–296.
68. Bewley A; on behalf of the Dermatology Working Group: Expert consensus: Time for a change in the way we advise our patients to use topical corticosteroids. Br J Dermatol 2008; 158:917–920.
69. Niemeier V, Kupfer J, Schill WB, et al. Atopic dermatitis—topical therapy: Do patients apply much too little? J Dermatolog Treat 2005; 16:95–101.
70. Wolkerstorfer A, Strobos MA, Glazenburg EJ, et al. Fluticasone propionate 0.05% cream once daily versus clobetasone butyrate 0.05% cream twice daily in children with atopic dermatitis. J Am Acad Dermatol 1998; 39:226–231.
71. Roeder A, Schaller M, Schäfer-Korting M, et al. Safety and efficacy of fluticasone propionate in the topical treatment of skin diseases. Skin Pharmacol Physiol 2005; 18:3–11.
72. Hebert AA, Cook-Bolden FE, Basu S, et al; Desonide Hydrogel Study Group. Safety and efficacy of desonide hydrogel 0.05% in pediatric subjects with atopic dermatitis. J Drugs Dermatol 2007; 6:175–181.
73. Lebwohl M. A comparison of once-daily application of mometasone furoate 0.1% cream compared with twice-daily hydrocortisone valerate 0.2% cream in pediatric atopic dermatitis patients who failed to respond to hydrocortisone: Mometasone furoate study group. Int J Dermatol 1999; 38(8):604–606.
74. Green C, Colquitt JL, Kirby J, et al. Clinical and cost-effectiveness of once-daily versus more frequent use of same potency topical corticosteroids for atopic eczema: A systematic review and economic evaluation. Health Technol Assess 2004; 8(47):iii,iv, 1–120.
75. Green C, Colquitt JL, Kirby J, et al. Topical corticosteroids for atopic eczema: Clinical and cost effectiveness of once-daily vs. more frequent use. Br J Dermatol 2005; 152:130–141.
76. Van Der Meer JB, Glazenburg EJ, Mulder PG, et al. The management of moderate to severe atopic dermatitis in adults with topical fluticasone propionate. Br J Dermatol 1999; 140:1114–1121.
77. Hanifin J, Gupta AK, Rajagopalan R. Intermittent dosing of fluticasone propionate cream for reducing the risk of relapse in atopic dermatitis patients. Br J Dermatol 2002; 147:528–537.
78. Berth-Jones J, Damstra RJ, Golsch S, et al. Twice weekly fluticasone propionate added to emollient maintenance treatment to reduce risk of relapse in atopic dermatitis: Randomised, double blind, parallel group study. BMJ 2003; 326:1367–1370.

79. Peserico A, Städtler G, Sebastian M, et al. Reduction of relapses of atopic dermatitis with methylprednisolone aceponate cream twice weekly in addition to maintenance treatment with emollient: A multicentre, randomized, double-blind, controlled study. Br J Dermatol 2008; 158:801–807.
80. Norris DA. Mechanisms of action of topical therapies and the rationale for combination therapy. J Am Acad Dermatol 2005; 53(1 suppl. 1):S17–S25.
81. Nakahara T, Koga T, Fukagawa S, et al. Intermittent topical corticosteroid/tacrolimus sequential therapy improves lichenification and chronic papules more efficiently than intermittent topical corticosteroid/emollient sequential therapy in patients with atopic dermatitis. J Dermatol 2004; 31:524–528.
82. Spergel JM, Boguniewicz M, Paller AS, et al. Addition of topical pimecrolimus to once-daily mid-potent steroid confers no short-term therapeutic benefit in the treatment of severe atopic dermatitis; a randomized controlled trial. Br J Dermatol 2007; 157:378–381.
83. Nilsson EJ, Henning CG, Magnusson J. Topical corticosteroids and *Staphylococcus aureus* in atopic dermatitis. J Am Acad Dermatol 1992; 27:29–34.
84. Stalder JF, Fleury M, Sourisse M, et al. Local steroid therapy and bacterial skin flora in atopic dermatitis. Br J Dermatol 1994; 131:536–540.
85. Clayton MH, Leung DYM, Surs W, et al. Altered glucocorticoid binding in atopic dermatitis. J Allergy Clin Immunol 1995; 96:421–423.
86. Herrscher RF, Kasper C, Sullivan TJ. Endogenous cortisol regulates immunoglobulin E–dependent late phase reaction. J Clin Invest 1992; 90:596–603.
87. Blotta MH, DeKruyff RH, Umetsu DT. Corticosteroids inhibit IL-12 production in human monocytes and enhance their capacity to induce IL-4 synthesis in CD4+ lymphocytes. J Immunol 1997; 158:5589–5595.
88. Krejci-Manwaring J, Tusa MG, Carroll C, et al. Stealth monitoring of adherence to topical medication: Adherence is very poor in children with atopic dermatitis. J Am Acad Dermatol 2007; 56:211–216.
89. Charman CR, Morris AD, Williams HC. Topical corticosteroid phobia in patients with atopic eczema. Br J Dermatol 2000; 142:931–936.
90. Zuberbier T, Orlow SJ, Paller AS, et al. Patient perspectives on the management of atopic dermatitis. J Allergy Clin Immunol 2006; 118:226–232.
91. Langeveld-Wildschut EG, Riedl H, Thepen T, et al. Modulation of the atopy patch test reaction by topical corticosteroids and tar. J Allergy Clin Immunol 2000; 106: 737–743.
92. Lee JH, Lee SJ, Kim D, et al. The effect of wet-wrap dressing on epidermal barrier in patients with atopic dermatitis. J Eur Acad Dermatol Venereol 2007; 21:1360–1368.
93. Foelster-Holst R, Nagel F, Zoellner P, et al. Efficacy of crisis intervention treatment with topical corticosteroid prednicarbat with and without partial wet-wrap dressing in atopic dermatitis. Dermatology 2006; 212:66–69.
94. Wolkerstorfer A, Visser RL, De Waard van der Spek FB, et al. Efficacy and safety of wet-wrap dressings in children with severe atopic dermatitis: Influence of corticosteroid dilution. Br J Dermatol 2000; 143:999–1004.
95. Nicol NH. Atopic dermatitis: The (wet) wrap-up. Am J Nurs 1987; 87(12):1560–1563.
96. Boguniewicz M, Nicol N. Conventional Therapy. In: Boguniewicz M, ed. Atopic Dermatitis. Immunol Allergy Clinics N Am 2002; 22:107–124.
97. Schnopp C, Holtmann C, Sybille S, et al. Topical steroids under wet-wrap dressings in atopic dermatitis—A vehicle-controlled trial. Dermatology 2002; 204:56–59.
98. Devillers AC, Oranje AP. Efficacy and safety of 'wet-wrap' dressings as an intervention treatment in children with severe and/or refractory atopic dermatitis: A critical review of the literature. Br J Dermatol 2006; 154:579–585.
99. Leyden JE, Marples RR, Kligman AM. *Staphylococcus aureus* in the lesions of atopic dermatitis. Br J Dermatol 1974; 90:525–530.
100. Leyden J, Kligman A. The case for steroid-antibiotic combinations. Br J Dermatol 1977; 96:179–187.
101. Lever R, Hadley K, Downey D, et al. Staphylococcal colonization in atopic dermatitis and the effect of topical mupirocin therapy. Br J Dermatol 1988; 119:189–198.

102. Abeck D, Mempel M. *Staphylococcus aureus* colonization in atopic dermatitis and its therapeutic implications. Br J Dermatol 1998; 139(suppl 53):13–16.
103. Larsen FS, Simonsen L, Melgaard A, et al. An efficient new formulation of fusidic acid and betamethasone 17-valerate (fucicort lipid cream) for treatment of clinically infected atopic dermatitis. Acta Derm Venereol 2007; 87:62–68.
104. Hung SH, Lin YT, Chu CY, et al. Staphylococcus colonization in atopic dermatitis treated with fluticasone or tacrolimus with or without antibiotics. Ann Allergy Asthma Immunol 2007; 98:51–56.
105. Gong JQ, Lin L, Lin T, et al. Skin colonization by *Staphylococcus aureus* in patients with eczema and atopic dermatitis and relevant combined topical therapy: A double-blind multicentre randomized controlled trial. Br J Dermatol 2006; 155:680–687.
106. Koning S, Verhagen AP, van Suijlekom-Smit LW, et al. Interventions for impetigo. Cochrane Database Syst Rev. 2004; (2):CD003261.
107. Parish LC, Jorizzo JL, Breton JJ, et al; SB275833/032 Study Team. Topical retapamulin ointment (1%, wt/wt) twice daily for 5 days versus oral cephalexin twice daily for 10 days in the treatment of secondarily infected dermatitis: Results of a randomized controlled trial. J Am Acad Dermatol 2006; 55:1003–1013.
108. Cookson BD. The emergence of mupirocin resistance: a challenge to infection control and antibiotic prescribing practice. J Antimicrob Chemother (1998) 41:11–18.
109. Niebuhr M, Mai U, Kapp A, Werfel T. Antibiotic treatment of cutaneous infections with *Staphylococcus aureus* in patients with atopic dermatitis: current antimicrobial resistances and susceptibilities. Exp Dermatol 2008; 17:953–957.
110. Albert MR, Gonzalez S, Gonzalez E. Patch testing reactions to a standard series in 608 patients tested from 1990 to 1997 at Massachusetts General Hospital. Am J Contact Dermat 1998; 9(4):207–211.
111. Williams JV, Vowels BR, Honig PJ, et al. *S. aureus* isolation from the lesions, the hands, and the anterior nares of patients with atopic dermatitis. Pediatr Dermatol 1998; 15:194–198.
112. Doebbeling BN, Reagan DR, Pfaller MA, et al. Long-term efficacy of intranasal mupirocin ointment. A prospective cohort study of *Staphylococcus aureus* carriage. Arch Int Med 1994; 154:1505–1508.
113. Gilani SJ, Gonzalez M, Hussain I, et al. *Staphylococcus aureus* re-colonization in atopic dermatitis: Beyond the skin. Clin Exp Dermatol 2005; 30:10–13.
114. Stalder JF, Fleury M, Sourisse M, et al. Comparative effects of two topical antiseptics (chlorhexidine vs KMnO$_4$) on bacterial skin flora in atopic dermatitis. Acta Derm Venereol Suppl (Stockh) 1992; 176:132–134.
115. Brockow K, Grabenhorst P, Abeck D, et al. Effect of gentian violet, corticosteroid and tar preparations in *Staphylococcus aureus*-colonized atopic eczema. Dermatology 1999; 199(3):231–236.
116. Akiyama H, Tada J, Toi J, et al. Changes in *Staphylococcus aureus* density and lesion severity after topical application of povidone-iodine in cases of atopic dermatitis. J Dermatol Sci 1997; 16(l):23–30.
117. Wohlrab J, Jost G, Abeck D. Antiseptic efficacy of a low-dosed topical triclosan/chlorhexidine combination therapy in atopic dermatitis. Skin Pharmacol Physiol 2007; 20:71–76.
118. Senti G, Steinmann LS, Fischer B, et al. Antimicrobial silk clothing in the treatment of atopic dermatitis proves comparable to topical corticosteroid treatment. Dermatology 2006; 213:228–233.
119. Gauger A, Fischer S, Mempel M, et al. Silver-coated textiles reduce *Staphylococcus aureus* colonization in patients with atopic eczema. Dermatology 2003; 207:15–21.
120. Juenger M, Ladwig A, Staecker S, et al. Efficacy and safety of silver textile in the treatment of atopic dermatitis (AD). Curr Med Res Opin 2006; 22:739–750.
121. Buonpane RA, Churchill HR, Moza B, et al. Neutralization of staphylococcal enterotoxin B by soluble, high-affinity receptor antagonists. Nat Med 2007; 13:725–729.
122. Back O, Scheynius A, Johansson SG. Ketoconazole in atopic dermatitis: Therapeutic response is correlated with decrease in serum IgE. Arch Dermatol Res 1995; 287:448–451.

123. Boguniewicz M, Schmid-Grendelmeier P, Leung DYM. Clinical Pearls: Atopic dermatitis. J Allergy Clin Immunol 2006; 118:40–43.
124. Bilsborough J, Leung DY, Maurer M, et al. IL-31 is associated with cutaneous lymphocyte antigen-positive skin homing T cells in patients with atopic dermatitis. J Allergy Clin Immunol 2006; 117:418–425.
125. Sonkoly E, Muller A, Lauerma AI, et al. IL-31: A new link between T cells and pruritus in atopic skin inflammation. J Allergy Clin Immunol 2006; 117:411–417.
126. Drake LA, Fallon JD, Sober A; Group DS. Relief of pruritus in patients with atopic dermatitis after treatment with topical doxepin cream. J Am Acad Dermatol 1994; 31(4):613–616.
127. Drake LA, Cohen L, Gillies R, et al. Pharmacokinetics of doxepin in subjects with pruritic atopic dermatitis. J Am Acad Dermatol 1999; 41(2 Pt l):209–214.
128. Groene D, Martus P, Heyer G. Doxepin affects acetylcholine induced cutaneous reactions in atopic eczema. Exp Dermatol 2001; 10(2): 110–117.
129. Sabroe RA, Kennedy CT, Archer CB. The effects of topical doxepin on responses to histamine, substance P and prostaglandin E2 in human skin. Br J Dermatol 1997; 137(3):386–390.
130. Weisshaar E, Heyer G, Forster C, et al. Effect of topical capsaicin on the cutaneous reactions and itching to histamine in atopic eczema compared to healthy skin. Arch Dermatol Res 1998; 290(6):306–311.
131. Rukwied R, Lischetzki G, McGlone F, et al. Mast cell mediators other than histamine induce pruritus in atopic dermatitis patients: A dermal microdialysis study. Br J Dermatol 2000; 142:1114–1120.
132. Nilsson H-J, Levinsson A, Schouenborg, J. Cutaneous field stimulation (CFS): A new powerful method to combat itch. Pain 1997; 71:49–55.
133. Bigliardi PL, Stammer H, Jost G, et al. Treatment of pruritus with topically applied opiate receptor antagonist. J Am Acad Dermatol 2007; 56:979–988.
134. Cooper KD, Kang K, Chan SC, et al. Phosphodiesterase inhibition by Ro 20–1724 reduces hyper-IgE synthesis by atopic dermatitis cells in vitro. J Invest Dermatol 1985; 84:477–482.
135. Butler JM, Chan SC, Stevens S, et al. Increased leukocyte histamine release with elevated cyclic AMP-phosphodiesterase activity in atopic dermatitis. J Allergy Clin Immunol 1983; 71:490–497.
136. Hanifin JM, Chan SC, Cheng JB, et al. Type 4 phosphodiesterase inhibitors have clinical and in vitro anti-inflammatory effects in atopic dermatitis. J Invest Dermatol 1996; 107:51–56.
137. Essayan DM, Huang S, Kagey-Sobotka A, et al. Differential efficacy of lymphocyte- and monocyte-selective pretreatment with a Type 4 phosphodiesterase inhibitor on antigen-driven proliferation and cytokine gene expression. J Allergy Clin Immunol 1997; 99:28–37.
138. Santamaria LF, Torres R, Giménez-Arnau AM, et al. Rolipram inhibits staphylococcal enterotoxin B-mediated induction of the human skin-homing receptor on T lymphocytes. J Invest Dermatol 1999; 113:82–86.
139. Bäumer W, Hoppmann J, Rundfeldt C, et al. Highly selective phosphodiesterase 4 inhibitors for the treatment of allergic skin diseases and psoriasis. Inflamm Allergy Drug Targets 2007; 6:17–26.
140. Ernst E. Adverse effects of herbal drugs in dermatology. Br J Dermatol 2000; 143(5):923–929.
141. Wood B, Wishart J. Potent topical steroid in a Chinese herbal cream. N Z Med J 1997; 110:420–421.
142. Allen BR, Parkinson R. Chinese herbs for eczema. Lancet 1990; 336:177.
143. Keane FM, Munn SE, du Vivier AWP, et al. Analysis of Chinese herbal creams prescribed for dermatological conditions. Br Med J 1999; 318:563–567.
144. Ramsay HM, Goddard W, Gill S, et al. Herbal creams used for atopic eczema in Birmingham, UK, illegally contain potent corticosteroids. Arch Dis Child 2003; 88:1032–1033.

145. Lim H, Son KH, Chang HW, et al. Inhibition of chronic skin inflammation by topical anti-inflammatory flavonoid preparation, Ato Formula. Arch Pharm Res 2006; 29:503–507.
146. Watanabe T, Kuroda Y. The effect of a newly developed ointment containing eicosapentaenoic acid and docosahexaenoic acid in the treatment of atopic dermatitis. J Med Invest 1999; 46(3–4):173–177.
147. Gehring W, Bopp R, Rippke F, et al. Effect of topically applied evening primrose oil on epidermal barrier function in atopic dermatitis as a function of vehicle. Arzneimittelforschung 1999; 49(7):635–642.
148. Berth-Jones J, Graham-Brown RA. Placebo-controlled trial of essential fatty acid supplementation in atopic dermatitis. Lancet 1993; 341(8860):1557–1560.
149. Patzelt-Wenczler R, Ponce-Poschl E. Proof of efficacy of Kamillosan(R) cream in atopic eczema. Eur J Med Res 2000; 5(4):171–175.
150. Tanno O, Ota Y, Kitamura N, et al. Nicotinamide increases biosynthesis of ceramides as well as other stratum corneum lipids to improve the epidermal permeability barrier. Br J Dermatol 2000; 143(3):524–531.
151. Soma Y, Kashima M, Imaizumi A, et al. Moisturizing effects of topical nicotinamide on atopic dry skin. Int J Dermatol 2005; 44:197–202.
152. Stücker M, Pieck C, Stoerb C, et al. Topical vitamin B12—A new therapeutic approach in atopic dermatitis-evaluation of efficacy and tolerability in a randomized placebo-controlled multicentre clinical trial. Br J Dermatol 2004; 150:977–983.
153. Di Marzio L, Centi C, Cinque B, et al. Effect of the lactic acid bacterium *S. thermophilus* on stratum corneum ceramide levels and signs and symptoms of atopic dermatitis patients. Exp Dermatol 2003; 12:615–620.
154. Horiuchi Y. Topical streptococcal preparation, OK-432, for atopic dermatitis. J Dermatol Treat 2005; 16:117–120.
155. Kimata H. Selective enhancement of production of IgE, IgG4, and Th2-cell cytokine during the rebound phenomenon in atopic dermatitis and prevention by suplatast tosilate. Ann Allergy Asthma Immunol 1999; 82:293–295.
156. Murakami T, Yamanaka K, Tokime K, et al. Topical suplatast tosilate (IPD) ameliorates Th2 cytokine-mediated dermatitis in caspase-1 transgenic mice by downregulating interleukin-4 and interleukin-5. Br J Dermatol 2006; 155:27–32.
157. Miyachi Y, Katayama I, Furue M. Suplatast/tacrolimus combination therapy for refractory facial erythema in adult patients with atopic dermatitis: A meta-analysis study. Allergol Int 2007; 56:269–275.
158. Moore C, Ehlayel MS, Junprasert J, et al. Topical sodium cromoglycate in the treatment of moderate-to-severe atopic dermatitis. Ann Allergy Asthma Immunol 1998; 81(5 Pt l):452–458.
159. Stainer R, Matthews S, Arshad SH, et al. Efficacy and acceptability of a new topical skin lotion of sodium cromoglicate (Altoderm) in atopic dermatitis in children aged 2–12 years: A double-blind, randomized, placebo-controlled trial. Br J Dermatol 2005; 152:334–341.
160. Dajee M, Muchamuel T, Schryver B, et al. Blockade of experimental atopic dermatitis via topical NF-κB decoy oligonucleotide. J Invest Dermatol 2006; 126:1792–1803.
161. Nakagami H, Tomita N, Kaneda Y, et al. Anti-oxidant gene therapy by NF kappa B decoy oligodeoxynucleotide. Curr Pharm Biotechnol 2006; 7:95–100.
162. De Vry CG, Valdez M, Lazarov M, et al. Topical application of a novel immunomodulatory peptide, RDP58, reduces skin inflammation in the phorbol ester-induced dermatitis model. J Invest Dermatol 2005; 125:473–481.
163. Pulvirenti N, Nasca MR, Micali G. Topical adelmidrol 2% emulsion, a novel aliamide, in the treatment of mild atopic dermatitis in pediatric subjects: A pilot study. Acta Dermatovenerol Croat 2007; 15:80–83.
164. Schachner L, Field T, Hernandez-Reif M, et al. Atopic dermatitis symptoms decreased in children following massage therapy. Pediatr Dermatol 1998; 15:390–395.

Franck Boralevi and Alain Taïeb

Pediatric Dermatology Unit and Department of Dermatology, Centre Hospitalier Universitaire of Bordeaux, Bordeaux, France

INTRODUCTION

Most of the patients with atopic dermatitis (AD) are children, and especially infants. The prevalence of the disease clearly varies according to the age, for example, in the United Kingdom where the prevalence is around 15% in children aged 13 to 14 years (1) and reaches peak incidence rate in infancy with 30% of affected children at 18 months (2). Several other reflections lead to consider infancy as a crucial period in AD. Infantile atopic eczema is the earliest manifestation of atopic disease; clinical features are rather different in this period than those usually seen later, and the management should be appropriate to age, taking into consideration not only the affected infant but also the parents' fears and expectations.

CLINICAL ASPECTS ACCORDING TO AGE

AD usually begins in infants aged three to six months, but may appear as soon as the first week of life (3). The first symptoms of the disease start before the sixth month of life in about 50% of patients. For the others, later onset of AD may appear throughout childhood or adulthood. Xerosis, scaling, localized erythema, or seborrheic-like lesions may be present from birth. The main skin features are represented by poorly demarcated and slightly edematous scaly erythematous patches, with a marked tendency for oozing or crusting during flares. The lesions are usually symmetrical on limb extensor aspects and facial convexities sparing constantly the tip of the nose and even the median part of the face (Fig. 1) (4). The site covered by napkins remains characteristically uninvolved, except in rare cases of diaper contact eczema, leading to a well-demarcated limit on the trunk and suggesting a protective local effect on disease expression (5,6). Less constantly, the scalp, forehead, and eyebrows may be involved early with well-demarcated seborrheic yellow scales and crusts. Without appropriate treatment, oozing lesions frequently lead to crusting (Fig. 2) and sometimes impetiginization. Nummular forms may appear since infancy, characterized by several or numerous well-demarcated discoid-type lesions, frequently covered with crusts (Fig. 3). Nipple eczema appears to be more frequent in those nummular forms.

Commonly present in older children, xerosis and flexural involvement can also be seen in infants. Minor forms seem to be frequent at this stage and not always recognized as AD, with limited involved areas, subauricular erosions or splits (Fig. 4), hypopigmented patches, and Dennie-Morgan infraorbital fold (Fig. 5) (4). In those minor forms, inflammatory lesions are not conspicuous and palpation only can mark the limits of abnormal rugose skin.

Pruritus is usually demonstrable in the first month of life causing sleep troubles. True scratching by hand is preceded in the second and third month of life by

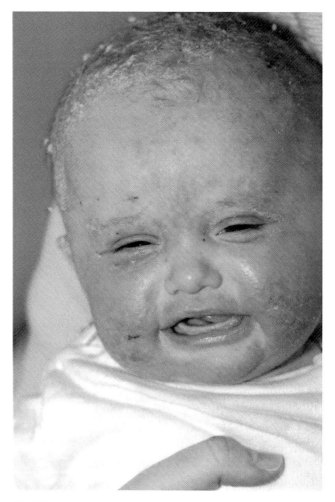

FIGURE 1 Symmetrical lesions on facial convexities, sparing constantly the tip of the nose.

equivalent movements such as rubbing the cheeks against the bed sheets or the mother's clothes, bed agitation with limbs, and trunk rubbing movements, leading also to sleep disturbance.

In young children, convexities are more rarely involved compared to the flexural areas, and skin xerosis tends to become more prevalent. Although clinical features and distributions lead to a wide spectrum of clinical forms, in a given patient, the pattern distribution of eczematous lesions is fairly constant with "bastion" areas, especially on flexures, hands, and face. As a consequence of chronic pruritus and scratching, lichenification may be observed from the second year of life, or earlier in black or Asian infants.

Descriptive items included into the SCORAD index appear useful to obtain an intensity score of AD in infancy (7). These items include erythema, edema or

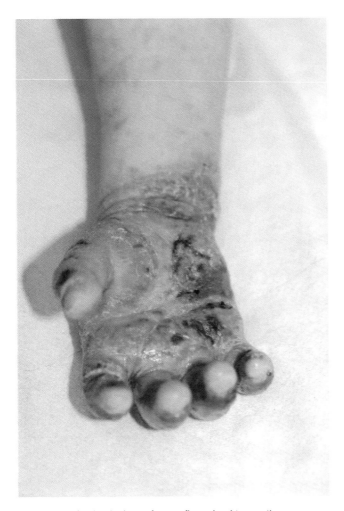

FIGURE 2   Oozing lesions of acute flares lead to crusting.

edematous papules, excoriations (an objective marker of pruritus), oozing, and/or crusting in relation with the acuteness of flares.

DIAGNOSTIC CRITERIA IN INFANTS

Several useful AD diagnostic criteria have been proposed in children, namely, those compiled by Hanifin and Rajka at the beginning of the 1980; the simpler derived U.K. Working Party criteria, which have been widely validated in children (8); and the criteria used in the ISAAC study restricted to simple items (1). However, there are no fully validated criteria for infants.

The use of the U.K. Working Party criteria does not make much sense in infancy, because the item of "onset under age two" is always positive in this age group. However, the authors of the original validation study suggested that they

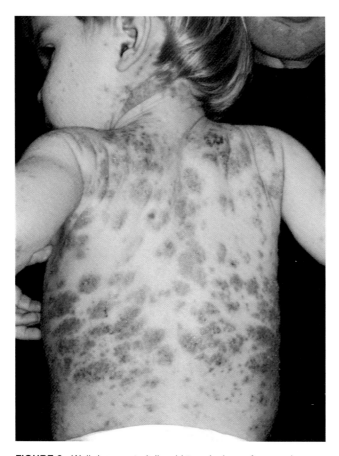

FIGURE 3 Well-demarcated discoid-type lesions of nummular eczema.

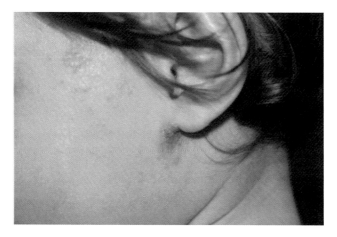

FIGURE 4 Sub-auricular split and localized eczema (minor form of AD).

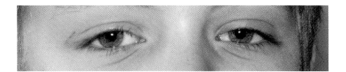

FIGURE 5   Dennie-Morgan infraorbital fold.

can be used in infants and they recommended that the identification of flexural dermatitis should be modified in infancy to include the outer arms or legs in order to
separate "seborrheic dermatitis of infancy" from AD. Later, an independent study
carried out to test a postal questionnaire version of the U.K. Working Party criteria in infants suggested that the distribution of dermatitis in infancy may be more
variable than previously thought. More than 40% of the children who had visible
dermatitis on at least one of the typical flexural sites did not also have dermatitis on
their cheeks, arms, or legs. The authors concluded that there is a need to refine the
U.K. Working Party criteria for infants.

The Hanifin and Rajka criteria are not easy to use in general practice and are
poorly appropriate to infants. As a consequence, an adaptation to infants (children
<2 years) of Hanifin and Rajka's criteria has been proposed in the early 1990 by
Sampson. Regarding those criteria, shown in Table 1(A), some remarks should be
made. Firstly, lichenified dermatitis is not a sensible criterion in very young children, because lichenification occurs generally at the end of the first year in Caucasian infants affected with moderate/severe eczema. Secondly, the minor criteria have not been selected adequately. Scalp involvement is not specific for AD,
because it appears as a very common feature in minor forms of pure seborrheic
dermatitis. Moreover, perifollicular accentuation is not so straightforward to diagnose, even by a seasoned clinician. In a case-control study performed in children
less than two years of age, only 7 out of 29 examined minor criteria have been met
in more than one-fourth of these infants. Those seven best minor criteria were xerosis (100%), course influenced by environmental factors (87%), facial erythema (54%),
skin reactions provoked by ingested food (39%), itch when sweating (34%), positive
skin prick test (29%), and hand eczema (28%). Because course influenced by external factor is particularly vague, facial erythema redundant with a major feature in
infants, prick testing beyond usual clinical examination, and itch when sweating is
not always testable in young children—a new modified and simplified set of criteria, partly adapted from the U.K. Working Party criteria, has been proposed, shown
in Table 1(B).

DIFFERENTIAL DIAGNOSIS AND SYNDROMIC FORMS

In infants, inflammatory skin disorders are largely dominated by AD, with a spectrum of clinical features that usually permit to identify the disease. However, several
differential diagnoses should be mentioned because the high frequency of AD cases
may blur the clinical acumen and lead to incorrect AD diagnoses.

Scabies is still a very prevalent condition, even in developed countries, and
may start from the first week of age. In our practice, scabies appear to be the main
differential diagnosis of AD; indeed, it is not so rare to rectify a diagnosis of AD

TABLE 1   Diagnostic Criteria for Infantile Atopic Eczema

(A) Modified Hanifin and Rajka's criteria for infants (Sampson, 1990)	
Major features	Family history of atopic dermatitis (9)
	Evidence of pruritic dermatitis
	Typical facial or extensor eczematous or lichenified dermatitis
	Napkin area and/or facial mouth/nose area is free of skin lesions
Minor features	Xerosis/ichthyosis/hyperlinear palms
	Periauricular fissures
	Chronic scalp scaling
	Perifollicular accentuation
(B) Criteria for atopic dermatitis in infants adapted from U.K. Working Party (Taïeb and Boralevi, 2006)	
Mandatory feature (10)	Evidence of relapsing itchy skin condition (duration more than 3 wk)
Other features (3 or more)	Head dermatitis leaving free mouth, nose, and orbital skin
	Pure extensor or mixed extensor/flexor dermatitis
	Absence of napkin area involvement
	Xerosis, diffuse
	Hand eczema
	Skin reactions following food ingestion
	History of atopic disease in a first-degree relative

loosely made, and to find that a scaly itchy dermatosis of several weeks or months duration was indeed scabies. In infantile scabies, face may be involved (Fig. 6) and some criteria should help the physician such as vesicles and pustules that involve the palms and soles, and purplish persistent nodules that involve the upper part of the trunk, especially the axillary areas. The other features that may be helpful to diagnose scabies are similar to those of adults, including shared pruritus between family members or relatives, scabious burrows, increased pruritus at night, or

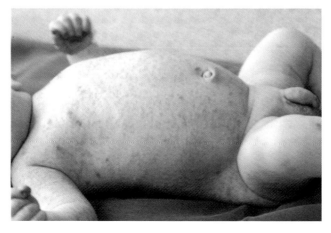

FIGURE 6   Infantile scabies. Eczema-like rash associated with specific lesions.

TABLE 2 Differential Diagnosis of Infantile Atopic Eczema

Conditions considered	Major differential points
Scabies	Palmoplantar involvement, scabious burrow, axillary nodules, familial pruritus
Acropustulosis of infancy	Plantar/lateroplantar and palmar involvement
Infantile seborrheic dermatitis and psoriasis	Bipolar rash with scalp and napkin area involvement, well-demarcated patches, involvement of major folds, no or mild pruritus
Langerhans cell histiocytosis	Papular and sometimes purpuric rash. Pruritus mild or absent. Biopsy
Miliaria rubra	Transient, heat induced, pruritus mild or absent
APEC (asymmetric perifexural exanthem of childhood)	May last up to 4 mo; Early asymmetric stage of eruption
Gianotti-Crosti syndrome	May include papulovesicular lesions on limbs and face, sometimes pruriginous Lymph nodes enlargement, virus induced
Keratosis pilaris	No pruritus, stable, palpation of lesions
Frictional lichenoid eruption of childhood	Elbows, dorsum of hands, seasonal variation, pruritus variable
Eosinophilic pustulosis of infancy	Starts mostly on scalp with recurrent crops of pustules. Associated hypereosinophilia

worsening lesions with topical steroids. Treatment of scabies with topical steroids may lead to the clinical presentation of erythrodermic/crusted scabies which may be uneasy to recognize and may disseminate further the disease to the community in a short period of time.

A list of common and less common differential diagnoses that may be mentioned in infancy is summarized in Table 2. Some of them are common, transient, and benign conditions, such as seborrheic dermatitis or miliaria rubra. A wrong diagnosis of AD is not prejudicial to the patients in those cases. APEC (asymmetric perifexural exanthem of childhood) and Gianotti-Crosti syndrome appear to be clinically different but may be mentioned here because in our practice such cases have been sometimes referred to us with a suspected diagnosis of AD. In cases seen at onset of symptoms, the major criterion of chronicity and relapsing course is lacking and the interpretation must remain cautious. In difficult cases, a biopsy should be taken, especially to rule out a case of Langerhans cell histiocytosis.

Thus, in all infants presenting with "eczema," a history needs to be obtained, and they must be examined thoroughly including growth assessment, mucous membranes inspection, lymph node and abdominal palpation, and pulmonary auscultation. If abnormal findings are encountered, such as growth or psychomotor retardation, unusual and/or repeated infections, unexplained fever, facial dysmorphism, purpura, specific investigations must be implemented to diagnose an inheritable disorder in which eczema-like lesions may be frequently observed. Those conditions are summarized in Table 3.

COMPLICATIONS
Cutaneous superinfections such as staphylococcal infections and eczema herpeticum are the most common and may require emergency procedures. The proneness to both types of superinfection has been related to an insufficient local production of antimicrobial peptides, namely, human β-defensins in staphylococcal

TABLE 3 Inheritable Disorders Associated with Atopic Eczema or Eczema-Like Lesions

Disorder	Inheritance (gene)	Main features
Hypohidrotic ectodermal dysplasia (Christ Siemens Touraine syndrome)	XLR or AR (ED1/EDA)	Hypohydrosis, hypotrichosis and microdontia/hypodontia/adontia
Wiskott Aldrich syndrome	XLR (WASP)	Purpura due to thrombocytopenia and small-sized platelets, recurrent infections due to T-lymphocytes dysfunction
Hyper-IgE syndrome (Job-Buckley syndrome)	Sporadic/AD (STAT-3)	Skin and scalp abcesses, pyogenic deep infections, coarse facies, high IgE level
Comel-Netherton syndrome	AR (SPINK5)	Ichthyosiform dermatosis, hair shaft abnormalities, infections, neonatal dehydratation
IPEX syndrome (immune dysregulation, polyendocrinopathy, enteropathy, X-linked)	AR (Foxp3)	Defective development of CD4+ CD25+ regulatory T cells, severe autoimmune enteropathy, thyroiditis, and type 1 diabetes
Dubowitz syndrome	AR	Craniofacial abnormalities, growth retardation, and mental retardation

Abbreviations: AR, autosomal recessive; AD, autosomal dominant; XLR, X-linked recessive.

infections and cathelicidin in herpes infection. Growth failure may be considered, especially in severe AD, with frequent monitoring of developmental milestones.

Staphylococcal Infections

Staphylococcus aureus constantly colonizes AD skin, as previously shown on involved and noninflammatory adult skin. The skin of infants and young children with AD also exhibits a striking susceptibility to staphylococcus colonization with a prevalence of 80% in two-year-old children. A linear increase in *S. aureus* counts with increasing severity of AD has been shown, indicating that it may play a role in the pathophysiology of AD. Indeed, the limits between acute weeping lesions and clinical impetigo are not easy to determine. Extensive oozing and crusting, even when *S. aureus* is found in bacteriologic examination of skin swabs, may be caused by severe AD flares and requires only topical treatment. Nevertheless, bullae suggest a diagnosis of bacterial superinfection and prompt a systemic treatment with antibiotics to avoid bacteremia and deep localizations.

TABLE 4 Graded Approach Situating Allergy Testing Within General Management of Infantile Atopic Eczema

Minor forms	SCORAD <15: emollients, counseling (including diet)
Moderate forms	SCORAD 15–40: id + topical steroids ± macrolactam derivatives ± anti-H1 and antibiotics during flares; allergy workup if more than 30 g/mo topical steroids
Severe forms	SCORAD >40: id + compliance assessment, hospitalization if needed, consider other treatments if no response to dermatologic treatments and allergen avoidance

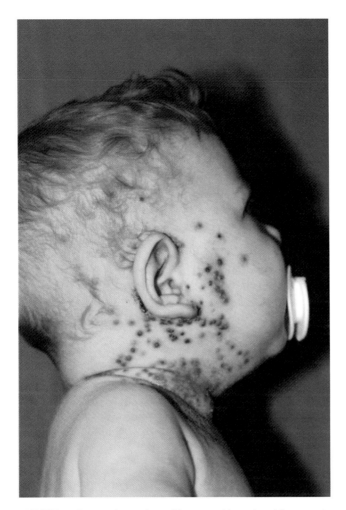

FIGURE 7 Eczema herpeticum. Monomorphic and rapidly extensive vesicles.

Eczema Herpeticum

Eczema herpeticum is a widespread herpes simplex virus infection that appears during primary infection or recurrence. Even when localized or mild lesions exist, eczema herpeticum may be considered as a potential life-threatening condition because cases of widespread and disseminated herpetic lesions complicated with dehydratation and death have been reported. Clinical features are characterized by a rapid change in the aspect of the skin with the presence of usually monomorphic extensive vesicles (Fig. 7), dome-shaped blisters and pustules in the eczematous areas. In infants, extensive vesicular lesions associated with severe systemic illness must lead to the prescription of an emergency appropriate for antiviral treatment. Herpes involvement should best be confirmed by rapid diagnostic tests.

Unlike herpes simplex infection, varicella and other herpesviridae infections are usually not more severe in infants with atopic eczema.

Growth Failure

Growth failure is usually correlated with severe atopic eczema and sleeplessness due to nocturnal pruritus. The monitoring of growth and development is mandatory as part of clinical evaluation of infants with atopic eczema. Other causes must be ruled out, such as intrauterine growth retardation, growth hormone deficiency, celiac disease, cystic fibrosis, etc. False-positive sweat tests have been already reported in this last setting. When infantile eczema is properly treated, growth and development resume a normal pattern. The role of topical steroids is frequently put forward but exceptionally causative of growth retardation.

Contact Dermatitis

Contact dermatitis is induced by skin contact with low-molecular-weight chemicals such as haptens. A higher prevalence of contact dermatitis has been previously reported in AD, but this particular association remains controversial since recent studies have shown that AD barrier genetic factors may modify susceptibility to contact allergens.

However, children and infants with AD should be investigated when unusual sites are involved or when the response to conventional treatment is poor, knowing they may develop contact dermatitis to various dressing accessories, namely, shoes, clothes, diaper, shin guards, or to topical products. The so-called Lucky Luke napkin dermatitis is a good example in infants, leading to localized eczema that features the area of contact.

PROGNOSIS

Until recently, AD was considered mostly as a pediatric disease, with usual recovery during later childhood except in a subgroup of patients. Later age at onset and females were thus considered as bad prognosis factors. Several more recent cohort studies have led to less optimistic results, showing that about 40% of infants will probably have persistent or recurrent AD features during childhood. Infantile severe cases are probably more prone to be long lasting, and asthma will develop in around 40% of infants with atopic eczema with at least one first degree relative with atopic disease—either AD, asthma, or allergic rhinitis.

MANAGEMENT

Management Plan to Communicate Efficiently with the Parents

A first attack of AD is a challenging situation for the child, his/her parents, and—certainly—for the doctor. Some items of rudimentary pathophysiology should be explained to the family, such as the primary epidermal barrier abnormalities that lead to more frequent sensitizations to indoor and outdoor allergens. Then, natural history should be discussed, stressing the chronicity of the disease and the recurrent flares that have not always clear allergic explanations. If the family has already been through Internet information, it may be useful to take some time to discuss about the information they found. And finally, it is equally important to assure the parents that this disease is, in most cases, controllable through correct treatment and that it has frequently a good prognosis. Early and proactive management is recommended to improve the quality of life and the outcome for patients with AD.

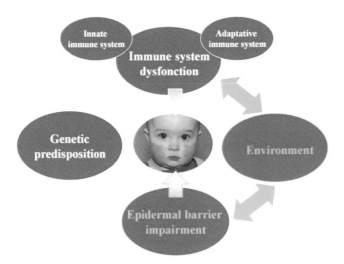

FIGURE 8 A simple figure that mentions the main outlines of the pathophysiology of AD may be useful to explain the disease to the parents.

Education and Compliance

The parents need to adhere to a therapeutic project delineated in common with the physician in charge. A specialized and dedicated management of infants with atopic eczema is often lacking, and the parents are frequently discouraged by previous unskilled counseling and contradictory views given on the situation of their child. Living with an infant with eczema may be a troublesome experience, due to lack of sleep in both infant and parents, as well as various worrisome effects on everyday life such as diet, time for treatment, stigmatization, etc.

Informing the family on the disease and its course, followed by an explanation on how to perform or better local treatments by a practical demonstration of skin care by a nurse on the child, is important to de-dramatize the situation. Explanations must be clear and specific on the various segments of care, and key points have to be repeated. Brochures, videos may help but cannot replace the time shared with the doctor and/or nurse. A priority for planning care is to assess previous treatments, especially amounts of topical steroids used and how they were used, and to check individually the patient's aggravating factors.

Following are the major points of the information given to the family:

1. *AD is not a mysterious disease*: Even though our knowledge of the pathophysiology remains incomplete and is continuously progressive, we should be able to stress some major mechanisms that lead to develop AD, if necessary, by using a simple diagram or figure that mentions the main outlines (Fig. 8). For example, it appears that explanations regarding, on one hand, the genetically determined primary epidermal impairment, and on the other hand, the close interactions with environmental factors, including allergens and microbial agents, may be easy to understand for the families. This educational approach seems important to avoid too frequent resort to alternative treatments such as faith practices.

2. *Atopic eczema is a chronic condition*: Its treatment must be identically chronic. This point must be clarified and repeated during the planning of therapy, whose aim is to improve significantly the cutaneous status of the child. The perspective of a cure can be discussed but is not the closest objective.

3. *Topical treatment is mandatory*: Local care allows to decrease the skin inflammation and to restore the cutaneous barrier compromised by the dermatitis. Inhaled steroids for asthma could be used as an example to persuade the family that local care is equivalent for skin of a long-term treatment.

4. *Topical corticosteroids are efficacious and do not harm when used properly under medical supervision*: Their inadequate use or under use is the major cause of both a feeling of helplessness and of rejection of local therapies in some families. Physicians share their part of responsibility in widespread corticophobia and in this suboptimal use of active treatments.

5. *In 2008, topical calcineurin inhibitors (TCI) may be considered as a safe and effective alternative treatment*: The therapeutic class of TCI, including tacrolimus and pimecrolimus, may be used as an alternative to topical corticosteroids, particularly in case of marked cutaneous atrophy—a rare finding in infants—or to treat facial lesions. In 2005, a few lymphoma (skin and nonskin) cases were reported in AD patients, leading to a FDA boxed warning regarding the use of topical calcineurin inhibitor. However, it is not possible to determine whether these cases represent more than would be expected in the population of patients with AD, as the exact exposure in terms of patient number is not known. Moreover, those cases were not EBV-positive B-cell lymphoma as it might be expected in immunosuppressed patients. Finally, preliminary results from long-term studies do not show an increased risk of malignancy compared to the general population.

6. *Alternatives to topical treatments associated to environment and if necessary diet control are limited*: They should be carefully weighted against conventional approaches based on the previous compliance to a basic skin therapy regimen. As it is the case for the use of systemic treatments, failure of an adequately administered topical treatment is of utmost importance for deciding allergy testing, which is best envisaged as a part of therapy or management leading, based on medically sound arguments to environmental or diet changes. In severe forms, hospital admission remains justified to complete education and perform adequately allergy or other tests.

7. *Information about aggravating factors must be given*: Explanations and counseling need to be adapted to the level of understanding of the family, in a relaxed, nontense atmosphere, where the family complaints should be taken seriously. A 45-minute visit is commonly required initially. However, even a long visit and brochures and video in addition are frequently not enough. A follow-up visit checking compliance to educational principles, with the help of a specialist nurse, is particularly useful. In case of management success, the family becomes autonomous and responsible, which is the best sign of a successful "transfer of technology."

Practical Implementation of Treatment

According to systematic reviews of treatments of atopic eczema, only few treatments are evidence based, and the reviews by Hoare et al. and Callen et al. are mandatory readings for those interested in this subject. The following section (11,12) is not evidence based but is based on personal experience and involvement in clinical research.

Decreasing Inflammation and Pruritus

Decreasing inflammation and pruritus is the major aim to help rapidly the patient. In most cases, topical treatments can treat efficiently atopic eczema flares and no systemic treatment is required.

Cleansing: The skin must be cleansed thoroughly to get rid of crusts and mechanically eliminate bacterial contaminants. The ideal cleanser should be very mild to avoid irritant dermatitis, and be very simple to avoid allergic dermatitis. Cleansers with or without antiseptics (the duration of action of antiseptics is very limited, thus mechanical cleansing is probably more important) can be used in non-irritant and low allergic formulae available in various galenic forms (soaps, syndets, aqueous solutions). In infants, it is easier to perform this first stage of gentle cleansing of skin on the nappy mattress rather than directly in the bathtub. A further cleansing followed by a rapid rinse is performed in the bath (33–34°C, not more than five minutes). The short duration of the bath is designed to avoid epidermal dehydration. Topical products are easy to apply on a skin, still lightly humid, gently dried by padding with a towel, avoiding energetic friction.

Topical antibiotics (e.g., sodium fusidate cream or mupirocine ointment) are not mandatory therapies, and in most cases it is safe to use corticosteroids directly in acute flares. However, when superinfection is obvious, the use of topical antibiotics may be useful. In the latter case, topical antibiotics should be applied for 5–7 days but not longer in order to avoid bacterial resistance.

Topical corticosteroid, in the potent or moderately potent range, may be used once daily until clearance or frank improvement (4–8 days in routine practice). Progressive interruption is not required. The amount of topical corticosteroid monthly applied is a relevant parameter to evaluate AD severity.

According to the current approval situation, topical calcineurin inhibitors can only be used as a second-line treatment in patients with insufficient improvement after topical corticosteroids. Pimecrolimus and tacrolimus, applied twice daily, proved to be effective with an overall good safety profile. A transient burning sensation of the skin is a frequent side effect that needs to be mentioned to the patients. Both pimecrolimus and tacrolimus have been tested in clinical trials in infants, but approval for individuals below 2 years of age has not been granted so far.

Tubular gauzes are most helpful to dress the young patient (after application of treatment) for the first days in severe cases requiring inpatient care. Tubifast® gauzes impregnated with topical corticosteroids have been mostly advocated by U.K. dermatologists, but their use is rather cumbersome and they have not been evaluated against standard care as outlined above. However, the use of wet-wrap dressings with diluted topical corticosteroids is a more efficacious treatment than wet-wrap dressings with emollients only.

Systemic treatment: There is a very limited access to systemic drug treatment in infants with atopic eczema. Oral antihistamines (anti-H1) are of questionable interest for long-term treatment of infantile atopic eczema, but may be helpful to decrease pruritus and permit sleep during flares. In this setting, sedative anti-H1 molecules such as hydroxyzine are frequently considered as more helpful than recent less sedative drugs.

Maintenance treatment includes intermittent use of topical corticosteroids or calcineurin inhibitors on inflammatory skin according to needs (pruritus, sleeplessness, new flare). Generally, a small amount of topical corticosteroids twice to thrice weekly (monthly amounts in the mean range of 15g), associated with a liberal use of emollients (monthly amounts in the range of 300–400g), allows a good maintenance with SCORAD values below 15 to 20. Such monthly amounts of even potent topical steroids in children below two years of age do not have adverse systemic or local effects. The need to use different potency of topical corticosteroids according to site treated or phase of treatment (induction/maintenance) is not currently the matter of a consensus among experts.

Improving the Cutaneous Barrier

Predisposing barrier anomalies have recently been demonstrated in AD, both in clinical and genetic studies, and may lead to easier early allergen introduction through the skin and more proneness to irritancy and subsequent cutaneous inflammation. Filaggrin null mutations and their consequences on epidermal impairment, on one hand, and a lack of important stratum corneum intercellular lipids or an inadequate ratio between compounds (cholesterol, essential fatty acids, ceramides), on the other hand, enhance transepidermal water loss and may favor AD development and asthma exacerbations. A better knowledge of this predisposing background should give access to nonimmunosuppressive and more specific barrier-improving topicals usable in infancy.

Currently, there are numerous available products composed of water, occlusive agents, humidifiers, tensioactive agents, preservatives, perfumes, etc. Their short-term efficacy have been demonstrated on TEWL and AD improvement, but no study has shown superiority of one product over the another. The cost of high-quality allergy-safe emollients refrains generally their use because such products are considered as nonprescription drugs, and the quantities needed are usually high (150–300 g/wk). Their direct use on inflamed skin is poorly tolerated, and it appears better to treat the acute flare first as outlined before applying moisturizers once or twice daily on the whole body.

Management of Aggravating Factors and Counseling

This time-consuming task is particularly important. The bottom line is to allow the child and family to have a life close to normal, avoiding unnecessary measures and putting too much constraint when avoidable. For example, it should be mentioned that all mandatory vaccines are safe, including those against measles in hen's egg allergy. Thus, the severity may guide the choices of the adviser (Table 4).

Identification and Avoidance of Allergens

The allergic part of AD remains a debated matter and some authors still doubt of its relevance relative to cutaneous symptoms, raising the question of the real need of allergy testing. Randomized controlled studies of avoidance interventions are lacking, or when performed (e.g., mattress encasings for HDM avoidance) provide conflicting results. Indeed, most opinions are derived of observational studies. In minor and moderate forms of AD, given the prevalence of the disease, the cost-effectiveness of allergy investigations and allergen avoidance measures must be taken into account and no systematic allergy testing should be performed. But in severe forms, for example, those resisting to conventional treatments, a comprehensive allergy workup is required to avoid blindly prescribed diets. A specialized management is thus highly recommended to choose the most appropriate test(s) and the allergens series to be used.

The help of a dietician is also needed to implement and assess avoidance diets in infants.

Food Allergens

About one-third of infants with moderate-to-severe AD have immediate reactions (e.g., urticarial rashes, gut symptoms, wheezing, etc.) to at least one major food allergen. Late reactions, namely, eczema worsening, occur rarely. The usual diagnostic approach is to perform skin-prick tests with commercial extracts or fresh foods after careful history taking, and, if positive, to propose single- or double-blind placebo-controlled oral food challenges (OFC) after a period of avoidance of incriminated foods. A clear history of immediate reaction is sufficient to bypass this procedure. In clinical practice, it is not possible to make clear conclusions concerning late reactions, and most data concerning food allergy in infants with AD are derived from immediate reactions. The benefit of avoidance diets following positive food challenges is variable, suggesting that if foods aggravate eczema, they represent only a fraction of the expression of the disease. It is noteworthy that food allergy symptoms may persist after clearance of eczema but that the reverse holds also true (tolerance to foods with persisting eczema). As simpler techniques need to be implemented to diagnose food allergy, the labial food challenge has been proposed to be used in outpatients, but gives poor sensitivity and specificity when compared to the OFC.

Contact Allergens

A bad or incomplete response to treatment or the need to increase amounts of topical steroids, the involvement of areas usually not involved in AD should prompt contact allergy testing. The interpretation of patch tests in infants is sometimes difficult, and irritant reactions are especially common with metals. A restricted battery usable in infants and children has been proposed, because of lack of space to test all products and of the possible risk of sensitizing patients.

Aeroallergens

Patch test positivity to pollens, house dust mite, and less frequently animal dander is surprisingly high in infants, averaging 80% in infants of less than one year of age. Clear positive reactions encourage both parents and physician to apply avoidance measures.

PREVENTION

Primary prevention is a major goal given the burden of disease and possible later respiratory involvement. In utero sensitization to allergens is poorly manageable, and at risk babies have been submitted to various interventions without frank success. Substitutes to mother's milk such as highly hydrolyzed casein or amino acids have been tested in controlled studies in high-risk infants, and may decrease the severity of symptoms without affecting sensitization profiles. Delaying the introduction of solid foods until six months is generally advocated by pediatricians keenly preoccupied by allergy because it has been shown that early solid feeding increases eczema and food allergy incidence. Cow's milk and egg avoidance in the first four months in mothers decreases atopic eczema, but most physicians are reluctant to implement such measures, which need dietician supervision. Probiotics, especially lactobacillus BB, given to at risk newborns have been shown to decrease by half the incidence of atopic eczema at age of two years, without decreasing allergen sensitization, possibly due to regulatory cytokine stimulation in the intestine (TGF β and IL10). Gamma linolenic supplementation in high-risk infants has also been tested and found beneficial. The presence of furred pets in the baby's environment is a matter of debate, since recent studies do not indicate an increased risk or rather a protective factor, but the definition of at risk groups in the studies needs possibly further improvement.

Secondary prevention is important when the diagnosis of AD is established. However, limited validated data exist suggesting a better short- and long-term outcome following interventions, concerning both the course of eczema and that of asthma/rhinitis.

REFERENCES

1. Worldwide variation in prevalence of symptoms of asthma, allergic rhinoconjunctivitis, and atopic eczema: ISAAC. The International Study of Asthma and Allergies in Childhood (ISAAC) Steering Committee. Lancet 1998; 351(9111):1225–1232.
2. Wadonda-Kabondo N, Sterne JA, Golding J, et al. A prospective study of the prevalence and incidence of atopic dermatitis in children aged 0–42 months. Br J Dermatol 2003; 149(5):1023–1028.
3. Boralevi F, Hubiche T, Leaute-Labreze C, et al. Epicutaneous aeroallergen sensitization in atopic dermatitis infants—Determining the role of epidermal barrier impairment. Allergy 2008; 63(2):205–210.
4. Thestrup-Pedersen K. Clinical aspects of atopic dermatitis. Clin Exp Dermatol 2000; 25(7):535–543.
5. Bonifazi E, Meneghini CL. Atopic dermatitis in the first six months of life. Acta Derm Venereol Suppl (Stockh) 1989; 144:20–22.
6. Aoki T, Kojima M, Adachi J, Okano M, et al. Effect of short-term egg exclusion diet on infantile atopic dermatitis and its relation to egg allergy: A single-blind test. Acta Derm Venereol Suppl (Stockh) 1992; 176:99–102.
7. Severity scoring of atopic dermatitis: The SCORAD index. Consensus Report of the European Task Force on Atopic Dermatitis. Dermatology 1993; 186(1):23–31.
8. Williams HC, Burney PJ, Hay RJ, et al. The U. K. Working Party's Diagnostic Criteria for Atopic Dermatitis. I. Derivation of a minimum set of discriminators for atopic dermatitis. Br J Dermatol 1994; 131(3):383–396.
9. Sampson H. Pathogenesis of eczema. Clin Exp Allergy 1990; 20:459–67.
10. Taieb A & Boralevi F. Atomic eczema in infants. In Ring J. Przybella B, Ruzicka T, ed. Handbook of atopic eczema 2nd ed. Springer, 2006; 45–53.
11. Hoare C, Li Wan Po A, William H. Systematic review of treatments for atopic dermatitis. Health Technol Assess 2000; 4:1–191.
12. Callen J, Chamlin S, Eichenfield LF, et al. A systematic review of the safety of topical therapies for atopic dermatitis. Br J Dermatol 2007; 156:203–21.

20 Specific Immunotherapy in Atopic Dermatitis

Thomas Werfel

Department Immunodermatology and Allergy Research, Hannover Medical School, Hannover, Germany

SUMMARY

Atopic dermatitis (AD) is one of the most frequent chronic inflammatory skin diseases with an increasing prevalence, affecting 10% to 20% of children and 1% to 3% of adults in industrialized countries. About 80% of adult AD patients belong to the subgroup with sensitizations against different aeroallergens and food allergens, which may be pivotal for eczema flare-ups and maintenance. Therefore, in addition to local and systemic therapy adjusted to the stage of the disease, the search for relevant trigger factors and consecutively their avoidance plays a crucial role in the reduction or even prevention of flare-ups. Although allergen-specific immunotherapy (SIT) is widely and most effectively used in allergy to insect venoms and allergic rhinitis, its use in AD is still controversially discussed. In recent clinical studies, it could be shown that SIT appears to be a promising approach for the treatment of patients with AD and leads to clinical improvement of eczema as well as subjective symptoms like pruritus and sleeplessness. Despite these encouraging data, the use of SIT as a therapeutic approach in the routine treatment of AD requires further evaluation in the near future.

THE ROLE OF ALLERGENS IN ATOPIC ECZEMA

AD is one of the most common skin diseases, which is characterized by a chronic course and intensive itching. AD belongs together with allergic rhinitis, conjunctivitis, and allergic bronchial asthma to the so-called atopic diseases.

Acute eczematous lesions are characterized by erythema, oozing, and crusting, whereas chronic lesions show thickened skin and papules. Pruritus and sleeplessness are further characteristics of AD. In addition to local and systemic therapy adjusted to the stage of the disease, the search for relevant trigger factors and consecutively their avoidance plays a crucial role in the reduction or even prevention of flare-ups. A causal therapy of AD is not available yet and the complexity of the disease leads to a polypragmatic therapeutic management (1,2).

The majority of patients are sensitized to inhalant or food allergens. Sensitizations to house dust mite allergens, which are detectable with specific IgE tests, are very common in adolescence and adult patients (1–3).

A T-cell–mediated delayed reaction is critical for the worsening of skin eczema, which can be triggered by the epicutaneous application of house dust mite or other protein allergens in sensitized patients (4,5). House dust mite antigens are able to penetrate into the skin where they are trapped via specific IgE, which is bound on high affinity Fc-receptors on Langerhans cells or other antigen presenting cells (APC). APC may subsequently present allergens to T-lymphocytes leading to a specific T-cell–proliferation and manifestation of skin eczema (6). Allergen-specific

T-cells have been shown both in acute reactions elucidated by the application of allergens onto the skin and in chronic skin lesions in AD in sensitized patients.

ALLERGEN-SPECIFIC IMMUNOTHERAPY

SIT represents the only specific treatment form that provides long-lasting amelioration of allergic symptoms. In most countries it is approved for patients with allergic rhinitis, mild asthma, and insect venom allergy. Administration of the allergens during SIT via both the subcutaneous and the sublingual routes has been established as long-term treatment. Overall, there is a longer practical experience available with subcutaneous SIT as compared to sublingual SIT. From current meta-analyses on the treatment of respiratory diseases with SIT, subcutaneous SIT appears to be more effective than that of sublingual SIT. On the other hand, no dangerous or fatal reactions have been described so far for sublingual SIT, which is not the case for subcutaneous SIT. Irrespective of the route of application, SIT reduces the symptoms of respiratory disease as well as the amount of medications required.

The main goal of SIT is to induce allergen-specific tolerance. The most important target cells addressed by SIT are T-cells, B-cells, APC, and different effectors cells (7). Decreased mediator released by mast cells and basophils has been observed upon the treatment with SIT and IgE-facilitated antigen presentation by dendritic cells has been shown to be impaired after SIT (8).

SIT has been described to generate allergen-specific T regulatory cells, including $CD4^+CD25^+$ T regulatory cells and inducible type 1 T-regulatory cells, which suppress proliferative responses to the specific allergen. Obviously, this is closely related to the development of allergen-specific tolerance.

Moreover, a change of cytokine polarization from Th2 towards Th1 has been observed during SIT, which is also regarded as a crucial event related to this form of therapy. This change of cytokine pattern may be related to the decrease of IgE and the increase of the amount and activity of blocking allergen-specific antibodies of the IgG1- and IgG4-type, which has further been observed as a phenomenon attending SIT (8).

In addition, increase of allergen-specific IgA2 in parallel to the increase of transforming growth factor-beta produced locally in the peripheral organs is suspected to contribute to the SIT-related induction of allergen-specific tolerance (9).

THE EFFECTS OF SPECIFIC IMMUNOTHERAPY IN AD

As mentioned above, SIT has proven to be effective mainly in respiratory IgE-mediated allergic diseases (10,11). The theoretical objection that SIT may lead to a deterioration of AD by boosting the cell-mediated immune response has somewhat hampered studies on the efficacy of SIT in AD in the past, although this has never been proven in controlled studies so far.

Darsow et al. recently reviewed a number of controlled studies that were performed in patients with not only respiratory allergy but also in patients who in addition suffered from AD. In these studies an improvement not only of allergic rhinitis and allergic asthma bronchiale but also of the skin condition was observed (12). Moreover, a number of open observational studies directly addressing AD published before 1990 pointed to a positive effect of SIT in AD (13–15).

Table 1 summarizes the most important case histories and series and controlled studies on SIT in AD.

TABLE 1 Case Reports and Clinical Studies Regarding Specific Immunotherapy for AD Patients

Authors	Type of publication	Number (age) of subjects	SIT procedure	Period of SIT	Study objective	Outcome
Di Prisco de Fuenmajor and Champion (13)	Controlled study	15 (6–14 yrs)	Subcutaneous		Clinical findings	Positive
Galli et al. (17)	Controlled study	42 in active group 18 in control group (0.5–12 yrs)	Oral	3 yrs	Clinical findings	Negative
Leroy et al. (16)	Double-blinded, placebo-controlled study	24 (17–61 yrs)	Intradermal injection of allergen–antibody complexes	1 yr	Clinical findings, Dpt-specific IgG	Positive
Mastrandrea et al. (22)	Cohort study	35	Sublingual	3 yrs	Clinical findings	Positive
Michils et al. (36)	Case report	1 (21 yrs)	First subcutaneous, second oral	1 st 6 wks, 2nd 7 mos	Clinical findings, total-IgE, specific IgE against dog epithelium	Positive
Mosca et al. (21)	Cohort study	41 and 48	Subcutaneous vs. sublingual	3 yrs	Clinical findings, drug consumption	Positive
Pacor et al. (23)	Study with control group	32	Subcutaneous	3 yrs	Clinical findings, skin-prick-test, total-IgE and Dpt-specific IgE	Positive, but no change in total-IgE
Pajno et al. (38)	Double-blinded, placebo-controlled study	56 (5–16 yrs)	Sublingual	18 mos	Clinical findings, topical steroid consumption	Positive for mild to severe AD, SCORAD <40
Petrova et al. (29)	Placebo-controlled study	99 (16–52 yrs)	Oral		Clinical findings	Positive
Ring (30)	Case report, placebo-controlled study	Monozygotic twins (10 yrs)	Subcutaneous	1 yr	Clinical findings	Positive
Silny and Czarnecka-Operacz (32)	Double-blinded, placebo-controlled study	20 (5–40 yrs)	Subcutaneous	1 yr	Clinical findings, total-IgE and Dpt-specific IgE	Positive, dropping of Dpt-specific IgE
Werfel et al. (34)	Double-blinded, placebo-controlled study	89 (18–55 yrs)	Subcutaneous	1 yr	Clinical findings, topical steroid consumption	Positive

The first double-blind placebo-controlled study which was reported to be effective in AD used allergen–antibody complexes (16), which have, however, not been used in clinical practice thereafter. It is still not known how these allergen–antibody complexes that contain autologous specific antibodies and house dust mite allergens work on a molecular or cellular basis. However, this study served as an early hint that the treatment approach with SIT might be beneficial in AD.

A further "early" unique study, which, however, provided negative results, was flawed by the ineffective oral route of extract administration (17). This study is sometimes cited because of the controlled design. It should, however, not be mixed-up with later studies using the sublingual route.

In 2006, Bussmann et al. conducted a systematic literature search in the databases MEDLINE, EMBASE, and CENTRAL (18) by using the key words "atopic dermatitis" or "atopic dermatitis" and "specific immunotherapy" or "hyposensitization" for the search. They combined their literature findings with a second search for "side effects" or "adverse events" and "atopic dermatitis" or "atopic eczema" and "specific immunotherapy" or "hyposensitization" and thus identified a total of 23 articles about studies on subcutaneous or sublingual allergen SIT in AE with different allergens (18).

Ten of these studies conducted between 1974 and 2006 were observational studies (13,14,19–25), 11 were controlled studies (16,17,26–34), and 2 were classified as case reports (35,36). Five placebo-controlled studies on subcutaneous allergen SIT were comparable (26,27,32–34) and used for a statistical meta-analysis. This showed a significant improvement of symptoms in patients with AD under SIT by using the inverse normal method or the inverse x2 method (37).

Moreover, a combined statistical analysis of seven comparable observational studies (13–15,19,20,23,24) showed a mean proportion of improvement of 71% of AD under SIT, in support of the hypothesis that SIT might represent a useful additional therapeutic option for a subgroup of patients with AD (18).

In the so far largest and most recent controlled study we investigated the clinical efficacy of a subcutaneously applied immunotherapy in patients with AD by using a double-blind placebo-controlled protocol (34). The study was a multicenter, double-blind trial with patients randomly assigned to treatment with SIT with ALK-depot SQ mites and maximum concentrations of 20 SQ-U (active placebo), 2000 SQ-U and 20000 SQ-U for one year. The double-blind design of the study was realized by a "blind observer" who evaluated the SCORAD.

Prior to the treatment we assessed the patients for inclusion/exclusion criteria. The inclusion criteria were: IgE-mediated sensitization against house dust mites (CAP RAST FEIA class $\geq$ 3), SCORAD score $>$ 40 points, age between 18 and 55 years, a chronic course of AD.

Patients were randomized into three dose groups for treatment with subcutaneous SIT with ALK-depot SQ Dermatophagoides pteronyssinus/farinae: group 1 ("active placebo"): constant dose of 20 SQ-U, group 2: maintenance dose of 2000 SQ-U, group 3: maintenance dose 20000 SQ-U. Therapy was started in all groups with 20 SQ-U. All injections were given at weekly intervals.

Treatment of AD was individually adapted to the clinical severity. Topical corticosteroids of European classes 1 to 3 and nonsedating antihistamines with a short half-life (cetiricine, loratadine) were allowed. Moreover, basic treatment of the skin with ointments was allowed.

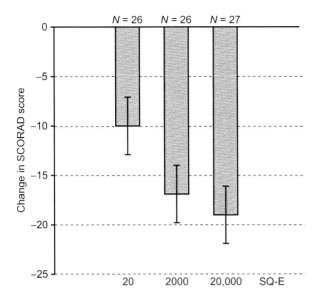

FIGURE 1 Changes from baseline to endpoint in SCORAD summary score at the end of treatment with specific immunotherapy versus baseline, mean (±SEM). *Source*: Adapted from Ref. 34.

There was a decline of the SCORAD score points in all study groups. The differences in the SCORAD between the baseline value and the values in the last three months of treatment were, significantly greater than that in groups 2 and 3 compared to group 1 (Fig. 1). The response rate as defined above was 66% in the pooled groups 2 and 3 and 46·2% in group 1.

The decline of SCORAD in the verum groups was significantly higher compared to placebo already after two months of treatment ($p < 0.05$). The differences between placebo and verum were maximal after six months of treatment ($p < 0.005$).

There was a significant difference in the application of topical corticosteroids with higher reduction in groups 2 and 3, but higher increase in group 1. Similar differences in favor of groups 2 and 3 were seen in the use of systemic antihistamines, but these were statistically less pronounced.

Markedly more patients assessed their skin to be improved or completely healed in groups 2 and 3 (61.5% and 70.4%, respectively) compared to group 1. The final assessment of the "blinded" physician confirmed a better skin condition at the end of therapy for patients from groups 2 and 3 compared to those from group 1.

Thus, allergen-SIT appears to be effective in patients with AD who are sensitized to house dust mite allergens and may be valuable in the treatment of this chronic skin disease.

SLIT FOR THE TREATMENT OF AD?

In addition to the approaches with subcutaneous application, there are also pilot studies on allergen SIT in patients with AD using the sublingual road of allergen administration with different therapeutic results (17,21,22,25). Due to different results of these studies, which cannot be directly compared due to different protocols no conclusion on the effect of SLIT on AD could be drawn in the meta-analysis published in 2006 (18).

In more recent controlled study using the sublingual route for allergen application, 56 children with AD sensitized against house dust mites were treated either with SLIT or placebo (38). The study included a build-up phase lasting 15 days and was conducted for a total of 18 months. Significant improvement measured by SCORAD in the active group was observable after 9 months of treatment, while lower use of rescue drugs in the active group was observable after 18 months. Subgroup analyses separating AD patients in patients with mild, moderate, or severe AD revealed a benefit from SLIT exclusively for children with mild-to-moderate variants of AD in this study. This is a difference to the findings using the subcutaneous route: Here, the skin of severely affected patients with AD also improved during SIT.

SIDE EFFECTS OF SIT IN STUDIES ON AD

In most studies the side effects of SIT were in most cases confined to local reactions and on the long run negligible.

In their systematic review Bussmann et al. (18) summarize the following side effects from single studies: severe exacerbation of AD were described in 2 of 15 children under SIT in one study (13) and worsening of the skin in 20% of the patients with AE was described in another study (32). A further study reported adverse reactions in 19.5% of patients with AD treated via the subcutaneous route and in 14.6% of patients with AD treated via the sublingual route (21).

With regard to side effects, it is worth noting that two patients of the active group in the most recent SLIT study being effective in mild AD (38) had to be excluded from the study due to intense generalized flush reactions occurring within one hour after sublingual allergen administration.

In particular, patients who were treated in the "active treatment" groups showed a good compliance with treatment in most clinical studies.

HOW DOES SIT WORK IN AD?

Allergen uptake by IgE receptor-bearing epidermal dendritic cells, followed by skin homing of cutaneous lymphocyte antigen-bearing T-cells, plays a central role in initiating the inflammatory process in the skin (39). Furthermore, recruitment of inflammatory cell subtypes induced by allergen challenges and directed by chemotactic signals is regarded as a causative factor for the development of the characteristic eczematous skin lesions (40). Allergen-specific T-lymphocytes and specific IgE play a key role in the initiation of these inflammatory processes.

Like in respiratory diseases, T lymphocytes are believed to be central target cells in SIT in AD. Whereas many in vitro or ex vivo studies are available for SIT in respiratory diseases or insect venom allergy, data on changes in cytokines, immunoglobulin serum levels, or chemokines or on cellular functions are rare for AD.

Three recent studies monitored the level of total and allergen-specific serum IgE (32,34,41) under SIT. In two of these studies using allergen extracts, total and allergen-specific IgE levels remained unchanged (32,34). In contrast, in one open-label study using HDM allergoid as treatment, a reduction of allergen-specific IgE after three months of SIT (and unchanged total serum IgE) has been reported (41). In this study, blocking IgG antibodies have also been evaluated, showing increasing levels of allergen-specific IgG4 already after three months in AD patients treated with SIT and a further increase after six months of treatment (41).

The same study investigated serum levels of chemokines, which go along with the disease activity such as interleukin-16 or thymus and activation-regulated chemokine (CCL17). Interestingly, in parallel to clinical improvement of the severity of the skin lesions, a decrease of serums of these chemokines was described. The authors conclude from their data that a SIT-related decrease of chemokine levels of the treated patients might generally reduce the disposition of AD patients to initiate inflammatory recruitment processes. They speculate that their observation might explain, in part, why even the treatment of a single sensitization in multisensitized AD patients would make sense, and putatively lead to improvement of the total clinical picture of these patients (41).

Two studies evaluated cytokine secretion pattern of T lymphocytes during SIT in AD. In this aspect, no significant changes were observable despite repetitive allergen challenge in SIT-treated AD patients (32,41).

During the chronification of eczema, a shift towards a TH1 cytokine pattern has been shown—this is probably relevant for not only the majority of nonspecific bystander T lymphocytes (42) but also within the allergen-specific compartment in the skin (43) in AD. Because SIT both leads to a shift from "TH2" towards "TH1" (in addition to its effects on T regulatory cells), the question can be raised why SIT should work in a TH1-polarized situation such as in chronic AD. This question is not answered yet. However, from the available clinical data it appears that on the longer runs even Th1-dominated chronic skin lesions can be influenced by allergen-SIT in sensitized patients with AD. The therapeutic effect is probably mediated by mechanisms that are effective rather in lymphatic organs bearing a Th2 milieu than that in the skin itself.

There is a high need of further studies on changes on the level of T-cells. These cells are closely related to rather specific mechanisms induced by SIT leading to activation of pathways, which result in the induction of tolerance towards a single allergen. In particular, the question if allergen-specific tolerance is mirrored by the induction of T regulatory cells in AD patients has to be addressed in further studies. Interestingly, the deregulation on the level of T regulatory cells has been reported in some recent studies on AD (44,45), which requires further evaluation in studies with SIT in this disease.

FUTURE DIRECTIONS OF SPECIFIC IMMUNOTHERAPY IN AD

Further double-blind placebo-controlled studies conducted in adults and children with AD by using different types of allergens are necessary. At least two studies fulfilling the criteria of randomized prospective phase III studies are currently being performed. Such studies are highly needed for a putative approval of SIT for the treatment of AD.

Further studies are also needed to evaluate which subgroups of patients with AD do benefit from SIT and which groups do not. Since most of the adults with AD are multisensitized, it is desirable to develop valuable readout criteria to select the most relevant allergens for SIT in individual patients in the future.

SIT cannot replace allergen avoidance or at least allergen reduction. In particular, during the build-up phase of SIT as well as during the allergen season, environmental control must still be recommended. Perennial allergens such as house dust mites should generally be reduced (also some conflicting results on the effects of encasing of bed mattresses have been published in the past). Future studies should address relation between allergen avoidance measures and the success rate of SIT in AD.

SIT has been shown to prevent further sensitizations in respiratory diseases. For AD it would be interesting particular in young patients if successful SIT is also preventive in that aspect and if—perhaps even more important—SIT can influence the so-called atopic march from AD to respiratory diseases.

REFERENCES

1. Akdis CA, Akdis M, Bieber T, et al. Diagnosis and treatment of atopic dermatitis in children and adults: European Academy of Allergology and Clinical Immunology/American Academy of Allergy, Asthma and Immunology/PRACTALL Consensus Report. Allergy 2006; 61:969–987.
2. Akdis CA, Akdis M, Bieber T, et al. Diagnosis and treatment of atopic dermatitis in children and adults: European Academy of Allergology and Clinical Immunology/American Academy of Allergy, Asthma and Immunology/PRACTALL Consensus Report. J Allergy Clin Immunol 2006; 118:152–169.
3. Werfel T, Kapp A. Environmental and other major provocation factors in atopic dermatitis. Allergy 1998; 53:731–739.
4. Ring J, Darsow U, Behrendt H. Role of aeroallergens in atopic eczema: Proof of concept with the atopy patch test. J Am Acad Dermatol 2001; 45:S49–S52.
5. Turjanmaa K, Darsow U, Niggemann B, et al. EAACI/GA2LEN position paper: Present status of the atopy patch test. Allergy 2006; 61:1377–1384.
6. Kluken H, Wienker T, Bieber T. Atopic eczema/dermatitis syndrome—a genetically complex disease. New advances in discovering the genetic contribution. Allergy 2003; 58:5–12.
7. Larche M, Akdis CA, Valenta R. Immunological mechanisms of allergen-specific immunotherapy. Nat Rev Immunol 2006; 6:761–771.
8. Akdis M, Akdis CA. Mechanisms of allergen-specific immunotherapy. J Allergy Clin Immunol 2007; 119:780–791.
9. Pilette C, Nouri-Aria KT, Jacobson MR, et al. Grass pollen immunotherapy induces an allergen-specific IgA2 antibody response associated with mucosal TGF-beta expression. J Immunol 2007; 178:4658–4666.
10. Malling HJ. Immunotherapy for rhinitis. Curr Allergy Asthma Rep 2003; 3:204–209.
11. Nelson HS. Advances in upper airway diseases and allergen immunotherapy. J Allergy Clin Immunol 2003; 111:S793–S798.
12. Darsow U, Fover I, Ping J. Spezifische Hyposensibilisierung bei atopischem Ekzem. Allergologie 2005; 28:53.
13. Di Prisco de Fuenmayor MC, Champion RH. Specific hyposensitization in atopic dermatitis. Br J Dermatol 1979; 101:697–700.
14. Zachariae H, Cramers M, Herlin T, et al. Non-specific immunotherapy and specific hyposensitization in severe atopic dermatitis. Acta Derm Venereol Suppl (Stockh) 1985; 114:48–54.
15. Seidenari S, Mosca M, Taglietti M, et al. Specific hyposensitization in atopic dermatitis. Dermatologica 1986; 172:229.
16. Leroy BP, Boden G, Lachapelle JM, et al. A novel therapy for atopic dermatitis with allergen–antibody complexes: A double-blind, placebo-controlled study. J Am Acad Dermatol 1993; 28:232–239.
17. Galli E, Chini L, Nardi S, et al. Use of a specific oral hyposensitization therapy to *Dermatophagoides pteronyssinus* in children with atopic dermatitis. Allergol Immunopathol (Madr) 1994; 22:18–22.

18. Bussmann C, Bockenhoff A, Henke H, et al. Does allergen-specific immunotherapy represent a therapeutic option for patients with atopic dermatitis? J Allergy Clin Immunol 2006; 118:1292–1298.
19. Grewe M. Hyposensibilisierung beim atopischen Ekzem. Allergo J 2000; 6:351–353.
20. Heijer A. Hyposensitization with aeroallergens in atopic eczema. Allergo J 1993; 2:3–7.
21. Mosca M, Albani-Rocchetti G, Vigini MA, et al. La vaccinoterapia sublinguale nella dermatite atopica. Ital Dermatol Venerol 1993; 128:79–83.
22. Mastrandrea F, Serio G, Minelli M, et al. Specific sublingual immunotherapy in atopic dermatitis. Results of a 6-year follow-up of 35 consecutive patients. Allergol Immunopathol (Madr) 2000; 28:54–62.
23. Pacor ML, Biasi D, Maleknia T. The efficacy of long-term specific immunotherapy for *Dermatophagoides pteronyssinus* in patients with atopic dermatitis. Recenti Prog Med 1994; 85:273–277.
24. Trofimowicz A, Rzepecka E, Hofman J. Clinical effects of specific immunotheraphy in children with atopic dermatitis. Rocz Akad Med Bialymst 1995; 40:414–422.
25. Zwacka G, Glaser S, Rieger B. Therapeutische Erfahrungen mit Pangramin-SLIT im Vergleich zu einer subkutanen Immuntherapie und zur symptomatischen medikamentoesen Behandlung bei Kindern mit Asthma bronchiale, Rhinokonjunktivts und atopischer Eczema. Allergologie 1996; 19:580–592.
26. Glover MT, Atherton DJ. A double-blind controlled trial of hyposensitization to *Dermatophagoides pteronyssinus* in children with atopic eczema. Clin Exp Allergy 1992; 22:440–446.
27. Kaufman HS, Roth HL. Hyposensitization with alum precipitated extracts in atopic dermatitis: A placebo-controlled study. Ann Allergy 1974; 32:321–330.
28. Noh GW, Lee KY. Blood eosinophils and serum IgE as predictors for prognosis of interferon-gamma therapy in atopic dermatitis. Allergy 1998; 53:1202–1207.
29. Petrova SI, Berzhets VM, Al'banova VI, et al. Immunotherapy in the complex treatment of patients with atopic dermatitis with sensitization to house dust mites. Zh Mikrobiol Epidemiol Immunobiol 2001; 1:33–36.
30. Ring J. Successful hyposensitization treatment in atopic eczema: Results of a trial in monozygotic twins. Br J Dermatol 1982; 107:597–602.
31. Silny W, Czarnecka-Operacz M, Silny P. Efficacy of specific immunotherapy in the treatment of children and youngsters suffering from atopic dermatitis. Part I. Evaluation of clinical score. Wiad Lek 2005; 58:47–55.
32. Silny W, Czarnecka-Operacz M. Spezifische Immuntherapie bei der Behandlung von Patienten mit atopischer Eczema. Allergologie 2006; 29:171–183.
33. Warner JO, Price JF, Soothill JF, et al. Controlled trial of hyposensitisation to *Dermatophagoides pteronyssinus* in children with asthma. Lancet 1978; 2:912–915.
34. Werfel T, Breuer K, Rueff F, et al. Usefulness of specific immunotherapy in patients with atopic dermatitis and allergic sensitization to house dust mites: A multi-centre, randomized, dose–response study. Allergy 2006; 61:202–205.
35. Chait I, Allkins V. Remission of life-long atopic dermatitis after hyposensitisation to house dust mite. Practitioner 1985; 229:609, 612.
36. Michils A, Farber CM, Van Vooren JP, et al. Sustained benefit of interferon-alpha therapy and oral hyposensitization in severe atopic dermatitis. Br J Dermatol 1994; 130:134–135.
37. Hedges L, Olkin I. Statistical Methods for Meta-Analysis. Orlando, FL: Academic Press, 1985.
38. Pajno GB, Caminiti L, Vita D, et al. Sublingual immunotherapy in mite-sensitized children with atopic dermatitis: A randomized, double-blind, placebo-controlled study. J Allergy Clin Immunol 2007; 120:164–170.
39. Kraft S, Kinet JP. New developments in FcepsilonRI regulation, function and inhibition. Nat Rev Immunol 2007; 7:365–378.
40. Homey B, Steinhoff M, Ruzicka T, et al. Cytokines and chemokines orchestrate atopic skin inflammation. J Allergy Clin Immunol 2006; 118:178–189.

41. Bussmann C, Maintz L, Hart J, et al. Clinical improvement and immunological changes in atopic dermatitis patients undergoing subcutaneous immunotherapy with a house dust mite allergoid: A pilot study. Clin Exp Allergy 2007; 37:1277–1285.
42. Cardona ID, Goleva E, Ou LS, et al. Staphylococcal enterotoxin B inhibits regulatory T cells by inducing glucocorticoid-induced TNF receptor-related protein ligand on monocytes. J Allergy Clin Immunol 2006; 117:688–695.
43. Verhagen J, Akdis M, Traidl-Hoffmann C, et al. Absence of T-regulatory cell expression and function in atopic dermatitis skin. J Allergy Clin Immunol 2006; 117:176–183.
44. Grewe M, Bruijnzeel-Koomen CA, Schopf E, et al. A role for Th1 and Th2 cells in the immunopathogenesis of atopic dermatitis. Immunol Today 1998; 19:359–361.
45. Werfel T, Morita A, Grewe M, et al. Allergen specificity of skin-infiltrating T cells is not restricted to a type-2 cytokine pattern in chronic skin lesions of atopic dermatitis. J Invest Dermatol 1996; 107:871–876.

21 Ultraviolet Phototherapy and the Management of Atopic Dermatitis

Travis Vandergriff and Heidi Jacobe
Department of Dermatology, University of Texas, Southwestern Medical Center, Dallas, Texas, U.S.A.

Atopic dermatitis (AD) is a common inflammatory disorder of the skin characterized by intense pruritus. In its acute phase, AD appears as erythematous patches and plaques with vesicles and oozing superficial erosions. Chronic AD is manifested as xerosis and thickening of the skin with prominence of skin lines known as lichenification. These changes result from repeated scratching and rubbing as patients attempt to relieve the itch. This so-called "itch–scratch cycle" is a major factor contributing to the chronicity of the disease.

A number of treatment options have been employed in the management of AD. Since their development in the 1950s, topical corticosteroids have been the mainstay of treatment. However, their long-term use is limited by the prevalence of adverse effects including epidermal atrophy, striae, telangiectasias, and suppression of the hypothalamic–pituitary–adrenal axis secondary to systemic absorption. These limitations make "steroid-sparing" agents an attractive alternative or adjunct therapy. Nonsteroidal treatment options of AD include emollients, topical calcineurin inhibitors such as pimecrolimus and tacrolimus, and oral immunomodulatory drugs like cyclosporine and azathioprine. These treatment modalities and their limitations are discussed in detail elsewhere in this text.

Ultraviolet (UV) phototherapy represents an important component of the armamentarium for treating AD. This nonpharmacologic modality has emerged as one of the most effective and well-tolerated treatments available for patients with AD. Herein, we address the role of UV phototherapy in the management of both acute and chronic AD.

A HISTORICAL PERSPECTIVE ON PHOTOTHERAPY

Phototherapy, the deliberate exposure of a patient to an external light source with the intention of treating a disease, has its origins in the medicinal practices of ancient Egyptians and Hindus (1). As early as 1400 BCE, Hindu patients with vitiligo were treated with plant extracts and exposure to sunlight (1). The medical use of sunlight is known as heliotherapy and was utilized in early 20th century Europe to treat a variety of disease ranging from psoriasis to rickets and tuberculosis (1).

The modern era of phototherapy began in Germany in 1894 when Lahmann constructed an artificial light source using a carbon arc lamp and used this device to treat a patient with lupus vulgaris (1). The technique was advanced by Danish dermatologist Niels Finsen who used concentrated UV radiation (so-called "chemical rays") to treat lupus vulgaris. His pioneering work in the field of phototherapy earned him the Nobel Prize in Physiology or Medicine in 1903.

In the 1960s and 1970s, chemical photosensitizing agents known as psoralens (8-methoxypsoralen and 5-methoxypsoralen) were extracted from plants and combined with UV phototherapy for the treatment of psoriasis. These agents may be applied topically or taken orally, and their combination with UV radiation therapy is known as photochemotherapy. The use of psoralens and ultraviolet A (UVA) is called PUVA and has been used since 1974 (1) for the treatment of a variety of skin diseases including AD, psoriasis, vitiligo, and cutaneous T-cell lymphoma.

Further advancements in phototherapy have been made possible by the development of compact light sources and filters capable of isolating specific wavelengths of UV radiation. Additionally, ongoing research into the biological effects of UV radiation has expanded our understanding of the mechanism of action, clinical utility, and limitations of UV phototherapy.

PHOTOBIOLOGY OF UV RADIATION

Radiation is the transfer of energy in the form of electromagnetic oscillations and particles (2). The electromagnetic spectrum is a continuum along which the various forms of radiation are categorized according to their wavelengths. It is the wavelength of the radiant energy that confers distinct biologic properties. At one end of the electromagnetic spectrum are γ-rays and x-rays with relatively short wavelengths. At the other end of the spectrum are radio waves with longer wavelengths. The spectrum of radiation that is visible to the human eye ranges from 400 to 800 nm, and in this range specific wavelengths determine the color of light (2). UV radiation is just outside of the spectrum that is visible to the human eye, and its wavelengths range from 100 to 400 nm. The spectrum of UV radiation is arbitrarily subdivided into three categories: ultraviolet A (UVA; wavelength 320–400 nm), ultraviolet B (UVB; wavelength 290–320), and ultraviolet C (UVC; wavelength 100–290nm) (2). The UVA spectrum may be further subdivided into UVA1 (wavelength 340–400 nm) and UVA2 (wavelength 320–340 nm). The biologic properties of UV radiation are the subject of intense research because of their implications ranging from therapy of skin diseases to cancer pathogenesis.

There are two primary mechanisms of action by which UV radiation exerts its effect in inflammatory disorders of the skin: induction of immunosuppression and initiation of apoptosis, or programmed cell death (3). UV radiation, specifically UVB, has been demonstrated to increase the production of interleukin (IL)-10 in locally irradiated skin (3). This cytokine exerts an anti-inflammatory effect by inhibiting the TH1 T-cell response and suppressing the production of interferon (IFN)-γ, a key cytokine in chronic AD (3,4). Additionally, UV radiation induces IL-4 production, leading to a decreased inflammatory TH1 response and a shift toward a more tolerogenic TH2 T-cell response (3).

UV radiation has been clearly demonstrated to induce apoptosis in keratinocytes and T-cells in irradiated skin (3). Furthermore, radiation in the UVA1 range decreases the density of both Langerhans cells and mast cells in the dermis and decreases the number of IgE receptors expressed on Langerhans cells (5). UV radiation leads to apoptosis by several different mechanisms. Direct damage to cellular DNA causes the formation of cyclobutane pyrimidine dimers, an intracellular trigger for apoptosis (3). UVB radiation also causes ligand-independent direct activation of T-cell death receptors including Fas and tumor necrosis factor (TNF) receptors (3). Finally, oxygen-free radical species formed by UV radiation lead to keratinocyte and T-cell apoptosis (3,6). Because of its longer wavelength, UVA1

TABLE 1 UV Phototherapy Modalities

Modality	Wavelength (nm)	Notes
PUVA	320–400	Combined UVA radiation with oral or topical photosensitizing psoralens
		Highest potential for carcinogenesis
UVA1	340–400	Newest UV modality
		Most efficacious in treatment of acute AD
		Unknown long-term potential for carcinogenesis
BBUVB	280–320	Acute adverse events rare
		Largely replaced by NBUVB
NBUVB	311	Acute adverse events rare
		Moderate potential for carcinogenesis
		Most efficacious treatment for chronic AD

Abbreviations: PUVA, psoralen-UVA; BBUVB, broad-band UVB; NBUVB, narrow-band UVB.

radiation penetrates deep into the dermis and exerts its anti-inflammatory and apoptotic effects on infiltrating T cells and Langerhans cells. UVA1 radiation has been demonstrated to cause direct and immediate induction of keratinocyte apoptosis within six hours of initial exposure, whereas UVB radiation–induced apoptosis occurs 24 to 48 hours after the exposure (7). The direct, ligand-independent apoptotic effect of UVA1 is mediated through the generation of singlet oxygen species, which damage the cellular mitochondrial membranes (8).

UV PHOTOTHERAPY AS TREATMENT FOR AD

In 1978, Morison et al. (9) published one of the first reports documenting the benefits of phototherapy (specifically, PUVA) for AD. This study was prompted by the historical observation that patients with severe AD often reported significant improvement during summertime exposure to sunlight. As technologic advances have been made, newer phototherapeutic modalities have been tested in patients with AD. The currently available modalities of UV phototherapy (Table 1) that have been investigated in patients with AD include PUVA, broad-band UVB (BBUVB; wavelength 280–320 nm), narrow-band UVB (NBUVB; wavelength 311 nm), combined UVA and UVB (UVAB), and UVA1. The UVA1 devices represent the most recently developed phototherapeutic modality.

Although case reports, case series, and reports of observations abound, relatively few randomized clinical trials have been performed to formally evaluate the different UV phototherapy modalities and their utility in treating AD. Furthermore, no standard clinical guidelines exist to aid clinicians managing AD with phototherapy. To address these deficiencies, we recently published a systematic review of the current medical literature regarding phototherapy and AD (10). Herein, we summarize the results of that study and review the most current clinical recommendations for the use of UV phototherapy in treating patients with AD.

When using phototherapy to treat any condition, the clinician must establish two main treatment parameters. First, the modality (i.e., wavelength of radiation) must be selected. The treating physician may choose to employ UVA, PUVA, BBUVB, NBUVB, UVA1, or a combination thereof. Second, the dosing regimen must be determined. The dose of UV phototherapy is measured in units of total energy delivered per unit of body surface area. Most commonly this is expressed as J/cm^2. A dosing schedule is determined by the frequency and duration of treatments, and a cumulative total dose may be calculated.

Published trials of phototherapy in AD may be divided into two groups: those that establish optimal wavelength modalities and those that establish optimal dosing regimens. Furthermore, some investigators treated patients with acute flares of AD, while others treated patients with chronic AD. Our review identified a total of nine studies eligible for inclusion. Of these nine, five studies (11–15) focused on severe, acute AD, while four studies (16–19) focused on chronic AD. Among the five trials involving acute AD, three (11–13) set out to establish optimal treatment modalities, while two (14,15) investigated treatment-dosing regimens. The four trials of phototherapy in chronic AD all were designed to establish the optimal wavelength. Two different standardized outcome measures were used by the study investigators to quantify patient responses to treatment. Some investigators used the system developed by Costa et al. (20), while others used the more ubiquitous SCORAD (21) index.

UVA1 IS THE OPTIMAL WAVELENGTH FOR TREATMENT OF ACUTE AD

UVA1 is the newest modality to be employed in the management of AD and appears to be the most efficacious for acute flares. In 1992, Krutmann et al. (11) demonstrated that high-dose UVA1 therapy (130 J/cm^2), as compared to conventional therapy with combined UVA and UVB (UVAB), achieves a more substantial improvement in the severity of symptoms as measured by the Costa scoring system. A later study by Krutmann et al., in 1998 (12), enrolled 53 patients hospitalized with severe, acute AD and randomized them into three distinct treatment groups. The first group was treated with high-dose UVA1 phototherapy, another group received only topical mid-potency corticosteroids, and a third group was treated with conventional UVAB phototherapy. After 10 treatments, UVA1 was clearly demonstrated to be superior to both treatment alternatives. Finally, von Kobyletzki et al. (13) investigated a novel UVA1 device designed to mitigate the enormous heat load generated by traditional UVA1 machines. This device, termed as the "UVA1 cold-light," was compared to traditional UVA1 machines and conventional UVAB in a study enrolling 120 patients with severe, acute AD. Based on outcomes measured via the SCORAD index, the UVA1 cold-light achieved superior results compared to conventional UVA1 and UVAB modalities immediately after three weeks of treatment and at one-month follow-up evaluations. Importantly, most of the therapeutic effect of UVA1 phototherapy was observed early in the course of treatment in all of these studies.

The clinical impact of these three studies is limited by the fact that different doses, treatment duration, and clinical scoring systems were used. Additionally, the criteria for defining both "acute" and "severe" AD differ between studies. Nonetheless, two important trends emerge. First, phototherapy with UVA1 achieves results faster than conventional UVAB when treating acute AD. The second and the most significant conclusion drawn from these studies is that UVA1 is more efficacious than either UVAB or topical corticosteroids for managing acute AD. Thus, when using phototherapy for the management of acute AD, UVA1 emerges as the optimal wavelength.

MEDIUM-DOSE UVA1 IS THE OPTIMAL DOSING REGIMEN FOR ACUTE AD

We identified two trials (14,15) specifically designed to compare alternative phototherapy dosing regimens for treating acute AD. UVA1 phototherapy may be administered in high doses (130 J/cm^2), medium doses (50 J/cm^2), or low doses (10 J/cm^2). Tzaneva et al. (14) enrolled 10 patients in a study to compare high-dose UVA1 to medium-dose UVA1. After three weeks of treatment, both high-dose and medium-dose regimens achieved similar results as indicated by reductions in SCORAD scores (34.7% and 28.2% reductions, respectively). There was no statistically significant difference demonstrated between the high-dose and the medium-dose regimens. Moreover, relapses or flares of AD began to appear approximately four weeks after the treatment cessation regardless of the dosing regimen employed. Kowalzick et al. (15) conducted a trial of 22 patients with acute AD. Half of the patients were randomized into a group receiving medium-dose UVA1, while the other half was randomized into a group treated with low-dose UVA1. Patients treated with medium-dose UVA1 had a 25.3% reduction in SCORAD scores after three weeks of treatment, while the low-dose regimen achieved only a 7.7% reduction in symptom severity. Again, most of the therapeutic results in both of these trials were achieved early in the course of treatment. The vast majority of results in both of these trials were observed within the first one to two weeks of treatment.

Analysis of these two trials leads to several important conclusions. First, medium-dose UVA1 is as effective as high-dose UVA1 but leads to significantly lower cumulative exposure to UV radiation. As the adverse effects of UV phototherapy are addressed later in this chapter, the benefits of minimizing total cumulative UV exposure become readily apparent. Further, medium-dose UVA1 is significantly superior to low-dose UVA1 for managing acute AD. The majority of therapeutic results will be observed within the first weeks of treatment regardless of the dosing regimen administered. It is also important to note that the clinical improvement achieved through UVA1 phototherapy appears to be short lived regardless of the dosing scheme. Although no absolute guidelines exist, UVA1 phototherapy for acute AD is typically administered five times weekly for a total of three weeks. Once the acute flare has been mitigated with UVA1 phototherapy, topical treatments are used to maintain disease suppression.

NARROW-BAND UVB IS THE OPTIMAL WAVELENGTH
FOR TREATING CHRONIC AD

The distinction between acute and chronic AD is more than just clinical. In fact, differences in pathogenesis have been observed. Acute AD is characterized histopathologically by a preponderance of mast cells and TH2 T-cells expressing IL-4, while TH1 T-cells expressing IFN-γ predominate in chronic AD. These distinctions are clinically significant in that different treatment modalities have different efficacies in acute and chronic AD. This statement holds true for phototherapy as well. Although UVA1 has been demonstrated as the optimal wavelength in managing acute AD, the same is not true of chronic AD.

Several controlled clinical trials (16–19) have been conducted to determine the optimal wavelength of UV phototherapy for patients with chronic AD. In two separate trials (16,17), Jekler and Larkö investigated the use of UV phototherapy for treating chronic AD. Their initial study (16) compared BBUVB to combined UVAB phototherapy. Statistically significant differences in favor of combined UVAB were demonstrated for three parameters: pruritus score, overall evaluation score, and total score (the sum of all measured variables in the outcome assessment tool) (16). No improvement was observed in the total body surface area involved by dermatitis. The second trial by Jekler and Larkö (17) enrolled 43 patients into two treatment arms comparing UVA to UVAB. Statistically significant results in favor of UVAB were again observed in both study arms as measured by healing score, overall evaluation score, and sum total score. From these two studies, it becomes apparent that modalities containing UVB are useful in managing the symptoms of chronic AD.

Two subsequent trials (18,19) further investigated the optimal wavelength of UV phototherapy for treating chronic AD by comparing NBUVB to different UVA modalities. Reynolds et al. (18) enrolled 69 patients, randomizing them into three separate treatment groups. One group received NBUVB phototherapy, another group received BBUVA, and a third group was treated with visible fluorescent light to serve as a control. Although patients in this trial were allowed to use mid-potency topical corticosteroids, their use was quantified and considered as part of the evaluation of treatment efficacy. While trends supportive of the superiority of NBUVB were seen in most measured parameters, statistically significant differences in favor of NBUVB over UVA were demonstrated for the mean reduction in the extent of disease and pruritus and for improvement in sleep. On follow-up evaluation three months after phototherapy, patients treated with NBUVB showed greater improvement in disease activity as compared to those treated with either UVA or visible light. A subsequent study led by Legat et al. (19) confirmed the advantages of NBUVB for treating chronic AD. This relatively small trial compared NBUVB to medium-dose UVA1 in nine patients with chronic AD. Treatment with NBUVB reduced Costa scores by 40%, while treatment with UVA1 did not achieve any statistically significant reductions. Furthermore, patients reported notably more improvement in disease severity with NBUVB. Taken together, these two trials demonstrate the superiority of NBUVB as compared to UVA modalities for managing chronic AD.

Unlike UVA1 phototherapy for acute AD, there is a significant variability in treatment parameters with NBUVB phototherapy and chronic AD. The regimen most often employed in the reviewed studies involves treatment three times weekly for eight weeks. However, the endpoint is often indistinct, and treatment requires sequential dose escalation and may continue indefinitely.

EVIDENCE-BASED CONCLUSIONS REGARDING PHOTOTHERAPY AND AD

The ability to generate conclusions by systematically reviewing the current medical literature regarding phototherapy and AD is limited by several important factors. First, as with review of medical literature, publication bias must be considered. Trials yielding positive results are more likely to be published (22). Also, the small sample sizes of most of the trials of phototherapy make for poor statistical power and rarely disclose any uncommon adverse effects (22). Finally, the variability of the parameters used in different trials must be taken into consideration. Investigators differ in the way they select patients for inclusion into their studies and in the way they administer treatments. Also, there is a certain degree of variability in outcome measurement despite the use of standardized scoring indices.

It is also critical to note that most studies of phototherapy and AD include adult patients rather than pediatric patients. AD is certainly more common in children than in adults, and results cannot always be extrapolated from adult studies to pediatric patients. Indeed, data regarding the efficacy and safety of phototherapy in children with AD is lacking.

These factors all conspire to minimize the ability to draw detailed conclusions about the reviewed studies. Therefore, detailed and specific therapeutic guidelines cannot be established based on the current medical literature, but several general principles are evident.

First, phototherapy with UVA1 is the optimal wavelength modality for treating acute AD. Because medium-dose therapy (50 J/cm^2) is equally as effective as high-dose therapy (130 J/cm^2) with less cumulative radiation exposure, medium-dose constitutes the optimal fluence for UVA1 phototherapy of acute AD. In addition, it is evident that the maximal clinical response will be seen within two weeks of beginning UVA1 phototherapy and that the results should not be expected to persist beyond two or three months. These observations have important clinical implications: patients should be counseled extensively so that their expectations about treatment efficacy and duration are realistic. Further, a plan should be in place for maintenance of the therapeutic response using emollients and standard topical therapies. It is also important to note that the use of UVA1 phototherapy is currently limited by access. The UVA1 devices are presently available in only a handful of academic medical centers in the United States and Europe. While the current data indicate that UVA1 phototherapy is the optimal wavelength for treating acute AD not adequately controlled by topical therapy, other modalities (e.g., NBUVB or UVAB) should still be considered when UVA1 is not available.

Second, phototherapy with UVB modalities, particularly NBUVB, should be used to manage chronic AD. In the absence of data specifying the most favorable dosing protocols in the treatment of AD, we anticipate that clinicians will continue to extrapolate from guidelines for managing psoriasis when treating chronic AD with UVB phototherapy. This situation is suboptimal and points to the need for further investigations.

GENERAL PRINCIPLES AND ADVERSE EFFECTS ASSOCIATED WITH PHOTOTHERAPY

Several factors must be considered before enrolling a patient into a phototherapy treatment program. Patients must be able to understand and carry out necessary safety precautions including the use of protective eye and genital shields when indicated. Additionally, they must be able to maintain body positioning and posture for several minutes at a time. In general, children too young to readily perform these tasks should not be considered candidates for phototherapy. Contraindications to phototherapy must also be considered. These include a past history of melanoma, photosensitive skin diseases (e.g., lupus erythematosus or polymorphous light eruption), genodermatoses associated with skin cancer (e.g., xeroderma pigmentosum, dysplastic nevus syndrome, or nevoid basal cell carcinoma syndrome), and past history of multiple nonmelanoma skin cancers.

As with any medical treatment, patients should be counseled prior to beginning phototherapy. The discussion should focus on the duration and modality of therapy, expected treatment outcomes, and potential adverse events. Patients with AD who choose to participate in phototherapy should do so after considering the benefits of therapy as well as the risks therein.

Adverse events (Table 2) associated with phototherapy may be considered either acute or chronic. Acute adverse events tend to be generated by a phototoxic or

TABLE 2 Adverse Events Associated with UV Phototherapy

Event	Relative risk
Acute	
Erythema with blistering	Rare overall. Occur in less than 1% of patients treated with UVB (21).
Induction of PMLE	
Pruritus	
Disease flare	
Reactivation of latent herpes virus infection	
Chronic	
Cutaneous SCC	Rate of SCC increases 25–250-fold with PUVA (22)
Cutaneous BCC	Rate of BCC increases 4–50-fold with PUVA (22)
Cutaneous malignant melanoma	Rate of melanoma increases 5-fold with PUVA
	Rate of NMSC increases by 40% with UVB (24)

Abbreviations: PMLE, polymorphous light eruption; SCC, squamous cell carcinoma; BCC, basal cell carcinoma; NMSC, nonmelanoma skin cancer.

photoallergic reaction to the UV radiation. The most common acute adverse event is erythema which, like a sunburn, may blister and peel (23). Less common acute reactions include pruritus or the induction of polymorphic light eruption (23). Patients with a history of mucocutaneous herpes virus infection, especially herpes labialis, should be warned that UV phototherapy may lead to reactivation of the latent virus (23). In some cases, patients may experience a flare of AD after beginning phototherapy. Overall, acute adverse events are rare. A recently published review estimated that less than 1% of patients undergoing treatment with UV phototherapy experience an acute adverse event (23). Avoidance of natural sunlight and other sources of UV radiation (e.g., tanning salons) is advisable to minimize the incidence of acute and chronic adverse events.

The primary chronic adverse event associated with UV phototherapy is the risk of carcinogenesis. As we move into the fourth decade of the field of phototherapy, epidemiologic data regarding the incidence of skin cancer in UV-irradiated patients is beginning to emerge. Most of this data pertains to patients treated for psoriasis, as this has historically been the most common indication for phototherapy. PUVA therapy significantly increases the risk of both cutaneous and genital squamous cell carcinoma (SCC) (24). In patients who have received PUVA therapy, the risk of cutaneous SCC is about 25 times that of a comparable general population (24). When high cumulative doses of PUVA are administered (greater than 400 treatments), the risk is 250 times higher than that of a matched, untreated population (24). In fact, more than half of patients receiving over 400 PUVA treatments will go on to develop cutaneous SCC (24). The increased incidence of basal cell carcinoma (BCC) in PUVA patients is also significant. In general, PUVA increases the risk of BCC by a factor of 4 (24). When over 500 treatments are administered, the increase is 50-fold (24). Unfortunately, the incidence of malignant melanoma also increases with the use of PUVA. With more than 250 PUVA treatments, a patient's risk of melanoma is increased by a factor of more than 5 (25).

UVB phototherapy appears to be less carcinogenic than PUVA (26). A literature review found no consistent evidence that UVB modalities increase the incidence of melanoma or nonmelanoma skin cancer (27). However, a recent study disclosed a moderate increase in the incidence of both SCC and BCC (26).

Patients receiving high cumulative doses of UVB (greater than 300 treatments) were observed to have a 40% increase in the incidence of nonmelanoma skin cancer when compared to patients receiving lower doses of UVB phototherapy (26).

Newer UV modalities such as UVA1 have not been in use for enough time to generate data regarding carcinogenicity. Unfortunately, these trends will only become evident with time, and extrapolations from PUVA and UVB data are imperfect at best. Therefore, patients should be made aware that higher cumulative doses of UVA1 may result in increased rates of skin cancer but that specific data is not yet available.

The safety profile of UV phototherapy may also be affected by certain patient comorbidities. Specifically, the safety of phototherapy in HIV-infected patients has been addressed (28). Experimental models have demonstrated that UV irradiation may lead to activation of the HIV virus (28). Additionally, an increase in viral antigenemia has been documented in several HIV-positive patients receiving phototherapy (28). However, there is currently no evidence that PUVA or UVB phototherapy lead to harmful effects in HIV-infected patients (28). Until larger randomized and controlled trials clarify the role of phototherapy in HIV-positive patients, the use of these treatments should be considered on a case-by-case basis with careful attention to the individual risks and benefits.

Another important consideration with phototherapy is the concomitant use of topical therapy, specifically topical corticosteroids, topical calcineurin inhibitors, and emollients. Most patients with AD will treat their disease topically prior to considering phototherapy and should be counseled on the appropriate use of topical therapy in combination with phototherapy. UV phototherapy and exposure to the heat generated by the machines often leads to xerosis, and it is important for patients to continue the liberal use of emollients. Although no data exists to either support or refute their safety in combination with phototherapy, topical corticosteroids are generally continued throughout the duration of phototherapy treatment.

Topical calcineurin inhibitors have emerged as an important steroid sparing agent for AD, but concerns regarding their potential to increase photocarcinogenicity have been raised. In fact, the patient information and package inserts for both pimecrolimus cream and tacrolimus ointment advise patients to avoid all forms of UV radiation while using the medication because their effect on photocarcinogenesis and DNA repair is unknown. It has been demonstrated that systemic calcineurin inhibitors including cyclosporine inhibit the removal of UV-induced pyrimidine dimers and inhibit UVB-induced keratinocyte apoptosis, thus making skin cells more susceptible to the carcinogenic properties of UV radiation (29). It is also known that the addition of systemic cyclosporine to PUVA therapy in psoriasis patients increases the incidence of squamous cell carcinoma by a factor of seven over PUVA alone (30). The same effect has not been demonstrated for topical use of calcineurin inhibitors. Mouse models have shown that topical tacrolimus ointment does not decrease the amount of UV radiation required to induce squamous cell carcinoma (31). In fact, one study demonstrated an 80% decrease in thymidine dimers induced by UVB radiation in mice pretreated with topical pimecrolimus cream (32). Long-term surveillance data and ongoing studies may further elucidate the effect of topical calcineurin inhibitors and photocarcinogenesis. Until then, it is prudent to advise patients to discontinue these medications while undergoing phototherapy.

SUMMARY AND FUTURE DIRECTIONS IN THE FIELD OF PHOTOTHERAPY AND AD

UV phototherapy represents an important treatment option in the management of AD. Based on a critical review of the medical literature, it appears that medium-dose UVA1 is the optimal modality for treating acute AD while UVB, specifically NBUVB, is the best method for treating chronic AD. Acute adverse events are rare, and patients should be counseled about the increased risk of skin cancer.

Both patients and clinicians stand to benefit greatly from future trials in which uniform methods of treatment, evaluation, and long-term follow-up are carefully employed. In order to allow for cross-comparison and comprehensive review, standardized trial protocols should be instituted. If future studies employed standardized fluences, cumulative exposures, UV wavelengths, and patient evaluation methods, we anticipate that comprehensive therapeutic guidelines could be established by systematically considering all study results. Additionally, careful long-term follow-up will allow for the evaluation of the carcinogenic effect of different UV phototherapy modalities. As our understanding of UV-related photobiology advances further, the application of UV phototherapy to AD and other diseases of the skin will continue to expand.

REFERENCES

1. Roelandts R. The history of phototherapy: Something new under the sun? J Am Acad Dermatol 2002; 46:926–930.
2. Kochevar IE, Pathak MA, Parrish JA. Photophysics, Photochemistry, and Photobiology. In: Fitzpatric TB, et al. Dermatology in General Medicine, 5th ed. New York, NY: McGrawHill, 1999; 220–229.
3. Weichenthal M, Schwarz T. Phototherapy: How does UV work? Photodermatol Photoimmunol Photomed 2005; 21:260–266.
4. Grewe M, Gyufko K, Krutmann J. Interleukin-10 production by cultured human keratinocytes: Regulation by ultraviolet B and ultraviolet A1 radiation. J Invest Dermatol 1995; 104:3–6.
5. Grabbe J, Welker P, Humke S, et al. High-dose ultraviolet A1 (UVA1), but not UVA/UVB therapy, decreases IgE-binding cells in lesional skin of patients with atopic eczema. J Invest Dermatol 1996; 107:419–422.
6. Mang R, Krutmann J. UVA-1 phototherapy. Photodermatol Photoimmunol Photomed 2005; 21:103–108.
7. Breuckmann F, von Kobyletzki G, Avermaete A, et al. Mechanisms of apoptosis: UVA1-induced immediate and UVB-induced delayed apoptosis in human T cells in vitro. J Eur Acad Dermatol Venereol 2003; 17:418–429.
8. Godar DE UVA1 radiation triggers two different final apoptotic pathways. J Invest Dermatol 1999; 112:3–12.
9. Morison WL, Parrish J, Fitzpatrick TB. Oral psoralen photochemotherapy of atopic eczema. Br J Dermatol 1978; 98:25–30.
10. Meduri NB, Vandergriff T, Rasmussen H, et al. Phototherapy in the management of atopic dermatitis: A systematic review. Photodermatol Photoimmunol Photomed 2007; 23:106–112.
11. Krutmann J, Czech W, Diepgen T, et al. High-dose UVA1 therapy in the treatment of patients with atopic dermatitis. J Am Acad Dermatol 1992; 26:225–230.
12. Krutmann J, Diepgen TL, Luger TA, et al. High-dose UVA1 therapy for atopic dermatitis: Results of a multicenter trial. J Am Acad Dermatol 1998; 38:589–593.
13. von Kobyletzki G, Pieck C, Hoffmann K, et al. Medium-dose UVA1 cold-light phototherapy in the treatment of severe atopic dermatitis. J Am Acad Dermatol 1999; 41:931–937.

14. Tzaneva S, Seeber A, Schwaiger M, et al. High-dose versus medium-dose UVA1 phototherapy for patients with severe generalized atopic dermatitis. J Am Acad Dermatol 2001; 45:503–507.
15. Kowalzick L, Kleinheinz A, Weichenthal M, et al. Low dose versus medium dose UV-A1 treatment in severe atopic eczema. Acta Derm Venereol 1995; 75:43–45.
16. Jekler J, Larkö O. Combined UVA–UVB versus UVB phototherapy for atopic dermatitis: A paired-comparison study. J Am Acad Dermatol 1990; 22:49–53.
17. Jekler J, Larkö O. Phototherapy for atopic dermatitis with ultraviolet A (UVA), low-dose UVB and combined UVA and UVB: Two paired-comparison studies. Photodermatol Photoimmunol Photomed 1991; 8:151–156.
18. Reynolds NJ, Franklin V, Gray JC, et al. Narrow-band ultraviolet B and broad-band ultraviolet A phototherapy in adult atopic eczema: A randomised controlled trial. Lancet 2001; 357:2012–2016.
19. Legat FJ, Hofer A, Brabek E, et al. Narrowband UV-B vs medium-dose UV-A1 phototherapy in chronic atopic dermatitis. Arch Dermatol 2003; 139:223–224.
20. Costa C, Rilliet A, Nicolet M, et al. Scoring atopic dermatitis: The simpler the better? Acta Derm Venereol 1989; 69:41–45.
21. Stalder JF, Taieb A. Severity scoring of atopic dermatitis: The SCORAD index. Consensus Report of the European Task Force on Atopic Dermatitis. Dermatology 1993; 186:23–31.
22. Ladhani S. The need for evidence-based management of skin diseases. Int J Dermatol 1997; 36:17–22.
23. Martin JA, Laube S, Edwards C, et al. Rate of acute adverse events for narrow-band UVB and Psoralen-UVA phototherapy. Photodermatol Photoimmunol Photomed 2007; 23: 68–72.
24. Nijsten TE, Stern RS. The increased risk of skin cancer is persistent after discontinuation of psoralen+ultraviolet A: A cohort study. J Invest Dermatol 2003; 121:252–258.
25. Stern RS, Nichols KT, Väkevä LH. Malignant melanoma in patients treated for psoriasis with methoxsalen (psoralen) and ultraviolet A radiation (PUVA). The PUVA Follow-Up Study. N Engl J Med 1997; 336:1041–1045.
26. Lim JL, Stern RS. High levels of ultraviolet B exposure increase the risk of non-melanoma skin cancer in psoralen and ultraviolet A-treated patients. J Invest Dermatol 2005; 124: 505–513.
27. Lee E, Koo J, Berger T. UVB phototherapy and skin cancer risk: A review of the literature. Int J Dermatol 2005; 44:355–360.
28. Breur-McHam J, Simpson E, Dougherty I, et al. Activation of HIV in human skin by ultraviolet B radiation and its inhibition by NFKB blocking agents. Photochem Photobiol 2001; 74(6):805–810.
29. Yarosh DB, Pena AV, Nay SL, et al. Calcineurin inhibitors decrease DNA repair and apoptosis in human keratinocytes following ultraviolet B irradiation. J Invest Dermatol 2005; 125:1020–1025.
30. Marcil I, Stern RS. Squamous-cell cancer of the skin in patients given PUVA and ciclosporin: Nested cohort crossover study. Lancet 2001; 358:1042–1045.
31. Lerche CM, Philipsen PA, Poulsen T, et al. Topical tacrolimus in combination with simulated solar radiation does not enhance photocarcinogenesis in hairless mice. Exp Dermatol 2008; 17:57–62.
32. Tran C, Lübbe J, Sorg O, et al. Topical calcineurin inhibitors decrease the production of UVB-induced thymine dimers from hairless mouse epidermis. Dermatology 2005; 211: 341–347.

22 Topical Immunomodulators: Topical Calcineurin-Inhibitors

Thomas A. Luger and Martin Steinhoff
Department of Dermatology, University of Münster, Münster, Germany

INTRODUCTION

The optimal disease management of atopic dermatitis (AD) involves several approaches including education, avoidance of trigger factors, topical agents such as emollients as well as anti-inflammatory compounds, UV-light, and finally for severe cases, systemic immunomodulating agents (1). The mainstay AD treatment in any case is the use of topical anti-inflammatory and immunomodulating drugs. For many years, corticosteroids, which have been introduced by Marion Sulzberger in the early 1950s for the topical treatment of eczema, were the only available and effective local therapy for AD (2). Despite the improved safety profile of novel corticosteroids, long-term application is still not suitable, especially in sensitive skin areas such as the face and intertriginous regions.

In the last years, several new drugs and biologic compounds have been developed for the treatment of inflammatory skin diseases. Among those the blockade of the calcineurin pathway in T lymphocytes with cyclosporin A (CyA) or tacrolimus (FK 506) proved to be a very effective immunomodulating strategy to prevent graft rejection and to treat immune-mediated diseases (3,4). The development of a topical formulation of CyA for the treatment of skin diseases unfortunately failed. However, topical formulations of both tacrolimus and other related calcineurin inhibitors (CIs) such as pimecrolimus (ASM 981) proved to be very effective for the treatment of AD (5). Therefore, the term topical calcineurin inhibitor (TCI) has been coined. Now tacrolimus ointment and pimecrolimus cream have been approved by the medical authorities of many countries for the treatment of this disease. In addition to pimecrolimus and tacrolimus, several other TCIs have been investigated in animal models but none of them is currently being developed for treatment of skin diseases.

In this chapter we will concentrate on the preclinical as well as clinical data of tacrolimus and pimecrolimus and outline novel therapeutic strategies, especially for the long-term management of AD. Finally, some emphasis will be given on the use of TCIs for the treatment of other inflammatory skin diseases.

TOPICAL CALCINEURIN INHIBITORS: MECHANISM OF ACTION

Four different CIs are in clinical use or are being developed for the topical and systemic treatment of immune-mediated and inflammatory diseases. These are cyclosporin A, tacrolimus, pimecrolimus, and voclosporin (ISA 247). CyA has been isolated from a fungus and was the first CI that is now widely used for the systemic treatment of several skin diseases such as severe AD and psoriasis (4). Voclosporin is a novel CI derived from CyA by a chemical modification with an improved safety

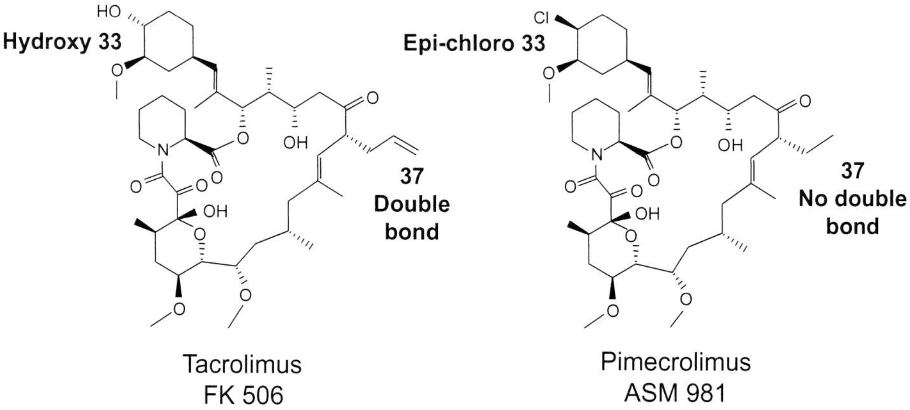

FIGURE 1 Molecular structures of tacrolimus and pimecrolimus.

and efficacy profile. In a recent phase III clinical trial, voclosporin was proven to be safe and effective for the treatment of moderate-to-severe psoriasis (6).

Although tacrolimus was firstly introduced as a systemic immunomodulating drug, pimecrolimus was primarily developed for the topical treatment of AD (7). Despite promising early-phase clinical trials in patients with AD and psoriasis, the development of an oral pimecrolimus preparation has been discontinued (8,9). According to their molecular structure, tacrolimus and pimecrolimus are different from CyA (Fig. 1). Tacrolimus is derived from *Streptomyces tsukubaensis*, whereas pimecrolimus was isolated from *Streptomyces hygroscopicus* var. *ascomycetus*. Both bind, though with different affinity, to a cytosolic immunophilin receptor, defined as FK-binding protein-12 (macrophilin-12), which is different from the cytosolic receptor for CyA designated as cyclophilin. After binding, the macrophilin complex associated with either tacrolimus or pimecrolimus inhibits a calcium-dependent serine-threonine phosphatase, defined as calcineurin. Because of dephosphorylation and nuclear translocation of a cytosolic transcription factor, the nuclear factor of activated T-cell protein (NF-ATp) is inhibited (10,11).

In Vitro Effects

Both tacrolimus and pimecrolimus inhibit Th1 as well as Th2 cell activation via suppressing the production of proinflammatory as well as immunomodulating cytokines such as interleukin-2 (IL-2), IL-4, IL-8, tumor necrosis factor alpha (TNF-α), interferon gamma (IFN-γ), and granulocyte-macrophage colony-stimulating factor (GM-CSF) (12). Furthermore, pimecrolimus was found to downregulate IL-5, IL-10, and IL-13 in CD4$^+$ as well as in CD8$^+$ T cells (13). Both topical pimecrolimus as well as tacrolimus were found to induce apoptosis in T lymphocytes but not in Langerhans cells (14). In addition to T-cells both tacrolimus and pimecrolimus inhibit mast cells as well as basophils to release mediators such as histamine and tryptase (15). Tacrolimus was also shown to downregulate cytokine production in eosinophils, basophils, and mast cells. Moreover, pimecrolimus and tacrolimus inhibit apoptosis of keratinocytes and T cells and suppress chemokine secretion by eosinophils as well as release of inflammatory mediators from mast cells (14,16).

Dendritic cells (DC) such as myeloid DC including Langerhans cells (LC) as well as inflammatory DC (IDEC), and plasmacytoid DC (pDC) play a crucial role in the pathogenesis of AD. Accordingly, LC and IDEC are present in atopic skin lesions and express the high affinity IgE receptor (FcεRI). LC occur in normal skin and contribute to a shift of the immune response towards Th2, whereas IDEC were only detected in inflamed skin and via producing IL-12 and IL-18 add to Th1 polarization. In contrast, pDC, which via the production of IFN-α have potent antiviral activity, are almost absent in AD skin (17). Therefore, several investigations have addressed the question whether TCIs have an effect on DC density or functions. Accordingly, pimecrolimus does not modify maturation as well as functions of DC's (18). Upon topical application of tacrolimus or pimecrolimus, the amount of epidermal CD1$^+$ IDEC was reduced (14,19). Contrary to corticosteroids, topical application of pimecrolimus was not able to alter the density of LC in the epidermis (20). Tacrolimus, however, was shown to decrease the T-lymphocyte–activating capacity of LCs and to modulate certain effects of IDECs such as the expression of to (FcεRI). In cultured LCs, tacrolimus was found to downregulate the expression of FcεRI, whereas corticosteroids increased its expression. Thus, effects of tacrolimus on DC in the skin may be of relevance for its beneficial property in the treatment of AD. Accordingly, during therapy with tacrolimus, the clinical improvement correlated positively with the decrease of the initially elevated number of CD1a$^+$ cells in the epidermis of AD lesions. The reduction of CD1a$^+$ cells was mainly due to a decrease in IDEC and not in LC density, suggesting a normalization of DC functions upon topical application with tacrolimus. Moreover, pimecrolimus like corticosteroids was found to deplete pDC in patients with AD (21). Whether this contributes to susceptibility of AD patients to skin infections needs to be explored.

In Vivo Effects

The anti-inflammatory capacities of tacrolimus and pimecrolimus have been investigated in several animal models of contact dermatitis. Both compounds block the elicitation phase of contact dermatitis, thereby diminishing the inflammatory activity. The in vitro evidence of a lesser immunosuppressive potential of pimecrolimus in comparison to tacrolimus has been supported in vivo by additional animal studies. Pimecrolimus in contrast to tacrolimus had no effect on the sensitization phase of allergic contact dermatitis and thus apparently did not impair a primary immune response. This has been further supported by a variety of other animal models of immune-mediated diseases. Using a localized rat model of "graft-versus-host reaction" pimecrolimus was significantly less effective than tacrolimus with respect to healing. In another rat model of kidney transplantation, pimecrolimus again was weaker in preventing graft rejection when compared to tacrolimus or cyclosporin. Moreover, upon investigation of the effect on T-helper-cell–assisted B-cell activation in rats, pimecrolimus turned out to be significantly less effective when compared to tacrolimus in vivo (22,23).

CLINICAL STUDIES WITH TOPICAL CALCINEURIN INHIBITORS

Both TCIs have been developed for the topical treatment of atopic dermatitis and are approved for this indication in many countries around the world. Tacrolimus can be obtained as 0.03% and 0.1% ointment (Protopic®), whereas pimecrolimus is available as a 1% cream (Elidel®, Aregen®, Isaplic®, Rizan®, Ombex®, and Velov®). In Europe, the United States, and many other countries tacrolimus ointment is approved for the treatment of moderate and severe atopic dermatitis in adults (0.1%) as well as in children (0.03%) ≥2-year old, and pimecrolimus cream (1%) is approved for mild and moderate cases of atopic dermatitis in adults and children ≥2-year old. In certain countries, pimecrolimus is approved for the therapy of atopic dermatitis regardless of age and severity of the disease. Several clinical trials verified both TCIs compounds to be highly effective and safe for the treatment of atopic dermatitis.

Pimecrolimus Cream
Short-Term Studies
In a three week proof of concept study, adults with moderate AD were treated with pimecrolimus 1% cream in comparison to vehicle once or twice daily. The twice-daily application resulted in a 71.9% improvement of the eczematous lesions, whereas an improvement rate of only 37.7% was observed in lesions, which were treated once daily. In areas treated with vehicle, the mean improvement was 10.3% or 6.2%, respectively (24). Subsequently, the efficacy of pimecrolimus 1% cream for the treatment of AD in adults, children, and infants has been proven in several clinical studies (24–26). As no significant drug-related side effects were observed in this study, pimecrolimus cream was applied twice daily in any of the following studies.

In order to evaluate the efficacy of pimecrolimus in comparison to corticosteroids, a randomized, double-blind, multicenter study was performed in 260 patients with AD. In a dose finding study, AD patients were treated three weeks with pimecrolimus cream at different concentrations (0.05%, 0.2%, 0.6%, and 1.0%), vehicle cream, or betamethasone-17-valerate cream 0.1%. According to this study, pimecrolimus 1% cream was most effective with a median eczema area and severity index (EASI) decrease of 47%. Betamethasone valerate treatment resulted in a median percent change from baseline of 78%. Furthermore, pruritus was shown to be effectively controlled by pimecrolimus within one week of treatment. No serious adverse events were reported in any of the treatment groups and a transient burning or a feeling of warmth in the treated areas was the most commonly observed side effects (26).

To further assess the efficacy and safety of a twice-daily application of pimecrolimus 1% cream in children (2–17 years) and infants (3–23 months) with mild, moderate, or even severe AD several multicenter clinical trials have been performed (25,27). A total of 403 children and 186 infants were included in these studies. After six weeks of treatment in the initial double-blinded phase, patients were continued on to an open-labeled 20-week extension phase. Both in children and infants, pimecrolimus cream 1% in comparison to vehicle proved to be highly effective in improving eczema as well as pruritus already after eight days of treatment. Treatment was well tolerated and no increased incidence of side effects including viral or bacterial infections has been reported (27). Therapeutic effects were independent of ethnic origin and disease severity (28). These results were confirmed in a recent double-blind study. During a four-week period of treatment, pimecrolimus cream reduced the mean EASI by 71.5% as compared to a decrease by 19.4% in the vehicle control group. The eczema reduction was statistically significant at day 4. Moreover, upon treatment with pimecrolimus, usually within two to four days a significant improvements of sleep loss and pruritus was observed (29,30). In a further study performed in infants ($n = 250$) and children ($n = 711$), the notion of pimecrolimus 1% cream being a safe and effective therapeutic option in children and infants was supported. Moreover, significantly more patients in the pimecrolimus group were maintained without corticosteroid therapy (31).

The poor efficacy of pimecrolimus cream in severe AD raised the question whether addition of topical pimecrolimus to a topical corticosteroid is of therapeutic benefit. This was evaluated in an exploratory two-week, double-blind, randomized within patient ($n = 45$) study with fluticasone propionate cream 0.05%. However, the efficacy of the treatment with the combination of fluticasone propionate and pimecrolimus was equivalent to that of fluticasone propionate and vehicle. These findings indicate that combination of pimecrolimus with a mid-potent topical corticosteroid has no additional therapeutic effect in the treatment of patients with severe AD (32).

There is evidence from several clinical studies indicating that pimecrolimus cream is particularly effective for the treatment of AD in sensitive areas of the skin such as face and neck. In a recent study, 200 patients aged 12 years or over with mild to moderate head and neck AD, intolerant of, or dependent on topical corticosteroids were randomized to either pimecrolimus cream or vehicle cream. After an initial six-week, a double-blind, randomized, vehicle-controlled phase, an additional six-week, open-label phase was conducted. In comparison to vehicle the treatment with pimecrolimus cream resulted in a higher percentage of patients being cleared or almost cleared of facial AD (47% vs. 16%, respectively). In these patients there was also evidence for a reversal of skin atrophy due to prior use of corticosteroids (33). In a further study using the same design, 200 children (2–12 years of age) were treated with pimecrolimus cream 1% or vehicle. Similarly, treatment with pimecrolimus cream resulted in a significant and fast improvement of eczema and pruritus (34). Finally, two four-week, randomized, double-blind, parallel-group studies performed in adult patients with perioral dermatitis were carried out. Accordingly, upon treatment with pimecrolimus cream, a rapid improvement of clinical symptoms such as eczema and pruritus as well as the quality of life of patients was observed (35,36).

Long-Term Studies

The efficacy of topical pimecrolimus in the long-term management of AD has been investigated in a number of studies with a follow-up period up to 12 months. In several multicenter, randomized, double-blind studies, 192 adults, 713 children (2–17 years of age), and 250 infants (3–23 months of age) were enrolled (37–39). Patients were randomized to apply twice-daily pimecrolimus cream 1% or vehicle cream upon the first signs of a flare (itching, eczema). In the case of uncontrolled flare, patients of both groups were allowed to use moderately potent topical corticosteroids until clearing. After 6 or 12 months of treatment, significantly lesser infants in the pimecrolimus group (67.6%) developed a severe flare requiring corticosteroids as compared to the vehicle therapy group (30.4%).

The efficacy of pimecrolimus treatment in infants was also reflected by a significant EASI reduction of 61.8% after six weeks and >80% after 12 months (38). Similar results were obtained with children, as after six months of treatment with pimecrolimus significantly more children remained without any flare (61%) in comparison to the control group (34.2%) (39). In a more recent study, the long-term control of AD with pimecrolimus cream was investigated in infants and young

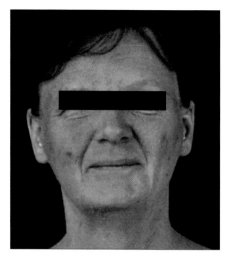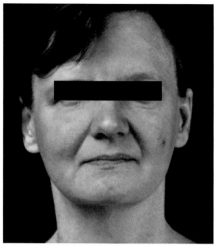

FIGURE 2   Patient with moderate AD before and 4 months after treatment with pimecrolimus cream 1%.

children for one year ($n = 91$) or two years ($n = 76$). Pimecrolimus treatment was safe and well tolerated and none of the patients had to discontinue therapy because of side effects. The incidence of systemic and skin infections including eczema herpeticum ($n = 2$) was not significantly higher in the pimecrolimus group (40,41). Among adults, 45% of the pimecrolimus-treated patients experienced no flare during the treatment period of six months compared to only 18.8% in the vehicle group. The mean time until the first flare was 144 days in the pimecrolimus group, while it was 26 days in the vehicle group-thus five-times faster in the latter group (37). The good efficacy and tolerability of pimecrolimus cream for the treatment of AD in children and adults have been confirmed by several recent clinical studies (42–44). In any of these long-term studies usually only two to three days after initiation of pimecrolimus treatment, a significant improvement of pruritus was noted (37–39). Moreover, several studies have shown that pimecrolimus treatment has a significantly greater beneficial effect on the quality of life in patients with AD (45–48).

Taken together, these long-term studies provide evidence that pimecrolimus cream 1% is effective for the treatment of mild, moderate, and severe AD in adults, children, and infants (Fig. 2). Pimecrolimus was safe and well tolerated during the entire study period-no clinically relevant drug-related systemic events occurred and no significant difference between treatment groups in terms of infections and application site reactions was observed. In addition, there was no evidence of systemic immunosuppression according to a comparable response to recall antigens (39). Thus, treatment with pimecrolimus 1% cream is safe and effective in the topical long-term management of AD.

There is evidence that lesions in the face and neck-which are often difficult to treat-respond even better to pimecrolimus treatment than eczematous lesions in other areas of the body. In a recent 24-week, controlled, double-blind, multicenter study, 140 patients, aged 2 to 17 years, with facial mild-to-moderate AD, it was evaluated whether treatment with pimecrolimus cream 1% versus vehicle can decrease the development of flares, thus necessitating the use of a topical corticosteroid such as prednicarbate. Patients in the pimecrolimus group suffered from significantly lesser flares, and the need for prednicarbate as a rescue medication was significantly reduced. Therefore, long-term intermittent treatment of facial AD in children and adolescents with pimecrolimus cream 1% was concluded to be highly effective and safe (49). Similar results were obtained in another study investigating 184 children with severe AD. Accordingly, the need of topical corticosteroids, especially on the head and the neck was significantly reduced upon use of pimecrolimus cream (50).

The question whether pimecrolimus 1% cream beyond controlled clinical trials would also provide an effective and safe long-term therapy for patients with mild-to-moderate AD was addressed in several open-label, observational studies involving a total of >9000 patients. In summary, the intermittent treatment of AD patients with pimecrolimus cream in a daily practice setting was generally effective, well-tolerated, and resulted in high percentage of patient satisfaction and the improvement of their quality of life (51–55).

Tacrolimus Ointment
Short-Term Studies
In a first placebo-controlled clinical study in patients with AD, a significant improvement of eczema and pruritus with tacrolimus ointment at three different concentrations (0.03%, 0.1%, and 0.3%) was reported after three weeks of treatment. Several subsequent short-term (3-12 weeks) clinical trials in patients with moderate-to-severe AD confirmed these findings. Taken together, tacrolimus ointment proved to be highly effective in improving the symptoms of AD (56). These results were confirmed by several subsequent studies by using different (3-12 weeks) treatment protocols for patients with moderate-to-severe AD. Moreover, the 0.1% formulation was found to be more efficient than tacrolimus 0.03% (57,58).

The efficacy of tacrolimus ointment in comparison to topical corticosteroids has been evaluated in several short-term controlled clinical trials. In adults with moderate-to-severe AD the effectiveness of tacrolimus ointment 0.1% was comparable to that of hydrocortisone butyrate ointment 0.1%, whereas tacrolimus ointment 0.03% was less effective (59). In children (2-15 years), both tacrolimus ointment preparations (0.1% and 0.03%) were superior to hydrocortisone acetate ointment 1% (60). There is evidence from one study in children that tacrolimus ointment 0.03% was more effective when compared to hydrocortisone acetate 1% (61). Moreover, in children with moderate disease state of AD, the once- or twice-daily application was equally effective whereas in severe cases the twice-daily treatment was superior (61). In a recent study in 265 children and adolescents with an acute flare of severe AD, tacrolimus ointment 0.03% has been compared with methylprednisone aceponate ointment 0.1%. Although efficacy and tolerability was similar in both treatment groups, methylprednisone aceponate was significantly superior to tacrolimus as far as EASI, itch, sleep, and tolerability was concerned (62). In a meta-analysis of 25 randomized controlled trials, tacrolimus ointment 0.1% was superior to hydrocortisone-acetate, -valerate 1%, or -butyrate 0.1%, whereas tacrolimus (0.03%) ointment 0.03% was as effective as hydrocortisone-acetate 1%, but less effective than that of hydrocortisone-butyrate 0.1% (63).

Several studies have been performed to compare the efficacy of the currently available topical formulations of CIs with each other. In a randomized clinical trial,

141 pediatric patients with moderate AD were treated either with pimecrolimus cream 1% or tacrolimus ointment 0.03% twice daily for six weeks. At the end of the study period the efficacy was similar in pimecrolimus as well as tacrolimus-treated patients and both therapeutic regimen were generally well tolerated. However, pimecrolimus cream 1% was reported for better formulation attributes as well as a superior local tolerability as compared to that of tacrolimus ointment 0.03% (64). In three multicenter, randomized, six-week studies, the efficacy and safety of tacrolimus ointment were compared to pimecrolimus cream in adult and pediatric patients with mild to very severe AD. All patients randomized to pimecrolimus received pimecrolimus cream 1% and adults as well as children with moderate-to-severe AD were treated with tacrolimus ointment 1% whereas children with mild disease received tacrolimus ointment 0.03%. In summary, tacrolimus ointment turned out to be more effective than pimecrolimus cream in children with moderate-and-severe disease and at week 1 in children with mild disease. Although in the two studies involving children there was no significant difference in the incidence of adverse events, including application site reactions, adults treated with tacrolimus experienced a higher number of local application site reactions at the beginning of the treatment (65). Therefore, tacrolimus ointment was concluded to be more effective with a faster onset of action than pimecrolimus cream in adults and children with AD, albeit adverse events such as burning and stinging were also more frequently observed in patients receiving tacrolimus ointment.

Long-Term Studies
Several long-term studies confirmed the efficacy and safety of tacrolimus ointment for the management of AD. In a multicenter, open label noncomparative trial, 316 adults with moderate-to-severe AD were treated with tacrolimus ointment 0.1% for six months ($n = 200$) or 12 months ($n = 116$). Medication was applied twice daily on all affected skin areas (5-60%) until one week after complete clearance and additional use of emollients without active ingredient were allowed (66). A total of 77.5% of the patients completed the study. After 12 months, an excellent improvement ($\geq90\%$) or total clearance of the symptoms was observed in 68.2% of those patients. More than 90% of these patients reported an improvement of at least 50% (Fig. 3).

In a more recent study, 972 adults with moderate-to-severe AD were treated with tacrolimus 0.1% ointment for six months in comparison to hydrocortisone acetate 1% for the face and hydrocortisone butyrate 0.1% for other areas. The overall efficacy of tacrolimus ointment 1% was found to be superior to that of corticosteroids, whereas the rate of adverse events was similar in both arms. However, a higher number of herpes simplex and bacterial infections were observed in patients treated with tacrolimus ointment (67). Most of these patients ($n = 672$) were enrolled in a two-year follow-up study, further supporting the high efficacy and safety of tacrolimus long-term treatment (68). These results have been confirmed by two long-term, open-label, noncomparative trials in adults as well as in children receiving tacrolimus either continuously or intermittently for up to four years. Accordingly, tacrolimus ointment proved to be highly effective for the management of pediatric and adult patients with no additional safety concerns after four years of continuous or intermittent treatment (69,70). In addition, no differences in the safety profile could be established between 0.03% and 0.1% formulation, and topical

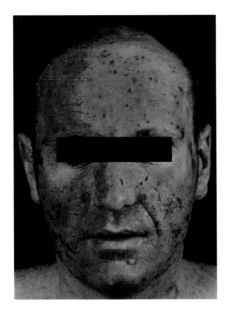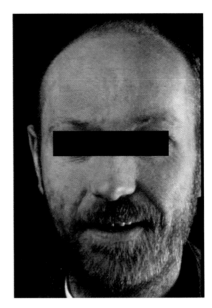

FIGURE 3 Patient with severe AD before and 6 months after treatment with tacrolimus ointment 0.1%.

tacrolimus treatment significantly improved the quality of life in children as well as in adults suffering from AD (71–73).

PHARMACOKINETIC PROFILE OF TOPICAL CALCINEURIN INHIBITORS

The profile of adverse events such as hypertension and nephrotoxicity of systemic CIs is well known. Therefore, the potential systemic exposure is a major concern when topical formulations of CIs are being developed. Accordingly, the capacity of both tacrolimus and pimecrolimus to penetrate into the skin and permeate through the skin was investigated in vitro using human cadaver skin. Although the quantity of pimecrolimus penetrating into the skin was similar to that of corticosteroids or tacrolimus, pimecrolimus was found to permeate significantly lesser through the skin in comparison to corticosteroids or tacrolimus (74). These findings indicate that the risk of systemic exposure ultimately associated with systemic side effects after the topical application of pimecrolimus is low and most unlikely (23). This was further supported by several pharmacokinetic studies performed in adults, children, and infants, which proved that after the topical use of pimecrolimus in patients with AD, blood concentrations were equally low regardless of age, severity of disease, and the body area treated. In 91% of the samples tested, pimecrolimus blood levels were below the limit of detection (>0.5 ng/mL) and in 99% of the cases the blood concentrations were below 2 ng/mL. This is considerably below the level of 10 to 15 ng/mL, which is required for a systemic anti-inflammatory effect (75). Moreover, in clinical trials it has been shown that blood levels of pimecrolimus in this range did not cause toxic adverse events (8,9). The low risk of systemic exposure after topical treatment with pimecrolimus was further confirmed by case reports demonstrating very low blood levels in children with Netherton's syndrome. Pimecrolimus blood levels in these patients remained low between 1.5 and 2 ng/mL and no accumulation was detected even after three months of daily application (76,77). These findings indicate that during the treatment with pimecrolimus cream 1%, the risk of systemic adverse events due to systemic exposure is negligible.

Blood tacrolimus levels were detected more frequently following topical application in patients with AD (78). In 67.1% of the patients, tacrolimus plasma levels remained below the level of quantification of 0.5 ng/mL. High blood levels (2–5 ng/mL) of tacrolimus were found in 3.7% of the cases and potentially toxic levels ($\geq$5 ng/mL) in 0.4% of these patients (79). In patients with a severe skin barrier dysfunction, as it is the case in Netherton's syndrome, extremely high blood concentrations (up to 20 ng/mL), which are known to possibly cause systemic adverse events, have been reported (80). However, usually very low and only transient blood levels of tacrolimus have been observed for tacrolimus, and circulating tacrolimus was no longer detectable upon restoration of the skin barrier function. In summary, the pharmacokinetic long-term studies did not show any evidence for a systemic accumulation, resulting in systemic adverse events after long-term treatment with pimecrolimus or tacrolimus (66,81–83).

The reason for the observed differences between tacrolimus and pimecrolimus, however, is not completely understood. One possible explanation may be the different structure, lipophilicity as well as content of lipophilic groups of these compounds. Moreover, pimecrolimus in contrast to tacrolimus has a high affinity for epithelial structures such as the skin but a low affinity for lymphoid organs (23). Recently, a higher binding capacity to not identified skin proteins of pimecrolimus in comparison to tacrolimus has been reported (84). These findings may provide an explanation for the lower permeation of pimecrolimus through the skin and the subsequent lower systemic exposure. In summary, the risk of systemic adverse events upon treatment with TCI is negligible with the exception of patients suffering from severe skin barrier defects such as those with Netherton syndrome.

SAFETY AND TOLERABILITY OF TOPICAL CALCINEURIN INHIBITORS

The safety and tolerability of tacrolimus ointment as well as pimecrolimus cream have been evaluated very carefully in several clinical trials. The most frequently observed local adverse event was a sensation of burning, stinging, and feeling of warmth, which in most cases only occurred transiently during the first few days of treatment and was regarded as mild to moderate (83,85). Transient itching was also noted in some children and adults following the application of tacrolimus ointment. Interestingly these local sensations occurred more frequently in adults and following a treatment with tacrolimus. Thus, the rate of burning after tacrolimus was ~30% in children versus ~47% in adults, whereas after pimecrolimus ~13% of children and ~16% of adults complained about this local adverse reactions (83,85). Recent data indicate that the burning, stinging, and itching following topical application of TCIs appear to be due to the release of preformed neuromediators from primary afferent nerve endings. Accordingly, a depletion of substance P (SP), which is known to cause burning, was observed in cutaneous nerves following the application of both tacrolimus and pimecrolimus (86). Moreover, after alcohol intake erythema and burning has been observed more frequently following tacrolimus therapy as compared to pimecrolimus treatment (87,88). Because neuropeptides such as SP may cause vasodilatation, the ethanol-induced flushing and burning may also be due to an additional or synergistic effect of TCIs plus alcohol activating the release of neuropeptides from afferent nerves.

An increased rate of bacterial or fungal skin infections was neither observed in adults nor in children following pimecrolimus (85). In long-term studies some patients receiving tacrolimus reported about an increased rate of bacterial skin infections during the first months of treatment. In addition, the risk of developing folliculitis or acne appeared to be increased in some young adults. However, within a few days after tacrolimus application, a decreased colonization with *Staphylococcus aureus* in the eczematous skin lesions was observed (89). This effect may be attributed to a normalization of the innate defence system in the skin. Accordingly, it has recently been shown that pimecrolimus was able to enhance the expression of antimicrobial peptides such as cathelicidin, beta-defensin-2, and beta-defensin-3 in cultured human keratinocytes (90). Furthermore, by using recall antigen tests it was shown that neither the treatment with pimecrolimus cream nor that with tacrolimus ointment was able to impair cellular immune responses (39). There is also one report on the normalization of the median multitest Merieux score after one year of tacrolimus ointment treatment, suggesting an improvement of the Th1 immune response (91). An increased risk to develop herpes simplex infections has been observed mostly in children after treatment with tacrolimus ointment or pimecrolimus cream. In addition, the incidence of eczema herpeticum was slightly elevated. However, none of the cases was reported causing a therapeutic problem (68,85). Thus, skin infections possibly related to TCIs may not be regarded as a major risk factor in patients with AD. However, cease of topical application with TCIs is recommended until a total clearance of the skin infections can be observed. Moreover, there is no evidence that the capacity to respond to vaccination with an appropriate antibody production is affected after topical pimecrolimus or tacrolimus therapy (40,92).

In contrast to corticosteroids, both tacrolimus as well as pimecrolimus did not suppress fibroblast functions such as collagen synthesis and therefore most importantly lack skin atrophogenicity (93,94). However, there is evidence from clinical trials that topical application of both tacrolimus and pimecrolimus may restore collagen synthesis and reverse the skin atrophy (33,95). Moreover, topical application of pimecrolimus was followed by a rapid restoration of the skin barrier and contrary to corticosteroids did not cause impairment of the epidermal barrier function (96). This may provide an additional explanation for the lack of tachyphylaxis upon treatment with topical CI. Finally, these advantageous effects of TCI's are important prerequisites for the long-term management of AD.

Risk of Malignancies

The use of systemic immunosuppressants such as CyA is well known to be associated with an increased risk for the development of UV-induced skin cancer (97,98). Therefore, it was necessary to carefully evaluate the potential risk of developing skin cancer after treatment with TCI's. Although the coincidence of nonmelanoma skin cancer (NMSC) has been reported in patients being treated with tacrolimus or pimecrolimus, a causal link between the occurrence of skin tumors and TCI therapy has not been established (83,85,99100). This was further supported by a case-control study in 5000 patients with AD—1000 with documented NMSC and 4000 controls. Accordingly, there was no evidence that the use of either tacrolimus or pimecrolimus is associated with an increased risk of NMSC. In contrast, there is a possibility of association for NMSC decreasing when the amount and potency of TCIs was increasing (99). In addition, there are several data from animal studies supporting the low potential of TCIs to contribute to the development of NMSC. Thus, in mice, topical tacrolimus treatment was found to inhibit the development of phorbol ester–induced skin tumors and in hairless mice it did not enhance solar radiation–stimulated photocarcinogenesis (101,102). Moreover, tacrolimus was able to suppress tumor growth factor beta-1 receptor (TGFβ1R) activation, which plays an important role in wound healing and tumor formation (103,104). Tacrolimus as well as pimecrolimus was also found to inhibit the UV-induced thymidin-dimer formation and thus prevents DNA damage (105,106). In addition, tacrolimus was able to prevent keratinocyte apoptosis (98). However, the question of tumor formation following long-term treatment with TCIs cannot be answered beyond doubt at present. Therefore, concomitant UV-therapy should be avoided and the patients should be instructed to apply UV-protective measurements.

Systemic immunosuppressing drugs are well known to increase the risk of lymphoma after organ transplantation, which is related to the level of immunosuppression achieved with the systemic administration of high doses (107). Cases of lymphoma have been reported in AD patients being treated with tacrolimus or pimecrolimus. However, an association between lymphoma and AD irrespective of the treatment is unclear. Therefore, a case-control study was performed to assess the risk of lymphoma associated with the use of topical corticosteroids and TCIs for treatment of AD. Among 293,253 patients 294 cases of lymphoma have been reported. No increased risk of lymphoma in patients treated with TCIs could be established, whereas the severity of AD appeared to be an important prediction factor associated with an increased risk of lymphoma (108).

TCIs are available for more than eight years for the treatment of AD and no data are available, indicating that the topical use of tacrolimus or pimecrolimus may increase the risk of malignancy. Based on a theoretical risk of malignancy derived from safety profiles, animal data, and reported cases of malignancy from clinical trials as well as postmarketing safety surveillance of oral CIs, the authorities in the United States and Europe have prompted the addition of a black-box warning to the prescribing information for tacrolimus ointment and pimecrolimus cream (109). However, in a press release from March 2006, the European Medicine Agency states that on the basis of available data it was not possible to conclude whether tacrolimus or pimecrolimus caused of skin cancer or lymphoma in the reported cases and that the benefit associated with the use of TCIs outweighs the risks.

CONCLUSION

With the launch of TCIs more than eight years ago, an innovative, effective, and safe treatment modality for AD was established. In addition to being highly effective in improving eczema and pruritus, the major advantage of tacrolimus and pimecrolimus in comparison to conventional therapies is their acceptable safety profile and tolerability. Therefore, TCIs proved to be the first anti-inflammatory compounds, which are suited as an effective, long-term management of AD. Moreover, several long-term studies have provided evidence that the intermittent treatment with tacrolimus ointment or pimecrolimus cream was associated with more flare-free days, less use of corticosteroids as a rescue medication, and a longer time period until the first relapse (39,110–113). Thus, the current recommendation is to

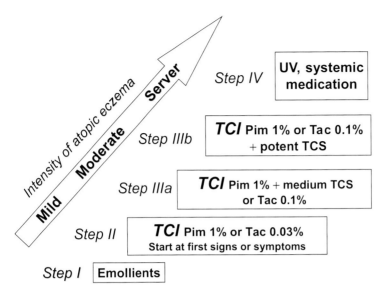

FIGURE 4 Treatment algorithm for atopic dermatitis based on the use of TCIs. *Abbreviations*: TCI, topical calcineurin inhibitor; TCS, topical corticosteroid; Pim, pimecrolimus; Tac, tacrolimus.

use tacrolimus or pimecrolimus as early as first signs of itching and eczema appear. It is currently being investigated whether proactive treatment with TCIs, especially in infants and children may even have a preventive effect on the development of the atopic march including skin and respiratory tract involvement (114).

These very promising results already have resulted in the introduction of a novel paradigm for the treatment of AD, which is aimed to reduce the need of other therapies frequently associated with severe side effects. Thus, upon the first signs of eczema and pruritus, patients should begin to use TCIs, and as soon as the symptoms have improved, the treatment may be continued with emollients only. If the disease cannot be controlled with TCI monotherapy, the intermittent use of other anti-inflammatory compounds such as topical corticosteroids is recommended. Finally, the use of UV-therapy and systemic immunosuppressants should be limited to severe AD, which cannot be controlled by topical treatment. On the other hand, after the improvement of very severe AD under systemic therapy, it may be considered, while tapering the systemic drug, to start TCIs and finally to control the disease with TCIs alone (1,115) (Fig. 4).

The good efficacy and safety profile of TCIs in the treatment of AD have resulted in numerous smaller clinical trials and case reports, investigating their efficacy in inflammatory skin diseases other than AD. Accordingly, both tacrolimus and pimecrolimus have been reported to improve seborrhoic eczema, psoriasis in children, the face and intertriginous areas, steroid-induced perioral dermatitis, steroid-induced rosacea, perianal dermatitis, chronic actinic dermatitis, granuloma annulare, lichen planus, lichen amyloidosus, lichen aureus and chronic actinic dermatitis, hand eczema, mucous lesions of lichen planus as well as lichen sclerosus et atrophicans, pyoderma gangraenosum, lupus erythematosus, dermatomyositis, bullous autoimmune diseases, and chronic graft-versus-host disease. The efficacy of TCIs in the treatment of vitiligo is controversial and UV-light may be additionally required. In contrast, treatment of alopecia areata in humans with TCIs was not effective (116,117).

One drawback of TCIs is the price, making long term therapy very expensive in comparison to conventional treatment modalities with corticosteroids. Therefore, the cost effectiveness of management of AD with TCIs has been analyzed in several studies. Although the results are still controversial, there is evidence from some studies comparing topical corticosteroids and previous standards of care that TCIs may be regarded as a cost-effective treatment option (118–120). However, the data are of limited value since only a few head-to-head comparative trials have been performed and no socioeconomic aspects have been taken into consideration. Thus, the currently available economical data are of limited value and further studies are required before eventually drawing any conclusions on the cost-efficacy of TCIs.

In conclusion, the introduction of topical CI as anti-inflammatory agents to combat inflammatory skin diseases has already changed our attitude for the therapy of atopic dermatitis and other inflammatory skin diseases. However, the future position of topical CI for the treatment of AD and other inflammatory skin diseases depends on further well-controlled clinical trials.

REFERENCES

1. Ellis C, Luger T, Abeck D, et al. International Consensus Conference on Atopic Dermatitis II (ICCAD II): Clinical update and current treatment strategies. Br J Dermatol 2003; 148(suppl 63):3–10.
2. Sulzberger MB, Witten VH, Smith CC. Hydrocortisone (compound F) acetate ointment in dermatological therapy. J Am Med Assoc 1953; 151(6):468–472.
3. Taylor AL, Watson CJ, Bradley JA. Immunosuppressive agents in solid organ transplantation: Mechanisms of action and therapeutic efficacy. Crit Rev Oncol Hematol 2005; 56(1):23–46.
4. Madan V, Griffiths CE. Systemic cyclosporin and tacrolimus in dermatology. Dermatol Ther 2007; 20(4):239–250.
5. Bornhovd E, Burgdorf WH, Wollenberg A. Macrolactam immunomodulators for topical treatment of inflammatory skin diseases. J Am Acad Dermatol 2001; 45(5):736–743.
6. Papp K, Bissonnette R, Rosoph L, et al. Efficacy of ISA247 in plaque psoriasis: A randomised, multicentre, double-blind, placebo-controlled phase III study. Lancet 2008; 371(9621):1337–1342.
7. Rappersberger K, Komar M, Ebelin ME, et al. Oral SDZ ASM981: Safety, pharmacokinetics and efficacy in patients with moderate to severe chronic plaque psoriasis. J Invest Dermatol 2000; 114(4):776.
8. Wolff K, Fleming C, Hanifin J, et al. Efficacy and tolerability of three different doses of oral pimecrolimus in the treatment of moderate to severe atopic dermatitis: A randomized controlled trial. Br J Dermatol 2005; 152(6):1296–1303.
9. Gottlieb AB, Griffiths CE, Ho VC, et al. Oral pimecrolimus in the treatment of moderate to severe chronic plaque-type psoriasis: A double-blind, multicentre, randomized, dose-finding trial. Br J Dermatol 2005; 152(6):1219–1227.
10. Marsland AM, Griffiths CE. The macrolide immunosuppressants in dermatology: Mechanisms of action. Eur J Dermatol 2002; 12(6):618–622.
11. Stuetz A, Baumann K, Grassberger M, et al. Discovery of topical calcineurin inhibitors and pharmacological profile of pimecrolimus. Int Arch Allergy Immunol 2006; 141(3):199–212.

12. Kalthoff FS, Chung J, Stuetz A. Pimecrolimus inhibits up-regulation of OX40 and synthesis of inflammatory cytokines upon secondary T cell activation by allogenic dendritic cells. Clin Exp Immunol 2002; 130(1):85–92.
13. Simon D, Vassina E, Yousefi S, et al. Inflammatory cell numbers and cytokine expression in atopic dermatitis after topical pimecrolimus treatment. Allergy 2005; 60(7):944–951.
14. Hoetzenecker W, Ecker R, Kopp T, et al. Pimecrolimus leads to an apoptosis-induced depletion of T cells but not Langerhans cells in patients with atopic dermatitis. J Allergy Clin Immunol 2005; 115(6):1276–1283.
15. Zuberbier T, Chong SU, Grunow K, et al. The ascomycin macrolactam pimecrolimus (Elidel, SDZ ASM 981) is a potent inhibitor of mediator release from human dermal mast cells and peripheral blood basophils. J Allergy Clin Immunol 2001; 108(2): 275–280.
16. Park CW, Lee BH, Han HJ, et al. Tacrolimus decreases the expression of eotaxin, CCR3, RANTES and interleukin-5 in atopic dermatitis. Br J Dermatol 2005; 152(6):1173–1181.
17. Bieber T. Atopic dermatitis. N Engl J Med 2008; 358(14):1483–1494.
18. Hoetzenecker W, Meingassner JG, Ecker R, et al. Corticosteroids but not pimecrolimus affect viability, maturation and immune function of murine epidermal Langerhans cells. J Invest Dermatol 2004; 122(3):673–684.
19. Schuller E, Oppel T, Bornhovd E, et al. Tacrolimus ointment causes inflammatory dendritic epidermal cell depletion but no Langerhans cell apoptosis in patients with atopic dermatitis. J Allergy Clin Immunol 2004; 114(1):137–143.
20. Meingassner JG, Kowalsky E, Schwendinger H, et al. Pimecrolimus does not affect Langerhans cells in murine epidermis. Br J Dermatol 2003; 149(4):853–857.
21. Hoetzenecker W, Meindl S, Stuetz A, et al. Both pimecrolimus and corticosteroids deplete plasmacytoid dendritic cells in patients with atopic dermatitis. J Invest Dermatol 2006; 126(9):2141–2144.
22. Alomar A, Berth-Jones J, Bos JD, et al. The role of topical calcineurin inhibitors in atopic dermatitis. Br J Dermatol 2004; 151(suppl 70):3–27.
23. Stuetz A, Grassberger M, Meingassner JG. Pimecrolimus (Elidel, SDZ ASM 981)—Preclinical pharmacologic profile and skin selectivity. Semin Cutan Med Surg 2001; 20(4):233–241.
24. Van Leent EJ, Graber M, Thurston M, et al. Effectiveness of the ascomycin macrolactam SDZ ASM 981 in the topical treatment of atopic dermatitis. Arch Dermatol 1998; 134(7):805–809.
25. Breuer K, Werfel T, Kapp A. Safety and efficacy of topical calcineurin inhibitors in the treatment of childhood atopic dermatitis. Am J Clin Dermatol 2005; 6(2):65–77.
26. Luger T, Van Leent EJ, Graeber M, et al. SDZ ASM 981: An emerging safe and effective treatment for atopic dermatitis. Br J Dermatol 2001; 144(4):788–794.
27. Eichenfield LF, Lucky AW, Boguniewicz M, et al. Safety and efficacy of pimecrolimus (ASM 981) cream 1% in the treatment of mild and moderate atopic dermatitis in children and adolescents. J Am Acad Dermatol 2002; 46(4):495–504.
28. Eichenfield LF, Lucky AW, Langley RG, et al. Use of pimecrolimus cream 1% (Elidel) in the treatment of atopic dermatitis in infants and children: The effects of ethnic origin and baseline disease severity on treatment outcome. Int J Dermatol 2005; 44(1):70–75.
29. Kaufmann R, Folster-Holst R, Hoger P, et al. Onset of action of pimecrolimus cream 1% in the treatment of atopic eczema in infants. J Allergy Clin Immunol 2004; 114(5):1183–1188.
30. Leo HL, Bender BG, Leung SB, et al. Effect of pimecrolimus cream 1% on skin condition and sleep disturbance in children with atopic dermatitis. J Allergy Clin Immunol 2004; 114(3):691–693.
31. Papp K, Staab D, Harper J, et al. Effect of pimecrolimus cream 1% on the long-term course of pediatric atopic dermatitis. Int J Dermatol 2004; 43(12):978–983.
32. Spergel JM, Boguniewicz M, Paller AS, et al. Addition of topical pimecrolimus to once-daily mid-potent steroid confers no short-term therapeutic benefit in the treatment of severe atopic dermatitis; a randomized controlled trial. Br J Dermatol 2007; 157(2):378–381.

33. Murrell DF, Calvieri S, Ortonne JP, et al. A randomized controlled trial of pimecrolimus cream 1% in adolescents and adults with head and neck atopic dermatitis and intolerant of, or dependent on, topical corticosteroids. Br J Dermatol 2007; 157(5):954–959.

34. Hoeger P, Lee KH, Jautova J, et al. The treatment of facial atopic dermatitis in children who are intolerant of, or dependent on topical corticosteroids: a randomized, controlled clinical trial. Br J Dermatol 2008; Nov 25 [Epub ahead of print].

35. Schwarz T, Kreiselmaier I, Bieber T, et al. A randomized, double-blind, vehicle-controlled study of 1% pimecrolimus cream in adult patients with perioral dermatitis. J Am Acad Dermatol 2008; 59(1):34–40.

36. Oppel T, Pavicic T, Kamann S, et al. Pimecrolimus cream (1%) efficacy in perioral dermatitis—Results of a randomized, double-blind, vehicle-controlled study in 40 patients. J Eur Acad Dermatol Venereol 2007; 21(9):1175–1180.

37. Meurer M, Folster-Holst R, Wozel G, et al. Pimecrolimus cream in the long-term management of atopic dermatitis in adults: A six-month study. Dermatology 2002; 205(3):271–277.

38. Kapp A, Papp K, Bingham A, et al. Long-term management of atopic dermatitis in infants with topical pimecrolimus, a nonsteroid anti-inflammatory drug. J Allergy Clin Immunol 2002; 110(2):277–284.

39. Wahn U, Bos JD, Goodfield M, et al. Efficacy and safety of pimecrolimus cream in the long-term management of atopic dermatitis in children. Pediatrics 2002; 110(1 Pt 1): e2.

40. Papp KA, Breuer K, Meurer M, et al. Long-term treatment of atopic dermatitis with pimecrolimus cream 1% in infants does not interfere with the development of protective antibodies after vaccination. J Am Acad Dermatol 2005; 52(2):247–253.

41. Papp KA, Werfel T, Folster-Holst R, et al. Long-term control of atopic dermatitis with pimecrolimus cream 1% in infants and young children: A two-year study. J Am Acad Dermatol 2005; 52(2):240–246.

42. Langley RG, Eichenfield LF, Lucky AW, et al. Sustained efficacy and safety of pimecrolimus cream 1% when used long-term (up to 26 weeks) to treat children with atopic dermatitis. Pediatr Dermatol 2008; 25(3):301–307.

43. Meurer M, Lubbe J, Kapp A, et al. The role of pimecrolimus cream 1% (Elidel) in managing adult atopic eczema. Dermatology 2007; 215(suppl 1):18–26.

44. Eichenfield LF, Thaci D, de PY, et al. Clinical management of atopic eczema with pimecrolimus cream 1% (Elidel) in paediatric patients. Dermatology 2007; 215(suppl 1):3–17.

45. Lee HH, Zuberbier T, Worm M. Treatment of atopic dermatitis with pimecrolimus—Impact on quality of life. Ther Clin Risk Manag 2007; 3(6):1021–1026.

46. McKenna SP, Whalley D, de PY, et al. Treatment of paediatric atopic dermatitis with pimecrolimus (Elidel, SDZ ASM 981): Impact on quality of life and health-related quality of life. J Eur Acad Dermatol Venereol 2006; 20(3):248–254.

47. Staab D, Kaufmann R, Brautigam M, et al. Treatment of infants with atopic eczema with pimecrolimus cream 1% improves parents' quality of life: A multicenter, randomized trial. Pediatr Allergy Immunol 2005; 16(6):527–533.

48. Meurer M, Fartasch M, Albrecht G, et al. Long-term efficacy and safety of pimecrolimus cream 1% in adults with moderate atopic dermatitis. Dermatology 2004; 208(4):365–372.

49. Zuberbier T, Brautigam M. Long-term management of facial atopic eczema with pimecrolimus cream 1% in paediatric patients with mild to moderate disease. J Eur Acad Dermatol Venereol 2008; 22(6):718–721.

50. Zuberbier T, Heinzerling L, Bieber T, et al. Steroid-sparing effect of pimecrolimus cream 1% in children with severe atopic dermatitis. Dermatology 2007; 215(4):325–330.

51. De BM, Morren MA, Boonen H, et al. Belgian observational drug utilization study of pimecrolimus cream 1% in routine daily practice in atopic dermatitis. Dermatology 2008; 217(2):156–163.

52. Ring J, Abraham A, de CC, et al. Control of atopic eczema with pimecrolimus cream 1% under daily practice conditions: Results of a >2000 patient study. J Eur Acad Dermatol Venereol 2008; 22(2):195–203.

53. Gollnick H, Luger T, Freytag S, et al. StabiEL: Stabilization of skin condition with Elidel-a patients' satisfaction observational study addressing the treatment, with pimecrolimus cream, of atopic dermatitis pretreated with topical corticosteroid. J Eur Acad Dermatol Venereol 2008; 22(11):1319–1325.
54. Luger TA, Gollnick H, Schwennesen T, et al. Safety and efficacy of pimecrolimus cream 1% in the daily practice: Results of a patient self-observation study in patients with atopic dermatitis. J Dtsch Dermatol Ges 2007; 5(10):908–914.
55. Sunderkötter C, Weiss JM, Bextermoller R, et al. Post-marketing surveillance on treatment of 5665 patients with atopic dermatitis using the calcineurin inhibitor pimecrolimus: Positive effects on major symptoms of atopic dermatitis and on quality of life. J Dtsch Dermatol Ges 2006; 4(4):301–306.
56. Ruzicka T, Bieber T, Schopf E, et al. A short-term trial of tacrolimus ointment for atopic dermatitis. European Tacrolimus Multicenter Atopic Dermatitis Study Group. N Engl J Med 1997; 337(12):816–821.
57. Cheer SM, Plosker GL. Tacrolimus ointment. A review of its therapeutic potential as a topical therapy in atopic dermatitis. Am J Clin Dermatol 2001; 2(6):389–406.
58. Rustin M. Tacrolimus ointment for the management of atopic dermatitis. Hosp Med 2003; 64(4):214–217.
59. Reitamo S, Rustin M, Ruzicka T, et al. Efficacy and safety of tacrolimus ointment compared with that of hydrocortisone butyrate ointment in adult patients with atopic dermatitis. J Allergy Clin Immunol 2002; 109(3):547–555.
60. Reitamo S, Van Leent EJ, Ho V, et al. Efficacy and safety of tacrolimus ointment compared with that of hydrocortisone acetate ointment in children with atopic dermatitis. J Allergy Clin Immunol 2002; 109(3):539–546.
61. Reitamo S, Harper J, Bos JD, et al. 0.03% Tacrolimus ointment applied once or twice daily is more efficacious than 1% hydrocortisone acetate in children with moderate to severe atopic dermatitis: Results of a randomized double-blind controlled trial. Br J Dermatol 2004; 150(3):554–562.
62. Bieber T, Vick K, Folster-Holst R, et al. Efficacy and safety of methylprednisolone aceponate ointment 0.1% compared to tacrolimus 0.03% in children and adolescents with an acute flare of severe atopic dermatitis. Allergy 2007; 62(2):184–189.
63. Ashcroft DM, Dimmock P, Garside R, et al. Efficacy and tolerability of topical pimecrolimus and tacrolimus in the treatment of atopic dermatitis: Meta-analysis of randomised controlled trials. BMJ 2005; 330(7490):516.
64. Kempers S, Boguniewicz M, Carter E, et al. A randomized investigator-blinded study comparing pimecrolimus cream 1% with tacrolimus ointment 0.03% in the treatment of pediatric patients with moderate atopic dermatitis. J Am Acad Dermatol 2004; 51(4):515–525.
65. Paller AS, Lebwohl M, Fleischer AB Jr, et al. Tacrolimus ointment is more effective than pimecrolimus cream with a similar safety profile in the treatment of atopic dermatitis: Results from 3 randomized, comparative studies. J Am Acad Dermatol 2005; 52(5):810–822.
66. Reitamo S, Wollenberg A, Schopf E, et al. Safety and efficacy of 1 year of tacrolimus ointment monotherapy in adults with atopic dermatitis. The European Tacrolimus Ointment Study Group. Arch Dermatol 2000; 136(8):999–1006.
67. Reitamo S, Ortonne JP, Sand C, et al. A multicentre, randomized, double-blind, controlled study of long-term treatment with 0.1% tacrolimus ointment in adults with moderate to severe atopic dermatitis. Br J Dermatol 2005; 152(6):1282–1289.
68. Reitamo S, Ortonne JP, Sand C, et al. Long-term treatment with 0.1% tacrolimus ointment in adults with atopic dermatitis: Results of a two-year, multicentre, noncomparative study. Acta Derm Venereol 2007; 87(5):406–412.
69. Reitamo S, Rustin M, Harper J, et al. A 4-year follow-up study of atopic dermatitis therapy with 0.1% tacrolimus ointment in children and adult patients. Br J Dermatol 2008; 159(4):942–951.
70. Hanifin JM, Paller AS, Eichenfield L, et al. Efficacy and safety of tacrolimus ointment treatment for up to 4 years in patients with atopic dermatitis. J Am Acad Dermatol 2005; 53(2)(suppl 2):S186–S194.

71. Remitz A, Harper J, Rustin M, et al. Long-term safety and efficacy of tacrolimus ointment for the treatment of atopic dermatitis in children. Acta Derm Venereol 2007; 87(1):54–61.
72. Drake L, Prendergast M, Maher R, et al. The impact of tacrolimus ointment on health-related quality of life of adult and pediatric patients with atopic dermatitis. J Am Acad Dermatol 2001; 44(1 suppl):S65–S72.
73. Kang S, Lucky AW, Pariser D, et al. Long-term safety and efficacy of tacrolimus ointment for the treatment of atopic dermatitis in children. J Am Acad Dermatol 2001; 44(1 suppl):S58–S64.
74. Billich A, Aschauer H, Aszodi A, et al. Percutaneous absorption of drugs used in atopic eczema: Pimecrolimus permeates less through skin than corticosteroids and tacrolimus. Int J Pharm 2004; 269(1):29–35.
75. Van Leent EJ, Ebelin ME, Burtin P, et al. Low systemic exposure after repeated topical application of pimecrolimus (Elidel, SD Z ASM 981) in patients with atopic dermatitis. Dermatology 2002; 204(1):63–68.
76. Henno A, Choffray A, De La BM. Improvement of Netherton syndrome associated erythroderma in two adult sisters through use of topical pimecrolimus. Ann Dermatol Venereol 2006; 133(1):71–72.
77. Oji V, Beljan G, Beier K, et al. Topical pimecrolimus: A novel therapeutic option for Netherton syndrome. Br J Dermatol 2005; 153(5):1067–1068.
78. Draelos Z, Nayak A, Pariser D, et al. Pharmacokinetics of topical calcineurin inhibitors in adult atopic dermatitis: A randomized, investigator-blind comparison. J Am Acad Dermatol 2005; 53(4):602–609.
79. Reitamo S. Topical immunomodulators for therapy of atopic dermatitis. In: Bieber T, Leung DY, eds. Atopic Dermatitis. New York, NY: Marcel Dekker, Inc., 2002.
80. Allen A, Siegfried E, Silverman R, et al. Significant absorption of topical tacrolimus in 3 patients with Netherton syndrome. Arch Dermatol 2001; 137(6):747–750.
81. Lakhanpaul M, Davies T, Allen BR, et al. Low systemic exposure in infants with atopic dermatitis in a 1-year pharmacokinetic study with pimecrolimus cream 1%. Exp Dermatol 2006; 15(2):138–141.
82. Paul C, Cork M, Rossi AB, et al. Safety and tolerability of 1% pimecrolimus cream among infants: Experience with 1133 patients treated for up to 2 years. Pediatrics 2006; 117(1):e118–e128.
83. Rustin MH. The safety of tacrolimus ointment for the treatment of atopic dermatitis: A review. Br J Dermatol 2007; 157(5):861–873.
84. Weiss HM, Fresneau M, Moenius T, et al. Binding of pimecrolimus and tacrolimus to skin and plasma proteins: Implications for systemic exposure after topical application. Drug Metab Dispos 2008; 36(9):1812–1818.
85. Langley RG, Luger TA, Cork MJ, et al. An update on the safety and tolerability of pimecrolimus cream 1%: Evidence from clinical trials and post-marketing surveillance. Dermatology 2007; 215(suppl 1):27–44.
86. Ständer S, Ständer H, Seeliger S, et al. Topical pimecrolimus and tacrolimus transiently induce neuropeptide release and mast cell degranulation in murine skin. Br J Dermatol 2007; 156(5):1020–1026.
87. Ogunleye T, James WD. Ethanol-induced flushing with topical pimecrolimus use. Dermatitis 2008; 19(2):E1–E2.
88. Knight AK, Boxer M, Chandler MJ. Alcohol-induced rash caused by topical tacrolimus. Ann Allergy Asthma Immunol 2005; 95(3):291–292.
89. Remitz A, Kyllonen II, Granlund H, et al. Tacrolimus ointment reduces staphylococcal colonization of atopic dermatitis lesions. J Allergy Clin Immunol 2001; 107(1):196–197.
90. Buchau AS, Schauber J, Hultsch T, et al. Pimecrolimus enhances TLR2/6-induced expression of antimicrobial peptides in keratinocytes. J Invest Dermatol 2008; 128(11):2646–2654.
91. Mandelin J, Remitz A, Virtanen H, et al. Recall antigen reactions in patients with atopic dermatitis treated with tacrolimus ointment for 1 year. J Allergy Clin Immunol 2008; 121(3):777–779.

92. Hofman T, Cranswick N, Kuna P, et al. Tacrolimus ointment does not affect the immediate response to vaccination, the generation of immune memory, or humoral and cell-mediated immunity in children. Arch Dis Child 2006; 91(11):905–910.
93. Queille-Roussel C, Paul C, Duteil L, et al. The new topical ascomycin derivative SDZ ASM 981 does not induce skin atrophy when applied to normal skin for 4 weeks: A randomized, double-blind controlled study. Br J Dermatol 2001; 144(3):507–513.
94. Reitamo S, Rissanen J, Remitz A, et al. Tacrolimus ointment does not affect collagen synthesis: Results of a single-center randomized trial. J Invest Dermatol 1998; 111(3):396–398.
95. Kyllonen H, Remitz A, Mandelin JM, et al. Effects of 1-year intermittent treatment with topical tacrolimus monotherapy on skin collagen synthesis in patients with atopic dermatitis. Br J Dermatol 2004; 150(6):1174–1181.
96. Cork M, Varghese J, Hadcraft J, et al. Differences in the effect of topical corticosteroids and calcineurin inhibitors on the skin barrier—Implications for therapy. J Invest Dermatol 2007; 127:45S.
97. Parrish JA. Immunosuppression, skin cancer, and ultraviolet A radiation. N Engl J Med 2005; 353(25):2712–2713.
98. Yarosh DB, Pena AV, Nay SL, et al. Calcineurin inhibitors decrease DNA repair and apoptosis in human keratinocytes following ultraviolet B irradiation. J Invest Dermatol 2005; 125(5):1020–1025.
99. Margolis DJ, Hoffstad O, Bilker W. Lack of association between exposure to topical calcineurin inhibitors and skin cancer in adults. Dermatology 2007; 214(4):289–295.
100. Naylor M, Elmets C, Jaracz E, et al. Non-melanoma skin cancer in patients with atopic dermatitis treated with topical tacrolimus. J Dermatolog Treat 2005; 16(3):149–153.
101. Lerche CM, Philipsen PA, Poulsen T, et al. Topical tacrolimus in combination with simulated solar radiation does not enhance photocarcinogenesis in hairless mice. Exp Dermatol 2008; 17(1):57–62.
102. Jiang H, Yamamoto S, Nishikawa K, et al. Anti-tumor-promoting action of FK506, a potent immunosuppressive agent. Carcinogenesis 1993; 14(1):67–71.
103. Lan CC, Kao YH, Huang SM, et al. FK506 independently upregulates transforming growth factor beta and downregulates inducible nitric oxide synthase in cultured human keratinocytes: Possible mechanisms of how tacrolimus ointment interacts with atopic skin. Br J Dermatol 2004; 151(3):679–684.
104. Yao D, Dore JJ Jr, Leof EB. FKBP12 is a negative regulator of transforming growth factor-beta receptor internalization. J Biol Chem 2000; 275(17):13149–13154.
105. Stern RS. Topical calcineurin inhibitors labeling: Putting the "box" in perspective. Arch Dermatol 2006; 142(9):1233–1235.
106. Gambichler T, Schlaffke A, Tomi NS, et al. Tacrolimus ointment neither blocks ultraviolet B nor affects expression of thymine dimers and p53 in human skin. J Dermatol Sci 2008; 50(2):115–122.
107. Opelz G, Dohler B. Lymphomas after solid organ transplantation: A collaborative transplant study report. Am J Transplant 2004; 4(2):222–230.
108. Arellano FM, Wentworth CE, Arana A, et al. Risk of lymphoma following exposure to calcineurin inhibitors and topical steroids in patients with atopic dermatitis. J Invest Dermatol 2007; 127(4):808–816.
109. Munzenberger PJ, Montejo JM. Safety of topical calcineurin inhibitors for the treatment of atopic dermatitis. Pharmacotherapy 2007; 27(7):1020–1028.
110. Sigurgeirsson B, Ho V, Ferrandiz C, et al. Pimecrolimus 1% cream in (paediatric) eczema: prevention of progression multi-center investigator study group. J Eur Acad Dermatol Venereol 2008; 22(11):1290–1301.
111. Gollnick H, Kaufmann R, Stough D, et al. Pimecrolimus cream 1% in the long-term management of adult atopic dermatitis: Prevention of flare progression. A randomized controlled trial. Br J Dermatol 2008; 158(5):1083–1093.
112. Wollenberg A, Reitamo S, Girolomoni G, et al. Proactive treatment of atopic dermatitis in adults with 0.1% tacrolimus ointment. Allergy 2008; 63(7):742–750.

113. Breneman D, Fleischer AB Jr, Abramovits W, et al. Intermittent therapy for flare prevention and long-term disease control in stabilized atopic dermatitis: A randomized comparison of 3-times-weekly applications of tacrolimus ointment versus vehicle. J Am Acad Dermatol 2008; 58(6):990–999.

114. Virtanen H, Remitz A, Malmberg P, et al. Topical tacrolimus in the treatment of atopic dermatitis—Does it benefit the airways? A 4-year open follow-up. J Allergy Clin Immunol 2007; 120(6):1464–1466.

115. Luger TA, Bieber T, Meurer M, et al. Therapy of atopic eczema with calcineurin inhibitors. J Dtsch Dermatol Ges 2005; 3(5):385–391.

116. Luger T, Paul C. Potential new indications of topical calcineurin inhibitors. Dermatology 2007; 215(suppl 1):45–54.

117. Wollina U. The role of topical calcineurin inhibitors for skin diseases other than atopic dermatitis. Am J Clin Dermatol 2007; 8(3):157–173.

118. Ellis CN, Kahler KH, Grueger J, et al. Cost effectiveness of management of mild-to-moderate atopic dermatitis with 1% pimecrolimus cream in children and adolescents 2–17 years of age. Am J Clin Dermatol 2006; 7(2):133–139.

119. Abramovits W, Boguniewicz M, Paller AS, et al. The economics of topical immunomodulators for the treatment of atopic dermatitis. Pharmacoeconomics 2005; 23(6):543–566.

120. Ellis CN, Drake LA, Prendergast MM, et al. Cost-effectiveness analysis of tacrolimus ointment versus high-potency topical corticosteroids in adults with moderate to severe atopic dermatitis. J Am Acad Dermatol 2003; 48(4):553–563.

23 Systemic Pharmacotherapy

Werner Aberer

Department of Dermatology, University of Graz, Graz, Austria

Klaus Wolff

Department of Dermatology, University of Vienna, Vienna, Austria

Thomas Bieber

Department of Dermatology and Allergy, University of Bonn, Bonn, Germany

INTRODUCTION

In the large majority of patients with mild-to-moderate forms, atopic dermatitis can be managed by the use of emollients, anti-inflammatory compounds such as topical corticosteroids or calcineurin inhibitors, phototherapy, avoidance of irritants, and treatment of infection (1,2). Time-honored, systemic treatments include antihistamines to suppress pruritus, systemic corticosteroids for the control of inflammation and pruritus, and, more recently, cyclosporine to suppress ongoing T-cell activation in this chronically relapsing disorder. This review will not only focus on antihistamines, corticosteroids, and cyclosporine but will also address other immunosuppressive and anti-inflammatory agents that have been employed to control atopic dermatitis or are presently being developed such as the biologics.

ANTIHISTAMINES

Antihistamines are among the most widely used drugs in the world and are prescribed in large quantities by dermatologists and general practitioners not only for atopic eczema but seemingly for pruritus of any cause (3). The rationale for their use in atopic dermatitis is to interrupt the itch–scratch–itch cycle. But even though early studies have reported increased histamine levels in normal and eczematous skin and that pruritus induced by intradermally administered histamine can be clinically suppressed with H1 receptor antagonists, the mechanism of itch in atopic dermatitis is still largely unknown. It is undisputed that antihistamines are antipruritic in certain conditions such as insect bites or urticaria, and the ongoing controversy on their use in atopic dermatitis therefore rests on the issue whether they are also antipruritic in this disease (4).

Clinical trials of antihistamines have been criticized for being inadequate in terms of study designs and sample size, and the outcomes are contradictory. Current recommendations and practices are based largely on the individual experience of patients and physicians.

First-Generation Antihistamines

These include ethanolamines, clemastine, piperazine derivatives, meclizine, phenothiazine derivatives, trimeprazine, chlorpheniramine, ethylene diamines, and alkylamines. The drowsiness and decline in performance have been the primary limitations of their daytime use, and when given at night, there may be "hangover" effects the following day. Because itch intensity often increases at night, the soporific effect of sedating formulations can be quite useful. Sedating antihistamines are therefore frequently used, especially at bedtime, to facilitate peaceful sleep.

Should patients with atopic dermatitis use these sedating agents? The prime argument against their use is that they have not been proven to relieve pruritus, but in the experience of most authors they have been useful by virtue of their soporific effect. A disadvantage is that they can only be used for short periods because tolerance is thought to develop quite quickly. Any of the standard antihistamines are essentially equally effective (or not): all cause sedation, impairment of cognitive function, diminished alertness, and slow reaction times. These drugs may also cause fatigue, lassitude, drowsiness, somnolence, weakness, dizziness, ataxia, and even narcolepsy or coma. Occasionally, paradoxical stimulatory effects such as insomnia, hyperreflexia, irritability, headaches, muscle twisting, nervousness, tremor, dyskinesia, dystonia, or seizures may occur. Neuropsychiatric and neurologic effects, dry mouth, and urinary retention have also been reported. Some first-generation H1 antagonists may cause gastrointestinal upset, appetite stimulation, inappropriate weight gain as well as rare cases of pancytopenia and jaundice after ingestion of trimeprazine.

Second- and Third-Generation Antihistamines

These include piperidine derivatives (e.g., terfenadine and astemizole), loratadine, azelastine, fexofenadine, cetirizine, and others. They are generally less sedating and produce considerably less impairment of cognitive and motor function than their earlier chemical cousins. The drowsiness and dry mouth associated with older, first-generation antihistamines resulted from significant penetration of these agents into the central nervous system (CNS). The chemical structures of the second-generation agents differ in that these newer agents are less lipophilic and bind to proteins to a greater extent, properties that prevent substantial CNS penetration. They are also more specific for the histamine receptor and do not appreciably block cholinergic receptors.

Some second-generation antihistamines are also not completely devoid of adverse CNS effects. The low sedating property of terfenadine, astemizole, loratadine, and others is well established (6). Pooled data from placebo-controlled clinical trials of cetirizine have indicated that while the incidence of sedation by cetirizine is lower than that with older antihistamines, it is higher than with the other second-generation antihistamines. As a result, the U.S. Food and Drug Administration (FDA) has classified cetirizine as "sedating" rather than nonsedating, and thus the full sedation precautions also apply to this drug. As terfenadine and astemizole were found to cause potentially serious arrhythmias, they have meanwhile been withdrawn from the market. The goal for the third generation of antihistamines was to develop therapeutically active metabolites that are devoid of cardiac toxicity. This group includes fexofenadine (the active metabolite of terfenadine), which was approved in 1996, norastemizole (the active metabolite of astemizole), and descarboethoxyloratadine (derived from loratadine).

Data on the clinical efficacy of the newer nonsedating agents are conflicting. Although several controlled clinical trials with cetirizine, loratadine, acrivastine, and terfenadine appear to support efficacy of these antihistamines in atopic dermatitis, an evidence-based review of the efficacy of antihistamines in relieving pruritus in atopic dermatitis (5) concluded that "little objective evidence exists to demonstrate relief of pruritus. The majority of trials are flawed in terms of the sample size or study design. Based on the literature alone, the efficacy of antihistamines remains to be adequately investigated. However, newer in vitro studies with some second- and third-generation antihistamines have revealed properties of some of these products that might broaden their spectrum for clinical use and also justify their administration to patients with atopic dermatitis.

Loratidine in vitro inhibits the release of histamine and leukotriene C4 (LTC4) from rodent mast cells, histamine and LTC4 from human basophils, and histamine, leukotrienes, and prostaglandin D2 from human skin tissue. It has also been shown to inhibit superoxide anion generation and eosinophil chemotaxis in vitro and eosinophil accumulation in nasal and bronchoalveolar lavage material after antigen challenge in vivo. In allergic subjects, blood flow to the skin was increased and late-phase reactions to both histamine and allergen skin-prick challenges were inhibited. Following these observations, loratadine 10 mg once daily has shown to reduce pruritus and rash more effectively than placebo and at least as well as hydroxyzine. Double-blind, randomized, placebo-controlled studies have meanwhile reproduced similar positive effects (6).

Cetirizine was shown in patients with severe reactions to insect bites to inhibit both the early and late inflammatory reaction as well as eosinophil infiltration and accumulation. In a double-blind, multicenter, placebo-controlled study, cetirizine gave a marked improvement of pruritus and the extent and activity of skin lesions. This was paralleled by a pronounced decrease in the number of blood eosinophils (7).

Diverse anti-inflammatory properties, such as the inhibition of mediator release and leukocyte chemotaxis, have been described for descarbethoxyloratadine, the active metabolite of loratadine, including cytokine synthesis and secretion from mast cells. Proven antihistaminic, anti-inflammatory (Th2 cytokines, chemokines, and adhesion molecules), and antiallergic (inhibition of mast cell products) activity has an enormous potential for treating the systemic aspects of allergic disease.

IgE-mediated hypersensitivity reactions and positive skin-prick tests to allergens are common in patients with atopic dermatitis and have been implicated in the pathogenesis of this disease. As treatment with antihistamines has convincing effects in IgE-mediated disease like allergic rhinitis or urticaria and in patients allergic to drugs or insect venoms, they should theoretically also exert effects in atopic dermatitis, where antigen exposure via the skin may induce local and systemic immune responses.

Conclusions

Critical reviews of the large body of clinical trials that refute or support the efficacy of antihistamines in relieving pruritus in patients with atopic dermatitis have summarized that there is no evidence to support the effectiveness of antihistamines in atopic dermatitis (5). An article by Henz et al. (4) on the effects of H1 receptor antagonists in pruritic dermatoses points to the differential effects on pruritus versus whealing and the low efficacy in atopic eczema as compared to urticaria. These authors suspect that different anti-inflammatory properties of H1 antagonists, such as the inhibition of mediator release and leukocyte chemotaxis, cytokine synthesis and secretion from mast cells, mediator release from leukocytes and others, "might have no impact on the chronic inflammatory processes in atopic dermatitis, where cytokines and growth factors may be more promising targets of itch therapy" (3).

On the other hand, there are millions of patients with atopic dermatitis who have tried to suppress their pruritus for years with antihistamines with supposedly good results, and many studies by renowned dermatologists claim to have proven efficacy of antihistamines in the treatment of atopic dermatitis. Can they all be wrong, and are we dealing with placebo effects? Juhlin (7) has analyzed many problems of such studies and concluded that "taking all clinical reports together, there is now evidence that the nonsedative or less-sedative antihistamines can reduce pruritus in patients with atopic dermatitis." However, high doses are required to reach substantial symptom relief (4).

Of course, evidence-based medicine certainly calls for new large, randomized, double-blind, placebo-controlled clinical trials to provide a definite answer. Such studies, however, may be difficult or even impossible to perform as most patients with atopic dermatitis take antihistamines because of associated IgE-mediated disease such as allergic rhinitis or asthma. In addition, the heterogeneity of atopic dermatitis with its many different provocative factors, like food allergy, infections, occupational irritants, and mite exposure, makes it difficult to identify patient cohorts comparable with regard to the extent and severity of eczema, level of IgE-associated symptoms, and compliance to perform such studies. The severity of disease has to justify treatment for a prolonged period of time, but then these patients apply topical corticosteroids that also relieve pruritus. Do we really need such a study? It is interesting that most expert clinicians dealing with atopic dermatitis indeed use antihistamines in their daily practice.

SYSTEMIC GLUCOCORTICOSTEROIDS
Glucocorticosteroids exert a wide range of anti-inflammatory and immunosuppressive effects and thus effectively reduce inflammation and pruritus in atopic dermatitis. Their use in atopic dermatitis is time honored, but large-scale controlled studies have never been performed. However, in contrast to the antihistamines, they have an undisputable, proven efficacy in atopic dermatitis. By understanding the properties and mechanisms of action, one can maximize their efficacy and safety as therapeutic agents, but it has to be noted that they should be employed only as a rescue treatment in this chronic disease.

Mode of Action
Systemic steroids decrease the synthesis of a number of proinflammatory molecules, including cytokines, interleukins (IL-1, IL-2, IL-6, and tumor necrosis factor), and proteases, largely through their effects on transcription. Some mediators of inflammation such as cyclooxygenase-2 are inhibited; some others such as lipocortin-1 are increased. Replication and movement of cells are suppressed, resulting in monocytopenia, eosinopenia, and lymphocytopenia (T-cells more than B-cells). Apoptosis of lymphocytes is induced, whereas the increase in circulating polymorphonuclear

leukocytes is related to demargination of cells from the bone marrow and inhibition of neutrophil apoptosis. Activation, proliferation, and differentiation of cells of the immune system are obtained either indirectly via modulation of mediator production or by direct suppression of cellular functions. Very high doses are needed to suppress antibody production of B lymphocytes and plasma cells, a disadvantage in atopic diseases where there is a high degree of IgE-mediated problems. On the other hand, granulomatous infectious diseases, such as tuberculosis, are prone to exacerbate and relapse during prolonged systemic treatment.

The multiplicity of biologic effects produced by glucocorticosteroids explains why currently there is no unifying hypothesis to explain the therapeutic efficacy of these agents.

Use in Atopic Dermatitis

Any decision to employ systemic glucocorticosteroids in atopic dermatitis should weigh expected benefits against potential side effects. In the small proportion of patients who do not respond to optimal skin care and topical management or when during an acute flare of severe atopic dermatitis more than 20% of the skin is affected, a decision to administer steroids systemically may be made (8,9). Systemic administration in atopic dermatitis thus represents a rescue treatment. Initial use of high doses of prednisone or prednisolone (1 mg/kg/day) maximizes the anti-inflammatory/immunosuppressive effects and allows more rapid tapering or conversion to an alternate day regimen. One should not taper too rapidly so as to minimize the risk of a steroid rebound, that is, a posttherapeutic exacerbation of disease to a more severe level. A simple approach, also easy for patients to follow, is to administer 60 mg daily for five days, to be followed by 40 and 20 mg for five days each. Treatment is continued by 20 mg on alternate days for another week and then stopped. A single daily dose given in the morning is preferable, as this regimen is thought to minimize hypothalamic–pituitary–adrenal suppression by mimicking the normal circadian rhythm of adrenal cortisol production. Topical glucocorticoids, ascomycins, or tacrolimus or other steroid-sparing agents should be continued during the taper to suppress rebound flaring, and hydration and moisturizers are needed to be continued or even intensified.

The literature is scarce on systemic steroid treatment in atopic dermatitis, and well-controlled studies have not been performed, obviously because of its empirically proven dramatic efficacy. Now that other systemic drugs like azathioprine and cyclosporine have proven effectiveness in atopic dermatitis, the use of systemic steroids is restricted to rescue treatment where a rapid response is required. This approach requires chronic retreatment leading to tachyphylaxis, cumulative long-term toxicity, and "steroid-addictive" behavior (10). Maintenance systemic glucocorticosteroid therapy has to be avoided in all instances.

Side Effects

The list of side effects is imposing and includes all the adverse events of topical corticosteroid therapy and multiple more significant sequelae like hypertension, gastric ulcers, osteoporosis, aseptic bone necrosis, and cataracts. Side effects on skin include atrophy and striae formation, possibly related to the antianabolic properties of glucocorticoids through suppression of proline hydroxylation and cross-linking of collagen, purpura from increased vascular fragility, formation of stellate pseudoscars, steroid acne, rosacea, perioral dermatitis, facial hypertrichosis, and initial masking and then worsening of cutaneous or systemic bacterial, fungal, or viral infections. Hypertriglyceridemia, altered lipid metabolism, hyperglycemia, gastritis, gastric ulcers, pancreatitis, potassium wasting, myopathy, posterior subcapsular cataracts, Cushingoid appearance, psychosis, pseudotumor cerebri, and growth retardation in children are all possible sequelae of prolonged systemic glucocorticoid administration.

Conclusions

In general, systemic steroids should be avoided in the management of a chronic, relapsing disorder such as atopic dermatitis. As rescue treatments they are justified but should never be administered on a long-term basis. If patients or parents demand immediate improvement of the disease and find topical therapy ineffective or impossible to perform, they have to be appropriately informed of the potential side effects of steroids and of the fact that dramatic improvement observed with systemic steroids may be and is frequently associated with an equally dramatic flare of atopic dermatitis following their discontinuation. Some patients and physicians have in the past preferred the use of systemic steroids over topical therapy, but with the availability of new topical drugs such as tacrolimus or ascomycins, this may become obsolete.

CYCLOSPORIN

Cyclosporin A (CsA) is a fungal peptide with powerful immunosuppressive activity. It effectively suppresses cell-mediated immune responses, particularly graft rejection, and the graft-versus-host reaction. A first report indicating the efficacy of this nonmyelosuppressive immunosuppressive agent in the management of severe atopic dermatitis was published in 1987 (11); several uncontrolled and placebo-controlled trials have been reported, studying the effects in children and adults, short-term and long-term safety, questions of dosage and different formulations, maintenance therapy and remission time, quality of life, disease markers like E-selectin or sCD30 levels in blood, and many others. Several workshop and consensus reports have been published (12–14). CsA is thus a drug for atopic dermatitis that has been carefully and extensively studied.

Regular CsA (marketed as Sandimmun®) has proven useful as a second-line treatment for severe atopic dermatitis in patients who do not respond to or cannot tolerate treatment with topical steroids or other modalities. However, its use has been somewhat hampered by high inter- and intrapatient variability in its bioavailability (15) and dose-dependent side effects. The use of CsA as a microemulsion (Sandimmun Neoral; Neoral®) in the treatment of dermatologic diseases was pioneered by Bourke et al. (16). Further investigations showed that Neoral has a better and more reproducible pharmacokinetic profile resulting in improved control of therapy and fewer adverse events. Data obtained in a randomized, double-blind, crossover study suggest that Neoral is an adequate replacement for Sandimmun, thanks to its high efficacy, its faster onset of action, and its better tolerability (15). The pharmacokinetic properties of Neoral provide for greater ease in individualizing dosage and maintaining CsA concentration within the therapeutic window (17). For conversion from the original formulation to the microemulsion formulation, a 1:1 dose-conversion strategy is recommended. It then may be necessary to make subsequent dose reductions in poor absorbers of conventional CsA to ensure that they are receiving the lowest effective dose. Careful safety monitoring is mandatory postconversion to comply with the safety guidelines (12).

Mode of Action
Peripheral blood eosinophilia frequently occurs in atopic dermatitis, and there is an increase of eosinophils and their products—the eosinophil cationic protein and eosinophil major basic protein—in atopic skin. These eosinophils are thought to be preactivated in the circulation as a result of exposure to the T-cell–mediated cytokines IL-3, IL-5, and GM-CSF. CsA probably acts by downregulating Th2 cells, which decreases IL-4 and IL-5, thereby lowering peripheral blood eosinophilia. Treatment of atopic dermatitis with CsA has also been shown to significantly reduce adhesion molecules that regulate leukocyte migration (E-selectin) (18) and CD30 (19), an activation marker of Th2 cell clones. Reduction of these factors significantly correlated with changes in disease activity parameters such as severity and extent of disease.

Patient Selection
CsA should at present only be used in adults and children (13,20) with severe atopic dermatitis that cannot be controlled by emollients, topical glucocorticosteroids, phototherapy, and/or photochemotherapy. The atopic dermatitis should be of sufficient severity in terms of extent of disease and/or effects on quality of life to justify the risks inherent in CsA treatment. These risks include nephrotoxicity, hypertension, and the consequences of immunosuppression. In children, CsA should be used with even more caution than in adults, in that only short-term treatment should be considered.

The treatment with CsA should only be installed by dermatologists having a large experience of managing atopic dermatitis in the specific age group, children, or adults, respectively, and comprehensive knowledge in the use of CsA in general. Close cooperation with a pediatrician or with the general physician of the patient and vice versa is recommended.

Before starting CsA therapy, patients should be clearly advised that this treatment necessitates close monitoring, is only symptomatic, and, based on the present state of knowledge, continuous treatment should not go beyond six weeks in children and one year in adults. Patients should also undergo a full physical examination with particular attention to skin neoplasms and blood pressure. Screening for gynecologic or prostate malignancy is strongly recommended according to published guidelines (14). Blood chemistry (blood count, serum bilirubin, liver enzymes, urea, creatinine on two occasions, potassium, uric acid, fasting lipids, and urinalysis for protein) should exclude potential contraindications for CsA therapy (Table 1). Pregnancy and lactation constitute contraindications (unless the potential benefits of CsA therapy outweigh the potential risks for the fetus or the baby). Drug interactions are numerous, some of them increasing CsA blood levels (Ca antagonists, antimycotics and antibiotics, corticosteroids, antiemetics, etc.), some lowering CsA levels (antiepileptics, barbiturates, some antibiotics, and somatostatin analogs), some increasing the risk of nephrotoxicity (aminoglycosides, NSAID, antimycotics and antibiotics, alkylating agents). CsA may raise blood levels of antigout agents, NSAID, cardiac glycosides, and corticosteroids. Concomitant therapy with systemic

TABLE 1 Contraindications for Use of Cyclosporin A

Previous or current malignancy (except basal cell carcinoma)
Premalignant conditions
Primary or secondary immunodeficiency
Severe renal and hepatic dysfunction
Uncontrolled hypertension
Serious infection
Drug or alcohol abuse
Lack of compliance with regular monitoring

Source: Adapted from Ref. 31.

corticosteroids, immunomodulating agents, or radiation therapy is contraindicated; concomitant use of topical corticosteroids is permitted and even encouraged in unstable situations.

Dosing and Treatment Regimens

There are still no conclusive data on the most appropriate starting dose of CsA. Although most authors use a starting dose of 5 mg/kg/day in adults, the guidelines edited by Concensus Conferences usually recommend to start at 2.5 mg/kg/day, to divide this dose into a morning and evening dose, and to adjust this dose by increasing with 1 mg/kg/day after every two weeks, up to a maximum dose of 5 mg/kg/day (14,20). This "hesitant" approach is not undisputed: 5 mg/kg/day will induce a more rapid remission, and short-term toxicity is normally a lesser problem than long-term toxicity, which is related to the duration of therapy and cumulative dose and not to the initial dose, when given with recommended levels. Early dose-finding studies indicated the superiority of starting with a high dose in clearing atopic dermatitis, in contrast to the crescendo regimen that entails a delay of clearing and thus often reduces the patient's confidence and compliance.

CsA should be stopped if patients do not respond after eight weeks of treatment, which is rarely the case when starting at 5 mg/kg/day. When skin lesions improve to an acceptable level, the CsA dose should be reduced in steps of 1 mg/kg every two weeks to the lowest effective dose. If clinical improvement continues, CsA should be discontinued to determine if therapy is still needed. However, present evidence indicates that the majority of patients will relapse after cessation of two-month treatment (21). Therefore, long-term therapy will inevitably have to be contemplated.

Whereas some authors recommend long-term therapy—up to one year—with the lowest dose providing adequate disease control, others plead for short-term cycles and to make every reasonable effort to limit the duration of CsA therapy cycles by returning to conventional means of treatment in between two cycles (22). Such a regimen would avoid or delay adverse effects, that is, nephrotoxicity and hypertension, and ultimately improve the long-term safety of CsA in the treatment of atopic dermatitis. Studies to prove the superiority of one approach over the other have not been performed.

In children, several studies were performed on an open basis with an initial dose of 5 mg/kg/day. Treatment was in most cases stopped after six weeks—not because of side effects but for safety precautions—although (limited) evidence from its use in transplantation, connective tissue disease, and diabetes mellitus would suggest that CsA is tolerated at least as well by children as by adults (12).

Body weight–independent dosing regimens of CsA were shown to be promising in transplant patients. In a double-blind study by Czech et al. (23), a total of 106 adults with severe atopic dermatitis were enrolled to receive either 2.2 mg/kg/day (low) or 4.2 mg/kg/day (high) of cyclosporine microemulsion. The results of this study suggest that weight-independent treatment is feasible in atopic dermatitis.

Safety Monitoring

In view of the potential toxicity of CsA, its use in atopic dermatitis must be carefully considered, monitored, and controlled. Follow-up investigations, including blood pressure estimations, serum creatinine, urinalysis, urea, and potassium, should be repeated every two weeks during short-term treatment and the dose reduction or withdrawal of CsA be considered, if adverse effects arise, depending on their severity. If serum creatinine rises to more than 30% above the patient's baseline on two consecutive occasions, CsA dose should be reduced by 25% to 50% for at least one month. Therapy can be continued if the serum creatinine level drops to less than 30% above the patient's baseline. Future therapy can only be started if serum creatinine values return to less than 10% above the patient's baseline. If the patient develops a mean diastolic blood pressure 95 mm Hg on two consecutive occasions, the CsA dose should be reduced by 25% to 50% or the hypertension should be treated with a calcium antagonist not interacting with CsA (e.g., nifedipine). Although continuous CsA treatment seems safe for up to one year, no renal biopsy studies are available as is the case in psoriasis patients.

Lymphadenopathy can develop in patients with severe atopic dermatitis. If it persists, lymphoma should be excluded by biopsy. Other side effects, like suspicious skin changes for tumors, skin infections including *Staphylococcus aureus* and herpes simplex, necessitate regular careful skin inspection. Tremor, hypertrichosis, gingival hyperplasia, or nausea should be recorded and treatment dose be adapted or stopped. Patients on long-term CsA should be warned of the risk of cutaneous malignancy following overexposure to solar radiation. There are no data on the predictive value of routine measurements of drug blood levels in atopic dermatitis, although this may be useful in detecting possible drug interactions or noncompliance—the latter potentially explaining some nonresponders (13). When the traditional oral formulation (Sandimmun) is prescribed at levels less than 5 mg/kg/day or Neoral less than 4 mg/kg/day, peak-trough measurements provide limited useful clinical information.

Response to Treatment and Evaluation of Efficacy

Physicians treating patients with the most severe forms of atopic dermatitis should not so much consider clinical improvement as success but concentrate more on patient satisfaction. The goal therefore is not to achieve complete clearing but marked improvement of the patient's symptoms. Different scoring systems have been developed in an attempt to reproducibly measure the signs and symptoms of atopic dermatitis and to assess the efficacy of therapeutic intervention. Ideally, such a scoring system should be quick, simple, and exhibit high inter- and intraobserver reproducibility. The two most popular systems are the SCORAD index and the SASSAD severity index, and patients on CsA should be regularly followed using such a system (24). In recent years more attention has been paid to the impact of dermatologic disease and therapeutic interventions on the patient's quality of life. The specialty-specific Dermatology Life Quality Index is simple and rapid and allows to objectively assess the subject's satisfaction with treatment (21,23).

In a representative paper (22), 43 patients with severe atopic dermatitis were closely followed after a six-week treatment period with CsA at 5 mg/kg/day. An almost maximal response to treatment was already apparent after two weeks of treatment. The overall efficacy of treatment was rated as very good or good by 37 of 42 patients after the first treatment cycle. Forty-two percent of the patients relapsed within two weeks and 71% six weeks after CsA was stopped. A second treatment period was performed, and the results were similar, most patients again responding favorably. But in contrast to the majority of patients who relapsed quickly, all seven patients who did not relapse after the first or second treatment period were still in remission after one year. This study confirms many similar ones demonstrating the efficacy of CsA in atopic dermatitis. It also suggests that CsA treatment may improve the long-term outcome of atopic dermatitis, although most patients initially relapsed a few weeks after CsA was stopped. It is also established that CsA reduces the pruritus in a subgroup of patients within two or three days and that in more than 50% of treated patients the skin improves within one to two weeks. In this well-responding group, the mean remission rate at month 6 is 70%.

Studies in children (20) have shown that at six weeks there was significant improvement from baseline of severity scores, proportion of skin surface affected, mean symptom scores for pruritus, irritability and sleep disturbance, and topical steroid requirement in almost all of the children. Of 27 children treated, 22 had complete clearing or marked improvement after six weeks; only one child completing treatment was considered to have shown no response. Quality of life improved for both the children and their families. Long remission after withdrawal of treatment was seen in some children, although most relapsed within a few weeks.

Side Effects

The potential side effects of CsA are substantial, the major limiting side effect being nephrotoxicity. Monitoring serum creatinine level seems to be a practical method of evaluating renal function, being easier and less error-prone than determinations of creatinine clearance or glomerular filtration rates. Although CsA nephrotoxicity is generally reversible if detected early, renal biopsies frequently show changes of interstitial fibrosis and less frequently irreversible glomerulosclerosis.

Cardiovascular side effects are of concern in patients receiving CsA for atopic dermatitis, and some patients have suffered myocardial infarction while ingesting the drug. CsA may worsen hypertension in those with preexisting blood pressure elevation, requiring alterations in antihypertensive regimens. It may also induce hypertension in normotensive individuals. Diet, exercise, and antihypertensive drug therapy may be necessary. CsA may also cause elevation of serum triglycerides and less frequently cholesterol. Among the most striking cutaneous side effects are hypertrichosis and gingival hyperplasia. Table 2 lists common adverse effects associated with CsA use.

One of the main concerns relates to possible long-term carcinogenicity. This concern is based on the general immunosuppressive activity of CsA and observations in long-term users such as graft recipients and psoriatic patients. In the latter, however, factors such as previous chemotherapy or long-term photo-chemotherapy may have played an important role as cocarcinogens, cofactors that are normally absent in atopic dermatitis patients.

TABLE 2 Adverse Effects of Cyclosporine A

System	Effects
Renal/electrolyte	Increase in blood-urea nitrogen and creatinine; decrease in glomerulum filtration and serum magnesium
Hematologic	Mild normocytic, normochromic anemia
Gastrointestinal	Nausea, vomiting, diarrhea, bloating
Hepatic	Elevated transaminases and alkaline phosphatase
Cardiovascular	Hypertension, hyperlipidemia
Mucocutaneous	Hypertrichosis, gingival hyperplasia
Constitutional	Fatigue, weight loss early in therapy
Neurologic	Encephalitis, tremor, paresthesias

Source: Adapted from Ref. 38.

CsA-induced carcinogenesis is of even greater importance in children. The effects of its prolonged administration are unknown in this age group, although considerable information is becoming available from its use in children after organ transplantation. There are almost no reports of CsA-related malignancies in children, and it is unlikely that short courses of the drug, as used in atopic dermatitis, could have a detrimental effect. In addition, patients receiving CsA following organ transplantation are much more intensely immunosuppressed. If, however, the patient with atopic dermatitis has signs of severe photodamage due to previous sunlight exposure, photo- or photochemotherapy, CsA therapy is to be avoided.

Conclusions

CsA has gained a place in treating difficult cases of atopic dermatitis in adults and in children (25–28). The available evidence suggests that short-term treatment with CsA is efficacious and safe in patients with recalcitrant disease not responding to classical treatment. Long-term treatment should only be considered in adults that do not respond to an eight-week therapeutic schedule. Quality of life measures improve significantly while patients are on the drug. Dermatologists are urged to use one of the available scoring systems (e.g., SCORAD) to assess extent, activity, and symptoms of atopic dermatitis before, during, and after therapeutic intervention with CsA.

Patients must be encouraged to maintain topical treatment with emollients and topical steroids during CsA therapy. It is also important to explain to the patient that a short course of CsA therapy is intended to induce a remission of the disease but that, at present, long-term remission, although reported in some patients, remains uncertain. There is no evidence for a rebound phenomenon after stopping CsA.

SYSTEMIC IMMUNOSUPPRESSANT DRUGS

Antimetabolites such as azathioprine, methotrexate, and cytotoxic drugs such as cyclophosphamide have been employed in patients with severe atopic dermatitis, and variable results have been reported (29). Azathioprine, because of its still widespread use in some countries, will be dealt with in more detail below. However, with none of these agents have controlled studies been performed. The excellent efficacy of CsA and the fact that this drug has been studied very carefully and its guidelines are available indicates that these drugs may become obsolete in the future. A few controlled studies have examined the effect of interferon-gamma in atopic dermatitis and efficacy was shown in a smaller proportion of patients; 45% of rIFN-gamma–treated patients, but also 21% of placebo-treated patients achieved greater than 50% improvement in physicians' overall response evaluations (30,31). Because interferon-gamma is not without side effects and its efficacy in no way matches that of CsA, this treatment has been abandoned. The same holds true for interferon-alpha (32) and interleukin-2 (33), of which all have been tried in limited numbers of patients.

Azathioprine
More than half of the dermatologists in the United Kingdom use azathioprine to treat severe atopic dermatitis (34,35), yet there is not one randomized controlled trial available to support its use. Several studies were therefore recently initiated in order to prove its efficacy and safety as compared to other immunosuppressive drugs (34,36,37). Tan et al. (34) point to uncontrolled studies involving small numbers of patients and leading to contradictory results. Their conclusion from the literature survey is that cyclosporin has potentially more side effects than azathioprine, but the latter is more cost-effective and easier to monitor, emphasizing the need for double-blind trials. Other authors also argue that azathioprine is an effective and cheaper alternative to cyclosporine in the treatment of severe adult atopic eczema, but that long-term toxicity remains unclear (36). Lear et al. (37) point to bone marrow suppression and its oncogenic potential; regarding the latter, a study comparing the incidence of cutaneous malignancy in renal allograft recipients who received cyclosporine or azathioprine showed no differences between the two drugs. In summary, azathioprine seems to be effective and is on the list of recommended systemic treatment modalities for severe forms of atopic dermatitis (38–40).

Mycophenolate Mofetil
Mycophenolate mofetil (MMF), an immunosuppressive agent that blocks the proliferative responses of T and B lymphocytes and is currently used to prevent rejection in renal transplant patients, has been used in the treatment of psoriasis, pemphigus vulgaris, bullous pemphigoid, pyoderma gangrenosum, and pompholyx (41). Trials in small numbers of patients suggest that MMF therapy may be beneficial for adult and children affected by atopic dermatitis (42–44) but call for controlled trials (45). Recent observations of staphylococcal septicemia complicating treatment of atopic dermatitis with MMF (41), however, call for a reconsideration of its use in atopic dermatitis, and its relative inefficacy in a small series of atopic dermatitis patients caused Hansen et al. (46) to conclude that MMF should be considered with cautions based on existing knowledge.

BIOLOGICS
Monoclonal antibodies, fusion proteins, and recombinant human proteins (so-called biologics) have been developed initially as new tools targeting key structures in the initiation of inflammation. Their effectiveness has been demonstrated in several chronic inflammatory diseases such as rheumatoid arthritis, chronic inflammatory bowel disease, and psoriasis. The use biologics, which modulate the T-cell response, therefore seems to be a reasonable approach in combating atopic dermatitis.

Anti–TNF-a Strategy

As TNF-a is a primary proinflammatory cytokine, which has been detected in tissue samples from atopic dermatitis patients (47), blocking this cytokine with TNF-a antagonists could be a useful treatment approach. However, both etanercept and infliximab show a rather moderate effect in the few cases reports published so far.

Anti–IL-5

Similar to anti–TNF-a strategy, blocking the Th2 cytokine IL-5 with the specific monoclonal mepolizumab did not prove to be clinically efficient in a placebo-controlled study, although the eosinophil count was significantly decreased in peripheral blood (48).

Anti-IgE

The humanized anti-IgE monoclonal antibody Omalizumab prevents its binding to the high-affinity receptor (FcεRI), leading to downregulation of IgE receptor density on effector cells and DC. In patients with atopic dermatitis, omalizumab reduced IgE transcription and increased IgG transcription in B cells, which correlated in some patients with a good treatment response. The limiting factor for its therapeutic use resides in the very high levels of IgE seen in patients with severe atopic dermatitis. Despite the meaningful rationale of the anti-IgE strategy in atopic dermatitis, the outcome of the clinical trials did not fulfill the hopes so far (49–52) and the results from case studies are contradictory. There is a great need for further clinical studies to better evaluate this therapy, especially in those patients who are characterized by high serum IgE.

Targeting B-Cells

Rituximab is a chimeric monoclonal directed against CD20, a structure expressed by precursor B cells and mature B cells, but not by plasma cells. A recently published surveillance study reported successful use of rituximab in atopic dermatitis patients (53). While total IgE dropped only slightly, the numbers of B-cells and T-cells were significantly reduced.

Targeting Adhesion Molecules

As other adhesion molecules, the CD11, a subunit of lymphocyte function associated antigen-1 (LFA-1), plays a key role in the migration of T-cells in tissues and in the immunologic synapse with antigen-presenting cells. Efalizumab is a recombinant, humanized monoclonal antibody, which targets the LFA-1 and has been successfully applied in psoriasis. A few studies have already shown that atopic dermatitis responds well to Efalizumab (54–56). This effect may be due to a kind of segregation of T-cells in the peripheral blood, a phenomenon that may also marked increase of circulating lymphocytes and of the cutaneous lymphocyte antigen (CLA) expressing CD4 T-cells in the blood. A relationship between successful treatment and a decrease in T-cells, CD11 a$^+$ dendritic cells (DC), and to a lesser extent CD206$^+$ DC and CD209$^+$ DC in the epidermis after six months has been reported (55,57). Since the clinical response to Efalizumab is rather delayed, this biologic may rather be used "in relay" to a more rapidly acting therapy such as CyA, especially in atopic dermatitis patients with low compliance. Double-blind placebo-controlled studies are awaited to clearly define the place of this interesting molecule in the therapeutic arsenal of atopic dermatitis.

DIVERSA

Specific Immunotherapy

Although the clinical response of allergen-specific immunotherapy (SIT) is proven in the treatment of allergic rhinitis and in allergic asthma, its use in atopic dermatitis has remained a matter of debate. This is due to the conflicting results from SIT in atopic dermatitis in the 1970, and the fear of exacerbation of the disease during allergen exposure. This was probably due to a rather unselected recruitment of atopic dermatitis patients without clear causality for the tested allergen. More recently, SIT was subjected to a kind of revival when a study published in 2006 with 89 adult patients showed that there was a significant reduction in SCORAD score after weekly injections for four months, especially in patients with severe atopic dermatitis (57). Randomized placebo-controlled trials with large numbers of carefully selected individuals are currently in progress to better reevaluate the efficacy of SIT in atopic dermatitis patients (58).

Intravenous Immunoglobulins

The immunomodulatory and anti-inflammatory effects of intravenous immunoglobulins (IVIG) are mainly mediated by the Fc-fragment of IgG, which interacts with complement receptors and Fc receptors, via the antigen-binding fragment and the variable region of the immunoglobulin (59). The mechanisms of effect include functional blocking of the Fc receptor on macrophages of the spleen, B, and T lymphocytes; inhibition of complement activation and related tissue damage by C3; modulation of production of cytokines and cytokine antagonists by monocytes, macrophages, and lymphocytes; inhibition of superantigen-mediated T-cell activation; and neutralization of antibodies and blocking Fas receptors by antibodies contained in the immunoglobulin concentrate. Based on the assumption that atopic dermatitis is a T-cell mediated, chronic inflammatory skin disease, with Th-2 predominance in early stages, IVIG has been given to downregulate T-cell function and IL-4 production. There may be an effect due to neutralization of antibodies in the chronic autoreactive form of atopic dermatitis. It is also possible that influencing *S. aureus* superantigens, altering migration of T lymphocytes to the epidermis by influencing skin-homing factors, or altering the expression of costimulatory molecules such as CD28 and CD40 or chemokines such as eotaxin, which plays a key role in eosinophil recruitment, could have a positive influence on atopic dermatitis. Although there are a few case reports and case series studies on IVIG therapy in atopic dermatitis, systematic studies are still needed. The results are mixed, but in general there is a better response in children, and in adults there is greater effectiveness when combined with other systemic therapies (59–63). Studies on the effectiveness of this therapy are needed, especially because of its high cost.

Extracorporeal Photophoresis

Extracorporeal photophoresis was originally developed for the treatment of cutaneous T-cell lymphoma. Treatment basically involves separating white blood cells from red blood cells and plasma in order to irradiate the white blood cells with UVA after exposing them to methoxsalen. This leads to binding between the pyrimidine bases of the DNA, preventing further cell proliferation (64). A positive effect of photophoresis on atopic dermatitis has been described in various studies (64–67) (Table 1). Treatment is time-consuming and expensive, however, and should be reserved for exceptional cases.

SUMMARY

The list of recommended substances for systemic treatment of patients suffering from atopic dermatitis is long, ranging from antihistamines, antibiotics, and corticosteroids to immunosuppressants, and from dietary supplements to unsaturated fatty acids and Chinese herbs and miscellaneous other treatment considerations. Many of them have been in traditional use for decades, several without having ever been tested in placebo-controlled trials, as is the case for systemic corticosteroids. Others, like cyclosporine, a relatively expensive and potentially toxic proprietary drug, have undergone well-controlled trials for the treatment of atopic dermatitis and have fulfilled expectations. More recently, the new family of target-designed drugs such as biologics has led to new hopes for modern and safety treatment. However, there are limited data on the use of biologics such as Efalizumab, although results from preliminary studies seem promising. Further randomized, double-blind, placebo-controlled studies are needed. Confirmation of the effectiveness of these drugs would provide an alternative for those patients who must discontinue immunosuppressive agents due to limited effectiveness or adverse effects. Allergen-specific immunotherapy can bring about long-term modulation of the immune response to the allergy trigger. It is not a suitable option for short-term therapy of eczema, but can be used for long-term stabilization of atopic dermatitis, which is triggered by a specific allergen. The results of studies, which are currently underway, are eagerly anticipated.

REFERENCES

1. Akdis CA, Akdis M, Bieber T, et al. Diagnosis and treatment of atopic dermatitis in children and adults: European Academy of Allergology and Clinical Immunology/ American Academy of Allergy, Asthma and Immunology/PRACTALL Consensus Report. Allergy 2006; 61:969–987.
2. Bieber T. Atopic dermatitis. N Engl J Med 2008; 358:1483–1494.
3. Greaves MW. Antihistamines in dermatology. Skin Pharmacol Physiol 2005; 18:220–229.
4. Henz BM, Metzenauer P, O'Keefe E, et al. Differential effects of new-generation H1-receptor antagonists in pruritic dermatoses. Allergy 1998; 53:180–183.
5. Klein PA, Clark RA. An evidence-based review of the efficacy of antihistamines in relieving pruritus in atopic dermatitis. Arch Dermatol 1999; 135:1522–1525.
6. Langeland T, Fagertun HE, Larsen S. Therapeutic effect of loratadine on pruritus in patients with atopic dermatitis. A multi-crossover-designed study. Allergy 1994; 49:22–26.
7. Juhlin L. Nonclassical clinical indications for H1-receptor antagonists in dermatology. Allergy 1995; 50:36–40.
8. Raimer SS. Managing pediatric atopic dermatitis. Clin Pediatr (Phila) 2000; 39:1–14.
9. Tay YK, Khoo BP, Goh CL. The profile of atopic dermatitis in a tertiary dermatology outpatient clinic in Singapore. Int J Dermatol 1999; 38:689–692.

10. Tofte SJ, Hanifin JM. Current management and therapy of atopic dermatitis. J Am Acad Dermatol 2001; 44:S13–S16.
11. van Joost T, Stolz E, Heule F. Efficacy of low-dose cyclosporine in severe atopic skin disease. Arch Dermatol 1987; 123:166–167.
12. Berth-Jones J, Graham-Brown RA, Marks R, et al. Long-term efficacy and safety of cyclosporin in severe adult atopic dermatitis. Br J Dermatol 1997; 136:76–81.
13. Camp RD, Reitamo S, Friedmann PS, et al. Cyclosporin A in severe, therapy-resistant atopic dermatitis: Report of an international workshop, April 1993. Br J Dermatol 1993; 129:217–220.
14. Naeyaert JM, Lachapelle JM, Degreef H, et al. Cyclosporin in atopic dermatitis: Review of the literature and outline of a Belgian consensus. Dermatology 1999; 198:145–152.
15. Zurbriggen B, Wuthrich B, Cachelin AB, et al. Comparison of two formulations of cyclosporin A in the treatment of severe atopic dermatitis. Aa double-blind, single-centre, cross-over pilot study. Dermatology 1999; 198:56–60.
16. Bourke JF, Berth-Jones J, Holder J, et al. A new microemulsion formulation of cyclosporin (Neoral) is effective in the treatment of cyclosporin-resistant dermatoses. Br J Dermatol 1996; 134:777–779.
17. Atakan N, Erdem C. The efficacy, tolerability and safety of a new oral formulation of Sandimmun–Sandimmun Neoral in severe refractory atopic dermatitis. J Eur Acad Dermatol Venereol 1998; 11:240–246.
18. Kagi MK, Joller-Jemelka H, Wuthrich B. Soluble E-selectin correlates with disease activity in cyclosporin A-treated patients with atopic dermatitis. Allergy 1999; 54:57–63.
19. Bottari V, Frezzolini A, Ruffelli M, et al. Cyclosporin A (CyA) reduces sCD30 serum levels in atopic dermatitis: A possible new immune intervention. Allergy 1999; 54:507–510.
20. Berth-Jones J, Finlay AY, Zaki I, et al. Cyclosporine in severe childhood atopic dermatitis: A multicenter study. J Am Acad Dermatol 1996; 34:1016–1021.
21. Salek MS, Finlay AY, Luscombe DK, et al. Cyclosporin greatly improves the quality of life of adults with severe atopic dermatitis. A randomized, double-blind, placebo-controlled trial. Br J Dermatol 1993; 129:422–430.
22. Granlund H, Erkko P, Sinisalo M, et al. Cyclosporin in atopic dermatitis: Time to relapse and effect of intermittent therapy. Br J Dermatol 1995; 132:106–112.
23. Czech W, Brautigam M, Weidinger G, et al. A body-weight-independent dosing regimen of cyclosporine microemulsion is effective in severe atopic dermatitis and improves the quality of life. J Am Acad Dermatol 2000; 42:653–659.
24. Kunz B, Oranje AP, Labreze L, et al. Clinical validation and guidelines for the SCORAD index: Consensus report of the European Task Force on Atopic Dermatitis. Dermatology 1997; 195:10–19.
25. Schmitt J, Schmitt N, Meurer M. Cyclosporin in the treatment of patients with atopic eczema—A systematic review and meta-analysis. J Eur Acad Dermatol Venereol 2007; 21:606–619.
26. Madan V, Griffiths CE. Systemic ciclosporin and tacrolimus in dermatology. Dermatol Ther 2007; 20:239–250.
27. Hijnen DJ, ten Berge O, Timmer-de Mik L, et al. Efficacy and safety of long-term treatment with cyclosporin A for atopic dermatitis. J Eur Acad Dermatol Venereol 2007; 21:85–89.
28. Leonardi S, Marchese G, Rotolo N, et al. Cyclosporin is safe and effective in severe atopic dermatitis of childhood. Report of three cases. Minerva Pediatr 2004; 56:231–237.
29. Akhavan A, Rudikoff D. Atopic dermatitis: Systemic immunosuppressive therapy. Semin Cutan Med Surg 2008; 27:151–155.
30. Hanifin JM, Schneider LC, Leung DY, et al. Recombinant interferon gamma therapy for atopic dermatitis. J Am Acad Dermatol 1993; 28:189–197.
31. Reinhold U, Kukel S, Brzoska J, et al. Systemic interferon gamma treatment in severe atopic dermatitis. J Am Acad Dermatol 1993; 29:58–63.
32. Rothe MJ, Grant-Kels JM. Atopic dermatitis: An update. J Am Acad Dermatol 1996; 35:1–13 [quiz 4–6].
33. Hsieh KH, Chou CC, Huang SF. Interleukin 2 therapy in severe atopic dermatitis. J Clin Immunol 1991; 11:22–28.

34. Tan BB, Lear JT, Gawkrodger DJ, et al. Azathioprine in dermatology: A survey of current practice in the U.K. Br J Dermatol 1997; 136:351–355.
35. Berth-Jones J, Takwale A, Tan E, et al. Azathioprine in severe adult atopic dermatitis: A double-blind, placebo-controlled, crossover trial. Br J Dermatol 2002; 147:324–330.
36. Buckley DA, Baldwin P, Rogers S. The use of azathioprine in severe adult atopic eczema. J Eur Acad Dermatol Venereol 1998; 11:137–140.
37. Lear JT, English JS, Jones P, et al. Retrospective review of the use of azathioprine in severe atopic dermatitis. J Am Acad Dermatol 1996; 35:642–643.
38. Hughes R, Collins P, Rogers S. Further experience of using azathioprine in the treatment of severe atopic dermatitis. Clin Exp Dermatol 2008; 33:710–711.
39. Meggitt SJ, Gray JC, Reynolds NJ. Azathioprine dosed by thiopurine methyltransferase activity for moderate-to-severe atopic eczema: A double-blind, randomised controlled trial. Lancet 2006; 367:839–846.
40. Murphy LA, Atherton D. A retrospective evaluation of azathioprine in severe childhood atopic eczema, using thiopurine methyltransferase levels to exclude patients at high risk of myelosuppression. Br J Dermatol 2002; 147:308–315.
41. Satchell AC, Barnetson RS. Staphylococcal septicaemia complicating treatment of atopic dermatitis with mycophenolate. Br J Dermatol 2000; 143:202–203.
42. Neuber K, Schwartz I, Itschert G, et al. Treatment of atopic eczema with oral mycophenolate mofetil. Br J Dermatol 2000; 143:385–391.
43. Murray ML, Cohen JB. Mycophenolate mofetil therapy for moderate to severe atopic dermatitis. Clin Exp Dermatol 2007; 32:23–27.
44. Heller M, Shin HT, Orlow SJ, et al. Mycophenolate mofetil for severe childhood atopic dermatitis: Experience in 14 patients. Br J Dermatol 2007; 157:127–132.
45. Grundmann-Kollmann M, Korting HC, Behrens S, et al. Successful treatment of severe refractory atopic dermatitis with mycophenolate mofetil. Br J Dermatol 1999; 141:175–176.
46. Hansen ER, Buus S, Deleuran M, et al. Treatment of atopic dermatitis with mycophenolate mofetil. Br J Dermatol 2000; 143:1324–1326.
47. Jacobi A, Antoni C, Manger B, et al. Infliximab in the treatment of moderate to severe atopic dermatitis. J Am Acad Dermatol 2005; 52:522–526.
48. Oldhoff JM, Darsow U, Werfel T, et al. Anti-IL-5 recombinant humanized monoclonal antibody (mepolizumab) for the treatment of atopic dermatitis. Allergy 2005; 60:693–696.
49. Lane JE, Cheyney JM, Lane TN, et al. Treatment of recalcitrant atopic dermatitis with omalizumab. J Am Acad Dermatol 2006; 54:68–72.
50. Krathen RA, Hsu S. Failure of omalizumab for treatment of severe adult atopic dermatitis. J Am Acad Dermatol 2005; 53:338–340.
51. Vigo PG, Girgis KR, Pfuetze BL, et al. Efficacy of anti-IgE therapy in patients with atopic dermatitis. J Am Acad Dermatol 2006; 55:168–170.
52. Forman SB, Garrett AB. Success of omalizumab as monotherapy in adult atopic dermatitis: Case report and discussion of the high-affinity immunoglobulin E receptor, FcepsilonRI. Cutis 2007; 80:38–40.
53. Simon D, Hosli S, Kostylina G, et al. Anti-CD20 (rituximab) treatment improves atopic eczema. J Allergy Clin Immunol 2008; 121:122–128.
54. Weinberg JM, Siegfried EC. Successful treatment of severe atopic dermatitis in a child and an adult with the T-cell modulator efalizumab. Arch Dermatol 2006; 142:555–558.
55. Hassan AS, Kaelin U, Braathen LR, et al. Clinical and immunopathologic findings during treatment of recalcitrant atopic eczema with efalizumab. J Am Acad Dermatol 2007; 56:217–221.
56. Takiguchi R, Tofte S, Simpson B, et al. Efalizumab for severe atopic dermatitis: A pilot study in adults. J Am Acad Dermatol 2007; 56:222–227.
57. Werfel T, Breuer K, Rueff F, et al. Usefulness of specific immunotherapy in patients with atopic dermatitis and allergic sensitization to house dust mites: A multi-centre, randomized, dose–response study. Allergy 2006; 61:202–205.
58. Bussmann C, Bockenhoff A, Henke H, et al. Does allergen-specific immunotherapy represent a therapeutic option for patients with atopic dermatitis? J Allergy Clin Immunol 2006; 118:1292–1298.

59. Jolles S, Hughes J, Rustin M. The treatment of atopic dermatitis with adjunctive high-dose intravenous immunoglobulin: A report of three patients and review of the literature. Br J Dermatol 2000; 142:551–554.
60. Gelfand EW, Landwehr LP, Esterl B, et al. Intravenous immune globulin: An alternative therapy in steroid-dependent allergic diseases. Clin Exp Immunol 1996; 104(suppl 1):61–66.
61. Jolles S, Hughes J. Importance of trial design in studies using high-dose intravenous immunoglobulin. Br J Dermatol 2003; 148:1284–1285 [author reply 5–6].
62. Paul C, Lahfa M, Bachelez H, et al. A randomized controlled evaluator-blinded trial of intravenous immunoglobulin in adults with severe atopic dermatitis. Br J Dermatol 2002; 147:518–522.
63. Noh G, Lee KY. Intravenous immune globulin (i.v. IG) therapy in steroid-resistant atopic dermatitis. J Korean Med Sci 1999; 14:63–68.
64. Sand M, Bechara FG, Sand D, et al. Extracorporeal photopheresis as a treatment for patients with severe, refractory atopic dermatitis. Dermatology 2007; 215:134–138.
65. Prinz B, Nachbar F, Plewig G. Treatment of severe atopic dermatitis with extracorporeal photopheresis. Arch Dermatol Res 1994; 287:48–52.
66. Prinz B, Michelsen S, Pfeiffer C, et al. Long-term application of extracorporeal photochemotherapy in severe atopic dermatitis. J Am Acad Dermatol 1999; 40:577–582.
67. Richter HI, Billmann-Eberwein C, Grewe M, et al. Successful monotherapy of severe and intractable atopic dermatitis by photopheresis. J Am Acad Dermatol 1998; 38:585–588.

Index

T - #1054 - 101024 - C48 - 229/152/24 [26] - CB - 9781420077988 - Gloss Lamination